CLINICAL NEUROPSYCHOLOGY
Theoretical Foundations for Practitioners

CLINICAL NEUROPSYCHOLOGY
Theoretical Foundations for Practitioners

Edited by

Mark E. Maruish
Strategic Advantage, Inc.

James A. Moses, Jr.
VA Palo Alto Health Care System
Stanford University School of Medicine

LEA LAWRENCE ERLBAUM ASSOCIATES, PUBLISHERS
1997 Mahwah, New Jersey

Lawrence Erlbaum Associates, Inc., Publishers
10 Industrial Avenue
Mahwah, New Jersey 07430

Library of Congress Cataloging-in-Publication Data

Clinical neuropsychology : theoretical foundations for practitioners / edited by Mark E. Maruish, James A. Moses, Jr.
p. cm.
ISBN 0-8058-1343-8
1. Clinical neuropsychology. 2. Neuropsychological tests.
3. Brain damage—Diagnosis. I. Maruish, Mark E. II. Moses, James A., Jr.
RC386.6.N48C528 1996
616.89—dc20 95-53118
CIP

Books published by Lawrence Erlbaum Associates are printed on acid-free paper, and their bindings are chosen for strength and durability.

Printed in the United States of America
10 9 8 7 6 5 4 3 2 1

Contents

Foreword

Arthur Benton

More rapidly than might have been anticipated, clinical neuropsychology is coming of age. I mean by this that it is evolving from what was largely a set of assessment procedures coupled with the diagnostic inferences to be drawn from them into a true discipline, conscious of its conceptual bases and concerned with the cognitive and neural mechanisms that mediate the behavior of normal individuals and patients with brain disease. This book, ably edited by Mark Maruish and James Moses, makes a distinctive contribution to this evolution in that it emphasizes these fundamental issues. At the same time, clinical and forensic practice, problems of training and organization, and the relationship of clinical neuropsychology to allied fields are also covered in considerable detail.

Without exception, each chapter in the volume provides a thoughtful and up-to-date analysis of the area it covers, and some are truly outstanding. *Clinical Neuropsychology: Theoretical Foundations for Practitioners* fills a clear need at this stage of development of the field. It is a valuable asset that will be welcomed by clinicians and researchers alike.

Preface

For nearly two decades, the level of interest, study, and practice devoted to clinical neuropsychology has enjoyed a rate of growth that may be unprecedented in the behavioral science field. The number of doctoral-level training programs with clinical neuropsychology tracks has increased dramatically. This has been accompanied by an increase in the number of predoctoral clinical psychology internships with neuropsychology rotations, and in the number of predoctoral internships and postdoctoral fellowships focused solely on clinical neuropsychological training. Membership in professional organizations such as the American Psychological Association's Division of Clinical Neuropsychology (Division 40), the National Academy of Neuropsychology (NAN), and the International Neuropsychological Society (INS) also has grown steadily. In addition, the number of journals that have been proliferated from the growing interest in and need for information in the area of clinical neuropsychology further reflect how far the field has progressed. However, it probably is the American Board of Professional Psychology's (ABPP's) acknowledgment of clinical neuropsychology as a speciality that most strongly identifies the field as being a discipline in its own right rather than being a subspecialty of clinical psychology.

With the emergence of clinical neuropsychology as one of the fastest growing specialties in the field of psychology comes the need for current and future practitioners to stay abreast of the most recent research in the field. The professional journals just mentioned more than adequately meet this need. At the same time, there also is a need to stay up-to-date on the current thinking on topics and issues that are important to the practice of the profession. For this reason, we set out to produce this volume. Drawing on the expertise of some of the leaders in the field, our intent was to provide the practitioner with a source for discussions of topics that are important to their ongoing development as clinical neuropsychologists but which generally are not addressed in the literature to any great degree.

We begin with a discussion of topics related to the emergence of clinical neuropsychology as a psychological specialty. First, the multidisciplinary origins and subsequent evolution of clinical neuropsychology as a professional specialty are detailed in the chapter by Meier. The rapid development of this clinical subspecialty has been made possible by concurrent, parallel advances in three related areas. Developments have been made in basic experimental neurobehavioral and cognitive research methodology. Advances in cognitive theoretical model building and psychometric assessment methods also have been contributory to the emergence of clinical neuropsychology as a specialty area. In addition, the development of sophisticated methods of neurobehavioral syndrome analysis have contributed to the emergence of clinical neuropsychology as a professional practice area. Meier presents a detailed, integrative survey of these key trends in experimental and clinical neuroscience during the past half-century, and he delineates the role of the clinical neuropsychologist as that of providing the integration and application of this multidisciplinary knowledge base to the syndrome analysis of neurobehavioral disorders.

Meier evaluates ongoing developments and controversies in the development and implementation of standards for neuropsychological training and professional practice. In particular, alternative models and standards for doctoral academic neuropsychological instruction, predoctoral and postdoctoral clinical training, professional credentialing, and board certification are presented. Meier himself has been a pioneering and leading figure in the development of each of these areas and thus is able to bring personal as well as professional expertise to the discussion.

Meier clarifies the boundaries of clinical neuropsychological practice and its evolving relationship to allied disciplines. He also discusses the development of specialty journals, professional societies, academic training programs, and advanced practice level specialty accreditation. These factors all have become increasingly important to the formal establishment and recognition of clinical neuropsychology as a professional practice specialty.

The interdisciplinary nature of clinical neuropsychology that Meier presents in the previous chapter is developed from the neurological viewpoint by Shuren. He illustrates the conceptual foundations of behavioral neurology and its conceptual and clinical relationship to clinical neuropsychology. His presentation begins with a historical overview of the development of neurobehavioral syndrome analysis. The historical origins and shortcomings of narrow localizationist and global holistic models of brain function are analyzed and shown to be incomplete. Refinements in the development of modular and integrative theories of functional brain systems are highlighted through discussion of the work of Penfield, Geschwind, and Sperry. Concepts from behavioral neurologic syndrome analysis also are shown to have influenced psychometric test development by clinical neuropsychologists.

Shuren defines the role of the behavioral neurologist as the diagnosis, medical treatment, and neurobehavioral analysis of neurologic disorders. He illustrates the integrated roles of the neurologic and mental status examinations in neurologic diagnosis and prognosis. Complementary methods of brain lesion localization and behavioral syndrome analyses using neurological and neuropsychological methods are described and clinically illustrated through case examples and clinical syndrome analyses. Throughout the chapter, Shuren advocates and models the complementary roles of behavioral neurology, clinical neuropsychology, and both basic and applied neuroscience to the analysis of neurobehavioral disorder.

Friedrich and Rader present an integrated model of modular cognitive processing that is based on complementary experimental and clinical behavioral analyses. The theory postulates specific modular cognitive components that may underlie complex information processing. This rigorous cognitive model often provides unique insight into complex neurobehavioral systems and syndromes. Friedrich and Rader's historical review of information processing models reveals that neurobehavioral theorists have postulated such hierarchically organized cognitive systems for over a century.

Friedrich and Rader discuss the analytic principles that guide current research trends in the development and validation of a general model of cognition. They present integrative research reviews of cognitive models of memorial processing, spatial perception, and visual imagery. These findings also have direct relevance to neurobehavioral modeling of neurologic functional system modeling. A fine-tuned theoretical basis for clinical syndrome analysis and standardized test development directly emerges from the model. The cognitive theory that they present also has proven to be useful in neural functional system modeling and in the analysis of specific cognitive deficit that is associated with discrete brain lesions.

In the first chapter of the "Issues in Neuropsychological Assessment" section, Pritchard presents an introductory overview of the field of forensic neuropsychology. He begins with a discussion on the differences between forensic and clinical neuropsychology. Noted here are differences between the two subspecialties in terms of their goals, the clients they serve, and the questions they address, as well as differences in the manner in which each arrives at decisions. The role of the neuropsychologist as an expert witness is discussed, both generically and with regard to what he or she has to offer the court.

Pritchard next presents a discussion of the types of questions commonly addressed in the field of forensic neuropsychology, including substantive questions of criminal, civil, and administrative law. Because it is an issue that must frequently be addressed, a discussion of malingering, or dissimulation, is presented. Issues related to training and general qualification standards and ethical considerations for forensic neuropsychologists are brought to bear, and desirable developments in the field are articulated. As an adjunct to the chapter, the reader also will find the American Psychological Association's *Specialty Guidelines for Forensic Psychologists* as the appendix.

In his chapter, Cripe reports that "The assessment of personality is one of the most important and challenging aspects of clinical neuropsychological practice" (p. 119). In tackling the topic of personality assessment of the brain-impaired, he addresses a number of issues that must be considered by clinical neuropsychologists and psychologists from other specialty areas who have occasion to assess such patients. These issues run the gamut of topics related to the general focus of his chapter. Issues related to personality, its neuroanatomical and neurophysiological bases, and methods of measuring personality also are presented. Particular attention to the use of the MMPI for personality assessment of the brain-impaired population is paid by the author. As an alternative to reliance on a single instrument such as the MMPI, Cripe enumerates specific guidelines for assessing the personality of the brain-impaired patient. Suggestions for areas of development in this field, including the area of new instrument development, also are provided.

The use of computers in psychological assessment is quite pervasive. Thus, any book dealing with the foundations of clinical neuropsychology would be wanting if it did not address the use of computerized test administration in neuropsychological assessment. For the purpose of this work, Kay and Starbuck first convey a historical perspective for computerized neuropsychological assessment. Next, they articulate the advantages of computerized test administration over the standard paper-and-pencil mode of administration. Conversions standard paper-and-pencil tests to computerized administration and tests specifically developed for administration via the computer are discussed. The authors go on to discuss in detail a number of commercially and publicly accessible batteries of neuropsychological tests. In closing the chapter, Kay and Starbuck present an evaluation of the current state of computerized neuropsychological test applications and convey predictions about future developments in this field.

In their chapter, Bigler, Porter and Lowry review the relationships of a wide variety of contemporary neuroimaging techniques to neurobehavioral syndrome analysis. They present brief overviews of the scientific basis and clinical indications for use of Computerized Tomographic Imaging, Magnetic Resonance Imaging, Single Photon Emission Computed Tomography, and Positron Emission Tomography. In addition, they discuss recent developments in Activation or Functional Magnetic Resonance Imaging, Magnetic Resonance Spectroscopy, Quantitative Electroencephalography, Brain (electrical activity) Mapping, and Magnetoencephalography. Extensive annotated illustrations are provided to allow one to compare the results of these neuroimaging methods.

Bigler and his colleagues also provide a detailed tabular overview of the literature that relates structural and functional brain imaging findings to cognitive function primarily in studies that have been published since 1989. They note that the literature published prior to that time very likely is based on technology that is now outmoded. To aid information location and retrieval, they have provided summaries of key articles in an extensive series of related tables that provides information on the neuroimaging method, neurobehavioral syndrome, lesion localization, patient sample, and neurobehavioral findings for each study.

Two chapters on the role of clinical neuropsychology in the treatment of brain-impaired patients follow next. First, Klonoff and her colleagues address one of the key components to the treatment and rehabilitation of persons with brain injuries, that is, cognitive retraining. In presenting an overview of the principle considerations and elements to this approach, the authors begin by stressing the importance of taking a milieu approach to cognitive retraining to enhance the patient's ability to apply gains made in the therapeutic setting to their functioning within the community. The role of neuropsychological assessment in identifying appropriate candidates also is presented. Related to this is the identification of patient characteristics whose presence increase the likelihood of success of cognitive remediation efforts.

In presenting their approach to treatment of the brain-injured patient, Klonoff et al. emphasize the importance of making the patient aware of his or her deficits. This is said to require "a sophisticated understanding of the patient's needs and capacity to flexibly shift and adapt treatment procedures" (p. 225). They show how interpreting the patient's performance, teaching compensatory strategies, and relating in-session observation to "real-life" behavior and situations can be helpful in accomplishing these goals. Also, general recommendations for remediation of deficits in specific areas of neuropsychological functioning (e.g., memory, attention, language) are given. In addition, the importance of working cooperatively with other rehabilitation disciplines—occupational therapy, speech therapy, recreational therapy—is discussed. Finally, the authors present a case study and preliminary empirical findings to address issues pertaining to outcome assessment and treatment efficacy of cognitive retraining exercises.

Schefft and his colleagues provide an extensive overview of the application and usefulness of self-regulation procedures that can be used with brain-injured patients. They first review factors that influence the use of self-regulation therapy. Included here is a discussion of the types of cognitive, behavioral, and emotional disabilities and handicaps brain-injured patients may present, as well as issues related to the evaluation of them. Next, various approaches to and models of treatment of these patients are reviewed. Included here are those models and approaches that are either self-regulatory or non-self-regulatory in their orientation.

In the final sections of their chapter, Schefft et al. present a detailed description of a self-regulation approach that has developed from work with a variety of psychiatric and neurologic populations. In describing the approach, the authors touch on the sources that influence or shape the dysfunctional behavior in brain-injured patients and draw the distinction between automatic versus controlled processing. They present a framework for the therapy process and outline strategies for achieving subgoals of therapy. Finally, future directions in this area are noted.

Diagnostic issues are covered in chapters by Goldstein and Csernansky et al. Goldstein's chapter begins by summarizing the shift of thinking about the etiology of mental illness from one in which mental disorders were viewed as having either a functional or organic basis to one in which biology serves as the basis of "most, if not all" (p. 306) mental disorders. Occurring along with this revolution in thinking has been a revolution in the direction of interests of some neuropsychologists. We now see a group of neuropsychologists focusing on the analysis of psychiatric disorders, either exclusively or in addition to the analysis of neurological disease. Goldstein notes how this change in focus likely began in the field of alcoholism, followed later by an interest in the neuropsychological aspects of schizophrenia. These areas of inquiry are explored, as are those of more recent research, including anxiety and mood disorders, personality and developmental disorders, attention-deficit hyperactivity, and autism.

In summarizing the state of affairs, Goldstein acknowledges how recent technologies have allowed for much of the recent work in the area of psychopathology. At the same time, they do not permit the definitive analysis of the neurobehavioral deficits that are associated with psychiatric disorders. Several methodological considerations are suggested to aid in future research planning. These include moving away from simplistic models of brain functioning, the state–trait aspect of the disorder, and symptomatic/diagnostic heterogeneity of diagnostic categories.

Csernansky, Black, and Faustman's chapter presents an overview of the *Diagnostic and Statistical Manual* (*DSM*) disorders in which significant cognitive deficits are their distinguishing characteristics. Beginning with a brief history of psychiatric nosology, the authors proceed to a discussion of the nosology of organic mental disorders, organized by a system of five classes. Class I disorders include those traditionally associated with brain damage (e.g., dementias, mental retardation, delirium). Class II disorders cover psychiatric symptoms associated with drug use (e.g., alcohol intoxication, delirium tremens). Indicative of Class III disorders are psychiatric syndromes which occur with other illnesses known to affect the brain. Examples include Tourette's syndrome and obsessive-compulsive disorder with encephalitis lethargica and schizophrenic-like psychosis with Wilson's disease. Class IV disorders lack consistent clinical–pathological correlational findings and include classic migraine headaches and tic disorders. Finally, Class V disorders include such severe disorders as schizophrenia, autism, and bipolar disorder. Although traditionally viewed as "functional" in nature, Class V disorders are now considered by many to be the result of brain abnormalities.

With the classification scheme defined, Csernansky et al. proceed with a presentation of neurological and neuropsychological findings for Class I and II disorders. The thrust of their presentation is on findings related to Alzheimer's disease, although other dementias (e.g., multi-infarct) and amnestic disorders also are addressed. In addition, findings for Class III disorders, (e.g., depression, mania, and anxiety that are secondary to a medical disease/disorder) are discussed.

The final two chapters of the book address issues in clinical neuropsychological research. In the first of the two chapters, Reynolds and Murdoch-James present an integrated discussion of basic test development psychometric principles. Principles of test domain sampling, item construction and analysis, target population selection, and the need for objectively quantified scoring system development are reviewed. Methods of qualitative and quantitative item scaling, test norm development, and demographic variable influence on level and pattern of component skill performance also are highlighted.

These presentations illustrate proper psychometric technique as well as common errors in neuropsychological test development. The basic principles and methods for establishment of content, construct, and criterion-related validity are reviewed, and examples of their application to neuropsychological test development are provided. Multivariate experimental design issues, base rate estimation, and actuarial analysis of classification accuracy shrinkage that occurs with cross-validation are highlighted. Much neuropsychological research has been compromised due to inattention to these principles.

In the final chapter, Krull and Adams address experimental design issues that are centrally relevant to neuropsychological research. They encourage conduct of hypothesis-driven rather than exploratory studies. Emphasis is placed on the evaluation and extension of theoretical models of neurobehavioral function. Key methodological issues include evaluation of sampling bias, base rate estimation, demographic variable matching, and careful control group composition. They also recommend use of explicit group inclusion and exclusion criteria, as well as consideration of the differential effects of fatigue on clinical and control groups. They note that performance pattern heterogeneity within a single diagnostic group often is overlooked. As a result, it may require the use of an experimental design in which disease progression staging is controlled in addition to demographic variable matching. Base rate analyses typically are lacking in neuropsychological research and should be included in actuarial classification studies.

Finally, Krull and Adams recommend refinement of neuropsychological experimental design to focus on modular patterns of cognitive performance rather than global intergroup performance level differences. They also call for analyses of functional systems or networks of related skills (see chapter 3, this volume) rather than on cognitive skills in isolation from each other.

We hope that the reader finds the information presented in this volume stimulating, informative, and useful as a tool for professional development. We also hope that it helps the reader obtain a better feel for where the field of clinical neuropsychology is, where it has come from, where it is going, and the potential problems and opportunities it faces as it continues to evolve and define itself. It is only through an awareness of where the profession has been and where it is going that its members can work to ensure that it develops in a manner that will help to further crystallize its identity and maximize the contributions it can make to both science and service.

1

The Establishment of Clinical Neuropsychology as a Psychological Specialty

Manfred J. Meier
University of Minnesota Medical School

Clinical neuropsychology has evolved as a specialized area of knowledge and practice with extensive intra- as well as interdisciplinary foundations. Considered from the perspective of the sociology of the professions, the specialty is characterized by activities in a number of scientific and professional domains. These domains can be seen as having laid the foundation for the practice of clinical neuropsychology, whose specialized mission encompasses roles that address psychological or behavioral manifestations of neurological, neuropathological, pathophysiological, and neurochemical changes in brain disease and the full range of aberrations in the central nervous system that may arise during development. The evolution of this mission has followed the characteristic course of scientifically based professional role functioning, insofar as the foundations in knowledge and practice have been derived not only from the discipline of psychology, but also from the various related disciplines within the traditional professions of medicine, education, and law.

Historically, three primary developmental domains appear to have provided the basis for this area of specialized knowledge and practice: basic experimental research in physiological and cognitive psychology, the development of quantitative and qualitative neuropsychological principles and procedures for clinical practice, and the syndromal analysis of the behavioral consequences of central nervous system lesions (Meier, 1992). The growth of the specialty has also been influenced by the introduction of formalized procedures for accrediting educational programs and individual competencies. The developmental process, based on a considerable expansion of interdisciplinary knowledge and practices during the past half-century, appears to be following a productive course. This is evidenced by the parallel development of participating organizations, publication of numerous books and journals, and the continued expansion of role applications beyond traditional neurological, neuropsychiatric, and rehabilitation settings into the forensic, educational, and vocational contexts.

HISTORICAL ANTECEDENTS

The historical foundations of this specialty are already sufficient to warrant a detailed historical account of its evolution. Such an account is beyond the scope of this chapter, which is designed to provide a general perspective by means of a review of major contributors in each of the three aforementioned converging lines of knowledge and practice. Even such a brief overview is insufficient to identify all major contributors so that the individuals identified here by no means constitute an exhaustive list. Although incomplete, such identifications may help to guide interested graduate students and practitioners in the field into the literature and to aid in formulation of career objectives. Extensive introductions to the prescientific, as well as the early scientific, literature of historical significance are available and should be read by the serious student or practitioner (Luria, 1966; Meyer, 1961). A review of modern clinical neuropsychology in general historical perspective, but not a detailed history, is also available (Meier, 1992). This section summarizes the developments within each of the three major developmental domains identified in the first paragraphs of this chapter.

Developments in Physiological, Comparative, and Cognitive Psychology

Karl Lashley (1929) was an extremely influential individual during his time. Publication of *Brain Mechanisms and Intelligence* resulted in the attribution of his intellectual leadership by many individuals who themselves subsequently became major figures in this domain. The doctrine of *strict localization of function* was widely held at that time; therefore, Lashley's finding that the behavioral consequences of experimentally induced brain lesions in rats were a direct function of the amount, rather than the location, of the tissue removed provided the basis for an opposing doctrine that incorporated *mass-action* principles into a theory of brain function. This work clearly forced an understanding of the nervous system as a functionally dynamic and resilient system, as opposed to a static and discretely differentiated "switchboard" conceptualization.

Although primarily an experimental psychologist, Lashley was known to rotate in clinical settings, such as at St. Elizabeth's Hospital in Washington, DC, and at laboratories engaged in the experimental analysis of higher cognitive functioning in primates, such as the Yerkes Primate Laboratory. Many physiological and comparative psychologists worked directly with Lashley, including Donald O. Hebb (1949), who subsequently engaged in interdisciplinary clinical research with Wilder Penfield at McGill University, where they set in motion a major series of research activities relating to the effects of removal of prefrontal or anterior/mesiotemporal tissue on intractable focal seizure disorders and, by extension, on higher cognitive and memory functioning. Hebb attempted to integrate the existing literature toward achieving an empirically based foundation for the *regional localization* doctrine that sought to formulate a rapprochement between the localizationistic and mass-action doctrines in the analysis of the behavioral consequences of cerebral lesions and ablations. His characterizations of cell assemblies and their functional relationships were similar to such concepts as the pluripotentiality of function and dynamic systems and subsystems as formulated by A. R. Luria (1966), the Russian psychologist and neurologist who is more widely acknowledged as having attempted to synthesize elements of strict localization and mass-action doctrine toward a general theory of higher cortical functioning. It was clear that the available empirical bases for formulating theoretical concepts were already sufficiently extensive to force consideration of more dynamic theories of higher cortical functioning.

Although Hebb's *behavior–cognition integration* was a major step toward a comprehensive theory of higher cortical functioning, there was an expanding experimental research literature that related to the effects of circumscribed cortical ablations on learning and problem-solving behavior which was expanding the empirical foundation for the analysis of brain–behavior relationships. One of the more noteworthy investigators in this area was Harry F. Harlow at the University of Wisconsin, who developed one of the first regional primate laboratories after World War II. Interestingly, Harlow is known primarily for his experimental studies of infant–maternal relationships in primates. However, the earlier work of his group is noteworthy for having provided perhaps the first experimental demonstration of a double dissociation of the effects of focal anterior and focal posterior cerebral lesions. The major experimental paradigm for isolating the effects of prefrontal regions was the *delayed reaction*, as described by Carlyle Jacobsen (1936). Visual-discrimination learning paradigms were introduced to isolate the effects of temporoparietal lesions. By demonstrating that solution of the oddity problem was affected by lesions in either the anterior or posterior association cortex (Harlow, Davis, Settlage, & Meyer, 1952), the double dissociation between delayed reaction and visual-discrimination deficits (as a function of the cephalocaudal location of the lesion) was set into even more dramatic relief. The nonspecificity of effect, therefore, and the higher position of the oddity problem function in the hierarchical organization of function in the cerebral hemispheres also were characteristic of the formation of learning sets.

It is perhaps unfortunate that Harlow abandoned this line of research in favor of the work on maternal surrogate–infant relationships for which he is most widely known. Harlow's research direction, however, was pursued in substantially greater depth by other physiological psychologists in subsequent decades. Among these, Mortimer Mishkin is known for having refined the experimental ablation approach, both methodologically and conceptually, thereby adding substantially to our knowledge of the regional localization of function in the prefrontal and inferotemporal cortex. Although Mishkin did not work directly with Harlow, there were relatively few physiological psychologists at that time and they were in ready communication with each other by means of the *Journal of Comparative and Physiological Psychology*. Mishkin worked with many on the Eastern seaboard, including Rosvold, Hebb, Sperry, Pribram, and Milner. Pribram is perhaps best known for his highly sophisticated theoretical formulations, but he was also a substantive empirical researcher as well as a neurosurgeon who was able to foster the development of neurosurgical skills among physiological psychologists at that time. He collaborated with Mishkin, who was helped on his career course to ultimately gain major professional recognition, including the Scientific Contribution Award from the American Psychological Association (APA; Mishkin & Pribram, 1954; Pribram, 1986).

The role of the temporal lobe in human learning and memory is now relatively well established. Mishkin and his associates have been able to introduce relatively refined experimental paradigms for studying the interaction between the amygdala and hippocampus in recognition memory and the independence of those structures in associative learning in primates. They have now identified separate pathways for object representation and for spatial vision connecting the occipital and inferotemporal cortices. They are exploring further the cognitive effects of interruptions in relationships between the cortex and the basal ganglia on stimulus–response learning. They are also elucidating the relationship between the cortex and the limbic system and their role in the mediation of stimulus–stimulus processing and learning (Mishkin, 1982; Mishkin & Petri, 1984; Mishkin & Ungerleider, 1983). Although this work may not have direct implications for comparable behavioral and cognitive processes in humans, it shows that where experimental analysis of behavior is feasible and the corresponding anatomical control can be achieved experimentally, theoretical refinements of potential significance for our understanding of human brain function can be achieved.

Hebb, of course, is well known for his positive influence on many students and colleagues in the late 1940s and 1950s. Among these, Brenda Milner at McGill University is perhaps the most notable. Her academic background was in experimental and comparative psychology after receiving the ScD degree at Cambridge. She had also worked with Oliver Zangwill at Cambridge as a graduate student, where she participated in construction of psychological tests and in radar research during World War II. She obtained the PhD in psychology at McGill, where she also participated in prepublication debates over Hebb's monumental 1949 volume. Her seminal article on the temporal lobes (Milner, 1954) was based on her PhD dissertation and her early work with Hebb and Penfield. A long series of important studies of the effects of prefrontal, anterotemporal, and mesiotemporal removals on learning and memory and on intractable focal (partial complex) seizures followed (Milner, 1964; Milner & Teuber, 1968). These carefully described studies reported perseveration and impairment in abstract reasoning and categorical thinking, as measured by the Wisconsin Card Sorting Test, as a consequence of prefrontal ablations. Dissociated from such deficits in the ability to shift set for the acquisition of a new sorting principle (conceptual flexibility), she also expanded on her earlier work implicating the anterior/mesiotemporal region in learning and recent memory functioning. Her findings about the effects of focal temporal lobe lesions have expanded remarkably on accounts of the neuroanatomical basis of mnestic deficits in Wernicke–Korsakoff Syndrome (Talland, 1966).

Milner (1967) has also been engaged in the study of cerebral dominance and the use of brief cognitive and memory testing procedures during specialized invasive procedures, such as the Wada Test. Her interlaboratory relationships with the group at the Massachusetts Institute of Technology (MIT) and the late Hans-Lukas Teuber has led to much collaborative work. In turn, she has also extended her interests by means of collaboration with Roger Sperry and his colleagues at the California Institute of Technology (Milner, Taylor, & Sperry, 1968). Among her many well-known students are Suzanne Corkin, Doreen Kimura, and Donald Taylor.

At the other end of what became known as the "MIT–McGill Axis" was the laboratory developed by Hans-Lukas Teuber, initially at New York's Bellevue Hospital and later at MIT. Teuber completed a doctoral degree in experimental psychology at Harvard University after he immigrated to the United States. While in the U.S. Navy, Teuber was assigned to the San Diego Naval Hospital, where he became associated with Morris Bender. Bender was among the few behavioral neurologists in this country who was interested in higher cortical functioning, especially the higher sensory processes, including visual perception, stereognosis, and tactile discrimination. These functions are now assessed routinely on a qualitative basis in a comprehensive neurological examination.

Teuber is remembered as a superb teacher and integrator of current knowledge, who had extraordinary extemporaneous speaking skills when he conveyed his rich theoretical conceptualizations that were based on a wide range of animal and human research in both clinical and experimental contexts. He had access to premorbid baseline data from group tests given in the military and, by means of contract research, was able to study the behavioral effects of penetrating missile wounds in veterans of World War II and Korea (Teuber, 1962, 1964, 1966). An engaging personality as well as the consummate communicator, he attracted large numbers of both students and colleagues.

Teuber's laboratory became engaged in numerous studies of visual field defects, somatosensory functioning, developmental complications of early brain lesions, problem-solving behavior, and many aspects of higher cognitive functioning, including studies of the conditional reaction (Weinstein, 1985). The works of his group on tactile sensitivity, two-point discrimination, point localization, pattern discrimination, roughness discrimination, spatial orientation, and body image are widely cited. His closest students and colleagues were Sidney Weinstein, Josephine Semmes, Mortimer Mishkin, Lila Ghent, and Stanley Battersby. The psychological component of cognitive neuroscience was initiated largely through his laboratory.

Following his untimely death, his influence continues at MIT, where Suzanne Corkin and her associates now represent that group on the McGill–MIT Axis. Activities of those two groups are well represented in the knowledge base for clinical neuropsychology as it relates to the effects of selected ablations and lesions on higher cortical functions in man. These more basic lines of neuropsychological research are being extended remarkably through the Society for Neuroscience and through the expansion of the neurosciences beyond the study of primary sensory and motor processes into the areas of sensory perception, attention, and problem-solving ability, as well as learning and memory. Such expansion has led to the *Journal of Cognitive Neuroscience*, edited by Michael Gazzaniga, Sperry's protegé, and published by MIT Press. The basic work conveyed through this journal includes frequent reference to clinical phenomena as a basis for conceptualizations that lead to specific experiments and theoretical formulations. A British journal, *Cognitive Neuropsychology*, expands on the neurobehavioral studies reported in cognitive neuroscience through an even more deliberate emphasis on clinical phenomena, such as the neurobehavioral syndromes, as a point of departure for the conduct of cognitive research.

Disciplinary boundaries in neuroscience are decidedly permeable, as can be inferred from the composition of the teams that report research results in these journals. The studies often require some integration of behavioral, neurophysiological, and neurochemical data so that cognitive neuroscience clearly has become an interdisciplinary venture. The recent body of knowledge in each area has already become so elaborate as to elude comprehensive knowledge on the part of the individual (scientist or practitioner), even within a particular discipline on a given subject. This will necessarily prompt permeability of disciplinary boundaries even more and require an increasingly interdisciplinary team approach to research.

Team approaches have long been acknowledged to be essential in basic, as well as more clinical, research. Such an approach is exemplified by the work of Roger Sperry and his group. Sperry received a master's degree in psychology at Oberlin and a PhD in zoology at the University of Chicago. He has been a major contributor to basic neurobehavioral research and the first Nobel Laureate with linkages to psychology. Sperry was also associated with Lashley while at the Yerkes Laboratories, where he began to study the selective growth of neural connections after the placement of highly circumscribed lesions. While studying with Paul Weiss, a neurophysiologist at the University of Chicago, Sperry (1958) wrote his doctoral dissertation on the reorganization of function following the surgical interchange of nerves and muscles in the frog. This work prompted modification of the neurological and neuropsychological concepts of central nervous system plasticity and the functional interchangeability of neural connections.

The work for which Sperry received the Nobel Prize involved the experimental analysis of the organization of lateralized cerebral functions using the corpus callosotomy paradigm, also known as the split-brain preparation (Sperry, Gazzaniga, & Bogen, 1969). This paradigm established the foundation for the multitude of related studies that followed and that have essentially confirmed many of the hypotheses derived from the clinical and experimental studies of the effects of focal lesions in either cerebral hemisphere. This research paradigm permitted the isolation of each cerebral hemisphere under controlled cognitive processing conditions to yield further experimental evidence that only the dominant cerebral hemisphere has access to word knowledge in confrontation naming, and that the nondominant cerebral hemisphere has a relative advantage for processing figural or nonverbal stimuli.

Development of Quantitative and Qualitative Neuropsychological Assessment Procedures

While physiological/experimental and cognitive neuropsychological research was being generated on the east coast, and to some extent on the west, a number of investigators, primarily in the midwest, were developing objective psychometric procedures that extended the assessment of higher cortical functions from standardized intelligence tests to specialized tests of perceptual, memorial, and abstract reasoning abilities as applied to individuals with known or suspected central nervous system lesions. The Wechsler and Binet scales were already in wide use and were being studied again, primarily in the midwest, for their sensitivity to the effects of lateralized lesions in the cerebral hemispheres. The marginal sensitivity of intelligence tests to the behavioral consequences of brain lesions, especially in neurologically "silent regions," led to the construction of adjunct procedures, the earliest of which was the Halstead Neuropsychological Test Battery.

Halstead received his doctorate from Northwestern University. His ties to neurology were largely made through Heinrich Klüver (a physiological psychologist) and Paul Bucy (a neurosurgeon). The initial motivation for Halstead's work came from the necessity to validate his theory of "biological intelligence" (Halstead, 1947). He was not highly concerned with clinical application (G. Goldstein, 1985; Reed, 1985). Halstead was impressed with the relative insensitivity of some tests of brain dysfunction in individuals with known neurological involvements, as compared to the potentially more powerful sensitivity of some other tests to intrinsic brain changes. He postulated two types of intelligence, one being instrumental in learned behavior and the other having an innate and fundamentally intrinsic organic basis, and thus more dependent on the integrity of the cerebral hemispheres. This latter, or *biological intelligence*, was hypothesized to decline after involvement of the prefrontal association cortex, the region of the cerebral hemispheres that is now believed to subserve *executive functions*. The distinction between these components of intelligence was similar to Hebb's (1949) Intelligence A and Intelligence B, and to Cattell's (1963) distinction between crystallized and fluid abilities.

Halstead can be regarded as having formed the first quantitative neuropsychological laboratory, and he set out to define and assess higher cortical functions in man, beginning in about 1936. His battery came into wide clinical use as a result of the amendations and extensive research generated by Ralph M. Reitan, one of Halstead's graduate students at the University of Chicago. Reitan (1964) has devoted his entire career to extending studies with this battery, which is now known as the Halstead–Reitan Neuropsychological Battery (HRNB), to a wide array of neurological populations by means of comparisons with groups of normal, psychiatric, and medical control subjects. The Halstead Impairment Index, a composite measure of outcomes defined by group differences on each of 10 subtests, continues to serve as the pivotal measure for interpreting test results on this test battery.

Tens of thousands of patients have now been assessed across numerous neuropsychological laboratories, especially those developed by Reitan's students, including Charles Matthews, Hallgrim Kløve, Homer Reed, James Reed, and Kathleen Fitzhugh-Bell. The HRNB is rarely used without the addition of procedures for the assessment of higher functions that are not sampled extensively by the HRNB. Owing to the paucity of effectively valid tests of planning and executive functions, adjunctive procedures often involve the use of the Wisconsin Card Sorting Test, the Porteus Maze Test, and verbal and figural associative fluency procedures to augment the Halstead Category Test (the primary basis for assessing such functions within the HRNB). The growing number of useful tests of verbal and nonverbal immediate and delayed memory has also led to the adjunctive assessment of such functions in this context, because the battery provides a less formal analysis of such functions than is considered necessary for a comprehensive neuropsychological evaluation. The HRNB does constitute an attempt to relate theory to practice, but it is primarily an empirically based set of procedures for inferring the presence of organic cerebral disease and its probable diffuse, focal locus, or both; analyzing the most likely etiological factors underlying the cognitive dysfunctions evidenced in the battery; and analyzing these findings for rehabilitation and recovery.

Another midwestern neuropsychologist, Arthur L. Benton, had his educational roots in the east, where he earned a PhD at Columbia University with Joseph Zubin and Carney Landis. He became involved in the assessment of manual test performances of psychiatric patients at the New York State Psychiatric Institute. Previous experience with Morris Bender at the San Diego Naval Hospital added to his biological orientation, because he had some opportunity to assess individuals with brain injuries during World War II. A noted historian and academician, Benton developed advanced knowledge of clinical/behavioral neurology, and also developed an interest in developmental phenomena and in speech and language (Benton, 1964, 1969). His first effort at developing a quantitative test resulted in the Benton Visual Retention Test, a measure of immediate figural recall (Benton, 1945). Initially identified as a clinical psychologist who directed a program at the University of Louisville and then at the University of Iowa, he did not become engaged heavily in neurobehavioral research until he joined the Neurology Department at the University of Iowa. It was here that his relationship with Robert Joynt and Maurice Van Allen helped him to launch a major program of neuropsychological research. Within this framework he was able to nurture and support a series of graduate students and visiting colleagues who became interested in developing their research and clinical skills in clinical neuropsychology. His subsequent record of research and development of procedures for assessing visuospatial judgment, visuoconstructional praxis, facial recognition, auditory perception, serial digit learning, cerebral dominance, developing language disorders, and language behavior are well known and have been identified selectively for didactic purposes (Costa & Spreen, 1985).

Benton's outstanding record in neuropsychology began in about 1958, when he was almost 50 years old. His record of achievement led the International Neuropsychological Society (INS) to establish an award in his name directed at recognizing research productivity in midcareer. Among those who trained or worked with Benton are Harold Bechtoldt, Don Shankweiler, Otfried Spreen, Harvey Levin, Kerry Hamsher, Nils Varney, and Julia Hannay. He also has influenced many of the best-known behavioral neurologists in the world, including Ennio DeRenzi (Italy), Amiram Carmon (Israel), Henry Hécean (France), Klaus Poeck (Germany), and Sumiko Sasanuma, a Japanese speech pathologist. To this partial sampling could be added the names of virtually all professionals who have had any contact with Benton, both within and outside of psychology and well beyond the geographic boundaries of the midwest. He received the Distinguished Professional Contribution Award of the APA in 1979. There does not appear to be anyone else whose work bridges the many domains in which Benton has functioned professionally and academically, including behavioral neurology, cognitive neuropsychology, neurolinguistics and aphasiology, developmental neuropsychology, clinical psychology, and experimental/physiological psychology. His name is legion as an integrator of knowledge within and between these domains.

American clinical neuropsychology is known for its large armamentarium of quantitative procedures (Filskov & Boll, 1986; Meier, Strauman, & Thompson, 1987). Muriel Lezak's (1995) comprehensive description of procedures and norms was a welcomed and necessary attempt to bring order to what had become a highly diverse collection of applicable quantitative procedures. A related development has been the identification of principles that incorporate qualitative criteria for analyzing the behavior of individuals when executing tasks that may also be subject to quantitative analysis. The work of the Boston University group, notably Harold Goodglass and Edith Kaplan, has contributed significantly to clinical practice by drawing deliberate attention to the processes underlying neuropsychological deficits. The Boston Diagnostic Aphasia Examination (Goodglass & Kaplan, 1983) is an example of an assessment instrument that depends as much on qualitative as it does on quantitative aspects of the protocol. Kaplan (1983) has modified the Wechsler Memory Scale to incorporate such qualitative considerations, and she has developed adjunctive qualitative analytic procedures for the Wechsler Adult Intelligence Scale–Revised to help delineate the processes underlying disturbances in brain functioning. The work of Goodglass and Kaplan has bridged clinical psychology, developmental psychology, neuropsychology, neurolinguistics, and behavioral neurology in ways that have contributed to both theory and practice (Jones & Butters, 1983). Among those who have worked in that tradition and who now are recognized for their many contributions are Nelson Butters, Sheila Blumstein, Edgar Zurif, Laird Cermak, and Marlene Oscar-Berman, who demonstrate how the Boston group has bridged the basic and applied worlds in the domains of language, learning and memory, and other higher cognitive functions (Goodglass, 1985).

This brief review of converging lines of experimental and clinical research in the history of clinical neuropsychology is intended to convey the evolution of a specialty that did not develop in isolation, but rather was decisively influenced by multiple fields within psychology and more broadly in the neurosciences. Some of the clinical applications that are most widely practiced today have been incorporated selectively into the armamentarium of the clinician. These concepts and procedural variations have some basis in the basic cognitive and experimental/physiological foundations of the specialty. Similarly, as clinical neuropsychological practices advance, particularly as a function of the study of amnesic and prefrontally lesioned patients, basic researchers in neuropsychology and the neurosciences have been able to ask more pertinent questions and to guide their research, in part, on clinical grounds.

Developments in Behavioral Neurology and Neuropsychiatry

Despite the strong linkages between American and European medicine during the late 19th and early 20th centuries, the interest within European neurology and psychiatry in the description and neuroanatomical bases of various behavioral syndromes was not characteristic of early American neurology and psychiatry. Following World War II, some European neurologists emigrated to the United States, such as Derek Denny-Brown who had trained with MacDonald Critchley in England. Denny-Brown ultimately located in Boston, where he began to influence younger neurologists. There was some interest in the neurology of behavior in North America through the neurosurgeon Wilder Penfield, who worked in experimental collaboration with Hebb and Milner at McGill University and, in addition, through Morris Bender, who collaborated with Teuber when he was at New York University.

A major work on the parietal lobes (Critchley, 1953) was widely read in the United States and Canada, as was the work of Kurt Goldstein, a neuropsychiatrist who had trained at Heidelberg and Breslau before leaving Germany for the United States in the 1930s. Goldstein had achieved considerable academic stature for his work on penetrating missile injuries after World War I, but he did not become known in the United States until the mid-1930s, when he began publishing a series of studies on the effects of frontal lobe lesions on abstract reasoning and categorical thinking, as reflected in performance on sorting tasks designed to measure loss of the abstract attitude and the ability to form concepts (K. Goldstein & Scheerer, 1941). Goldstein was engaged primarily in private practice in this country and was a conceptualizer who engaged philosophical and psychodynamic issues, organismic psychology, psychoanalysis, and Gestalt theory. However, he is best known in neuropsychology for his work on abstract reasoning and categorical thinking in association with penetrating brain injuries and schizophrenia. He also was among the first investigators to explore cognitive functions that transcended primary sensory and motor functions. He investigated the assumption of particular cognitive sets, the conceptual flexibility required to shift cognitive sets as prompted by changes in environmental feedback, and the ability to maintain simultaneous or compound cognitive sets. His work complemented methodologically the procedures developed by Weigl in Germany, and helped to lay the foundation for the development of the Wisconsin Card Sorting Test as a means of assessing the ability to abstract from the common properties in a test situation the essential principles for guiding actions and decisions.

Goldstein's work is an example of the permeability of interdisciplinary boundaries. He relied heavily on relatively formalized psychometric procedures and worked with psychologists, but was formally trained in medicine. The interest in this area of assessment remains extremely strong because it constitutes one of the few methodologies with some demonstrated sensitivity to the effects of prefrontal cortical involvement. The definitive assessment of the effects of prefrontal lesions remains relatively elusive, however, given the inconsistency with which even these more sensitive measures can identify the presence of frontal lobe disease, though some progress toward improved construct validity of inferences derived from attentional tasks is being achieved (Stuss, 1991).

The 19th century European literature on the neurology of aphasia was relatively unknown in this country until Norman Geschwind (1965) published a summary of that work. Norman Geschwind served a residency with Denny-Brown and Fred Quadfasel at the Boston Veterans Administration Medical Center. Geschwind had earlier been influenced by the mass-action views of higher cortical functioning of the British neurologists, such as Hughlings Jackson and Henry Head. Bent on obtaining a deeper knowledge of 19th century European behavioral neurology, Geschwind secured a Moseley scholarship and spent 3 years at Queen Square Hospital in London, where he immersed himself in that literature. He subsequently reversed direction theoretically and became an advocate of a relatively strict localizationistic view, at least as it is applied to clinical phenomena during the acute and subacute phases of cerebrovascular accidents of a relatively localized nature.

In his theoretical formulations (Geschwind, 1965) and in his many highly articulate presentations around the country, he brought to the attention of North American neurologists, psychiatrists, and psychologists the symptomatic features or syndromes associated with the white-matter disconnection of selected structures in the brain. He began a collaborative relationship with Harold Goodglass and Edith Kaplan at the Boston Veterans Administration Medical Center, where they developed a major program of research and a set of procedures for assessing aphasia that are now widely taught in the training programs of various disciplines (Damasio, 1985; Goodglass, 1986). Geschwind went on to describe anatomical asymmetries between the cerebral hemispheres that contradicted traditional views of structural equivalence of the hemispheres (Geschwind & Levitsky, 1968). He also came to recognize mechanisms that facilitated recovery and that required some deviation from a strict localizationistic view of CNS functioning. His research interests expanded considerably into the epidemiology of dyslexia before his untimely death in 1985. In the course of his brief but extremely productive career, he inspired numerous protégés to high levels of clinical and academic achievement, including Martin L. Albert, D. Frank Benson, Antonio Damasio, Kenneth Heilman, and Alan Rubens.

European neurology and North American psychology and medicine became increasingly connected after World War II. In France, Henry Hécean and F. Lhermitte came to prominence as a result of their extensive neurobehavioral research and their publications, along with Jean De Ajuriaguerra. *Neuropsychologia* was an early journal, edited by Hécean, whose relationship to American neuropsychology was mediated largely by Arthur Benton and Brenda Milner. He had done research with both Benton and Milner on the lateralized specialization of function in the cerebral hemispheres, the epidemiology of aphasic syndromes and other neurobehavioral syndromes, and the psycholinguistic analysis of aphasia (Albert, 1984). He was a collaborator of Oliver Zangwill in England and, accordingly, he was instrumental in relating the growing French and Anglo American literatures. Similarly, Ennio DeRenzi in Milan established the journal *Cortex*. Like Hécean, DeRenzi was closely associated with Benton, with whom he spent some time as a postdoctoral associate at the University of Iowa. These individuals provide another relevant context in which Benton's contribution to interdisciplinary collaboration was influential.

Perhaps the most widely read European neurologist is A. R. Luria, who had a PhD in psychology (1936), as well as an MD (1943) from the Moscow Medical Institute. He is well known for his major text, *Higher Cortical Functions in Man* (Luria, 1966). Distinctions between psychology, psychiatry, and neurology were less well-defined in European medicine before World War II, partly because Luria, like many others, began his clinical practice in psychoanalysis, the predominant movement within the clinical domain of numerous disciplines. His research initially was focused on the isolation of unconscious processes underlying motor responsivity. The prescribed Soviet materialistic psychology of that time prompted a shift into a study of human reflexes. Social psychological interests were diverted into more ideologically benign areas. This was to the good fortune of neuropsychology, because his contributions were clearly path-finding and path-determining for neuropsychology, considered from a broad interdisciplinary perspective. Vygotsky, another major Russian psychologist, influenced Luria through his cultural–historical theory of cognitive functioning, which proposed that perception, attention, and memory are converted into socially structured cognitive functions through learning. Therefore, Luria developed an interest in the symbolic operations underlying the very highest mental functions and became launched on an intensive course of clinical and experimental investigation.

Luria was instrumental in placing numerous neuropsychological papers from around the world on the program of the International Congress of Psychology held in Moscow in 1966. He was unable to travel outside the Soviet Union due to political constraints, but he was permitted to communicate with colleagues in England and, through them, with colleagues elsewhere in the world. His text includes a remarkable breadth of content and depth of knowledge of the world literature for an individual who was so isolated. He became a major conceptualizer of the existing literature, and he became best known for his sophisticated elaboration of the general regional localization theory of higher cortical functions, which attempts to integrate the localizationistic and the mass-action/equipotentiality doctrines. Through his extensive study of the consequences of brain injuries during World War II, he achieved a level of conceptual formulation that carried the theory of higher cortical functioning toward the level that is now being attained in cognitive neuroscientific research. Luria's formulations of the concept of functional neural systems and their behavioral analysis through qualitative and quantitative test procedures, and through the analysis of symptom configurations for inferring the regional localization of the primary disease process, are now well accepted. The concept of *pluripotentiality* (or redundancy of function) at different levels of the nervous system has had explanatory value for the analysis of recovery of function after acute cerebral injury.

Perhaps more than any other individual in the history of clinical neuropsychology, Luria has facilitated the integration of basic and clinical research. In accord with the more quantitative American emphasis in the assessment of higher cortical functions, his work prompted various individuals to formalize procedures he described in analyses of individual cases for large-sample research and for diagnostic and rehabilitation application (Christensen, 1975; Golden, Hammeke, & Purisch, 1980).

CLINICAL NEUROPSYCHOLOGY: WHAT IS IT?

The foregoing historical overview indicates that the knowledge underlying neuropsychological practice has been derived from multiple disciplinary and interdisciplinary sources over the past half-century or more. The major empirical and theoretical domains have been the basic experimental research in physiological, comparative, and cognitive psychology; the development of quantitative and qualitative neuropsychological principles and procedures for clinical application; and the descriptive syndromal analysis of the behavioral consequences of localized and diffuse neuropathological processes. The primary role of the clinical neuropsychologist is the integration of knowledge and practice across these domains. This professional function is reflected in the current definition of a clinical neuropsychologist as put forth by the Division of Clinical Neuropsychology of the American Psychological Association (Division 40 Task Force, 1989a).

The use of the designation *clinical neuropsychologist* is complicated by the fact that individuals of numerous disciplines identify themselves by the use of this term, yet there is no statutory authority within state licensing laws that isolates this role from the other roles of the various professions involved, including psychology, various medical specialties, and the speech and language professions. As nonstatutory credentialing procedures have been developed (e.g., American Board of Clinical Neuropsychology/American Board of Professional Psychology), some confusion has arisen with respect to the eligibility of individuals from disciplines other than psychology to be examined for the professional clinical neuropsychology credential. Even within psychology, state licensing statutes do not embrace specialty licensure considerations, although some states are attempting to enact legislation that will empower state licensing boards to examine in specialized areas of psychology such as neuropsychology (Mendoza, 1993).

A general definition of what constitutes clinical neuropsychological practice is necessarily very broad, as suggested by the Division 40 definition which also attempts to incorporate criteria for training and supervised experience (Division 40 Task Force, 1989a). Such definitions must necessarily be augmented by the delineation of roles and responsibilities that are encompassed by that definition. This task has been performed by the APA Division 40 Task Force on Education, Accreditation, and Credentialing (TFEAC), a continuing policy-oriented body that was established initially in 1977 by the International Neuropsychological Society (INS), and subsequently was cosponsored by INS and Division 40 of APA before becoming the sole responsibility of Division 40 in about 1982.

The rationale for recognition of a new specialty was derived from the scientific and professional products of the various supporting organizations of which INS and Division 40, through the efforts of the TFEAC, provided a leading role. These organizations generated the basic and clinical knowledge foundation through various experimental, cognitive, physiological, developmental, and applied activities, and through the proliferation of research into the psychological processes affected by the pathophysiological processes that determine the nature and extent of neuropsychological deficits in neurologic and psychiatric disorders. Setting aside for the moment the special problems that must be addressed when clinical neuropsychology is defined in terms of its practice by specialists in other disciplines, such as behavioral neurologists and speech pathologists, it seems reasonably clear that the scientific and professional activities of psychologists in clinical neuropsychology are being integrated into a progressively more definable and expanding area of specialization within psychology (Benton, 1987; Costa, 1983; Division 40 Task Force, 1987; Meier, 1981; Rourke, 1991). The discussion that follows focuses on the specialized functions of psychologists as clinical neuropsychologists.

The first and still fundamental practice of clinical neuropsychology is the evaluation of psychological and behavioral disturbances associated with organic central nervous system dysfunction. The clinician is required to establish a comprehensive database of historical and current general medical and surgical, neurological, pharmacological, developmental, and psychosocial factors underlying the presenting problem. Included in this database is the entire complement of specialized neural diagnostic procedures such as neural imaging, electroencephalography, and brain-mapping techniques. An assessment strategy is derived from the database and referral issues and requires knowledge of the various neuropsychological protocols, test procedures, and inventories that are available through a rapidly expanding literature. This function includes the application of fixed batteries at their current stage of validation and the design of flexible test batteries based on an understanding of the probable primary processes that may be affected by the underlying disease process. The assessment goal is to address relevant neurobehavioral aspects of higher psychological functioning that are considered to be central to understanding the cognitive strengths and deficits of the individual.

The following assessment functions were identified by the Divison 40 Task Force (1987):

- Differential diagnosis between psychogenic and neurogenic syndromes and disorders (e.g., depression vs. dementia).
- Differential diagnosis between two or more suspected etiologies of cerebral dysfunction (e.g., neoplasm vs. cerebral vascular accident).
- Delineation of spared and impaired functions secondary to an episodic event (e.g., cerebral vascular accident, head trauma, infection).
- Establishment of baseline measures to monitor progressive cerebral disease or recovery processes (e.g., neoplasm, demyelinating disease, head injury).
- Comparison of pre- and postneuropsychological functioning following pharmacologic, surgical and behavioral interventions (e.g., drug trials, tissue excision, shunts, revascularization, language, or cognitive therapy).
- Assessment of cognitive and affective status for the formulation of rehabilitation strategies and the design of remedial interventions.

Competency in clinical neuropsychology requires the knowledge and skills to comprehend and integrate information in numerous areas of psychological science and the clinical neurosciences, including:

- Selected aspects of functional neuroanatomy, neuropathology, and pathophysiology.
- Disorders of attention, sensory, perceptual, conceptual thinking, language, memory, and voluntary and involuntary motor and affective processes.
- Neurological and related diseases, including their manner of presentation, course, and treatment.
- CNS effects of systemic disorders.
- Child development and ontology of neuropsychological processes.

- Expected decrements in neuropsychological processes as a function of normal aging.
- Behavioral pathology and psychopharmacology.
- Psychophysiological principles underlying behavioral pathology.
- Sociocultural factors as codeterminants of behavior.
- Principles of personality assessment and interviewing skills.
- Principles of test administration and interpretation relating to both fixed and flexible neuropsychological batteries.
- Principles of cognitive remediation and derivation of specific intervention strategies.

It is immediately evident that the assessment role in clinical neuropsychology includes the derivation of intervention strategies and, by implication, an intervention role. Because clinical neuropsychologists are ordinarily specializing from a generic applied base, either in clinical, counseling, or school psychology, they have already acquired a foundation in assessment and intervention that is being extended by means of specialized training and supervised experience into the neurobehavioral domain, when it is broadly defined. A search for a core curriculum that will ensure the development of neuropsychological competency necessarily would include cognitive, physiological, and experimental psychology; differential psychology, abnormal psychology, and life-span developmental psychology. The curriculum would also include relevant areas of clinical neuroscience, including clinical neurology, behavioral neurology, and specialized neurodiagnostic technologies as a basis for refinement of skills to extend competency into increasingly more specialized activities. The latter would appear to include design and validation of new neuropsychological procedures to extend applications in behavioral analysis and modification, learning disorders, psychopharmacology, psychophysiology, remedial interventions, behavior genetics, psycholinguistics, personality, and psychopathology (functional and organic). Therefore, clinical neuropsychology as practiced by psychologists would build on a knowledge base that includes other disciplines as well as subdisciplines within psychology. Members of the subdisciplines of psychology involved in this knowledge base do not ordinarily practice clinical neuropsychology unless, of course, they have taken steps to acquire the generic applied, as well as the specialized, knowledge and clinical skills that comprise a full competency in the specialty.

Parameters of Practice in Clinical Neuropsychology

Clinical neuropsychology has evolved as a specialized area of knowledge and application and is increasingly recognized as having distinct disciplinary and interdisciplinary features. It is noteworthy that within the discipline of psychology, clinical neuropsychology has not received uniform recognition as a specialty, owing largely to the characteristic lag between developments in the field and modification of APA policies to address those changes. APA has recognized this problem for many years and has charged committees and boards within the organization to pursue a rationale for the identification and continued recognition of new specialties. It has been more than a decade since the APA Subcommittee on Specialization (SOS) of the APA Board of Professional Affairs submitted its first report. The SOS report was subsequently revised in the form of a manual (Sales, Bricklin, & Hall, 1984) that included a proposed set of principles and procedures which a new specialty might address to establish its case for initial identification and continued recognition as a specialty.

Clinical neuropsychology had been evolving through an identifiable sequence of developments and was the first area of practice to provide an organized response to the SOS manual. It was hoped that the APA would devise procedures for review of such a claim by appropriate organizational and interorganizational bodies. This hope did materialize, so there is now a formal mechanism for the recognition of new specialties within the APA. The Commission for the Recognition of Specialties and Proficiencies in Professional Psychology (CRSPPP) was established by the APA in 1995 to receive and process petitions by sponsoring organizations in support of an emerging area of practice to be recognized as a specialty or as a proficiency. The Division 40 Planning Committee (chaired by the author) then prepared a petition package for submission to the CRSPPP, following guidelines modeled largely after the earlier deliberations of the SOS, in support of claims by Division 40 that clinical neuropsychology meets the CRSPPP criteria for a specialty. CRSPPP unanimously approved this petition in April, 1996. This endorsement has now been forwarded to the Council of Representatives for further action and movement through the APA governance structure.

An important contribution of the SOS was the identification of four parameters of specialized practice that characterize a specialty and help to differentiate a given specialty from preexisting and other emerging specialties; that is, *problems*, *procedures*, *populations* and *settings*. The SOS also elaborated conceptually the distinction between generic and specialized competencies and proposed that any specialized competency must be built on a generic applied core as well as basic knowledge of psychology. Generic applied competency requires a foundation in psychological science with a predominantly clinical emphasis, although such training may be attained through other generic avenues if a clinical internship is included. The generic base for clinical neuropsychology was expected to include the structure and process of interviewing, intellectual abilities, aptitude, interest and personality measurements, selected psychotherapy and counseling interventions, consultation skills, and a consumer/patient educational orientation. Specialized competency was deemed to include comprehensive history taking, definition of clinical problems/issues to be addressed, establishment of problem- and goal-oriented records, proficiency in goal attainment scaling as a basis for intervention, quality assurance and service systems evaluation, application of a wide range of neuropsychological assessment procedures to multiple populations served by neuropsychologists, test construction and validation, remedial and supportive intervention design and implementation, individual and agency consultation, and consumer education skills. Such specialized competency was expected to be achieved by means of sets of skills anchored to the four parameters of practice that the SOS identified.

Clinical neuropsychologists function primarily based on referrals from health, education, and legal professionals; agencies and institutions; and in response to needs of other service systems (e.g., courts, schools, extended rehabilitation and general care facilities, military installations, chemical treatment facilities). Primary employment settings are estimated to be almost equally divided between hospital medical centers, private practice, a combination of (salaried) hospital- or clinic-based employment, and private practice (Putnam & DeLuca, 1990, 1991). The four parameters of practice identified by the SOS have implications for distinguishing between specialties and proficiencies and for the definition and assessment of competency.

Problems Confronted

Referrals for clinical neuropsychological assessment typically include, but are not limited to, the following: differential diagnoses between psychogenic and neurogenic syndromes; differential diagnoses between two or more suspected etiologies of cerebral dysfunction; elucidation of spared and impaired functions secondary to a cerebral cortical or subcortical event; establishment of neurobehavioral baseline measures for monitoring progressive cerebral disease or recovery; comparison of pre- and postpharmacologic, surgical, or behavioral interventions; and assessment of higher cortical functions for the formulation of rehabilitation strategies. Intervention problems include design of procedures for utilizing available functions to compensate for an impaired function, retraining of the impaired function to a higher level of adaptive effectiveness, and environmental (ecological) manipulations to enhance adaptive effectiveness.

Populations Served

Adult neurological populations include cerebrovascular accidents, neoplasms, infectious and inflammatory diseases, degenerative diseases, head trauma, demyelinating disease, and various forms of dementing illness. Psychiatric populations of primary interest include somatoform disorders of pseudoneurologic character; depression as a component of, a diagnostic alternative to, or both to be differentiated from dementia; and psychosis as a pseudodementing disorder or as a differential diagnostic entity to be distinguished from behavioral disturbances in selected neurological populations such as partial complex seizure disorder.

General medical and surgical populations include older individuals who may have some neuropsychological deficits associated with an early dementing illness that may complicate medical or surgical management; candidates for kidney transplant or dialysis; candidates for cardiac surgery, including transplants; and chronic pain patients with a neurological versus functional basis.

Children with learning disabilities with a possible neurologic basis are referred from pediatricians, pediatric neurologists, and the schools, in addition to a marked expansion of neuropsychological evaluation and treatment of pediatric neurological patients. Growing referral populations include the chemically dependent (especially polydrug users and alcoholics), AIDS dementia cases, and victims of environmental toxin exposures.

Settings

Practice is prevalent in health science centers and associated teaching hospitals, community hospitals and clinics, rehabilitation institutes, military hospitals, Veterans Administration Medical Centers, and private practices.

Services and Procedures

Primary services include neuropsychological assessment, cognitive remediation and intervention, agency and institutional consultation, education and counseling for individuals and families, and selected psychotherapies or behavioral therapies as appropriate for neurologically involved individuals. A growing armamentarium of procedures is available for neuropsychological assessment (Lezak, 1995) and for cognitive remediation and intervention (Meier, Benton, & Diller, 1987).

The APA subsequently put a second group to work on the new specialty issue; namely, the Task Force on Scope and Criteria of Accreditation, which issued a report in June of 1989 that called for the establishment of procedures for recognizing new specialties. These procedures are currently under consideration and should result in more formal procedures for recognizing new specialties. Clinical neuropsychology stands at the top of the list for such recognition and has been invited to work through Division 40 and other interested organizations, such as the American Board of Professional Psychology, for early consideration. Therefore, clinical neuropsychology is likely to become the first formally recognized new specialty based largely on the work of the TFEAC and its liaison activities with the SOS/BPA and the Board of Educational Affairs (BEA) of APA. The American Board of Clinical Neuropsychology (ABCN), through its relationship with the American Board of Professional Psychology (ABPP), has become a leader in the development of knowledge and competency-based examining procedures. ABPP has been prompted by ABCN to provide leadership for the specification of criteria for postdoctoral programs, which probably will become the major source for advanced specialization training of clinical neuropsychologists in the future.

EDUCATIONAL MODELS

Predoctoral Level

The TFEAC has produced guidelines for predoctoral programs, doctoral internships, and postdoctoral education and training (Division 40 Task Force, 1987). Analysis of predoctoral options suggested five potential models for curriculum design (Meier, 1981). All require inclusion of courses and supervised practicum experiences in the critical knowledge and skill areas identified earlier. Representative curriculum outlines are available elsewhere.

Model I—Complete Intradepartmental Curriculum. This model would have all aspects of the curriculum, including psychological, neuropsychological and clinical neuroscience components, provided by a Department of Psychology graduate faculty in an applied (usually clinical) program. Only departments without access to a major health sciences center would be expected to attempt to apply this model. Such departments would necessarily be geographically remote and have limited clinical training opportunities. However, they might have access to a network of clinical facilities with qualified clinical supervisors that would be required to develop a definitive program. The likelihood of such a program meeting future accreditation requirements seems questionable given the knowledge and skill agendas outlined earlier.

Model II—Interdepartmental Supporting Program. Although the basic psychological science and generic clinical core courses would be provided by a graduate department of psychology, an interdepartmental supporting program (or minor), usually in a medical school located in a major health sciences center, would complement the curriculum through clinical neuroscience courses and supervised neuropsychological practicum (e.g., University of Iowa, University of Minnesota). This model adds one year to a characteristic clinical or other appropriate departmentally-based generic applied program and assumes inclusion of an internship with generic and specialty activity foci. A 2-year internship (one generic and one specialized) is usually necessary for definitive competency development as recommended for the future in all applied areas at the Gainesville Conference on Internship Training (Belar et al., 1989). A 1-year internship with generic and specialized components could be followed by 1 year of formal specialized postdoctoral training in this model.

Model III—Autonomous Designated Program. A comprehensive predoctoral curriculum designed to produce a fully competent clinical neuropsychologist has been attempted by a few departments. Such programs are notable for their independence of other applied programs, including clinical programs, within the sponsoring psychology department (e.g., University of Houston, Queens College of the City University of New York). Such programs are not eligible for accreditation review and approval under current APA policies. This may account, at least in part, for their small number. Another important factor is the need to establish a generic competency base before or while acquiring specialized competency, which presents a difficult challenge for such programs unless the curriculum is lengthened by at least 1 year. It is noteworthy that the Houston program has been integrated with the APA-Accredited Clinical Program in that department to form a track, much like programs at the University of Windsor and University of Memphis.

Model IV—Simultaneous Pursuit of PhD and PsyD Degrees. Although conceptually interesting, no examples of this model have been identified. In addition to being unrealistic to meet the needs of most students interested in clinical neuropsychology, the model does not circumvent the need for generic as well as specialized competency development. However, a conceptual analysis of the model yields a better understanding of the academic requirements for developing research in contrast to clinical competencies in a given specialty (Meier, 1981).

Model V—Integrated Clinical Neuroscience Curriculum. A few universities have integrated relevant departmental resources into a clinically oriented, but largely basic, neuroscience curriculum. A core curriculum in neuroscience is pursued by students from different disciplines, including psychology. The primary goal of such programs is the production of clinical neuroscientists with an interdisciplinary orientation (e.g., University of California–Berkeley, Stanford University, University of Minnesota). Psychology students in such a curriculum who wish to acquire clinical neuropsychological competency are still confronted with the need for supervised generic clinical and specialized neuropsychological education and training. Such considerations apply as well to graduate students in experimental, physiological, cognitive and developmental psychology who sometimes enter the clinical neuropsychological arena without generic clinical or specialized clinical neuropsychological backgrounds. They may feel entitled to function in applied roles on the basis of their academic credentials, but then naively (yet in good faith) attempt to enter professional practice. Clinical neuropsychology continues to embrace the scientist–practitioner approach to training and practice, but appreciates that different orientations and competencies are involved in research and practice roles.

Predoctoral Internship Level

Like predoctoral programs in the (de facto) traditional specialties (e.g., clinical, counseling, school psychology), predoctoral internships are accredited by the APA. However, accreditation applies to the designated specialty and not to any specialized tracks within the internship. Accreditation, therefore, has only generic clinical implications for the competencies being developed. The primary goal of the internship is to ensure competency for entry into professional practice. Most jurisdictions then require 2 years of supervised applied experience for licensure. This renders most internships incomplete for specialized competency development. Many internships are providing substantial rotations in neurologic, psychiatric, and rehabilitation settings and they are preparing people very well for a formal postdoctoral specialty training year or two (e.g., University of Florida, University of Michigan). Accreditation criteria require that at least one half of the internship be devoted to generic clinical activities. Other than a 2-year internship format, internship experience does not appear to be sufficient for specialized competency attainment. Internships can provide an introduction to specialty practice, but they are increasingly followed by postdoctoral training (Meier, 1987).

Postdoctoral Level

The TFEAC anticipated that doctoral education-training would become the primary basis for establishing specialized competency in clinical neuropsychology. Although there has been some increase in the number of clinical psychology programs with specialized tracks in neuropsychology, the number of complete predoctoral programs have not increased significantly. Instead, most of the growth in training activities has occurred at the postdoctoral level. This is due, in part, to the absence of accreditation mechanisms for neuropsychological specialization at the doctoral and internship levels. More importantly, there appears to be wide recognition of a need to establish generic applied knowledge and skills before embarking on specialized competency attainment. The SOS Principles and Procedures documents appear to have anticipated this development by distinguishing between generic and specialized competencies and emphasizing the interdependency between them. In addition, the doctoral and internship levels have been pressed to provide adequate generic applied preparation within the traditional time frame, and cannot readily provide more than introductory specialized knowledge and practicum experience. Because most licensure statutes require 2 years of supervised postdoctoral experience, the predisposition to seek postdoctoral training is further increased. Add to such factors the marked increase in knowledge and application that is dramatically apparent when one attends a major professional meeting (e.g., INS, APA Division 40), and the need for postdoctoral training becomes even more compelling.

This rapid specialty development probably accounts for the growth in postdoctoral training opportunities that is reflected in the recent establishment of the Association of Postdoctoral Programs in Clinical Neuropsychology (APPCN). This association evolved from the Midwest Neuropsychological Consortium, a group of programs directed by ABPP/ABCN Diplomates in clinical neuropsychology that are largely located in large health sciences centers. The APPCN adheres to the TFEAC Guidelines for Postdoctoral Training (Division 40 Task Force, 1987). Formalization of postdoctoral training guidelines is proceeding further through initiatives from the American Board of Professional Psychology (ABPP), which sponsored an interorganizational meeting in 1991 that resulted in the establishment of the Interorganizational Council for Accreditation of Postdoctoral Programs in Psychology (IOCAPP). This group of organizations includes ABPP, APA, the National Register, APPIC, the Canadian Register, the Association of State and Provincial Psychology Boards (ASPPB), and representatives from ABPP specialty boards or associations of postdoctoral programs such as the APPCN. The impetus for this development came from ABPP at the suggestion of the American Board of Clinical Neuropsychology (ABCN) representative (Manfred Meier) on the ABPP Board of Trustees. APPIC and APA have now conducted postdoctoral conferences to define standards for postdoctoral education and training. The development of postdoctoral program standards by the APPCN and new specialty recognition by APA should lead to the accreditation of clinical neuropsychology postdoctoral programs in the near future.

It is assumed that clinical neuropsychology programs at all training levels (predoctoral, internship, or postdoctoral) have as a primary goal the development of clinical competence. Therefore, the distinguishing feature of such programs is their emphasis on training for clinical practice. The scientist–practitioner model that is widely endorsed as the primary basis for developing such skills calls for the establishment of research competency as well. The scientist component of that model could be extended to require development of a competency for utilizing research findings in clinical practice rather than mastery of an advanced level of research competency, which may well require more basic psychological and cognitive neuroscience preparation than postdoctoral clinical neuropsychological programs can provide.

There also is the issue of subspecialization, which appears to be following a pediatric/adult/geriatric compartmentalization. All levels of training would be expected to provide a life span developmental perspective through appropriate courses and practicum experiences; therefore, it may be premature for individuals to consider developmental stage subspecialization through entirely separate training programs that do not provide much overlap between age groups in their training activities. Nevertheless, subspecialized interests will inevitably arise and favor relative subspecialization in, for example, the pediatric as contrasted with the adult, or later adult, age groups. Considered from the standpoint of the four parameters of practice, the developmental dimension appears to pervade populations and settings which then present somewhat different constellations of problems and procedures for providing clinical services. It seems reasonable to require of any curriculum the introduction of a definitive developmental component which could then serve as a point of departure for guiding individuals into subspecialized areas. The ABCN/ABPP examination permits the candidate to elect child or adult cases for corresponding components of the examination and for work sample production purposes. Therefore, a subspecialized component is already interwoven into the formal credentialing procedure.

The differentiation of specific professional knowledge and practice skill requirements in these areas may be sufficient to warrant the election to pursue subspecialized competency at about the time the person receives the doctoral degree. By that time, those interests should have congealed sufficiently. Postdoctoral programs would then be expected to differentiate those elements of their respective curricula sufficiently to help the interested candidate for the program to estimate the likelihood that her or his needs can be met. Certainly, the major postdoctoral training programs are already being identified as having relative strengths and emphases in the pediatric or adult domains or both. Detailed program brochures are now being developed utilizing the guidelines for program content, and are being distributed by the APPCN. Predoctoral and internship programs are listed in the *Directory of the Association of Psychology Postdoctoral and Internship Centers* (APPIC). Postdoctoral programs in clinical neuropsychology are also listed annually in *The Clinical Neuropsychologist*, as collated by Lloyd Cripe. Postdoctoral program criteria and a list of membership programs in the APPCN are available from Thomas Hammeke, Chair of the Organizing Committee for that organization.

In addition to these developments in postdoctoral education, groups are forming to define similar criteria for predoctoral and internship-level training. For this reason, specific recommendations with regard to program content and direction are not provided in this chapter. The interested reader should find considerable access to the available information through literature citations offered here. There is obviously major movement in training, following the important work of the TFEAC and relatively extensive analyses of curriculum considerations and projections for the future (Bornstein, 1988; Costa, 1983; Division 40 Task Force, 1987; Meier, 1981, 1987; Rourke, 1991).

RECOGNITION OF NEUROPSYCHOLOGY AS A PSYCHOLOGICAL SPECIALTY

The slow, but deliberate, progress within APA toward recognition of new specialties attests to the greater differentiation of roles and responsibilities, based on their advancing knowledge and practice within the discipline of psychology. Clinical neuropsychology was the first new specialty in 28 years to be recognized by the American Board of Professional Psychology (ABPP). The last previous specialty to be recognized by ABPP was school psychology, preceded by counseling and clinical psychology, both of which were recognized for credentialing when ABPP was founded in 1947.

Further evidence of recognition of clinical neuropsychology has been the proliferation of professional and scientific organizations that have served an integrative role for this remarkable expansion of its basic and applied scientific knowledge that guides clinical practice. A parallel development has been the virtual explosion of major texts and journals that are devoted largely to clinical neuropsychological issues.

Scientific and Professional Organizations

There were no organizational mechanisms to provide a forum for clinical neuropsychology until the formation of the International Neuropsychological Society (INS) in the 1960s. The INS initially met as a relatively small and informal group, usually at APA meetings, and did not expand remarkably until the 1970s (Smith, 1980). Its continued rapid growth has led to a current multidisciplinary membership that exceeds 3,000. The INS growth curve spurted with the New Orleans meeting in 1973, which was the first year that INS offered a comprehensive scientific program. Arthur Benton was president of INS at that time and he deemed it appropriate to forge ahead with a major program, given the expanding knowledge base for neurobehavioral theory and clinical practice. He appointed a program committee of international stature, chaired by Paul Satz, that attracted numerous program submissions from major contributors to the field at that time. The INS remained primarily a North American organization, but gradually extended its mission and scope to include a European branch.

Aaron Smith was the key figure in the establishment of INS, and he worked effectively to maintain the organization in its formative years as editor of the *INS Bulletin*, which he established. He subsequently received a Distinguished Service Award from the INS for his many professional contributions, including the editorship of this periodical, which served as the central organizational device for clinical neuropsychology as the specialty was beginning to achieve formal recognition, well before INS and other subsequent organizations became more structured (Butters, Benton, Goodglass, Rourke, & Bakker, 1984). The INS went on to adopt its first official journal, the *Journal of Clinical Neuropsychology*, which later became the *Journal of Clinical and Experimental Neuropsychology*, edited by Louis Costa and Byron Rourke. Although this is an independent journal, it has served as the official journal of the INS for the purpose of publishing the abstracts of the two annual meetings of the association. INS has recently decided to publish its own organizational journal.

Because the readiness to establish a Division of Clinical Neuropsychology within APA was lacking at that time, due largely to the novelty of the specialty and, as yet, its lack of wide recognition, INS remained the major vehicle for individuals and groups that were interested in clinical neuropsychological theory, research, and practice. Growth was reflected in an annual attendance exceeding 600, and a membership that reached 2,000 by 1980. By then, the INS had become more widely international as well as interdisciplinary. Clinical neuropsychologists, experimental and physiological psychologists, behavioral neurologists, psychiatrists, neurosurgeons, physiatrists, speech pathologists, and professionals from assorted rehabilitation disciplines were joining INS in substantial numbers. Nevertheless, disciplinary composition of the INS remained approximately 90% psychologists; the remainder of the membership came from all of the other disciplines. However, the variegated composition of INS fostered both an interdisciplinary and an international orientation in its membership.

The differentiation of roles and responsibilities and the differing educational and professional perspectives of such a diverse set of interests made it difficult for the INS to consider the professional issues confronting North American clinical neuropsychologists in the 1970s. Nevertheless, at Arthur Benton's recommendation, the INS Board of Governors established the Task Force on Education, Accreditation, and Credentialing which was chaired by the present author. It was charged with developing guidelines for predoctoral, internship, and postdoctoral training; guidelines for the credentialing of individual competencies; and the formulation of a proposal for accreditation of educational programs at various levels. These guidelines and recommendations were intended to encourage more systematic educational efforts and the establishment of external review procedures for assessing both the competence of individual practitioners and the effectiveness of educational programs.

North American clinical neuropsychology was confronted with the responsibility for moving such indirect regulatory procedures in a direction that would encourage more deliberate preparation for research and practice which was, until then, provided by individuals who had little formal educational preparation or supervised clinical experience in neuropsychology. Most claims to professional competency were based on limited workshop and conference activities by practitioners who were lacking formal training and supervised experience. These ends are now being achieved, as evidenced by the advent of numerous formal postdoctoral training programs and the expansion of clinical neuropsychological training opportunities within predoctoral and internship programs. There has been, however, less than the anticipated expansion of formal predoctoral programs of an exclusively neuropsychological nature.

The *Journal of Clinical Neuropsychology* was an immediate success and, combined with the already established *Neuropsychologia* and *Cortex* that were being published in Europe, the appearance of the new journal gave impetus to INS and the formation of other neuropsychological organizations in the scientific and professional communities. It quickly became evident that educational and professional issues would need to be processed within nations by members of the interested disciplines, and not through the INS. The TFEAC continued its work but encouraged groups to be formed that would permit the pursuit of such issues by nation and by discipline. This led to the formation in 1979 of a Steering Committee, chaired by Louis Costa and independent of INS, for the purpose of establishing a division within APA. This required the overcoming of significant political barriers because clinical neuropsychology was not formally recognized as a specialty by APA, and it was considered by many psychologists within APA to be a subspecialty of limited scope within the specialty of clinical psychology. Resistances were also encountered from the Division of Physiological and Comparative Psychology (Division 6), but the proposal for a new division passed the Council of Representatives in 1980, following considerable debate. With the proliferation of new divisions within APA, there was a natural resistance to further expansion. However, there was no rationale for a restrictive, reactionary attitude, and the relatively democratic governance procedures of APA prevailed to ensure a place for the specialty within that large organization. This series of events led to the formation of another journal, *The Clinical Neuropsychologist*, in 1987, which has served as the unofficial journal for Division 40 for the purpose of publishing the Division's abstracts of presentations at APA meetings.

The relatedness of INS and Division 40 as organizations was reflected in a proposal from INS to share responsibility for future planning and growth by inviting Division 40 to serve as a cosponsor of the TFEAC. As Division 40 matured and demonstrated that it could effectively address the professional issues and problems confronting clinical neuropsychology in the United States and Canada, the INS withdrew from the TFEAC and encouraged Division 40 to exercise sole managerial control. The first formal position statement from the Task Force was issued jointly in an attempt to define clinical neuropsychology as a specialty, generate models for predoctoral educational preparation, and delineate the knowledge base for establishing individual clinical competence (Meier, 1981). Subsequently, the Task Force developed guidelines for internship and postdoctoral programs which are being elaborated by the Association of Postdoctoral Programs in Clinical Neuropsychology (APPCN), thus setting the stage for the ultimate accreditation of programs at various levels (Division 40 Task Force, 1987). The TFEAC has now generated guidelines for doctoral, predoctoral internship, and postdoctoral training (Division 40 Task Force, 1987); entry into the specialty (Bornstein, 1988); continuing education (Bornstein, 1988; Meier, 1987); use of nondoctoral personnel (Division 40 Task Force, 1989b); computer-assisted neuropsychological evaluation (Matthews, 1987); and computer-assisted neuropsychological rehabilitation and cognitive rehabilitation (Matthews, Harley, & Malec, 1991).

A third major professional organization, the National Academy of Neuropsychology (NAN), was established independently of these developments in the late 1970s by a few individuals who used the organization primarily as a vehicle for presenting continuing education workshops to the many clinical practitioners who endeavored to expand their clinical skills. Continuing education, primarily for clinical practitioners, has become the primary role of NAN, which has added poster sessions to its programs in recent years. NAN has shown some recent interest in addressing educational and professional issues, but has not done so deliberately, emphasizing workshop activities in the course of its growth into an organization of over 2,000 individuals. It published a newsletter for some years and more recently established the *Archives of Clinical Neuropsychology* as its official journal. NAN has clearly moved beyond its initial mission and facilitates practitioner focus on clinical issues through continuing education, workshop activities, and poster sessions. The formats of INS and Division 40 meetings emphasize symposia, platform and poster presentations, and a limited selection of continuing education workshop activities.

Collectively, the INS, APA Division 40, and NAN provide an ample organizational framework for pursuing almost any configuration of neuropsychological interests. Furthermore, APA provides access to developments in cognitive and physiological psychology as these specialties relate to clinical neuropsychology. The American Psychological Society (APS) offers opportunities for acquiring basic psychological knowledge as it relates to cognitive psychology, as does the Society for Neuroscience for those with primarily research interests. There is also a ground swell of interest at the local level, as evidenced by the formation of numerous city, county, state, and regional organizations in North America, and counterpart groups around the world. The latter are gaining access to these organizations, particularly INS, through the conduct of regional meetings such as that organized by a group of neuropsychologists from the Pacific Rim nations that was held in Australia in 1992. There has also been an effort to develop a world federation of neuropsychological societies, the impetus for which has come from psychologists in underdeveloped nations who need assistance in attending meetings of the aforementioned organizations and in developing their own organizations. The socialization of clinical neuropsychology as a specialty, as represented by all these organizational developments, is an inevitable consequence of the healthy growth of a vital human activity.

Credentialing Boards

Just as the deliberations of the TFEAC stimulated the formation of a Steering Committee for the establishment of a Division of Clinical Neuropsychology within APA, its efforts also gave impetus to the formation of a Steering Committee to establish the American Board of Clinical Neuropsychology (ABCN), chaired by the present author. As President of the ABCN, I was charged to negotiate a formal arrangement with the American Board of Professional Psychology (ABPP) to achieve recognition of clinical neuropsychology as a new specialty within the ABPP structure. The ABPP had served as the credentialing board for the evaluation of advanced competence in the specialties of clinical, counseling, school, and industrial/organizational psychology, since its inception in 1947. The ABPP Board of Trustees in 1982 agreed to the arrangement and assigned the ABCN with the responsibility for establishing eligibility criteria and an effective competency-based examination for the attainment of diplomate status in clinical neuropsychology. Therefore, the ABCN was permitted to function as an autonomous examining board, but was accountable to the ABPP Board of Trustees for the relevance of its eligibility criteria and the effectiveness of its competency-based examination. This was achieved by localizing administrative activities in the ABPP central office and through ABCN representation on the ABPP Board of Trustees, where the activities of ABCN could be monitored by the overarching board. In turn, ABCN could also influence the other areas of practice being credentialed under the jurisdiction of ABPP. The resulting interactions over the next decade have led to the examination of individuals credentialed by ABCN through ABPP, beginning with the initial ABCN board, which was examined by ABPP Diplomates in one or more of the other specialties who themselves were also examined, all with ABPP participation. The ABCN has now credentialed over 250 individuals. Its success has also contributed to change within the ABPP governance structure, insofar as ABPP has moved from a regionally controlled diplomating board to a specialty-centered diplomating board in which each specialty of ABPP is now required to form an autonomous credentialing board. These boards have been formed and are responsible to ABPP for quality assurance and continued monitoring of the specialty boards' activities. Moreover, the diplomates of each specialty board are forming membership organizations to separate membership from credentialing functions and, thereby, to minimize the potential for conflicts of interest between boards and members.

There now exist 10 credentialing boards under the umbrella of the ABPP Board of Trustees (BOT). The BOT is made up of representatives from the following participating boards: Clinical Psychology, Counseling Psychology, School Psychology, Industrial/Organizational Psychology, Clinical Neuropsychology, Forensic Psychology, Family Psychology, Health Psychology, Behavioral Psychology, and Psychoanalysis. Clinical neuropsychology was the first new specialty added to the ABPP roster since school psychology was added as a diplomate specialty in 1974. It is interesting that with the establishment of ABCN, there quickly followed the addition of the Forensic, Family, Health, and Behavioral Psychology specialty boards. It is also noteworthy that the expansion of ABPP in the last decade has compelled a change within ABPP from a regional to a specialty-oriented organizational structure in which each specialty is constituted as an independent board for conduct of the examinations. In part, this change was prompted by ABCN's effective application of the assessment center approach to competency evaluation. Therefore, ABCN is contributing to increased standardization of procedures within and between specialties relative to level of difficulty, reliability, and validity for the assessment of competence.

The ABCN also was instrumental, through its representative on the ABPP/BOT, in fostering a stronger linkage between developments in the accreditation of educational programs, particularly postdoctoral programs, and development of competency at an advanced level as assessed by means of the ABCN examination. ABPP now regards formal postdoctoral preparation in a given specialty as both desirable and deserving of a shorter time lag following the award of the doctoral degree before becoming eligible to take the ABPP examination through the specialty boards. A distinguishing feature of ABCN's initial presentation to ABPP (before any examinations in clinical neuropsychology were given) was a document from the TFEAC that addressed the SOS manual toward describing how the assessment center approach could be applied to the evaluation of clinical competence. After meeting ABPP's general requirements as well as ABCN's eligibility criteria, applicants are asked to submit two work samples, the structure for which is clearly defined in manuals that have been developed to serve both the potential examinee and the work sample reviewers. With the approval of the work sample for defense, an oral examination is then carried out using the assessment center model (Bray, 1984; MacKinnon, 1975; Moses & Byham, 1977). The examination process is monitored by the ABPP through its liaison operations with constituent boards; it is implemented by the ABCN (Bieliauskas & Matthews, 1987, 1990).

The ABCN examination now also includes an objective knowledge evaluation that was developed in cooperation with the Professional Examination Service. This examination makes use of the format and test construction procedures that have been applied in the national psychology licensure examination. This objective examination is designed to screen candidates for general neuropsychological knowledge before they enter the work sample phase so that the oral examination phase should be reached only by individuals who are clearly ready to demonstrate advanced professional competence based on definitive clinical and theoretical knowledge. All of these activities are monitored through the ABPP/BOT and, therein, by the various other specialties that are represented on the BOT, which thus ensures profession-wide participation in the verification of procedural quality and effectiveness. The reciprocally beneficial effects of ABPP's change to a federated board organizational structure should increase the effectiveness of each specialty of psychology as specialty practice standards within the profession become more clearly defined and differentiated.

Accordingly, ABPP can be regarded as the first organization to recognize clinical neuropsychology as a specialty. All of the aforementioned professional and scientific organizations have contributed to the identity of the specialty in accord with their respective missions. The relationship of ABCN to ABPP has placed the competency examination process into an organizational framework that extends beyond these two organizations to include the entire configuration of organizations and regulatory bodies that define the profession of psychology.

A major locus of organizational interaction has been the establishment of the Interorganizational Council for the Accreditation of Postdoctoral Programs in Professional Psychology (IOCAPPP), also known as the "IOC." This council was established as a result of a meeting in Minneapolis of various organizations invited by the ABPP in September of 1991. The other participating organizations were the Association of State and Provincial Psychology Licensing Boards (AASPB), the National Register of Health Services Providers in Psychology (NR), the Association of Psychology Postdoctoral and Internship Centers (APPIC), the APA through its Board of Professional Affairs and Accreditation Committee, and representatives of the specialties and appropriate educational organizations such as the Association of Postdoctoral Programs in Clinical Neuropsychology (APPCN). The latter group has now met a number of times and has produced a model for the accreditation of postdoctoral programs for neuropsychological specialization. The model includes a program Self-Study Form and a Site Visit Evaluation Form, both of which are available through the Chair of APPCN. These forms were developed by the Midwest Consortium of Postdoctoral Programs in Clinical Neuropsychology, the forerunner of the APPCN. In addition, APPIC sponsored a major conference on postdoctoral accreditation in Ann Arbor, Michigan, in 1992. Because the APA also sponsored a conference on related issues that was held in Norman, Oklahoma, in January of 1994, a definitive interorganizational movement toward postdoctoral program accreditation is in progress.

As the initiator of the interorganizational conference that led to the formation of the IOC, ABPP is clearly committed to making its competency evaluation procedures for the determination of advanced competence reflect the knowledge and skill components that will help to set directions for the continued evolution of postdoctoral, as well as predoctoral and internship, training programs. The cooperative activities of these various organizations toward the generation of standards of practice and for establishment of the basis of competence in professional knowledge and practice have clearly led to continued effectiveness of ABCN; for example, as a specialty board in clinical neuropsychology.

Given this extensive developmental history, ABCN can be characterized as endorsing the scientist–practitioner model for the practice of clinical neuropsychology. That model would apply in the broadest sense to include not only the practitioner as a producer of research, but also the practitioner as a consumer of research. Therefore, the model does not preclude a nonresearcher from achieving advanced professional competence. On the contrary, the majority of individuals entering the ABCN credentialing process are not researchers or members of an intellectually elite group of clinical neuropsychologists; rather, they are commonly graduates of clinical programs with years of professional experience that have been supplemented by selected continuing education activities.

ABCN would appear to have introduced an orderly and professionally endorsed competency-based examination procedure for the specialty with the support, supervision, and assistance of ABPP and, indirectly, of the various organizations with which ABPP has established a dialogue. Accordingly, the effectiveness of ABCN and its relevance to the individual who claims advanced competence (or the necessary competence for effective professional practice) in clinical neuropsychology are subject to the scrutiny of the entire profession of psychology through the ABPP and, indirectly, through ABPP's associated network of regulatory organizations. Therefore, ABCN has stood the test of peer review at the organizational level so that its procedures and policies carry endorsements from legitimate sources outside of the specialty as well as those within the specialty. A list of ABCN/ABPP diplomates is published in the APA Directory. It is this characteristic that distinguishes the ABCN/ABPP credentialing procedure from others that have been introduced, such as that of the American Board of Professional Neuropsychology (ABPN), which was originally established in 1982.

The ABPN Board members initially awarded their diploma to an unknown number of individuals, believed to approach 200, on the basis of a credentials review. The nature of this review does not appear to have been published or shared in any formal manner with the profession. Following an initial spurt of such credentialing activity, there appears to have been a cessation of ABPN work for a number of years before a cadre of individuals was activated to resume these credentialing activities. Descriptions of these activities are currently portrayed in a brochure that is available from the ABPN (American Board of Professional Neuropsychology, 1994). The brochure calls for the submission of a completed application package, followed by work samples if the application is approved, and an oral examination, which is described as consisting of testing in the areas of core knowledge, the work samples, and ethics. This general description is preceded by a statement of purpose and a history of the ABPN, including reference to the period of inactivity "during reassessment of the need for ABPN's continued existence." Initially, the informal impression originally conveyed was that this credential was to be directed at the journeyperson level professional. The more recently described activities are alleged to assess advanced competence and "the pursuit of excellence in the practice of neuropsychology." Therefore, ABPN has issued two different diplomas. The initial diploma was awarded to a group of unexamined individuals, and a later diploma issued only to a group of examined individuals (J. A. Moses Jr., personal communication, May 12, 1994).

There appears to be a "continuing education requirement" as a means of maintaining the ABPN credential. This is a laudatory feature if it is enforced. However, the brochure also refers to "candidate preparation workshops," which are "offered by members of the Examination Committee." Such workshops could place an examination committee in a conflict of interest if, for example, the examination committee subsequently is responsible for performing the examinations. If an examination committee were not so responsible, it would still be functioning in a role that could artificially increase the number of individuals reaching a particular criterion level of performance through coaching or other revelations in the course of these workshops.

It has been argued informally by proponents of this approach that the credential is more relevant for the practice of clinical neuropsychology than is the ABCN/ABPP credential, which has been perceived as having greater relevance for academicians. In any case, it is difficult to regard the ABCN and ABPN diplomas as equivalent measures of professional excellence or advanced competence (given the profession-wide evaluative framework within which only the ABCN functions). One reaches this conclusion based on the evidence even when one applies a more limited definition of competence as the necessary competence for effective practice (versus highly effective practice). Even a cursory review of the history of these two boards leads to the conclusion that the credentials issued by them are not comparable. Any suggestion that they are comparable could be very misleading to the aspiring clinical neuropsychologist who is seeking verification of her/his claim to advanced professional competence as well as to consumers of clinical neuropsychological services who are unlikely to have knowledge of the history of the potentially confusing credentialing configuration in clinical neuropsychology at this time.

Another board whose brochure has been distributed nationally is known as the American Board of Vocational Neuropsychology. The initial brochure invites members of various disciplines, at subdoctoral as well as doctoral levels of preparation, to apply for board certification. The brochure is available to potential applicants (American Board of Vocational Neuropsychology, 1994). The activities of that board appear to fall outside the purview of this chapter, which is exclusively directed at issues that confront psychologists at the doctoral level.

Books and Journals

There has been a remarkable expansion of the number of journals and books that have appeared in the literature over the past few decades. There is now an immense pool of research findings to assist in the interpretation of test results and to ensure that neuropsychological theories of cognitive and personality functioning will continue to stimulate objective clinical and basic research activity. The publication of *Cortex* was quickly followed by *Neuropsychologia* in Europe. Luria's (1966) comprehensive integration of the available empirical knowledge with regional localization theory also constituted a major stimulus within an already expanding literature.

Many neuropsychological articles appeared in the 1950s in medical and psychological journals in the United States and Europe. Many of those journals continue to publish neuropsychological research, even as the number of journals that are devoted exclusively to neuropsychology increases. The number of journals whose primary editor is a psychologist (clinical or cognitive/experimental) has now reached at least 15. Also, there are at least 30 journals edited by nonpsychologists, usually specialty physicians and speech pathologists, that have been identified as publishing neuropsychological research. Similarly, the number of relevant books has increased geometrically over the past decade in each empirical domain.

The large number of books that are directly related to the practice of clinical neuropsychology is much too extensive to be listed here. Requests for a representative sampling of such books is made frequently by graduate students, postdoctoral fellows and practitioners in the field. A representative sampling of such books is offered in Appendix A.

It is likely that an alternate listing of books in the same areas, but with different authors, could be identified. This group of books is intended to convey the breadth and depth of knowledge and application in clinical neuropsychology. It seems extremely likely that any individual who has a working knowledge of the major subjects in these volumes and who can convert that knowledge into clinical practice would have no difficulty demonstrating the necessary competence for highly effective practice.

Similarly, representative journals for individuals interested in pursuing substantive knowledge of both theory and practice in clinical neuropsychology are listed in Appendix B.

SUMMARY AND FUTURE DEVELOPMENT OF CLINICAL NEUROPSYCHOLOGY

This chapter has been organized to present a historical perspective for the development of clinical neuropsychology. The discussion has been focused on the primarily professional issues confronting clinical neuropsychology as it enters early, and perhaps even middle, adulthood in its development as a specialty. This process is occurring at a time when opportunities for education and the actualization in practice of effective professional competence are likely to be progressively more difficult to achieve. In many situations professional specialty training activities, particularly postdoctoral training programs, have been instrumental in establishing practice positions in the very institutions in which the advanced training has occurred, or in institutions that are networked with the training programs. Common examples of this process include state hospitals, the Department of Veterans Affairs, the military, community hospitals, private practice groups, the schools, and the legal system. Maintenance of training activities and the promotion of new positions, either in the public or the private sector, will depend on the continued availability of a significant cost–benefit ratio return for the services provided by clinical neuropsychologists.

The key to anticipating the future of clinical neuropsychology lies in the effects of national health reform on reimbursement for clinical services. As with the medical and allied health professions, clinical neuropsychology will need to adapt to changing conditions and undergo significant transformations in roles and procedures. There has always been a lag between the available basic and applied research in psychology and the level of application in practice. Professional service is commonly provided by clinicians who often have neither the time nor the skills to achieve a ready conversion of research knowledge to clinical practice. Practice, as a consequence, tends to remain relatively resistant to change, as is evidenced by the wide range of up-to-date knowledge and professional competence that is found among individuals who practice clinical neuropsychology. Everyone who has been in the field for any period of time has witnessed this variation, which is difficult to document objectively. In turn, that difficulty prompts the development of objective evaluation procedures, such as the ABCN examination, to determine individual levels of competence for professional practice. Furthermore, the scientific knowledge base on which clinical practice depends is expanding on a multidisciplinary basis so that interdisciplinary boundaries are becoming blurred, at least as they are related to the establishment of the necessary knowledge base for effective clinical practice.

Clinical neuropsychologists can no longer function competently without a working knowledge of behavioral neurology and cognitive neuroscience. The appended array of books and journals underscores the categorical scope of knowledge that is relevant to the practice of the specialty of clinical neuropsychology and the growing interdisciplinary emphasis in investigation, evaluation, and treatment of impaired brain functioning. The political, economic, and scientific/professional context of the times dictates the expectation that neuropsychological services will probably need to be provided at both a lower cost and a higher level of professional effectiveness in the future. Lower costs are likely to be dictated by national health reform because available resources will have to reach the entire population and not only those who are currently insured. Greater effectiveness will probably be necessitated by the increased competition for existing resources among the health professions, of which psychology is obviously not the most powerful. Clinical neuropsychologists, hopefully, will adapt to these changes by increasing the efficiency of their techniques and the transmission of the interpretations of findings by means of advances in computer-assisted technology and in telecommunications. Program evaluation research also likely will be required more of clinical neuropsychologists to demonstrate the effectiveness of particular assessment procedures, interventions, and therapies.

Although psychology has been grappling with the many implications of its own socialization as a profession, a gap between developments in the specialty of clinical neuropsychology and recognition of this specialty by the parent discipline appears to be closing since APA has established its own journal in neuropsychology, has initiated formal steps to recognize clinical neuropsychology as a specialty, and is moving toward the accreditation of specialty training programs in clinical neuropsychology, probably beginning at the postdoctoral level, which is the most characteristic level for the professional preparation of clinical neuropsychologists. The astounding growth of clinical neuropsychology, as a function of developments in the discipline as well as in other fields of knowledge and application, will require continued curriculum planning and revision and continued upgrading of objectives and program evaluation criteria in the areas of education, accreditation, and credentialing. The initiatives described earlier have produced curriculum models, external credentialing through board certification, and a foundation for the accreditation of specialty education programs. Convergence of the aforementioned developments will necessarily require a definitive interdisciplinary orientation and increased technological sophistication in order to pursue the necessary knowledge and competence for effective practice in a cost-efficient, yet increasingly more competent, manner. Because clinical neuropsychology has demonstrated great promise and is likely to be the first new practice specialty to be recognized as APA moves in that direction, it should fare well in the future, at least as well as other specialties within psychology.

Clinical neuropsychologists are already engaged in reflections about the future and foresee major challenges in efforts of practitioners in the specialty to apply an already formidable body of basic and applied knowledge to actualize the possibilities presented by technological advances in this and other fields. Rourke (1991) enunciated a set of predictions regarding directions for research and application during this decade. He foresaw an expansion of research into the normal development of cognitive processes that are relevant to an understanding of brain–behavior relationships, the parallel monitoring of neurophysiological and behavioral phenomena, analysis of the component processes measured by neuropsychometric procedures, refinements in the statistical and mathematical analysis of neuropsychological data, the elucidation of personality and psychosocial factors to variation in neuropsychological performances, cognitive rehabilitation, credentialing, and other issues. The potential for further growth in the specialty that is suggested by his reflections and by the developments in recent decades point toward future actualization of the earlier expectations that experimental and clinical neuropsychology would become a major productive force within the discipline of psychology in the 21st century (Costa, 1983).

ACKNOWLEDGMENTS

This chapter is heavily dependent on the work of the INS/APA Division 40 Task Force on Education, Accreditation, and Credentialing (TFEAC), which was chaired by the author from 1976 to 1985. Although the Chair wrote numerous sections and organized and edited the reports that emanated from the TFEAC during that period, he was ably assisted by many of its members. Particularly active in the development of documents were Kenneth Adams, Linas Bieliauskas, Thomas Boll, Louis Costa, Edith Kaplan, Charles Matthews, Steven Mattis, Paul Satz, Byron Rourke, Daniel Sheer (deceased), and Barbara C. Wilson.

REFERENCES

Albert, M. L. (1984). Henry Hécean, M. D., neurologist–neuropsychologist. *Archives of Neurology*, *41*, 458–459.

American Board of Professional Neuropsychology. (1994). (Advertisement). *APA Monitor*, *25* (6) 67.

American Board of Vocational Neuropsychology. (1994). (Advertisement). *APA Monitor*, *25* (66) 67.

Belar, C. D., Bieliauskas, L. A., Larson, K. G., Mensh, I. N., Poey, K., & Roehlke, H. J. (1989). National conference on internship training in psychology. *American Psychologist*, *44*, 60–65.

Benton, A. L. (1945). A visual retention test for clinical use. *Archives of Neurology and Psychiatry*, *54*, 212–216.

Benton, A. L. (1964). Contributions to aphasia before Broca. *Cortex*, *1*, 314–327.

Benton, A. L. (1969). Development of a multilingual aphasia battery: Progress and problems. *Journal of the Neurological Sciences*, *9*, 39–48.

Benton, A. L. (1987). Evolution of a clinical specialty. *The Clinical Neuropsychologist*, *1*, 5–8.

Bieliauskas, L. A., & Matthews, C. G. (1987). American board of clinical neuropsychology: Policies and procedures. *The Clinical Neuropsychologist*, *1*, 21–28.

Bieliauskas, L. A., & Matthews, C. G. (1990). American board of clinical neuropsychology update, 1990. *The Clinical Neuropsychologist*, *4*, 337–343.

Bornstein, R. A. (1988). Entry into clinical neuropsychology: Graduate, undergraduate and beyond. *The Clinical Neuropsychologist*, *2*, 213–220.

Bray, D. W. (1984, August). *Assessment centers for research and application*. Psi Chi Distinguished Lecture delivered at the meeting of the American Psychological Association, Toronto, Canada.

Butters, N., Benton, A., Goodglass, H., Rourke, B. P., & Bakker, D. J. (1984, November). A testimonial to the bulletin and its editor Aaron Smith. *The INS Bulletin*, 75–76.

Cattell, R. B. (1963). Theory of fluid and crystallized intelligence: An initial experiment. *Journal of the Neurological Sciences*, *9*, 39–48.

Christensen, A. L. (1975). *Luria's neuropsychological investigation* (2nd ed.). Copenhagen: Munksgaard.

Costa, L. (1983). Clinical neuropsychology: A discipline in evolution. *Journal of Clinical Neuropsychology*, *5*, 1–11.

Costa, L., & Spreen, O. (Eds.). (1985). *Studies in neuropsychology: Selected papers of Arthur Benton*. New York: Oxford University Press.

Critchley, M. (1953). *The parietal lobes*. London: Edward Arnold.

Damasio, A. R. (1985). Norman Geschwind. *Archives of Neurology*, *42*, 500–504.

Division 40 Task Force. (1987). Reports of the Task Force on Education, Accreditation, and Credentialing. *The Clinical Neuropsychologist*, *1*, 22–29.

Division 40 Task Force. (1989a). Definition of a clinical neuropsychologist. *The Clinical Neuropsychologist*, *3*, 22.

Division 40 Task Force. (1989b). Guidelines regarding the use of nondoctoral personnel in clinical neuropsychological assessment. *The Clinical Neuropsychologist*, *3*, 23–24.

Filskov, S. B., & Boll, T. J. (Eds.). (1986). *Handbook of clinical neuropsychology* (2nd ed.). New York: Wiley.

Geschwind, N. (1965). Disconnexion syndromes in animals and man. *Brain*, *88*, 237–294, 585–644.

Geschwind, N., & Levitsky, W. (1968). Human brain: Left–right asymmetries in temporal speech region. *Science*, *161*, 186–187.

Golden, C. J., Hammeke, T. A., & Purisch, A. D. (1980). *Manual for the Luria–Nebraska Neuropsychological Battery*. Los Angeles: Western Psychological Series.

Goldstein, G. (1985). The history of clinical neuropsychology: The role of some American pioneers. *International Journal of Neuroscience*, *25*, 273–275.

Goldstein, K., & Scheerer, M. (1941). Abstract and concrete behavior. *Psychological Monographs*, *53* (Whole No. 39).

Goodglass, H. (1985). Aphasiology in the United States. *International Journal of Neuroscience*, *25*, 307–311.

Goodglass, H. (1986). Norman Geschwind (1926–1984). *Cortex*, *22*, 7–10.

Goodglass, H., & Kaplan, E. (1983). *The assessment of aphasia and related disorders*. (2nd ed.) Philadelphia: Lea & Febiger.

Halstead, W. C. (1947). *Brain and intelligence: A quantitative study of the frontal lobes*. Chicago: University of Chicago Press.

Harlow, H. F., Davis, R. T., Settlage, P. H., & Meyer, D. R. (1952). Analysis of frontal and posterior association syndromes in brain-damaged monkeys. *Journal of Comparative and Physiological Psychology*, *45*, 410–429.

Hebb, D. O. (1949). *The organization of behavior*. New York: Wiley.

Jacobsen, C. F. (1936). Studies of cerebral functions in primates: I. The functions of the frontal association areas in monkeys. *Comparative Psychology Monographs*, *13* (3, Whole No. 63), 3–60.

Jones, B. P., & Butters, N. (1983). Neuropsychological assessment. In M. Hersen, A. E. Kazdin, & A. S. Bellack, *The clinical psychology handbook* (pp. 377–396). New York: Pergamon.

Kaplan, E. F. (1983). Process and achievement revisited. In S. Wapner & B. Kaplan (Eds.), *Toward a holistic developmental psychology* (pp. 143–156), Hillsdale, NJ: Lawrence Erlbaum Associates.

Lashley, K. (1929). *Brain mechanisms and intelligence*. Chicago: University of Chicago Press.

Lezak, M. D. (1995). *Neuropsychological Assessment* (3rd ed.). New York: Oxford University Press.

Luria, A. R. (1966). *Higher cortical functions in man*. New York: Basic Books.

MacKinnon, D. W. (1975). An overview of assessment centers. (Tech. Rep. No. 1). Greensboro, NC: Center for Creative Leadership.

Matthews, C. G. (1987). Division 40: Task force report on computer-assisted neuropsychological evaluation. *The Clinical Neuropsychologist*, *2*, 161–184.

Matthews, C. G., Harley, J. P., & Malec, J. F. (1991). Guidelines for computer-assisted neuropsychological rehabilitation and cognitive mediation. *The Clinical Neuropsychologist*, *5*, 3–19.

Meier, M. J. (1981). Education for competency assurance in human neuropsychology. In S. B. Filskov & T. J. Boll (Eds.), *Handbook of clinical neuropsychology* (pp. 754–781). New York: Wiley.

Meier, M. J. (1987). Continuing education: An alternative to respecialization in clinical neuropsychology. *The Clinical Neuropsychologist*, *1*, 9–20.

Meier, M. J. (1992). Modern clinical neuropsychology in historical perspective. *American Psychologist*, *47*, 550–558.

Meier, M. J., Benton, A. L., & Diller, L. (Eds.). (1987). *Neuropsychological Rehabilitation*. New York: Guilford.
Meier, M. J., Strauman, S., & Thompson, W. G. (1987). Individual differences in neuropsychological recovery: An overview. In M. J. Meier, A. L. Benton, & L. Diller (Eds), *Neurological rehabilitation* (pp. 71–110). Edinburgh, Scotland: Churchill Livingstone.
Mendoza, J. E. (1993, October). *Clinical neuropsychology specialty licensure designation: Proposed regulations for the state of Louisiana*. Paper presented at the 13th annual conference of the National Academy of Neuropsychology, Phoenix, AZ.
Meyer, V. (1961). Psychological effects of brain damage. In H. J. Eysenck (Ed.), *Handbook of abnormal psychology* (pp. 529–565). New York: Basic Books.
Milner, B. (1954). Intellectual function of the temporal lobes. *Psychological Bulletin, 51*, 42–62.
Milner, B. (1964). Some effects of frontal lobectomy in man. In J. M. Warren & K. Akert (Eds.), *The frontal granular cortex and behavior* (pp. 313–334). New York: McGraw-Hill.
Milner, B. (1967). Brain mechanisms suggested by studies of the temporal lobes. In C. H. Milikan & F. L. Darley (Eds.), *Brain mechanisms underlying speech and language* (pp. 122–132). New York: Grune & Stratton.
Milner, B., Taylor, R., & Sperry, R. W. (1968). Lateralized suppression of dichotically presented digits after commissure section in man. *Science, 161*, 184–186.
Milner, B., & Teuber, H. L. (1968). Alteration of perception and memory in man: Reflections on methods. In L. Weiskrantz (Ed.), *Analysis of behavior change* (pp. 268–375). New York: Harper & Row.
Mishkin, M. (1982). A memory system in the monkey. *Philosophical Transactions of the Royal Society, B298*, 85–95.
Mishkin, M., & Petri, H. L. (1984). Memories and habits: Some implications for the analysis of learning and retention. In L. R. Squire & N. Butters (Eds.), *Neuropsychology of memory* (pp. 287–296). New York: Guilford.
Mishkin, M., & Pribram, K. H. (1954). Visual discrimination performance following partial ablations of the temporal lobe: I. Ventral vs. lateral. *Journal of Comparative and Physiological Psychology, 47*, 14–20.
Mishkin, M., & Ungerleider, L. G. (1983). Contribution of striate inputs to the visuospatial functions of parieto–preoccipital cortex in monkeys. *Behavioral Brain Research, 6*, 55–77.
Moses, J. L., & Byham, W. C. (Eds.). (1977). *Applying the assessment center method*. New York: Pergamon.
Pribram, K. H. (1986). Nonlocality and localization in the primate brain. In S. B. Filskov & T. J. Boll (Eds.), *Handbook of clinical neuropsychology* (Vol. 2, pp. 606–651). New York: Wiley.
Putnam, S. H., & DeLuca, J. W. (1990). The TCN professional practice survey: Part I: General practices of clinical neuropsychologists in primary employment and practice settings. *The Clinical Neuropsychologist, 4*, 199–243.
Putnam, S. H., & DeLuca, J. W. (1991). The TCN professional practice survey: Part II: An analysis of the fees of neuropsychologists by practice demographics. *The Clinical Neuropsychologist, 5*, 102–124.
Reed, J. (1985). The contributions of Ward Halstead, Ralph Reitan and their associates. *International Journal of Neuroscience, 25*, 289–293.
Reitan, R. M. (1964). Psychological deficits resulting from cerebral lesions in man. In J. M. Warren & K. Akert (Eds.), *The frontal granular cortex and behavior* (pp. 295–312). New York: McGraw-Hill.
Rourke, B. R. (1991). Human neuropsychology in the 1990s. *Archives of Clinical Neuropsychology, 6*, 1–14.
Sales, B., Bricklin, P. & Hall, J. (1984). *Manual on specialization: Principles proposed to the board of professional affairs*. Washington, DC: American Psychological Association.
Smith, A. (1980, June). How the INS began. *The INS Bulletin*, 3–4.
Sperry, R. W. (1958). Physiological plasticity and brain circuit theory. Behavior and evolution. In H. F. Harlow & C. N. Woolsey (Eds.), *Biological and biochemical bases of behavior* (pp. 401–424). Madison: University of Wisconsin Press.
Sperry, R. W., Gazzaniga, M. S., & Bogen, J. E. (1969). Interhemispheric relationships: The neocortical commissures, syndromes of hemisphere disconnection. In P. J. Vinkon & G. W. Bruyn (Eds.), *Handbook of clinical neurology* (Vol. 4, pp. 273–290). Amsterdam: North Holland.
Stuss, D. T. (1991). Interference effects on memory function in postleukotomy patients: An attentional perspective. In H. S. Levin, H. M. Eisenberg, & A. L. Benton (Eds.), *Frontal lobe function and dysfunction* (pp. 157–172). New York: Oxford University Press.
Talland, G. A. (1966). *Deranged memory*. San Diego, CA: Academic Press.
Teuber, H.-L. (1962). Effects of brain wounds implicating right and left hemisphere in man: Hemisphere differences and hemisphere interaction in vision, audition, and somesthesis. In V. B. Mountcastle (Ed.), *Interhemisphere relations and cerebral dominance* (pp. 203–208). Baltimore: Johns Hopkins University Press.
Teuber, H.-L. (1964). The riddle of frontal lobe function in man. In J. M. Warren & K. Akert (Eds.), *The frontal granular cortex and behavior* (pp. 410–444). New York: McGraw-Hill.
Teuber, H.-L. (1966). In J. C. Eccles (Ed.), *Brain and conscious experience* (pp. 182–216). New York: Springer.
Weinstein, S. (1985). The influence of Hans-Lukas Teuber and the psychological laboratory on the establishment and development of neuropsychology. *International Journal of Neuroscience, 25*, 277–288.

APPENDIX A

Adams, K. M., & Rourke, B. P. (1992). *The TCN guide to professional practice in clinical neuropsychology*. The Netherlands: Swets & Zeitlinger.

Benton, A. L., Hamsher, K. D., Varney, N. R., & Spreen, O. (1983). *Contributions to NP Assessment*. Oxford.

Bornstein, R. A., & Brown, G. G. (1991). *Neurobehavioral aspects of cerebrovascular disease*. New York: Oxford University Press.

Filskov, S. B., & Boll, T. J. (1981, 1986). *Handbook of clinical neuropsychology* (Vols. 1 & 2). New York: Wiley.

Finger, S., & Stein, D. G. (1982). *Brain damage and recovery*. New York: Academic Press.

Goldstein, G., & Ruthven, L. (1983). *Rehabilitation of the brain damaged adult*. New York: Plenum.

Goodglass, H., & Kaplan, E. F. (1983). *The assessment of aphasia and related disorders* (2nd ed.) Philadelphia: Lea and Febiger.

Grant, I., & Adams, K. M. (1985). *Neuropsychological assessment of neuropsychiatric disorders*. New York: Oxford University Press.

Hécean, H., & Albert, M. L. (1978). *Human neuropsychology*. New York: Wiley.

Heilman, K. M., & Valenstein, E. (1993). *Clinical neuropsychology* (3rd ed.). New York: Oxford University.

Levin, H. S., Benton, A. L., & Grossman, R. G. (1982). *Neurobehavioral consequences of closed head injury*. New York: Oxford.

Lezak, M. D. (1995). *Neuropsychological assessment* (3rd ed.). New York: Oxford University Press.

Luria, A. R. (1980). *Higher cortical functions in man*. (2nd ed.). Basic Books.

Margolin, D. I. (1992). *Cognitive neuropsychology in clinical practice*. New York: Oxford University Press.

Meier, M. J., Benton, A. L., & Diller, L. (1987). *Neuropsychological rehabilitation*. New York: Guilford.

Reitan, R. M., & Davison, L. A. (1974). *Clinical neuropsychology: Current status and applications*. New York: Hemisphere.

Reitan, R. M., & Wolfson, D. (1985). *The Halstead–Reitan neuropsychological test battery*. (2nd ed.) Tucson: Neuropsychology Press, 1993.

Rourke, B. P. (1991). *Neuropsychological validation of learning disability subtypes*. New York: Guilford.

Rourke, B. P., Bakker, D. J., Fisk, J. L., & Strang, J. D. (1983). *Child neuropsychology*. New York: Guilford.

Squire, L. R., & Butters, N. (1984). *The neuropsychology of memory*. New York: Guilford.

Strub, R. L., & Black, F. W. (1988). *Neurobehavioral disorders: A clinical approach*. Philadelphia: Davis.

APPENDIX B

Archives of Clinical Neuropsychology
Brain and Cognition
Brain and Language
Clinical Neuropsychology
Cortex
Developmental Neuropsychology
Journal of Clinical and Experimental Neuropsychology
Neuropsychologia
Neuropsychology Review
Neuropsychology
The Clinical Neuropsychologist

2

Interdisciplinary Relationships: Behavioral Neurology

Jeffrey E. Shuren
University of Cincinnati College of Medicine

The study of the human mind has stirred the imagination of mankind for centuries. Although scientists have explored it, philosophers have argued about it, Hollywood has filmed it, and advertising has exploited it, the understanding of the mind still remains our most compelling, elusive, and challenging quest. In our current semantics *mind* is often replaced by *cognition, mental function, behavior,* or *mentation.* For the purposes of this chapter I use the term *behavior* to represent the functions of the human brain and its interactions with the environment and the rest of the body. Behavior implies the possibility for objective and subjective observation and investigation that are the bases for the disciplines I discuss.

The study of behavior may be approached through a myriad of different philosophies and methodologies. In this chapter I explore one of these fields, behavioral neurology, and focus on its interaction with neuropsychology. Behavioral neurology is the study of behavior that results from neurologic dysfunction. It uses nonstandard methods of investigation, whereas neuropsychology studies such altered behavior through the use of standardized measurement techniques. However, the differences and similarities between these two disciplines cannot be explained in such an oversimplified manner. The answers lie not only in the practices of today but stem from the history of each respective field.

HISTORICAL PERSPECTIVES

The first attribution of behavior to the brain was made by Herophilus (300 B.C.) and later by Galen (130–200 A.D.; Young, 1990). This view was not widely held, however. Instead, behavior was attributed to the spirit, an entity that remained separate from the body. It was Franz Joseph Gall (1758–1828) who first ascribed specific behaviors to specific regions of the brain. He championed the cause for the use of neuroanatomical studies in understanding the function of specific brain loci and was the first to fractionate and classify behavior. These claims were challenged by Pierre Flourens, who instead proposed that the cerebral hemispheres worked as a single unit. His conclusions were based on his studies with birds in whom brain function recovered regardless of the site of neural injury. Behavioral disturbances did not arise until a critical mass of brain tissue was damaged (Flourens, 1824, translated in von Bonin, 1960). Although most of Gall's conclusions and the field of phrenology were later disproved, his basic principles of investigation still form the cornerstone of behavioral neurology research. It was here that behavioral neurology was born.

The prevailing mood of the scientific community, however, was not ready for behavioral localization. In 1861, Ernest Auburtin, who had been strongly influenced by the work of Gall, argued in favor of his mentor Bouillaud's (1825) contention that the center for speech production lay in the frontal lobes in opposition to Gratiolet, who viewed the brain as working as a single entity (Benson, 1993; Critchley, 1979). On April 18, 1861, Paul Broca, after speaking with Auburtin, described his patient Leborgne to the Anthropological Society of Paris (Critchley, 1979). Leborgne could only say the word "tan" and at autopsy had a stroke that primarily affected the posterior portions of the left middle and inferior frontal gyri. Several weeks later, Broca reported a second patient with similar clinical and anatomical findings. Broca's clear presentations and reputation succeeded in reestablishing the principle that specific behaviors can be localized to specific brain regions. At the time, strokes were considered progressive lesions; therefore, speech production was attributed to the posterior one third of the inferior frontal gyrus (Broca's area, where the area of infarction was greatest), although the strokes of Broca's patients extended beyond the frontal lobe. Even Broca later noted that some patients who developed aphasia had lesions involving the insula or areas adjacent to but sparing the inferior frontal gyrus (Clarke, 1896). In 1867, Ange Duval proposed that the left hemisphere was the repository of language. Broca came to a similar conclusion subsequently and thereby set off the still present controversy of hemispheric specialization and dominance. (These same points had been made previously by Marc Dax in 1836 but remained in obscurity at the time; see Critchley, 1979 for a discussion on the Broca–Dax controversy.)

Broca's contributions, however, extend beyond the resurgence of brain-behavior localization and the importance of the left hemisphere in language. With Broca the *lesion-method* (the localization of brain function through the anatomic study of brain lesions) gained acceptance as a tool for understanding brain–behavior relationships. The lesion method became the first and foremost tool of behavioral neurology, a field not yet conceived even by its forebearers.

The second tool of behavioral neurology was introduced by Carl Wernicke in 1874. In that year Wernicke published a series of cases in which he outlined a model of language organization. Within this model, there was a motor language center that when damaged would produce the speech production deficits described by Broca; a sensory language center that when damaged would result in comprehension deficits (Wernicke's aphasia); and a pathway between them that when damaged would, he predicted, result in a third aphasia in which repetition was impaired (conduction aphasia). Wernicke came to these conclusions using the *symptom-complex method,* whereby clinical deficits that co-occur are grouped together as a single manifestation of brain injury. For example, Wernicke's aphasia is a symptom complex of fluent, paraphasic speech, poor repetition, and impaired auditory comprehension (Albert, Goodglass, Helm, Rubens, & Alexander, 1981). Wernicke's model was subsequently expanded by Lichtheim (1885), who first described a conduction aphasic and added the transcortical aphasias to a growing list of aphasia syndromes.

The late 19th century saw a flourishing of behavioral localizationists and heralded the age of the "diagram makers" (Shallice, 1988); for example, hemiachromatopsia (Verrey, 1888), visual agnosia (Lissauer, 1890), prosopagnosia (Wilbrand, 1892). New syndromes were described based on clinical observations and autopsy studies of lesion location from which models of brain function were conceived. These early schema depicted the brain as a serial processor wherein one brain locus performed one function and then transmitted that information to the next locus or center. The work of these investigators formed the basis of and the groundwork for current neuropsychological information-processing models.

A third tool that also gained ascendency during this time period was the single case study. Most of the original behavioral syndromes were based on the examination of a single patient. Today the debate over the efficacy of single case studies still continues.

Although the late 1800s were marked by a prolific outpouring of data favorable to behavioral localization, there was strong opposition to the claims of its supporters. The localizationists based their conclusions on the assumption that each behavior was controlled by one brain center and that the behavior following brain injury represented normal brain function minus the behavior performed by the lesioned center. Jackson (1958), however, posited that the behavior demonstrated by the brain-damaged patient represented compensation by the still viable brain. The brain was also not a serial processor composed of separate centers but a hierarchic processor. Other prominent clinicians of the time, such as Freud (1953) and Bergson (1896), offered further arguments against brain localization. The data presented by the localizationists was often insufficient to support their claims and patients who were purported to be pure cases (demonstrate an isolated deficit) often displayed multiple deficits. The now-famous debate in Paris between Marie, who opposed, and Déjerine, who supported, localization (Cole & Cole, 1971) heralded the end of the diagram makers.

From the turn of the century to the 1960s, the general view of the neurologic community was that the brain functioned as a whole. Lashley (1929) proposed the theory of *mass action,* which held that the amount of behavioral dysfunction was related to the amount of brain that was injured. All association cortices functioned equally (Lashley, 1950). The study of a series of patients rather than a single case became the dominant approach. The use of clinical observation and "bedside" tests—the implements of clinical neurology—for behavioral assessment was criticized for its lack of objectivity and precision. Subjects were now assessed with more standardized and quantifiable tests (e.g., Head, 1926). The use of normal matched controls was introduced (Rylander, 1939). However, the criteria used by these investigators for selecting patients were often too broad (e.g., brain damaged but able to comply with testing) and the theoretical claims made were often based on methodologically flawed testing. However, with the use of standardized testing, psychologists were asked to evaluate patients to assess behavior.

By the end of World War II, psychological testing was common. The principle concern of psychologists at that time was whether or not there was brain damage (organic brain syndrome). Halstead (1947), at the University of Chicago, advocated the use of objective, quantifiable measures to assess the location of brain injury and the nature of the deficit. His student, Ralph Reitan, organized and added to his mentor's tests to produce the Halstead–Reitan Neuropsychology Battery (Boll, 1980). The definitions of localization and nature of the deficit that were used were broad (e.g., language deficit, left hemisphere). However, their battery represented the first marriage of standardized, measurable behavioral testing with brain-behavior localization, which comprise the foundations of neuropsychology. Subsequently, Arthur Benton advocated assessing specific behaviors with specific, more sensitive tests, many of which, at the time, he had designed (see Benton, Hamsher, Varney, & Spreen, 1983).

Although a holistic view of brain function dominated the first half of the 20th century, localization studies were still performed (e.g., Penfield and colleagues' studies of brain function through direct electrical stimulation of the cerebral cortex, Penfield & Rasmussen, 1950; Penfield & Roberts, 1959, and Sherrington's, 1977, studies on reflexes). Behavioral neurology lay dormant during these years with rare exceptions (e.g., Critchley, 1953; Kleist, 1934).

In 1965, interest in behavioral neurology was rekindled through the work of Geschwind, who published a series of old and new cases with distinct behavioral syndromes that resulted from the disconnection of one brain center from another (e.g., optic aphasia arose from a lesion disconnecting visual input to the language system). He resurrected the original theories and models of the behavioral neurologists of the late 1800s and used them as the basis for forming testable hypotheses of brain–behavior relationships. Geschwind's collaborators in psychology and speech pathology used these theories to develop standardized tests for the assessment of behavior. For example, the Wernicke–Lichtheim model was used as the basis for aphasia research (Goodglass & Kaplan, 1972), out of which came the Boston Diagnostic Aphasia Examination for the assessment of aphasia type and lesion localization through the use of both quantitative and qualitative measures. The collaboration of Geschwind (a behavioral neurologist) with psychologists and speech pathologists demonstrated the clinical and academic utility of interactive work between the three fields. Moreover, he reintroduced the single case study and demonstrated its importance in behavioral research.

Meanwhile, Sperry (1968) and his colleagues in the 1960s provided evidence in support of differences in hemispheral processing through the examination of split-brain patients. Behavioral neurology also underwent a resurgence in Europe and Asia. Neuropsychology was also reborn, by such people as Benton (1959), Milner (1966), Goodglass (1968), Luria (1966), Kinsbourne (1971), and Warrington (Warrington & James, 1967). Teuber (1955) introduced the concept of *double dissociation,* which states that if two behaviors are performed by one system, damage to that system should produce deficits in both behaviors. However, if there exists Subject A who demonstrates deficits in the first behavior but not the second whereas Subject B shows deficits in the second behavior but not the first, the two behaviors must be performed by two different systems (or components of the same system). This concept of dissociations proved to be an important tool of neuropsychology and behavioral neurology. Neuropsychological assessment became further fine-tuned over time as behaviors were fractionated into component features.

With the arrival of newer neuroimaging techniques (e.g., computerized tomography and later magnetic resonance imaging), the emphasis of neuropsychology shifted from lesion localization to diagnosing disease etiology (e.g., head trauma, Alzheimer's disease), behavior management, and behavior rehabilitation (Tranel, 1992). Behavioral neurology also benefited from modern technological advances. The advent of better imaging of brain anatomy through computed tomography (CT) and magnetic resonance imaging (MRI) and functional imaging with single photon emission computed tomography (SPECT), positron emission tomography (PET), and activation MRI has allowed behavioral neurologists to make anatomic correlations of behavior while the patient is still alive.

Today, the boundaries between behavioral neurology and neuropsychology are not as clear as they once were. Some neurologists have acquired training in neuropsychology and use standardized measures in research and to supplement bedside testing, whereas some neuropsychologists have gained expertise in neuroanatomy and neuroimaging. However, the basic tools and principles of behavioral neurology remain the same: The study of brain–behavior relationships in patients with neurologic illness using the lesion method and the symptom-complex method through a marriage of qualitative bedside testing and a knowledge of medicine, neuroanatomy, neurochemistry, and neuroimaging. Whereas the lesion method has remained almost the sole domain of behavioral neurology, the symptom complex method has been used by both behavioral neurology and neuropsychology. Both methods rely heavily on determining associations and, more importantly, dissociations between different behaviors and between different behaviors and brain loci. In the remaining sections of this chapter, I discuss the advantages and limitations of each approach.

QUALITATIVE ASSESSMENT

The purpose of the behavioral neurologic examination is to diagnose the underlying illness(es), characterize the behavioral manifestations, give a prognosis, and prescribe medical treatment if warranted. Often ancillary blood, imaging, and, sometimes, cerebrospinal fluid studies must be obtained before making a final diagnosis, but the examination will still determine which studies are necessary.

At the core of a behavioral neurologic evaluation is the use of qualitative, nonstandardized measures to assess behavior. It is a subjective evaluation relying on the clinical judgment and experience of the examiner, much as is the elemental neurologic exam (testing of cranial nerve function, motor strength, tone, reflexes, coordination, gait, and sensation), which is the standard assessment tool used by all neurologists. The behavioral neurologic exam, therefore, is only as good as the clinician who performs it. The neuropsychological examination also requires the skill of the clinician to select the appropriate tests and to interpret the test results; however, the data used is quantifiable and standardized, thereby requiring far less subjective interpretation on the part of the examiner.

The behavioral neurologic examination begins with taking the history and observing the patient as he interacts with the examiner and family members. Through open-ended ("Why did you come to see me today?") and pointed ("Are you depressed?") questions, the examiner may be able to determine the duration of the illness and the type of behavioral changes that have become manifest (e.g., memory loss, personality changes, getting lost while driving, changes in mood). An acute onset suggests a vascular event, whereas a gradual deterioration over several years is more consistent with a neurodegenerative disease, such as Alzheimer's disease. The presence of systemic illnesses may directly or indirectly contribute to the patient's behavior (e.g., atherosclerotic heart disease leading to cardioembolic strokes or cerebral hypoperfusion from poor cardiac output), as may medications taken by the patient. A history of similar behavioral changes in other family members suggests a hereditary illness such as Huntington's disease.

After the history is taken, an elemental neurologic exam is performed. Together, the history and neurologic exam findings may help in the assessment of the patient's behavior, whereas a characterization of the patient's behavior may assist in either narrowing or broadening the field of possible etiologies and anatomic localization of the disease process. For example, on the elemental neurologic exam the patient has a very mild left hemisensory loss consistent with right hemispheral or brainstem injury. On behavioral examination, the patient has a left hemispatial attentional neglect consistent with right parietal injury. However, the patient also has a verbal amnesia, thereby suggesting left hemispheral injury as well. The findings on the elemental neurologic examination may also guide the mental status exam. If a left inferior visual field defect is present, the examiner will closely examine right parietal function.

The mental status examination may vary from neurologist to neurologist but the goal of the examination and often the key features remain the same: to assess behavior in a brief period of time. A comprehensive behavioral examination may require 20 to 45 minutes. In contrast, a comprehensive neuropsychological assessment requires several hours to complete at a cost of several hundred dollars. The behavioral examination includes an assessment of the patient's orientation, memory, language, visuoconstructive skills, visuospatial skills, and executive function. However, it also often includes an evaluation of skills not routinely assessed on neuropsychological testing (e.g., right–left orientation, finger localization) and skills for which adequate neuropsychological (quantifiable, standardized) testing has not been developed (e.g., spatial attention, praxis, emotional processing). Conversely, there are aspects of behavior that do not readily lend themselves to quick, bedside testing (e.g., abstraction, judgment) and hence may not be clearly assessed in a mental status examination. Behavioral neurologists may also supplement their examination with neuropsychological tests if indicated or refer the patient to a neuropsychologist for further evaluation.

Another aspect of behavior that neither bedside tests nor neuropsychological measures assess is the impact of the impaired behavior on the patient's daily life. Patients do not complain of difficulty copying intersecting pentagons or performing serial subtractions. The patient with frontal lobe injury may perform well on structured testing yet be unable to perform adequately at work. The right hemisphere damaged patient may understand what it is to be happy, sad, or angry, but not be able to discern the anger in his wife's voice.

The components of the behavioral examination are, by definition, not standardized. Judgments about behavior are based on how patients perform and the type of errors they make. One of the tests often used to assess memory is the recall of three words at a short (5-minute) and a long (20-minute) delay. Recent studies suggest that performance by normal subjects may vary, based in part on the age of the subject and the type of words used (high frequency versus low frequency), and performance may not correlate well with standarized tests. Even if a statistically significant correlation existed between the performance of a group of normal or brain-injured subjects on three-word recall and a standardized memory test (e.g., Wechsler Memory Scale, Wechsler, 1945; California Verbal Learning Test, Delis, Kramer, Kaplan, & Ober, 1987), the correlation is not necessarily valid for a single subject (see Cullum, Thompson, & Smernoff, 1993, for a review). However, the mental status examination is used in the office and in the hospital to evaluate individual patients.

An analysis of the correlation between objective performance on three-word recall and a standardized verbal-memory test also fails to assess the subjective elements of the test. Elderly patients with normal memory for their age may fail to recall the three words; however, when asked to recall the words they were told to remember, they may spontaneously say, "Oh yes, the three words you told me" or "You mean the three words I repeated back to you" or "You distracted me by having me subtract sevens," thereby demonstrating insight into the test and recollection of the test instructions. Patients with memory loss secondary to Alzheimer's disease may instead say, "What words?" or, "You did not ask me to remember anything," or give the names of items from a different part of the examination. Some patients with memory loss make confabulatory responses. Therefore, observation of patients and qualitative aspects of their responses may give better insights into their behavior than their objective performance on a bedside test.

Another test that is often used is to have the patient draw a clock and place the hands at 10 past 11. On this test the type of errors made may help to identify and localize the site of dysfunction. The patient may fail to write in the numbers on the left side of the clock, place the hands of the clock in the wrong location, and so on (Freedman, Kaplan, & Delis, 1994; Grossi, Modafferi, Pelosi, & Trojano, 1989; Rouleau, Salmon, Butters, Kennedy, & McGuire, 1992). In this instance test performance has a greater correlation with the presence (but not necessarily the absence) of as well as the location of neural injury. Second, data on both normal and brain-damaged populations, although limited, has been collected. However, neither the three-word recall test nor the clock drawing test allow for quantitative measurement of behavior, nor has the reliability of retest performance been measured. Instead, both tests may (or may not) demonstrate the presence of behavioral abnormalities (e.g., amnesia, hemispatial neglect). In contrast to neuropsychological tests, performance on these, as on many of the bedside tests used by behavioral neurologists, do not demonstrate that the subject being tested is "normal." Indeed, most bedside tests may be adequate measures of abnormal but not normal function.

Attempts to incorporate multiple bedside tests into a single standardized method of behavioral assessment have met with limited success. The Mini-Mental State Examination (Folstein, Folstein, & McHugh, 1975) has been used as a screening test for the presence of dementia. However, patients with dementia may perform within the normal range and test scores cannot be translated into an accurate account of what behavioral deficits are present. Modifications of this test have been made that show moderate correlation with the Wechsler Adult Intelligence Scale and good test–retest reliability (Stern, Sano, Paulson, & Mayeux, 1987). However, this and similar tests cannot adequately decipher the components of abnormal behavior, nor can they replace the expertise of a trained clinician.

I have not made these points to argue that bedside testing is inadequate for the assessment of behavior. In the acute setting, when a patient evaluation must be made quickly or when patients are not capable of participating in long testing sessions, there is no alternative to using bedside tests. Often times, the use of neuropsychological testing in the office is not practical from the standpoint of either time or cost. The use of short bedside tests avoids patient fatigue, which may influence performance. Some patients may also be too impaired to comply with neuropsychological testing but may nevertheless be assessable by a simpler bedside evaluation. However, at other times, an adequate evaluation of a patient cannot be made without neuropsychological testing. In most instances the mental status exam can be used to determine whether or not a more extensive evaluation of behavior by neuropsychological testing is required and what aspects of behavior should be assessed.

The behavioral neurologic exam, therefore, incorporates historical material with the findings on elemental neurologic exam and performance on the mental status exam. The final assessment of patient's behavior is not based on their performance on any single test but on their performance on and throughout all testing. As in the case of neuropsychological measures, bedside tests assess more than one particular behavior and impaired performance may result from deficits in various mental functions. For example, poor performance on the 3-word recall test may result from poor memory (either encoding or retrieval), attention, or lexical access/retrieval. Alternatively, dysfunction in one process (e.g., sustained attention) may cause impaired performance on multiple tests (e.g., memory, calculations, auditory comprehension).

The purpose of the mental status examination is to form a gestalt of the patient's behavior and, in light of the history, elemental neurologic examination, blood tests, neuroimaging findings, and so on, come to a diagnosis of the patient's illness. Knowledge of the disease process will aid in determining whether or not the patient will benefit from cognitive rehabilitation or medical intervention. The patient with speech output deficits that results from a stroke may benefit from melodic intonation therapy or bromocriptine (Albert, Bachman, Morgan, & Helm-Estabrooks, 1988), whereas a patient with similar deficits from Pick's disease would not be a suitable candidate for these therapies because of the progressive nature of the disease. Second, knowing what the underlying disease is can give insight into patients' behavior (e.g., the amnesia of Huntington's disease results from retrieval deficits) as well as prognosis for recovery or progression.

The findings from a behavioral neurologic examination have limited value when considered separately. They are like flecks of color in a pointilist painting that together create a coherent whole.

In the following cases I hope to illustrate some of the previous points:

Case 1. JW was a 34-year-old lawyer who developed a mild tremor when using his hands. He had difficulty organizing his thoughts and attributed this to his being concerned and self-conscious of the tremor. There was a family history of essential tremor (inherited tremor without known cause and without other sequelae). He went to see a behavioral neurologist who found a normal examination. The neurologist thought JW had an essential tremor but, because JW's wife was concerned about his performance at work, the neurologist referred JW to a neuropsychologist. On neuropsychological testing, JW had a Wechsler Adult Intelligence Scale–Revised (WAIS–R; Wechsler, 1981) full-scale IQ of 110. On the Nelson Adult Reading Test (NART; Nelson & O'Connell, 1978), JW had a baseline IQ of 125. JW performed within low normal range on the Wechsler Memory Scale–Revised (WMS–R; Wechsler, 1987) and in the high normal range on the Multilingual Aphasia Examination (MAE; Benton & Hamsher, 1976) and Judgment of Line Orientation (JLO; Benton, Hannay, & Varney, 1975). On the Wisconsin Card Sorting Test (WCST; Berg, 1948; Grant & Berg, 1948) JW completed five categories and made many perseverative errors. The neuropsychologist concluded that JW had deficits in planning with mild memory deficits secondary to distractibility consistent with damage to the frontal lobes or frontal connections. Based on the combination of tremor with frontal deficits, the neurologist ordered serum copper and ceruloplasmin levels. The copper level was elevated and the ceruloplasmin level was low, consistent with Wilson's disease (deposition of copper in the basal ganglia and liver; Wilson, 1912). The neurologist placed JW on penicillamine to try to prevent further copper deposition and subsequent neurologic decline.

In this case the mental status testing of the behavioral neurologist was not sensitive to the behavioral abnormalities manifested by JW. However, in conjunction with a neuropsychological evaluation, the correct diagnosis was made, thus allowing appropriate treatment to be initiated early in the disease course before further cerebral injury occurred.

Case 2. RV was a 68-year-old woman who noted that her vision had gradually become blurred over 2 months. Her ophthalmologist found that she had normal vision. Her internist performed a neurologic examination, the results of which were normal, and therefore sent her to a neuropsychologist for a thorough evaluation. On the WAIS–R RV had a verbal IQ of 98, a performance IQ of 90 and a full-scale IQ of 95. Her baseline IQ according to her performance on the NART was 100. She performed within low–normal range on the WMS–R, normal range on the WCST, and low–normal range on the JLO. RV demonstrated impaired copying of the Rey–Osterrieth Complex Figure (ROCF; Osterrieth, 1944; Rey, 1941), primarily in reproducing the overall configuration of the design with relatively good reproduction of the internal details. The neuropsychologist concluded that RV had focal right parietal damage, probably secondary to a focal process such as stroke or tumor, and therefore referred her to a behavioral neurologist.

RV had a normal elemental neurologic examination, but on mental status testing the neurologist observed that RV was slow to look at targets, had mild difficulty with eye–hand coordination (when given a page filled with Xs she had difficulty pointing to the center of some of the Xs), and, when given pictures of various scenes to describe (e.g., people playing on a beach, a wedding), she tended to "overlook" some items in the pictures. The rest of her mental status exam was normal. The neurologist concluded that she had the features of a mild Balint's syndrome (asimultanagnosia, optic ataxia, and ocular apraxia; Balint, 1909). He ordered a CT scan of the brain which demonstrated widening of the parieto–occipital sulci bilaterally consistent with mild posterior cortical atrophy. The neurologist concluded that RV had early onset Alzheimer's disease.

This patient developed visuospatial deficits that fell outside the purview of current neuropsychological measures but were detected by observation and bedside tests. The findings on the behavioral neurologic examination with the neuroimaging results led to the diagnosis.

Case 3. LM was a 55-year-old male dentist who noted progressive difficulty using his tools and memory loss over a 24-month period, necessitating retirement from his practice. His family practitioner was concerned about Alzheimer's disease. He ordered a CT scan of the brain, which was normal, and then referred LM to a neuropsychologist. On the WAIS–R he had a full-scale score of 100 with a baseline IQ on the NART of 115. He performed in the mildly impaired range on the WMS–R in the immediate and delayed sections of both the logical memory and visual reproduction subtests. He had a mild anomia on both the visual naming subtest and the controlled oral word-association subtest of the MAE, but performed within normal range on the remainder of the test. He showed poor copying of the ROCF, had mildly impaired performance on the JLO, and made many perseverative errors on the WCST. The neuropsychologist concluded that the findings were consistent with Alzheimer's disease and referred the patient to a behavioral neurologist to complete the evaluation.

On elemental neurologic examination the neurologist observed that LM had a magnetic grasp with both hands (reached for objects placed in close proximity to him and then failed to relinquish his hold until the object was taken from him) and mild cogwheel rigidity. On mental-status testing LM had limited insight into his deficits. He was amnestic, anomic, and echopraxic, with impaired visuospatial and visuoconstructive skills. LM also demonstrated a profound ideomotor apraxia. The neurologist concluded that the constellation of apraxia, magnetic grasp, cogwheel rigidity with a mild amnesia, anomia, echopraxia, and impaired visuospatial and visuoconstructive skills was most consistent with corticobasal degeneration (Lang, Riley, & Bergeron, 1994; Rebeiz, Kolodny, & Richardson, 1968). Because this disease causes prominent basal ganglia degeneration (as well as cortical and thalamic degeneration), the neurologist started LM on deprenyl, a MAO–B inhibitor that has been shown to slow the rate of progression of Parkinson's disease. The neurologist followed LM on deprenyl in conjunction with the neuropsychologist.

Mild parkinsonian features (e.g., cogwheel rigidity) can occur in Alzheimer's disease. However, in Case 3, the presence of a profound ideomotor apraxia with only mild changes in memory and language suggested a diagnosis of corticobasal degeneration. Although several elements of LM's behavior could not be assessed by current neuropsychological measures, the use of standardized, quantifiable neuropsychological tests allowed the neurologist to follow LM's course on deprenyl. Therefore, optimal patient care required the combined efforts of both the behavioral neurologist and the neuropsychologist. The utility of neuropsychological testing for assessing behaviors over time can and has been applied to drug studies and assessing the outcome of neurosurgical procedures (e.g., the effects of surgical resection of a seizure focus in an epileptic patient).

The behavioral neurologic examination has several advantages over a neuropsychological evaluation: (a) It requires less time to perform and hence suffers less from the effects of patient fatigue. (b) The tests used are often simple and therefore may be used on some patients who are too impaired to comply with neuropsychological testing. (c) It is less expensive. (d) The exam focuses on the types of errors made rather than the number of errors made. (e) It may assess aspects of behavior that neuropsychological testing cannot currently evaluate. (f) The exam integrates a knowledge of neurology (medical perspective) with a knowledge of brain behavior (neurological and neuropsychological perspective).

There are several disadvantages that the behavioral neurologic exam has when compared with a neuropsychological evaluation: (a) It is not standardized—normal performance is often highly variable and therefore subjects can make errors and yet be cognitively normal. (b) The tests used are simplistic and hence subjects may not make any errors though they are cognitively impaired. (c) The tests are not quantitative; therefore, they cannot be used to measure the amount of behavioral dysfunction or to follow the rate of decline or improvement secondary to disease progression or medical intervention. (d) Some aspects of behavior often are not sensitive to bedside tests. (e) The behavioral neurologic examination relies heavily on the skills of the examiner, which makes it very subjective and difficult to analyze, compare, or teach.

THE LESION METHOD

Since the time of Broca, the lesion method has remained the hallmark of behavioral neurologic research. This method relies on two key premises: (a) anatomy correlates with function, and (b) damage to one locus in the brain results in normal behavior minus the function(s) performed by the damaged locus. As we have learned, neither premise is absolutely correct. However, there are still advantages to using the lesion method as the study of frontal lobe function illustrates.

Harlow (1848, 1868) first described the now-famous case of Phineas Gage, a 25-year-old foreman who was considered a good worker and father until a tamping iron went through his skull, damaging both ventromedial frontal lobes. Subsequently, Gage retained much of his previous skills but his personality changed. He became argumentative and abusive until "he was no longer Gage." Brickner (1936) described a 39-year-old man who developed headaches and profound lethargy. He was operated on by Walter Dandy, the famous neurosurgeon, who discovered a large meningioma compressing both frontal lobes. Dandy had to remove large sections of both frontal lobes. Following surgery the patient appeared to have preserved memory and intellectual capacities without deficits in primary motor or sensory functions. However, his behavior changed such that he had a shallow affect, appeared hypomanic, made socially inappropriate comments, and had poor planning skills. These two cases, as well as well other cases from the time, suggested that the frontal lobes are important for personality but play little role in general intellectual abilities.

Anatomic studies of the brain (carried out primarily in monkeys) demonstrated that there were cytoarchitectonic differences between various regions of the frontal lobe (as well as other areas of the brain; Brodmann, 1909). The dorsomedial nucleus of the thalamus was shown to have spatially organized afferent projections to prefrontal cortex (the medial part of the nucleus projects to orbitofrontal cortex, whereas the lateral part projects to the upper frontal pole; Walker, 1938). Therefore, it was conceptually possible at the time that lesions to different regions of prefrontal cortex would produce different changes in behavior rather than a single "frontal lobe syndrome" as might be expected based on the cases of Harlow and Brickner. Indeed, Cummings (1985), based on several clinico–anatomic studies, described three distinct behavioral syndromes that correlate respectively to injury to three distinct prefrontal regions. The orbitofrontal syndrome is marked by disinhibition; the patient is emotionally labile, impulsive, and distractible with a shallow affect, poor social judgment, and a tendency to make socially inappropriate comments. The frontal convexity syndrome (secondary to injury to dorsolateral frontal lobe) is marked by apathy; the patient lacks initiative and motivation, has difficulty maintaining or shifting behavioral set and inhibiting incorrect responses, shows a tendency to respond to external stimuli rather than internal drives (stimulus bound), has an impaired ability to abstract and reason, and does not learn from mistakes. The medial frontal syndrome is marked by akinesia; the patient has limited spontaneous movement and speech.

In a series of papers, Starkstein, Robinson, and colleagues (Robinson, Bosotn, Starkstein, & Price, 1988; Robinson & Szetela, 1981; Starkstein & Robinson, 1989; Starkstein, Robinson, & Price, 1987) described various affective disorders secondary to stroke. They reported that the closer a stroke approached the anterior pole of the brain (frontal lobe or subcortical structures deep to the frontal lobe, such as the caudate nucleus), the greater the likelihood that the patient would develop depression. Depression was also more common immediately following left hemisphere strokes, whereas an increase in depression following right hemisphere strokes was observed at 6 months poststroke (Åström, Adolfsson, & Asplund, 1993). When injured, the cortical site most commonly associated with depression was the fronto–opercular region. In contrast, mania was most commonly observed following orbitofrontal or basolateropolar temporal lobe injury on the right side.

The studies conducted by Starkstein, Robinson, and colleagues and those reviewed by Cummings used patient observation and correlated behavior with structural damage as determined by autopsy or CT scans. Supportive data has also been derived using blood flow imaging techniques (e.g., SPECT, PET) in subjects without apparent structural abnormalities in the frontal lobes. Baxter et al. (1989) found that left prefrontal hypometabolism was the most severe abnormality detected on PET imaging in patients with unipolar or bipolar depression or major depression with obsessive–compulsive disorder. Blood flow and glucose metabolism studies are useful in that they may demonstrate areas of diminished function. However, they do not by themselves determine whether or not the observed decrease or alteration in function is secondary to injury to the area of hypoperfusion/hypometabolism or structures to which the involved area connects. These techniques also have poor resolution, limited cerebral localization capabilities, and are fraught with methodological difficulties (see Démonet, Wise, & Frackowiak, 1993; Mazziotta et al., 1985; Rezai, Kirchner, Armstrong, Ehrhardt, & Heistad, 1988; Sergent, Zuck, Lèvesque, & MacDonald, 1992, for a discussion of some of the advantages and disadvantages of these techniques). However, when combined with CT, MRI, and autopsy studies, these techniques may prove to be helpful adjunctive measures.

These examples of the lesion method have suggested that the frontal lobes play an important role in personality, mood, planning and motivation, and that different areas of the frontal lobes subserve different functions. Early studies of frontal lobe lesion patients assumed that the frontal lobes had isolated and separable functions. Although the frontal lobes may receive information from and send information to various cerebral structures, each structure was considered to be part of a relay. Damage to one structure could impair frontal function by depriving the frontal lobes of particular inputs, but not because the processing of the frontal lobes were themselves directly affected. This conception was used to understand the function of all cerebral structures. However, this view is currently falling out of favor. The following examples using the lesion method are meant to illustrate this change in thinking and the reasoning behind the change.

Neglect is the failure to report, respond, or orient to stimuli that cannot be explained by primary sensory or motor deficits (Heilman, Watson, & Valenstein, 1993). Neglect may result from inattention or unawareness of a stimulus (attentional—sensory—neglect) or an inability to orient, prepare, initiate, or maintain movement towards a stimulus (intentional—motor—neglect). Neglect occurs more frequently after right hemisphere injury. Patients may demonstrate attentional neglect, intentional neglect, or both (Bisiach, Geminiani, Berti, & Rusconi, 1990; Coslett, Bowers, Fitzpatrick, Haws, & Heilman, 1990). Hemispatial neglect (neglect for items in one half of a particular spatial plane) has been reported following dorsolateral frontal lobe lesions in monkeys (Bianchi, 1895) and in man (Heilman & Valenstein, 1972). Watson, Miller, and Heilman (1978) trained monkeys to respond with the right hand when touched on the left and with the left hand when touched on the right. Following unilateral frontal arcuate gyrus lesions, the monkeys showed contralateral neglect without motor weakness. When touched on the contralesional (neglected) side they moved the ipsilesional hand, but when touched on the ipsilesional side they did not move the contralesional hand. These findings could not be explained by an attentional deficit. Instead, the authors posited that the frontal lobes play a role in motor intention.

Reports using the lesion method have demonstrated a greater frequency of intentional neglect following right frontal lesions, whereas attentional neglect more commonly follows right parietal lesions. Intentional neglect has also been reported following damage to structures that have connections to the dorsolateral frontal lobe. These papers include reports of lesions to the centromedian–parafascicular (intralaminar) nuclei of the thalamus in monkeys (Watson et al., 1978) and in man (Bogousslavsky, Miklossy, Deruaz, Regli, & Assai, 1986; this patient also had damage to the dorsomedial, ventroposteromedial, ventroposterolateral, and ventrolateral thalamic nuclei), the ventral tegmental area in rats (Marshall, 1979), and the putamen in rats. Similar disturbances in intention have also been reported after temporoparietal damage in monkeys (Valenstein, Van den Abell, Watson, & Heilman, 1982). Both left hemispatial attentional neglect and proximal intentional neglect have been described following a right parietal lesion in man (Gold, Shuren, & Heilman, 1994). Conversely, both intentional and attentional deficits have been described following frontal lesions in monkeys (Deuel & Farrar, 1993).

Although the initial studies using the lesion method to evaluate the role of the frontal lobes in spatial attention suggest that the frontal lobes mediate intention, the results of more recent studies using the same method in both animals and man draw us to a different conclusion: Damage to structures that connect to each other may produce identical or similar deficits. Therefore, the structures that connect to the frontal lobes do not function only as relays to pass information on to the frontal lobes (serial processing); rather, all the connected structures function together as a processing network with distributed but interconnected components (e.g., parallel distributed processing—PDP; although PDP is still a theoretical construct for cerebral processing, it explains more aspects about neural processing and plasticity than older theories invoking serial processing. I return to this point later in the chapter). Therefore, the use of the lesion method has contributed not only to our understanding of the frontal lobes but also to our knowledge of how the brain is functionally organized and the way in which it processes.

The concept of neural networks is further demonstrated by the work of Goldman-Rakic and colleagues on working memory (dynamic short memory store in which information can be retrieved to be worked on or for immediate use; Baddeley, 1990). The caudal principal sulcus in the dorsolateral frontal lobe of monkeys is important for spatial working memory. Lesions to the dorsolateral frontal lobes of monkeys will result in impaired performance on spatial delayed-response tasks in which the monkey is shown a target and then must make a visual saccade to the site opposite from the one at which the target was presented (Goldman-Rakic, 1987). Similar deficits in spatial memory also result from lesions to the hippocampal formation (Zola-Morgan & Squire, 1985) or dorsomedial nucleus of the thalamus (Isseroff, Rosvold, Galkin, & Goldman-Rakic, 1982), structures with which the dorsolateral frontal lobes connect (Goldman-Rakic & Porrino, 1985; Goldman-Rakic, Selemon, & Schwartz, 1984). Studies have also been performed in nonlesioned monkeys using neural discharge recordings or PET imaging. Activity was recorded from prefrontal neurons (Fuster & Alexander, 1971) and hippocampal neurons (Watanabe & Niki, 1985) in monkeys on spatial memory tasks. Increased metabolism was also detected on PET imaging in the dorsolateral frontal lobes, mediodorsal thalamus, anterior thalamus, and hippocampus of monkeys on tasks of spatial working memory but not on sensory-motor control tasks (Friedman & Goldman-Rakic, 1988; Friedman, Janas, & Goldman-Rakic, 1990). Goldman-Rakic has interpreted the results of the lesion method, cell recording, and PET imaging studies as consistent with processing by parallel distributed networks (Roland & Friberg, 1985).

A modern-day Karl Lashley may take these reports as evidence that brain function is not localized, but rather is spread evenly throughout the hemispheres. However, the work of Deuel and Farrar (1993) in the monkey demonstrated that an anatomic structure may contribute to multiple networks and may contribute in different ways, or at least to a different extent than another structure of the network. They removed unilateral sections of periarcuate (dorsolateral frontal) or inferior parietal cortex in monkeys and then assessed their performance on several tasks of spatial attention. The monkeys demonstrated evidence of contralateral intentional neglect, attentional neglect, or both when either the frontal or parietal cortex was removed. The type of errors made was dependent on the tasks employed and not on the lesion location.

Complementary research by Alexander, DeLong, and Strick (1986) has shown that different subregions of a brain structure may participate in different neural networks. Therefore, a particular function may be spread across a multiple but limited number of brain structures with different aspects of a function localized to a fewer number of brain structures. The challenge is for the clinician to try to differentiate different aspects of a behavior and use this knowledge to better localize the site(s) of brain injury that the patient has sustained. A complementary approach is to use the presence of multiple behaviors (to which a particular brain region may contribute) to clinically localize the site of neural injury, as is currently performed in both behavioral neurology and neuropsychology.

Damasio and Damasio (1989) have noted that the lesion method's utility is dependent on how insightful is the testing used (whether it be standardized or experimental) to assess the behavior, how accurate are the hypotheses on which the testing and subsequent conceptualizations are based, how well the observers can integrate neural processing with behavioral processing, and how well the anatomy can be defined by the procedure being used. As the study of frontal lobe function has shown, the level of sophistication of the neuropsychological testing administered, the hypothetical constructs used to drive research and to conceptualize the neural processing of behavior both anatomically and functionally, and the anatomical resolution of imaging techniques have grown as our knowledge, technology, and insights have grown.

At present, the lesion method is used in conjunction with neuroimaging, MRI in particular. Neuroimaging allows brain–behavior relationships to be determined while the patient is still alive. In this way, behavior may be directly correlated with a lesion through temporal association. If we were limited only to the evaluation of brain anatomy at autopsy, it would be difficult to decipher the role of multiple lesions in the brain, as no temporal association could be made. The process leading to death may also add to the number of neural insults or extend the patient's original lesion, thus confounding the clinico–pathological findings.

The use of neuroimaging studies, on the other hand, has its own drawbacks. The degree of resolution depends on the type of lesion. Certain infiltrative brain tumors may spread beyond its presumed borders as outlined on a CT scan or MR image (e.g., astrocytomas). Strokes, the most common lesion used in brain–behavior correlation studies, may not be imaged fully or may not be recognized at all depending on their location, how soon after the stroke the scan is obtained (e.g., strokes may disappear on CT between 1 and 4 weeks after onset;

Becker, Desch, Hacker, & Pencz, 1979; Kinkel, 1992), the size of the stroke (small vessel strokes are often not imaged), and whether or not a scan slice was made through the level of the stroke (MR can resolve brain structures to approximately 0.5 millimeters, although newer methodologies are starting to visualize intracortical structures; e.g., cell columns and myelin septa; Damasio, Kuljis, Yuh, Van Hoesen, & Ehrhardt, 1991). The region of ischemic insult may extend beyond the area imaged to distal sites in the same vascular territory producing microinfarctions. Although a stroke can involve subcortical structures in isolation, microinfarctions may occur distally in the cortex that are not detected on a neuroimaging study, but do produce clinically evident changes in behavior.

The type of lesion causing the behavior is important as well. Patients with tumors in the left hemisphere who were matched with patients with strokes of similar size and in similar locations had less severe language deficits than their stroke counterparts (Anderson, Damasio, & Tranel, 1990). Lesion localization may also be difficult using current neuroimaging techniques. To determine the location of a lesion in the brain, various neuroanatomical landmarks may need to be identified (e.g., the frontal lobe begins anterior to the central sulcus, a structure that is sometimes difficult to identify even at autopsy). At least two and usually three planes of imaging are required to accurately map a lesion (see Damasio & Frank, 1992). The need for accurate identification of neuroanatomical landmarks is even more important when using SPECT or PET imaging because of the poor resolution of these techniques. Damasio and colleagues (material presented at the Decade of the Brain plenary session of the 45th annual meeting of the American Academy of Neurology, April 1993) administered simple visual stimuli to a patient during a PET scan. The patient demonstrated increased metabolism in regions consistent with visual association cortex but not with primary visual (calcarine) cortex. However, when an MRI scan was obtained and matched with the PET scan images, it was evident that the patient's calcarine cortex turned superiorly and was indeed the area of increased metabolism detected on PET imaging. Had adequate anatomic mapping not been performed using identification of cerebral landmarks as a guide, erroneous conclusions might have been drawn. Interindividual differences between the anatomic locations for the neural processing of different behaviors (Varney, Damasio, & Adler, 1989) make it difficult to ascribe brain–behavior correlations from a single-case study without corroborative data or multiple single-case studies.

When a syndrome is complex and results from a large lesion, it is not possible to investigate the various components of the syndrome or to ascertain the contribution of each of the anatomical sites involved. The lesion method can be used to analyze the individual contributions of each anatomical site to the syndrome, can enrich our knowledge of the syndrome, and give insights into the interaction and joint processing by the different neural structures involved (i.e., the whole is more than the sum of its parts). Using the lesion method and CT imaging, Alexander, Naeser, and Palumbo (1990) examined patients with individual strokes affecting one or more neural sites that together result in Broca's aphasia. They concluded that lesions restricted to the frontal operculum affect speech initiation, those restricted to the lower motor cortex produce dysarthria, and lesions involving the subcortical and periventricular white matter result in the production of phonemic paraphasias and agraphia. When damage occurred to these structures and the medial subcallosal fasciculus, Broca's aphasia was produced.

The lesion method also has a clinical utility. Although similar behaviors can result from damage to different anatomic components of a network, the prognosis for recovery may differ. Impaired production of spontaneous speech can result from lesions involving any one of various sites in cortical or subcortical dominant frontal lobe. Naeser, Palumbo, Helm-Estabrooks, Stiassny-Eder, and Albert (1989) have shown that patients with impaired spontaneous speech production secondary to lesions involving two subcortical white matter areas (the most medial and rostral section of the subcallosal fasciculus and the periventricular white matter deep to the lower motor and sensory cortex for the mouth) have a lesser chance for recovery than patients with similar deficits resulting from lesions in other neural sites. The size of the lesion is also important for recovery of language and other neurologic functions. In general, the larger the lesion size, the poorer the prognosis for recovery (Bushnell, Gupta, Mlcoch, & Barnes, 1989).

The lesion method and the current neuroimaging techniques used to implement this method still remain important clinical and research tools. However, caution must be exercised when interpreting neuroimaging studies in the context of brain–behavior relationships.

The lesion method may be enhanced today by looking at performance in patients with lesions involving different structures of a neural network and looking at differences in performance. The work of Posner and colleagues on spatial attention is one example (see Posner & Petersen, 1990). In a series of papers, Posner and his collaborators have suggested that the visual attentional system is capable of *disengaging* attention from one stimulus, *shifting* attention to a different spatial location, and then *engaging* another stimulus. According to these researchers, disengaging, shifting, and engaging are performed by the parietal lobes, superior colliculi, and thalami, respectively.

It is important to recognize that using brain-impaired subjects in lesion-behavior analysis studies may not reflect normal brain function, as discussed earlier in this chapter. Further refinement of old technologies and the development of new technologies may help to redress these shortcomings of the lesion method.

THE SYMPTOM-COMPLEX METHOD

The symptom-complex method dates back at least to Wernicke. The underlying principle of the method is that symptoms that tend to co-occur result from injury to the same anatomic area (localizationist approach), the same underlying cognitive process (functional system approach), or to the same underlying disease (pathophysiologic approach). Although using this method can lead to erroneous associations, the conclusions drawn are testable hypotheses. If two symptoms are thought to co-occur and subsequently patients are found in whom each symptom occurred in isolation, there would be a double dissociation; that is, the two symptoms are functionally distinct. Alternatively, if two symptoms always co-occur, their presence may aid in lesion localization or they may give insight into the underlying processing they share.

For example, consider the case of Gerstmann's syndrome. In 1940, Josef Gerstmann (his concepts were reported in German in 1930) described a constellation of symptoms (acalculia, agraphia, finger agnosia [localization], right–left disorientation) that he attributed to a disturbance of the body schema resulting from left angular gyrus injury. Subsequently, the "Gerstmann syndrome" attracted harsh criticisms (Benton, 1961). Several questions were raised: (a) Are the components of the syndrome closely linked or are they dissociable? (b) Does the syndrome occur in isolation or are other deficits part of the complex? (c) Does the syndrome result from isolated left angular gyrus injury? (d) Is there one underlying mechanism for the syndrome? (e) What does each component of the syndrome represent clinically? (f) Is it practical to group these symptoms as a syndrome? What each component of the syndrome truly represented was altered over time to be overinclusive (e.g., finger agnosia secondary to position sense deficits) or remained too broad and undefined (e.g., acalculia and agraphia; Critchley, 1966). Right–left disorientation occurs in normal men and women (Harris & Gitterman, 1978; Wolf, 1973). Gerstmann's syndrome rarely occurs in isolation and is often associated with aphasia (Poeck & Orgass, 1966) or constructional apraxia (Kinsbourne &

Warrington, 1962). Each component of the syndrome could occur in isolation. Moreover, there was a correlation between the number of components present and the size of the lesion, suggesting that Gerstmann's syndrome represented one of many concurrent deficits (Heimburger, DeMeyer, & Reitan, 1964). The syndrome not only results from single lesions but also from more diffuse processes (e.g., alcoholism, lead poisoning, carbon monoxide toxicity, degenerative diseases, various psychotic states; Critchley, 1966). Components of the syndrome, finger agnosia and dysgraphia (probably spatial agraphia), have been observed following right hemisphere injury (Poeck & Orgass, 1966) and the full Gerstmann syndrome has been reported following a left posterior thalamic lesion (Santos, Cope, & Keller, 1991). Each component of the syndrome can arise from different mechanisms (Benton & Sivan, 1993). Damage to the angular gyrus may produce various deficits besides those observed in Gerstmann's syndrome (e.g., alexia, ideomotor apraxia, aphasia, constructional apraxia; Benson & Cummings, 1982).

Recently, evidence has been garnered to support the existence of a distinct Gerstmann's syndrome (see Benton, 1992, for a review). Roeltgen, Sevush, and Heilman (1983) described a 62-year-old man who demonstrated all four features of the syndrome without evidence of aphasia, constructional apraxia, alexia, topographical disorientation, or amnesia. A CT scan of the head showed an infarct involving the superior angular gyrus, the posterior supramarginal gyrus with minimal extension into the posteroinferior part of the superior parietal lobule. This case was the first clear example of an isolated Gerstmann's syndrome secondary to a focal parietal lesion. Morris, Lüders, Lesser, Dinner, and Hahn (1984) subsequently described a 17-year-old boy with epilepsy who underwent electrocortical stimulation of his left parietal lobe. Stimulation of one site in the region between the angular and supramarginal gyri produced agraphia, acalculia, and finger agnosia, whereas stimulation to an adjacent site produced right–left disorientation in a boy who did not previously have any of these symptoms. Stimulation to nearby sites produced combinations of some of the Gerstmann symptoms with other deficits (e.g., anomia, alexia, constructional apraxia). This case serves as further evidence for the existence of this syndrome with isolated dominant angular gyrus/supramarginal gyrus dysfunction. As pointed out by Roeltgen et al. (1983), isolated Gerstmann's syndrome may be rarely observed because the occurrence of a small lesion in the appropriate site is uncommon. Although Gerstmann's assertions of the existence and localization of the symptom complex that he described have been affirmed, there is no conclusive data that supports damage to a single process as the underlying mechanism.

Gerstmann's report of his symptom complex led to testable hypotheses that have been borne out by careful research. Most of the supportive data that had been accumulated required modern technological advances (CT, refined cortical stimulation techniques). Although Gerstmann's symptom complex is rare in isolation, its components are not. Today, Gerstmann's syndrome remains of clinical utility for anatomic localization. By assessing for the components of the syndrome as well as other features of dominant parietal dysfunction (apraxia, aphasia, etc.), the yield of identifying dominant parietal injury increases. (This still remains a theoretical and anecdotal issue, as no formal study of the diagnostic yield of testing for all the components of Gerstmann's syndrome has been undertaken using modern neuroimaging techniques and standardized assessment.) The greater the number of Gerstmann syndrome features present and the more isolated the deficits, the more likely the lesion involves dominant parietal lobe. However, when syndrome features occur in isolation, the diagnostic yield is poor.

Gerstmann's syndrome is only a minor victory for the symptom-complex method. Although the presence of the full tetrad is of localizing significance, the syndrome in isolation is rare and there is no known functional unity (at present) between the four components.

The symptom-complex method has been used in other instances not always with success (e.g., deep dysphasia; see Shallice, 1988, for a critique). Today, the symptom-complex method remains essential for the diagnosis of dementia etiology. Often the clinician is confronted with a patient who has experienced intellectual impairment in the absence of abnormal findings on the physical examination, elemental neurologic examination, or laboratory studies. Diagnosis often rests on the history and mental status examination. For example, a 75-year-old with progressive amnesia and anomia with a normal elemental neurologic examination and laboratory findings has probable Alzheimer's disease, whereas a 55-year-old with progressive personality changes, disinhibition, hyperorality, and roaming behavior with a normal elemental neurologic examination and laboratory and imaging studies likely has Pick's disease (Cummings & Benson, 1992; Mendez, Selwood, Mastri, & Frey, 1993).

In some cases it is a combination of characteristic findings on mental status examination and elemental neurologic examination that defines the disease. A 70-year-old who develops psychotic behavior followed by slowed gait and increased tone with normal laboratory and imaging studies likely has diffuse Lewy body disease (Burkhardt et al., 1988; Crystal, Dickson, Lizardi, Davies, & Wolfson, 1990). Finally, a symptom complex may not be characteristic of only one disease but may at least limit the field of possibilities and thereby guide the evaluation. A 50-year-old man develops agitation, fluctuations in his level of arousal, visual hallucinations, and paranoid delusions. The latter may suggest a psychosis, and agitation could result from a stroke. However, when accompanied by fluctuations in level of arousal and visual hallucinations, the most likely diagnosis is delirium secondary to a toxic-metabolic etiology.

The symptom-complex method remains an important tool in neurologic diagnosis, in understanding brain function, and in localizing sites of neural injury by clinical examination. As was the case with the lesion method, the symptom-complex method is least successful when the observer/experimenter makes unjustified assumptions, uses poor theoretical constructs, lacks insight into neural processing, or uses inadequate examination techniques. Unfortunately, the errors of the experimenter are often attributed to the failings of the underlying method rather than to the shortcomings of the experimenter.

BEHAVIORAL NEUROLOGY AT THE CROSSROADS

The behavioral neurologists of old relied on clinical acumen and autopsy studies to explore brain–behavior relationships and the clinico–anatomic manifestations of neurologic diseases. The behavioral neurologists of today have access to a wider range of investigative tools that have both challenged (e.g., serial processing) and confirmed (e.g., Gerstmann's syndrome) the dogma of days past and have revealed new insights into brain function, organization, and the impact of disease. The study of autism is a case in point.

Autism is a developmental disorder affecting primarily social and emotional skills and, in many children, intellectual abilities as well (see Dawson, 1989, for a discussion of some of the problems in defining this disorder). Early theories invoked a cold social environment as the cause of autism (Bettelheim, 1959). Subsequently, Kanner (1943, 1971) advocated an organic etiology for the disorder. In 1982, Maurer and Damasio published their clinical insights into autism from a behavioral neurologist's standpoint. As the basis for their arguments, they used an analogy approach. If the clinical manifestations of autism were similar to known neurologic illnesses, then the underlying anatomic substrate affected in the known diseases may be the area(s) affected in autism. Maurer and Damasio observed that autistic patients tended to be bradykinetic with flexed posture, masked facies, impaired righting reflex, sometimes mild rigidity, and limb dystonia. These findings are also seen in patients with Parkinson's disease, a neurodegenerative disease of the substantia nigra and putamen (components of the basal ganglia; Adams & Victor, 1989). Autistic patients demonstrated impaired facial movement with emotion but not to volition (voluntary-mimetic dissociation), which can occur following injury to mesial frontal lobe, temporal lobe, neostriatum (caudate and putamen), insula, or thalamus (Hopf, Müller-Forell, & Hopf, 1992). Mutism, echolalia, stereotypic language, and dysprosody were present in autistic patients as well. These deficits often result from mesial frontal lobe damage or damage to structures with which the mesial frontal lobes are connected (Alexander, Benson, & Stuss, 1989). Deficits in planning, orienting to environmental stimuli, and compulsive behaviors, as well as lack of empathy frequently result from injury to the frontal lobe or its connections (Hymas, Lees, Bolton, Epps, & Head, 1991; Shallice, 1988). The authors concluded that autism may result from dysfunction in structures in mesial frontal and temporal lobes as well as the striatum—structures that are phylogenetically related.

PET and SPECT studies in autistic patients have shown cerebral cortical dysfunction (Daura et al., 1984; Minshew, 1991). MRI studies, on the other hand, have demonstrated posterior cerebellar vermal hypoplasia and hyperplasia (Courchesne, Townsend, & Saitoh, 1994). Autopsy cases have not demonstrated consistent cortical findings (Coleman, Romano, Lapham, & Simon, 1985; Williams, Hauser, Purpura, DeLong, & Swisher, 1980). Instead, abnormally small, densely packed neurons have been found in the amygdala, hippocampus, mammillary bodies, medial septal nucleus, and diagonal band of Broca (Bauman & Kemper, 1985). In the cerebellum loss of Purkinje cells and a decreased number of granule cells in neocerebellum and archicerebellum have been reported (see Bauman, 1991). Retrograde neuronal loss was not demonstrated in the inferior olive with which the cerebellum connects. Because the inferior olive projects to the cerebellum after 30 weeks of gestation, the cerebellar abnormalities reported in autistic patients must arise prior to this time (Bauman & Kemper, 1989). The cerebellum is thought to play a role in behavior (Schmahmann, 1991). Cerebellar damage may result in executive dysfunction (as shown by neuropsychological assessments of patients with cerebellar lesions) that is similar to behavioral disturbances resulting from frontal lobe injury (Appollonio, Grafman, Schwartz, Massaquoi, & Hallett, 1993) and consistent with behavior described in autism.

The original insights form behavioral neurologic observations that autism results from mesial frontal, mesial temporal, and neostriatal dysfunction were in part supported by PET, SPECT, and histopathologic data and in part disproved by histopathologic data. However, the executive function deficits described in autistic patients and initially posited to follow from mesial frontal dysfunction may occur from abnormalities in other structures with which it is connected, such as the cerebellum. This finding represents further evidence in support of the existence and importance of functional neural networks. Furthermore, any theory that attempts to explain the function of a neural structure must explain all of the relevant data. Indeed, the presence of cerebellar abnormalities may explain the presence of at least some "frontal" deficits. Through a marriage of behavioral neurology, neuropsychology, neuroanatomy, and neuroimaging, greater insights into autism and into the function of specific neural structures were obtained than those that resulted through the efforts of any one of these disciplines in isolation.

Neuropharmacology has added to our knowledge of neural function and organization. Studies on the effects of various drugs and of neurotransmitter pathways in different psychiatric patient populations has rekindled interest in the biologic basis of psychiatric illnesses (Elliott, 1986). In neurology, similar studies have advanced our knowledge of different diseases and their treatment. An example can be found in the case of Parkinson's disease.

The predominant site of neural injury in Parkinson's disease is the dopamine-producing cell complex of the substantia nigra, pars compacta. Fewer dopamine-producing cells are lost in the ventral tegmental area of the midbrain. This abnormality results in depletion of dopamine in the putamen/caudate nucleus (nigrostriatal pathway) and in limbic areas (cingulate, entorhinal cortex, hippocampus, nucleus accumbens, parolfactory gyrus) and neocortex (frontal, temporal, occipital; mesolimbic pathway; Agid, Javoy-Agid, & Ruberg, 1987). The role of dopamine in behavior has been studied, in part, by assessing the effects of levodopa on behavior in patients with Parkinson's disease. Gotham, Brown, and Marsden (1988) evaluated "frontal" function in patients with Parkinson's disease both on and off levodopa. Patients showed worsened performance on an alternating word fluency test when off levodopa, worsened performance on a visual–visual conditional associative learning test and a self-ordered pointing test when on levodopa, and equally poor performance on the Wisconsin Card Sorting Test when on or off levodopa. Attention, arousal, and mood were not affected by the presence or absence of levodopa and hence these were not the mechanisms responsible for test performance. Instead, the systems important for some tasks may have had more dopamine depletion (test performance would improve with levodopa secondary to adequate levels of dopamine) than systems important for other tasks (test performance would deteriorate with levodopa secondary to elevated levels of dopamine). Alternatively, some systems may be intrinsically more sensitive to dopamine.

Regardless, the data suggest that neurotransmitters may have optimal levels at which a particular brain function is best performed and that increases or decreases of the neurotransmitter from its optimal level may produce adverse effects on that brain function. Second, the optimal level of a neurotransmitter may differ between neural systems or between brain functions. These findings support the existence of functional neural systems based, in part, on commonality of the neurotransmitter used rather than structural similarities and connectivity. Therefore, in this example, the integration of behavioral neurology, neuropsychology, and neuropharmacology led to greater insights into the behavioral effects of a drug (levodopa), the effects of depletion and replacement of a neurotransmitter (dopamine) on behavior, and insights into similarities and differences of the processes assessed by different neuropsychological measures. For example, if performance on three tasks is enhanced on two of the tasks and worsened on one of the tasks after administering levodopa, then the two tasks in which performance was enhanced may share the same processing system or components of that system.

Computer modeling has offered a new avenue for testing hypotheses of brain function and for exploring neuropsychological models of neural processing. In recent years, *parallel distributed processing* (PDP) models have been used to try to simulate neural processing. A PDP model is based on a large array of processing units, each performing a simple function, and each interconnected with many of the other units. The units act as a single system whose processing power lies within the strength of the connections between the units rather than the additive effect of each unit operating in isolation. Processing occurs in parallel rather than in a serial fashion. Information is not stored within individual units; instead, it is the pattern of activation across the array that is the representation. Learning is the achievement of the appropriate connection strengths so that the correct pattern of activation is generated under the appropriate conditions (McClelland & Rumelhart, 1986).

Many of the criticisms of PDP point out the current limitations of these models. However, PDP models can be used to develop "explanatory" theories in which a set of general principles (ones that underlie multiple neural systems) independently motivated but constrained by neurobiologically relevant data is formulated, rather than "descriptive" theories in which an explanation limited to empirical data is derived (Seidenberg, 1993). PDP models can provide alternative explanations of specific neural functions and of the broad principles common to multiple functions (e.g., Farah & McClelland, 1991; Patterson,

Seidenberg, & McClelland, 1989). Such theories may or may not prove to be correct, but they represent testable hypotheses constrained by, but not limited to, the empirical data drawn from normal and brain-impaired subjects. PDP models can also be "lesioned" to try to simulate or predict neural behavior, a luxury that is not possible with human subjects.

For example, Rumelhart and McClelland (1986) presented their network with 10 cycles of 10 high-frequency verbs (8 irregular, 2 regular), followed by 190 cycles of 410 medium-frequency verbs. The network was then assessed on 86 low frequency verbs it had not encountered before. The network showed a U-shaped learning curve in generating past-tense irregular verbs in which it first produced learned irregular verbs correctly, then made regularization errors (e.g., *know* became *knowed* rather than *knew*), and finally produced the past tense of the irregular verbs correctly. The performance of the network mimicked the performance of young children who learn the past tense of verbs in a similar manner. Therefore, the network performed in a way that was neither predicted nor for which it had been programmed, but one that partially replicated normal brain function (see Pinker & Prince, 1988, for a critical analysis).

FUTURE DIRECTIONS

The German philosopher Georg Hegel (1956) proposed that history is a continuous interplay of thesis, antithesis, then synthesis. Put simply, the pendulum must swing both ways before changing course. Recently, this same evolution has begun in neuropsychology. Whereas traditionally behavioral neurologists have focused on the qualitative aspects of behavior (e.g., the types of errors made) and neuropsychologists have focused on the assessment of the quantitative aspects of behavior (e.g., the number of errors made), a melding of these two disciplines has been undertaken in the past decade. Several neuropsychologists, spearheaded by Edith Kaplan, have developed the *process approach* to neuropsychological assessment (Kaplan, 1983, 1990; Milberg, Hebben, & Kaplan, 1986). Arguing, as did Werner (1956), that different subjects may achieve the same score on a standardized test but arrive at their answers using different strategies, these neuropsychologists have proposed that recording the strategy used and the kinds of errors made would enhance lesion localization, diagnostic accuracy, monitoring the course of functional recovery or decline, and recommendations for treatment. In contrast to the approach of behavioral neurologists, the qualitative aspects of behavior would be quantified.

For example, the Block Design subtest of the WAIS–R is a timed test that assesses visuospatial processing. Scoring is pass–fail. Full credit is given only if the design correctly matches the template and is executed within the alotted time frame. Therefore, a subject who constructs the design correctly but is too slow in his execution (e.g., Parkinson's disease) will be given a score of zero. Kaplan and colleagues have found that patients with single lesions will tend to start the design in the hemiattentional field ipsilateral to the lesion and will make a greater number of errors in the hemiattentional field contralateral to the lesion. Moreover, patients with focal right hemispheric lesions demonstrate a greater tendency to break the square configuration in their designs than do patients with focal left hemispheric lesions. Therefore, Kaplan and colleagues have suggested that the Block Design subtest be administered without time constraints and that the number of instances of broken configuration, right-side starting positions (normal right-handed subjects start on the left side), and total number of errors be recorded. They further recommended that scoring can be expanded such that one point is given for each correctly positioned block. In a 2 × 2 design, scoring would range from 0 to 4, whereas in a 3 × 3 design, scoring would range from 0 to 9. These broader scoring criteria may enhance the diagnostic utility of the Block Design subtest.

In this chapter, I have not sought to dwell on the various differences between behavioral neurology, neuropsychology, and other disciplines (e.g., neurophysiology, neurochemistry); they are in continual flux. Instead, through examples, I have tried to illustrate the advantages and disadvantages of each discipline in isolation and of the greater benefits achieved through their combined interactions. In the future the progressive synthesis of the behavioral neurological and neuropsychological approaches to the analysis of brain–behavior relationships in conjunction with the ever-growing sophistication of modern radiologic imaging should lead to greater insights into neural processing and the sequelae of neural injury. Through continued collaborative efforts between these disciplines, we will pursue the conquest of neural space more successfully. As these fields continue to grow and expand, the only limitations to their potential successes appear to be those of the human mind itself.

REFERENCES

Adams, R. D., & Victor, M. (1989). *Principles of neurology.* New York: McGraw-Hill.

Agid, Y., Javoy Agid, F., & Ruberg, M. (1987). Biochemistry of neurotransmitters in Parkinson's disease. In C. D. Marsden & S. Fahn (Eds.), *Movement disorders 2* (pp. 166–230). London: Butterworths.

Albert, M. L., Bachman, D. L., Morgan, A., & Helm-Estabrooks, N. (1988). Pharmacotherapy for aphasia. *Neurology, 38,* 877–879.

Albert, M. L., Goodglass, H., Helm, N. A., Rubens, A. B., & Alexander, M. P. (1981). *Clinical aspects of dysphasia.* New York: Springer-Verlag.

Alexander, G. E., DeLong, M. R., & Strick, P. L. (1986). Parallel organization of functionally segregated circuits linking basal ganglia and cortex. *Annual Review of Neuroscience, 9,* 357–381.

Alexander, M. P., Benson, D. F., & Stuss, D. T. (1989). Frontal lobes and language. *Brain and Language, 37,* 656–691.

Alexander, M. P., Naeser, M. A., & Palumbo, C. (1990). Aphasia after lesions including the frontal operculum. *Neurology, 40,* 353–362.

Anderson, S. W., Damasio, H., & Tranel, D. (1990). Neuropsychological impairments associated with lesions caused by tumor or stroke. *Archives of Neurology, 47,* 397–405.

Appollonio, I. M., Grafman, J., Schwartz, V., Massaquoi, S., & Hallett, M. (1993). Memory in patients with cerebellar degeneration. *Neurology, 43,* 1536–1544.

Åström, M., Adolfsson, R., & Asplund, K. (1993). Major depression in stroke patients: A 3-year longitudinal study. *Stroke, 24,* 976–982.

Baddeley, A. (1990). *Human memory: Theory and practice.* Boston: Allyn & Bacon.

Balint, R. (1909). Seelenlähmung des "schauens," optische ataxie, räumliche störung der aufmerksamkeit. *Monatsschrift für Psychiatrie und Neurologie, 25,* 5–81.

Bauman, M. L. (1991). Microscopic neuroanatomic abnormalities in autism. *Pediatrics, 87,* 791–796.

Bauman, M. L., & Kemper, T. L. (1985). Histoanatomic observations of the brain in early infantile autism. *Neurology, 35,* 866–874.

Bauman, M. L., & Kemper, T. L. (1989). Abnormal cerebellar circuitry in autism? *Neurology, 39* (Suppl.), 186.

Baxter, L. R., Schwartz, J. M., Phelps, M. E., Mazziotta, J. C., Guze, B. M., Selin, C. E., Gerner, R. H., & Sumida, R. M. (1989). Reduction of prefrontal cortex glucose metabolism common to three types of depression. *Archives of General Psychiatry, 46,* 243–250.

Becker, H., Desch, H., Hacker, H., & Pencz, A. (1979). CT fogging effect with ischemic cerebral infarcts. *Neuroradiology, 18,* 185–192.

Benson, D. F. (1993). Aphasia. In K. M. Heilman & E. Valenstein (Eds.), *Clinical neuropsychology* (3rd ed., pp. 17–36). New York: Oxford University Press.

Benson, D. F., & Cummings, J. L. (1982). Angular gyrus syndrome simulating Alzheimer's disease. *Archives of Neurology, 39,* 616–620.

Benton, A. L. (1959). *Right–left discrimination and finger localization: Development and pathology.* New York: Hoeber-Harper.

Benton, A. L. (1961). The fiction of the Gerstmann syndrome. *Journal of Neurology, Neurosurgery, and Psychiatry, 24,* 176–181.

Benton, A. L. (1992). Gerstmann's syndrome. *Archives of Neurology, 49,* 445–447.

Benton, A. L., & Hamsher, K. deS. (1976). *Multilingual aphasia examination* (Manual, Rev. 1978). Iowa City: University of Iowa.
Benton, A. L., Hamsher, K. deS., Varney, N. R., & Spreen, O. (1983). *Contributions to neuropsychological assessment*. New York: Oxford University Press.
Benton, A. L., Hannay, H. J., & Varney, N. R. (1975). Visual perception of line direction in patients with unilateral brain disease. *Neurology, 25,* 907–910.
Benton, A. L., & Sivan, A. B. (1993). Disturbances of the body schema. In K. M. Heilman & E. Valenstein (Eds.), *Clinical neuropsychology* (pp. 123–140). New York: Oxford University Press.
Berg, E. A. (1948). A simple objective test for measuring flexibility in thinking. *Journal of General Psychology, 39,* 15–22.
Bergson, H. (1896). *Matière et mémoire*. Paris: Alcan.
Bettelheim, B. (1959). Joey: A "mechanical boy." *Scientific American, 200,* 116–127.
Bianchi, L. (1895). The functions of the frontal lobes. *Brain, 18,* 497–522.
Bisiach, E., Geminiani, G., Berti, A., & Rusconi, M. L. (1990). Perceptual and premotor factors of unilateral neglect. *Neurology, 40,* 1278–1281.
Bogousslavsky, J., Miklossy, L., Deruaz, J. P., Regli, F., & Assai, G. (1986). Unilateral left paramedian infarction of thalamus and midbrain: A clinico–pathological study. *Journal of Neurology, Neurosurgery, and Psychiatry, 49,* 686–694.
Boll, T. J. (1980). The Halstead–Reitan neuropsychological battery. In S. B. Filskov & T. J. Bell (Eds.), *Handbook of clinical neuropsychology* (pp. 577–607). New York: Wiley-Interscience.
Bouillaud, J. B. (1825). Recherches cliniques propres à démontrer que la perte de la parole correspond à la lésion des lobules anterieurs du cerveau. *Archives Générales de Medicine, 8,* 24–45.
Brickner, R. M. (1936). *The intellectual functions of the frontal lobes: Study based upon observation of a man after partial bilateral frontal lobectomy.* New York: Macmillan.
Brodmann, K. (1909). *Vergleichende lokalisationslehreder grosshirnrinde*. Leipzig: Barth.
Burkhardt, C. R., Filley, C. M., Kleinschmidt-DeMasters, B. K., de la Monte, S., Norenberg, M. D., & Schneck, S. A. (1988). Diffuse Lewy body disease and progressive dementia. *Neurology, 38,* 1520–1528.
Bushnell, D. L., Gupta, S., Mlcoch, A. G., & Barnes, W. E. (1989). Prediction of language and neurologic recovery after cerebral infarction with SPECT imaging using N-isopropyl-*p*-(I 123) iodoamphetamine. *Archives of Neurology, 46,* 665–669.
Clarke, T. E. (1896). The comparative anatomy of the insula. *Journal of Comparative Neurology, 6,* 59–100.
Cole, M. F., & Cole, M. (Eds.) (1971). *Pierre Marie's papers on speech disorders*. New York: Hafner.
Coleman, P. D., Romano, J., Lapham, L., & Simon, W. (1985). Cell counts in cerebral cortex in an autistic patient. *Journal of Autism and Developmental Disorders, 15,* 245–255.
Coslett, H. B., Bowers, D., Fitzpatrick, E., Haws, B., & Heilman, K. M. (1990). Directional hypokinesia and hemispatial inattention in neglect. *Brain, 113,* 475–486.
Courchesne, E., Townsend, J., & Saitoh, O. (1994). The brain in infantile autism: Posterior fossa structures are abnormal. *Neurology, 44,* 214–223.
Critchley, M. (1953). *The parietal lobes*. London: Edward Arnold.
Critchley, M. (1966). The enigma of Gerstmann's syndrome. *Brain, 89,* 183–198.
Critchley, M. (1979). *The divine banquet of the brain*. New York: Raven.
Crystal, H. A., Dickson, D. W., Lizardi, J. E., Davies, P., & Wolfson, L. I. (1990). Antemortem diagnosis of diffuse Lewy body disease. *Neurology, 40,* 1523–1528.
Cullum, C. M., Thompson, L. L., & Smernoff, E. N. (1993). Three-word recall as a measure of memory. *Journal of Clinical and Experimental Neuropsychology, 15,* 321–329.
Cummings, J. L. (1985). *Clinical neuropsychiatry.* New York: Harcourt Brace Jovanovich.
Cummings, J. L., & Benson, D. F. (1992). *Dementia: A clinical approach*. Boston: Butterworth-Heinemann.
Damasio, H., & Damasio, A. R. (1989). *Lesion analysis in neuropsychology.* New York: Oxford University Press.
Damasio, H., & Frank, R. (1992). Three-dimensional in vivo mapping of brain lesions in humans. *Archives of Neurology, 49,* 137–143.
Damasio, H., Kuljis, R. O., Yuh, W., Van Hoesen, G. W., & Ehrhardt, J. (1991). Magnetic resonance imaging of human intracortical structure in vivo. *Cerebral Cortex, 1,* 374–379.
Daura, R., Rumsey, J., Grady, C., Kessler, R., Rapoport, S. I., Rapoport, J. L., & Cutler, N. (1984). Cerebral glucose metabolism in adult autism. *Neurology, 34* (Suppl.), 117.
Dawson, G. (1989). *Autism: Nature, diagnosis, and treatment*. New York: Guilford.
Delis, D. C., Kramer, J. H., Kaplan, E., & Ober, B. A. (1987). *California verbal learning test*. San Antonio, TX: The Psychological Corporation.
Démonet, J. F., Wise, R., & Frackowiak, R. S. J. (1993). Language functions explored in normal subjects by positron emission tomography: A critical review. *Human Brain Mapping, 1,* 39–47.

Deuel, R. K., & Farrar, C. A. (1993). Stimulus cancellation by macaques with unilateral frontal or parietal lesions. *Neuropsychologia, 31,* 29–38.

Elliott, F. (1986). Historical perspective on neurobehavior. In R. M. Restak (Ed.), *The psychiatric clinics of North America: Neuropsychiatry* (pp. 225–239). Philadelphia: W. B. Saunders Company.

Farah, M. J., & McClelland, J. L. (1991). A computational model of semantic memory impairment: Modality-specificity and emergent category-specificity. *Journal of Experimental Psychology, 120,* 339–357.

Folstein, M. F., Folstein, S. E., & McHugh, P. R. (1975). "Mini-mental state": A practical method for grading the mental state of patients for the clinician. *Journal of Psychiatric Research, 12,* 189–198.

Freedman, M., Kaplan, E., & Delis, D. C. (1994). *Clock-drawing: A neuropsychological analysis.* New York: Oxford University Press.

Freud, S. (1953). *On aphasia.* New York: International Universities Press.

Friedman, H. R., & Goldman-Rakic, P. S. (1988). Activation of the hippocampus and dentate gyrus by working memory: A 2-deoxyglucose study of behaving rhesus monkeys. *Journal of Neuroscience, 8,* 4693–4706.

Friedman, H. R., Janas, J., & Goldman-Rakic, P. S. (1990). Enhancement of metabolic activity in the diencephalon of monkeys performing working memory tasks: A 2-deoxyglucose study in behaving rhesus monkeys. *Journal of Cognitive Neuroscience, 2,* 18–31.

Fuster, J. M., & Alexander, G. E. (1971). Neuron activity related to short-term memory. *Science, 173,* 652–654.

Gerstmann, J. (1940). Syndrome of finger agnosia, disorientation for right and left, agraphia and acalculia. *Archives of Neurology and Psychiatry, 44,* 398–408.

Geschwind, N. (1965). Disconnexion syndromes in animals and man. *Brain, 88,* 237–294, 585–644.

Gold, M., Shuren, J., & Heilman, K. M. (in press). Proximal intentional neglect: A case study. *Journal of Neurology, Neurosurgery, and Psychiatry, 57,* 1395–1400.

Goldman-Rakic, P. S. (1987). Circuitry of primate prefrontal cortex and regulation of behavior by representational memory. In F. Plum (Ed.), *Handbook of physiology: The nervous system: Vol. 5. Higher functions of the brain* (pp. 373–417). Bethesda, MD: American Physiological Society.

Goldman-Rakic, P. S., & Porrino, L. J. (1985). The primate mediodorsal (MD) nucleus and its projection to the frontal lobe. *Journal of Comparative Neurology, 242,* 535–560.

Goldman-Rakic, P. S., Selemon, L. D., & Schwartz, M. S. (1985). Dual pathways connecting the dorsolateral prefrontal cortex with the hippocampal formation and parahippocampal cortex in the rhesus monkey. *Neuroscience, 12,* 719–743.

Goodglass, H. (1968). Studies in the grammar of aphasics. In S. Rosenberg & J. H. Koplin (Eds.), *Developments in applied psycholinguistics research* (pp. 177–208). New York: Macmillan.

Goodglass, H., & Kaplan, E. (1972). *The assessment of aphasia and related disorders.* Philadelphia: Lea & Febiger.

Gotham, A. M., Brown, R. G., & Marsden, C. D. (1988). "Frontal" cognitive function in patients with Parkinson's disease "on" and "off" levodopa. *Brain, 111,* 299–321.

Grant, D. A., & Berg, E. A. (1948). A behavioral analysis of degree of reinforcement and ease of shifting to new responses in a Weigl-type card-sorting problem. *Journal of Experimental Psychology, 38,* 404–411.

Grossi, D., Modafferi, A., Pelosi, L., & Trojano, L. (1989). On the different roles of the cerebral hemispheres in mental imagery: The "o'clock test" in two clinical cases. *Brain and Cognition, 10,* 18–27.

Halstead, W. C. (1947). *Brain and intelligence: A quantitative study of the frontal lobes.* Chicago: University of Chicago Press.

Harlow, J. M. (1848). Passage of an iron bar through the head. *Boston Medical and Surgical Journal, 39,* 389–393.

Harlow, J. M. (1868). Recovery from the passage of an iron bar through the head. *Publications of the Massachusetts Medical Society, 2,* 327–347.

Harris, L. J., & Gitterman, S. R. (1978). University professors' self-descriptions of left–right confusability: Sex and handedness differences. *Perceptual Motor Skills, 47,* 819–823.

Head, H. (1926). *Aphasia and kindred disorders of speech.* Cambridge, England: Cambridge University Press.

Hegel, G. W. F. (1956). *Philosophy of history* (J. Sibree, Trans.). New York: Dover Publications.

Heilman, K. M., & Valenstein, E. (1972). Frontal lobe neglect in man. *Neurology, 22,* 660–664.

Heilman, K. M., Watson, R. T., & Valenstein, E. (1993). Neglect and related disorders. In K. M. Heilman & E. Valenstein (Eds.), *Clinical neuropsychology* (pp. 279–336). New York: Oxford University Press.

Heimburger, R. F., DeMeyer, W., & Reitan, R. M. (1964). Implications of the Gerstmann syndrome. *Journal of Neurology, Neurosurgery, and Psychiatry, 27,* 52–57.

Hopf, H. C., Müller-Forell, W., & Hopf, N. J. (1992). Localization of emotional and volitional facial paresis. *Neurology, 42,* 1918–1923.

Hymas, N., Lees, A., Bolton, D., Epps, K., & Head, D. (1991). The neurology of obsessional slowness. *Brain, 114,* 2203–2233.

Isseroff, A., Rosvold, H. E., Galkin, T. W., & Goldman-Rakic, P. S. (1982). Spatial memory impairments following damage to the mediodorsal nucleus of the thalamus in rhesus monkeys. *Brain Research, 232,* 107–113.

Jackson, J. H. (1958). On affectations of speech from disease of the brain. In J. Taylor (Ed.), *Selected writings of John Hughlings Jackson* (pp. 155–183). New York: Basic Books.

Kaplan, E. (1983). Process and achievement revisited. In S. Wapner & B. Kaplan (Eds.), *Toward a holistic developmental psychology* (pp. 143–156). Hillsdale, NJ: Lawrence Erlbaum Associates.

Kaplan, E. (1990). The process approach to neuropsychological assessment of psychiatric patients. *Journal of Neuropsychiatry, 2,* 72–87.

Kanner, L. (1943). Autistic disturbances of affective contact. *Nervous Child, 2,* 217–250.

Kanner, L. (1971). Follow-up study of eleven autistic children originally reported in 1943. *Journal of Autism and Childhood Schizophrenia, 1,* 119–145.

Kinkel, W. (1992). Computerized tomography in clinical neurology. In R. J. Joynt (Ed.), *Clinical neurology* (Vol. 1, pp. 1–115). Philadelphia: J. B. Lippincott.

Kinsbourne, M. (1971). Cognitive deficit: Experimental analysis. In J. L. McGaugh (Ed.), *Psychobiology: Behavior from a biological perspective* (pp. 285–348). New York: Academic Press.

Kinsbourne, M., & Warrington, E. K. (1962). A study of finger agnosia. *Brain, 85,* 47–66.

Kleist, K. (1934). *Gehirnpathologie.* Leipzig: Barth.

Lang, A. E., Riley, D. E., & Bergeron, C. (1994). Cortical-basal ganglionic degeneration. In D. B. Calne (Ed.), *Neurodegenerative diseases* (pp. 877–894). Philadelphia: W. B. Saunders.

Lashley, K. S. (1929). *Brain mechanisms and intelligence.* Chicago: University of Chicago Press.

Lashley, K. S. (1950). In search of the engram. *Symposia of the Society for Experimental Biology, 4,* 454–482.

Lichtheim, L. (1885). On aphasia. *Brain, 7,* 433–484.

Lissauer, H. (1890). Ein fall von seelenblindheit nebst conem beitrage zur theorie derselben. *Archiv für Psychiatrie, 21,* 222–270.

Luria, A. R. (1966). *Human brain and psychological processes.* New York: Harper & Row.

Marshall, J. F. (1979). Somatosensory inattention after dopamin-depleting intracerebral 6-OHDA injections: Spontaneous recovery and pharmacological control. *Brain Research, 177,* 311–324.

Maurer, R. G., & Damasio, A. R. (1982). Childhood autism from the point of view of behavioral neurology. *Journal of Autism and Developmental Disorders, 12,* 195–205.

Mazziotta, J. C., Huang, S.-C., Phelps, M. E., Carson, R. E., MacDonald, N. S., & Mahoney, K. (1985). A noninvasive positron computed tomography technique using oxygen-15-labeled water for the evaluation of neurobehavioral task batteries. *Journal of Cerebral Blood Flow and Metabolism, 5,* 70–78.

McClelland, J. L., & Rumelhart, D. E. (1986). *Parallel distributed processing, Vol. 1.* Cambridge, MA: MIT Press.

Mendez, M. F., Selwood, A., Mastri, A. R., & Frey, W. H. II (1993). Pick's disease versus Alzheimer's disease: A comparison of clinical characteristics. *Neurology, 43,* 289–292.

Milberg, W. P., Hebben, N., & Kaplan, E. (1986). The Boston process approach. In I. Grant & K. M. Adams (Eds.), *Neuropsychological assessment of neuropsychiatric disorders* (pp. 65–86). New York: Oxford University Press.

Milner, B. (1966). Amnesia following operations on the temporal lobes. In C. W. M. Whitty & O. L. Zangwill (Eds.), *Amnesia.* London: Butterworth.

Minshew, N. J. (1991). Indices of neural function in autism: Clinical and biological implications. *Pediatrics, 87,* 774–780.

Morris, H. H., Lüders, H., Lesser, R. P., Dinner, D. S., & Hahn, J. (1984). Transient neuropsychological abnormalities (including Gerstmann's syndrome) during cortical stimulation. *Neurology, 34,* 877–883.

Naeser, M. A., Palumbo, C. L., Helm-Estabrooks, N., Stiassny-Eder, D., & Albert, M. L. (1989). Severe nonfluency in aphasia: Role of the medial subcallosal fasciculus and other white matter pathways in recovery of spontaneous speech. *Brain, 112,* 1–38.

Nelson, H. E., & O'Connell, A. (1978). Dementia: The estimation of premorbid intelligence levels using the New Adult Reading Test. *Cortex, 14,* 234–244.

Osterrieth, P. A. (1944). Le test de copie d'une figure complexe. *Archives de Psychologie, 30,* 206–356.

Patterson, K., Seidenberg, M., & McClelland, J. (1989). Dyslexia in a distributed, developmental model of word recognition. In R. Morris (Ed.), *Parallel distributed processing* (pp. 131–181). New York: Oxford University Press.

Penfield, W., & Rasmussen, T. (1950). *The cerebral cortex of man: A clinical study of localization of function.* New York: Macmillan.

Penfield, W., & Roberts, L. (1959). *Speech and brain mechanisms.* Princeton, NJ: Princeton University Press.

Pinker, S., & Prince, A. (1988). On language and connectionism: Analysis of a parallel distributed processing model of language acquisition. *Cognition, 28,* 73–193.

Poeck, K., & Orgass, B. (1966). Gerstmann's syndrome and aphasia. *Cortex, 2,* 421–437.

Posner, M. I., & Petersen, S. E. (1990). The attention system of the human brain. *Annual Review of Neuroscience, 13,* 25–42.

Rebeiz, J. J., Kolodny, E. H., & Richardson, E. P. (1968). Corticodentatonigral degeneration with neuronal achromasia. *Archives of Neurology, 18,* 20–33.

Rey, A. (1941). L'examen psychologique dans les cas d'encéphalopathie traumatique. *Archives de Psychologie, 28*(112), 286–340.

Rezai, K., Kirchner, P. T., Armstrong, C., Ehrhardt, J. C., & Heistad, D. (1988). Validation studies for brain blood flow assessment by radioxenon tomography. *The Journal of Nuclear Medicine, 29,* 348–355.

Robinson, R. G., Bosotn, J. D., Starkstein, S. E., & Price, T. R. (1988). Comparison of mania with depression following brain injury: Causal factors. *American Journal of Psychiatry, 145,* 172–178.

Robinson, R. G., & Szetela, B. (1981). Mood change following left hemispheric brain injury. *Annals of Neurology, 9,* 447–453.

Roeltgen, D. P., Sevush, S., & Heilman, K. M. (1983). Pure Gerstmann's syndrome from a focal lesion. *Archives of Neurology, 40,* 46–47.

Roland, P. E., & Friberg, L. (1985). Localization of cortical areas activated by thinking. *Journal of Neurophysiology, 53,* 1219–1243.

Rouleau, I., Salmon, D. P., Butters, N., Kennedy, C., & McGuire, K. (1992). Quantitative and qualitative analyses of clock drawings in Alzheimer's and Huntington's disease. *Brain and Cognition, 18,* 70–87.

Rumelhart, D. E., & McClelland, J. L. (1986). On learning the past tense of English verbs. In J. L. McClelland & D. E. Rumelhart (Eds.), *Parallel distributed processing* (Vol. 2, pp. 216–271). Cambridge, MA: MIT Press.

Rylander, G. (1939). Personality changes after operations of the frontal lobes. *Acta Psychiatrica et Neurologica Scandanavia, 20* (Suppl.), 13–327.

Santos, C. C., Cope, M. L., & Keller, K. (1991). Gerstmann syndrome secondary to posterior left thalamic lesion. *Annals of Neurology, 30,* 474.

Schmahmann, J. D. (1991). An emerging concept: The cerebellar contribution to higher function. *Archives of Neurology, 48,* 1178–1187.

Seidenberg, M. S. (1993). Connectionist models and cognitive theory. *Psychological Science, 4,* 228–235.

Sergent, J., Zuck, E., Lèvesque, M., & MacDonald, B. (1992). Positron emission tomography study of letter and object processing: Empirical findings and methodological considerations. *Cerebral Cortex, 2,* 68–80.

Shallice, T. (1988). *From neuropsychology to mental structure.* Cambridge, England: Cambridge University Press.

Sherrington, C. S. (1977). *The integrative action of the nervous system.* New Haven, CT: Yale University Press.

Sperry, R. (1968). Mental unity following surgical disconnection of the cerebral hemispheres. *The Harvey Lecture Series, 62,* 293–323.

Starkstein, S. E., & Robinson, R. G. (1989). Affective disorders and cerebral vascular disease. *British Journal of Psychiatry, 154,* 170–182.

Starkstein, S. E., Robinson, R. G., & Price, T. R. (1987). Comparison of cortical and subcortical lesions in the production of post-stroke mood disorders. *Brain, 110,* 1045–1059.

Stern, Y., Sano, M., Paulson, J., & Mayeux, R. (1987). Modified Mini-Mental State Examination: Validity and reliability. *Neurology, 37* (Suppl.), 179.

Teuber, H. L. (1955). Physiological psychology. *Annual Review of Psychology, 9,* 267–296.

Tranel, D. (1992). Neuropsychological assessment. In J. Biller & R. G. Kathol (Eds.), *The psychiatric clinics of North America: The interface of psychiatry and neurology* (pp. 283–299). Philadelphia: W. B. Saunders.

Valenstein, E., Van den Abell, T., Watson, R. T., & Heilman, K. M. (1982). Nonsensory neglect from parietotemporal lesions in monkeys. *Neurology, 32,* 1198–1201.

Varney, N. R., Damasio, H., & Adler, S. (1989). The role of individual difference in determining the nature of comprehension defects in aphasia. *Cortex, 25,* 47–55.

Verrey, D. (1988). Hémiachromatopsie droite absolute. *Archives d'Ophthalmologie, 8,* 289–301.

von Bonin, G. (1960). *Some papers on the cerebral cortex.* Springfield, IL: Charles C. Thomas.

Walker, A. E. (1938). *The primate thalamus.* Chicago: University of Chicago Press.

Warrington, E. K., & James, M. (1967). Disorders of visual perception in patients with localized cerebral lesions. *Neuropsychologia, 5,* 253–266.

Watanabe, T., & Niki, H. (1985). Hippocampal unit activity and delayed response in the monkey. *Brain Research, 325,* 241–254.

Watson, R. T., Miller, B. D., & Heilman, K. M. (1978). Nonsensory neglect. *Annals of Neurology, 3,* 505–508.

Wechsler, D. (1945). Astandardized memory scale for clinical use. *Journal of Psychology, 19,* 87–95.

Wechsler, D. (1981). *WAIS–R manual.* New York: Psychological Corporation.

Wechsler, D. (1987). *Wechsler memory scale–revised.* New York: Psychological Corporation.

Werner, H. (1956). Microgenesis and aphasia. *Journal of Abnormal and Social Psychology, 52,* 347–353.

Wernicke, C. (1874). *Der aphasische symptomenkomplex.* Breslau: Cohn & Weigert. (Translated in Eggert, G. H., [1977]. *Wernicke's works on aphasia: A sourcebook and review.* New York: Mouton.)

Wilbrand, H. (1892). Ein fall von seelenblindheit und hemianopsie mit sectionsbefund. *Deutsches Zeitschrift für Nervenheilkunde, 2,* 361–387.

Williams, R. S., Hauser, S. L., Purpura, D. M., DeLong, G. R., & Swisher, C. N. (1980). Autism and mental retardation. Neuropathologic studies performed in four retarded persons with autistic behavior. *Archives of Neurology, 37,* 749–752.

Wilson, S. A. K. (1912). Progressive lenticular degeneration: A familial nervous disease associated with cirrhosis of the liver. *Brain, 34,* 295–509.

Wolf, S. M. (1973). Difficulties in right–left discrimination in a normal population. *Archives of Neurology, 29,* 128–129.

Young, R. M. (1990). *Mind, brain and adaptation in the nineteenth century.* New York: Oxford University Press.

Zola-Morgan, S., & Squire, L. R. (1985). Medial temporal lesions in monkeys impair memory on a variety of tasks sensitive to human amnesia. *Behavioral Neuroscience, 99,* 22–34.

3

Component Process Analysis in Experimental and Clinical Neuropsychology

Frances J. Friedrich
Stephen D. Rader
University of Utah

Imagine that you have been asked to evaluate a patient with a reading disorder, a patient similar to the case described by Caramazza and Hillis (1991). According to that report, patient HW is capable of reading certain words when they are used as nouns (e.g., There is a *crack* in the mirror.), but not when they are used as verbs (e.g., Do not *crack* the nuts in here.) How can it be that this patient's reading performance could be so different for the same word when used in different grammatical contexts? Similarly, what of the type of patient described by Saffran and Marin (1977), who might see the word "crocus" but read it as "tulip"? How are we to understand these kinds of deficits?

It certainly is not enough to label these two cases as language disorders and leave it at that—it is clear that language disorders can take a wide variety of forms. In every cognitive domain, including language, visual perception, memory, attention, and abstract reasoning, it is possible to find intriguing examples of dissociations within a specific cognitive function or otherwise curious distortions of the normal process. The message these cases send is clear, and not surprising to researchers and clinicians in the field of neuropsychology: within any given cognitive function, a whole range of things can go wrong; conversely, a specific deficit in memory, attention, or language can manifest itself in a variety of interesting ways. How, then, are we to approach and make sense of this diversity of disorders? To what extent can the experimental literature tell us what kind of impairments may occur and how they reflect underlying brain processes? To what extent can the clinical literature help us develop models of cognitive functioning that can account for both normal and impaired performance?

In recent years, there has been an interesting and useful convergence of approach within the experimental and clinical branches of neuropsychology. In both areas, we can see an increasing use of *component processes analysis* both in developing models of cognitive functions and in developing assessment techniques to identify the nature of various deficits. In this chapter, we attempt to lay out the framework for this type of approach, and then demonstrate how it may apply in three different domains: memory, spatial attention, and visual imagery. These examples show, we hope, how experimental and clinical perspectives can be integrated within a powerful and clarifying framework.

TRENDS IN COGNITIVE PSYCHOLOGY

Although the specific issues of interest in cognitive psychology have changed over the years, the information-processing approach has been a major influence in shaping the questions asked and methodologies employed in many domains. Consequently, the primary focus of the field has been to identify the processes that underlie complex cognitive functions and to characterize the nature of the information used in those processes; that is, the internal representations or codes (Posner, 1978). For example, Sternberg (1966, 1969) had a profound impact on the development of modern cognitive psychology with his work on a stage model of short-term memory scanning processes. The basic assumption was that specific and discrete stages of processing, including encoding, comparison, decision, and motor response processes could be isolated and that the effects of different factors, such as the quality of visual information or the size of the memory set, could be "localized" within a particular stage. The validity of serial stage models has since been debated, with increasing emphasis on parallel, interactive, and cascading processes (e.g., Marslen-Wilson & Welsh, 1978; McClelland, 1979; McClelland & Rumelhart, 1981). Nevertheless, the goal of understanding a complex cognitive function in terms of component processes, and, more specifically, the time course of those processes, remains a central focus of the field and one that has proved to be particularly well suited for relating mental processes to brain structures and processes (e.g., Farah, 1984; Friedrich, 1990b; Kosslyn, 1987; Posner, 1978; Posner, Petersen, Fox, & Raichle, 1988).

The nature of the internal codes used in these processes has also been of prime importance in the development of cognitive models. A single stimulus may give rise to a number of different types of representations, such as visual, phonological, motor, and semantic codes, each of which can be demonstrated to have a functional independence of the others (Posner, 1978). Although the distinctions between different codes and their relation to separable neural systems have been most fully developed with respect to language processing (e.g., Coltheart, 1985; Posner, Petersen, et al., 1988), the same principles apply to models of memory (e.g., Kesner, 1991), visual imagery (e.g., Kosslyn, 1987), and spatial processing (Kolb & Whishaw, 1985).

In recent years, computational models and, more specifically, neural network models, have played an increasingly important role both in how cognitive models are conceptualized and in clarifying the relationship between mind and brain processes. In some cases, although not all, these computational models are compatible with traditional information processing models; they provide a computational architecture and a "microstructure" analysis of cognition that attempts to account for how processes may actually be implemented. Often, a process described at a macrostructure level, such as word recognition, is seen as an emergent property of the microstructure processes (e.g., McClelland, Rumelhart, & Hinton, 1987). Some assumptions of these models, however, such as the parallel and interactive nature of processing, may not be compatible with certain information processing models.

One reason that these models have captured the attention of so many cognitive neuropsychologists is that they seem to provide a "language" that can be used to describe processes at both a cognitive and a neural level. Certainly, scholars have attempted to relate mind and brain processes for many centuries, primarily by identifying a region of the brain responsible for a particular function. However, knowledge of specific neural processes, such as how cells communicate, and cognitive processes, such as word recognition or response selection, seemed to bear little relation to one another. Neural network models have encouraged cognitive psychologists to think in terms of excitatory and inhibitory processes as the basis for cognitive operations, and they have provided a means to evaluate how highly interactive systems (of which we assume the brain is one) operate.

TRENDS IN CLINICAL NEUROPSYCHOLOGY

Historical accounts of the development of neuropsychology often begin with Broca, who in 1861 made a case for localization and lateralization of the language function (Caplan, 1987). Indeed, although there have been periodic disputes between proponents and opponents of localization, descriptions of mind–brain relations in the field of neurology typically have been driven by attempts to identify a specific structure responsible for a particular function. Clinical categorizations of deficits reflected a syndrome-based approach: describing deficits in terms of the constellation of symptoms that result from a specific brain lesion (see Heilman & Valenstein, 1985).

Even from the early days of neuropsychology, however, another approach to describing deficits anticipated the formal emergence of information processing theories by nearly a century. In the 1870s Carl Wernicke, taking what was at the time an antilocalization position, described the language system in terms of a variety of different types of representations and processes, including visual word forms, word sound representations, word meaning, and the pathways linking them (Margolin, 1991). The neurologist John Hughlings Jackson (1874/1915) speculated at length about the nature of abstract mental representations and how they might relate to more basic sensory-motor representations. Jackson argued that concepts may be multiply represented, in increasingly abstract forms, and that the different types of lesions (discrete or diffuse) would have effects at different levels of this hierarchical structure. More recently, Luria (1973) reexamined the notions of functional systems and localization, arguing that a functional system consists of a complex of component processes, which can be reconfigured in a variety of ways in order to complete a cognitive task. Rather than being narrowly localized, mental functions "must be organized in systems of concertedly working zones, each of which performs its role in the complex functional system, and which may be located in completely different and often far distant areas of the brain" (p. 31).

The lasting impact of Wernicke, Jackson, and Luria derives in part from the fact that their goal was to understand not just what part of the brain is responsible for what type of activity, but to understand the *nature* of thought processes, how knowledge is represented, and at what level of the functional system the deficit occurs as a result of the brain injury.

The same type of tension between "where" a function is localized and "how" it unfolds has been recapitulated in recent years as more formalized approaches to neuropsychological assessment have emerged (Lezak, 1983). From one view, batteries have been developed with the goal of predictive accuracy in determining the presence or location of brain damage; typically, cut-off points on scaled indices are used to differentiate between brain-injured and other populations. Alternatively, standardized tests have been modified or extended in order to reveal the nature of deficits and their functional consequences (Kaplan, 1988; Lezak, 1983; Milberg, Hebben, & Kaplan, 1986). This type of process approach focuses on the qualitative performance of the patient and the pattern of scores in order to clarify how a patient attempts to solve the specific cognitive task. As a result, any deficits revealed can be better interpreted in the context of models of cognitive functioning and in terms of how the impairment will affect daily functioning (Milberg et al., 1986).

For example, Kaplan (1988) has demonstrated that impaired performance on the Block Design test of the WAIS, typically treated as an indication of a right-hemisphere lesion, can result from either right- or left-hemisphere lesions. A key consideration is the sequence of construction and the nature of errors when they occur—patients with right-hemisphere lesions tend to start working on the right side of the design (in contrast to neurologically intact right-handers) and to make errors that violate the overall configuration of the design, whereas left-hemisphere lesion patients tend to begin on the left and make featural errors on the right side of the design. Therefore, both types of patients might receive poor scores on this subtest, but for very different reasons. Moreover, these patterns of errors make sense in the context of current models of spatial attention and visual–spatial organization, described later in this chapter.

Therefore, although the immediate goals and techniques used in clinical and experimental investigations of cognitive functions may appear to be quite different, in recent years there has been a remarkable and exciting convergence of approach. The development of many cognitive models is being influenced by dissociations between processes, as demonstrated by brain-injured patients, and the development and interpretation of some neuropsychological assessment devices is being guided by these models and by a functional system approach. The manner in which this approach has developed has, of course, differed from one domain to another; we consider first the current models and the potential usefulness of a component process approach in the area of memory.

MODELS OF MEMORY

Although some arguments have been made for unitary models of memory (e.g., Melton, 1963), most recent models have treated memory as consisting of multiple systems, storing information in different forms and for different durations. Neuropsychological studies have had a profound influence on the field, providing striking evidence of the functional independence of short-term and long-term memory systems, as well as multiple dissociations within each system. This work is forcing us to think in terms of many different types of memory representations, as well as multicomponent storage systems.

Short-Term/Working Memory

In 1890, James described two memory stores: primary memory, which holds information in conscious awareness, and secondary memory, which holds information on a more permanent basis once it is dismissed from conscious awareness. The relationship between these two forms of memory was formalized in several multistore models in the 1960s (e.g., Atkinson & Shiffrin, 1968; Waugh & Norman, 1965). From this view, information has to be held in the short-term store (STM) for a period of time in order to be successfully transferred to the long-term store (LTM); memories retrieved from the LTM are read back into STM and conscious awareness.

Patients with anterograde amnesia, who retain an intact STM (as measured by digit span) but who show a severely impaired capacity to store new information for longer periods of time, fit rather nicely into this type of multiple memory system. Such a dissociation demonstrates that STM can operate independently of more permanent storage. However, these sequential models, in which LTM depends on rehearsal in STM, predict that an impairment in STM should have consequences for LTM. Recent descriptions of patients with selective STM deficits, provide even stronger evidence for the independence of the two memory systems and call into question the dependence of long-term storage on short-term rehearsal processes (e.g., Shallice & Warrington, 1970; Warrington & Shallice, 1969; see Vallar & Shallice, 1990, for a recent review of STM deficits). That is, the ability to acquire new information, at a normal learning rate, appears to remain intact in the face of a severely impaired digit span.

Early investigations of STM deficits also showed a dissociation within the STM system: Auditory–verbal span could be impaired, whereas visual span remained relatively unaffected (e.g., De Renzi & Nichelli, 1975; Shallice & Warrington, 1970; Warrington & Shallice, 1969). At about the same time, studies with neurologically intact populations demonstrated the independence of visual and auditory STM processes using dual-task paradigms (e.g., Brooks, 1968).

One of the most influential models to emerge from this fractionation of STM is the *working memory model*, which consists of three main components: an articulatory loop, a visual–spatial scratchpad, and a central executive (Baddeley, 1986, 1992; Baddeley & Hitch, 1974). From this view, the central executive acts as an attentional control system, constrained by limited-capacity attentional resources and responsible for strategy selection and integrating information from various sources. The articulatory and visual–spatial "slave" systems operate relatively automatically and independently to maintain speech-based and visual–spatial representations. In addition, the articulatory loop has two components, based on different codes or representations of speech: a nonarticulatory phonological store and an articulatory rehearsal loop.

The basis for a multicomponent model of working memory comes from a variety of sources, including evidence from both normal and neurological populations (see Baddeley, 1992, for a recent review). Initial work in this area focused on evidence that working memory is more than what is measured by digit span; that is, although working memory must have one component devoted to rehearsing and refreshing speech-based information, other functions can also be carried out, sometimes concurrently. As the nature of the articulatory loop has been investigated in more detail, evidence has emerged supporting a distinction between phonological and articulatory components of the loop. For example, irrelevant spoken material disrupts immediate serial recall, suggesting that speech has automatic access to the phonological store (Salame & Baddeley, 1982). Articulatory suppression (uttering an irrelevant sound or word) also disrupts immediate recall, but has a more widespread effect on material presented visually than aurally, suggesting that visual material must be converted to a phonological form through an articulatory process (Baddeley, Lewis, & Vallar, 1984). Moreover, patients with reduced verbal spans differ in important ways, some showing patterns that suggest a deficit in phonological storage (e.g., Friedrich, Glenn, & Marin, 1984; Martin, 1987; Vallar & Baddeley, 1984) and others showing patterns consistent with a rehearsal deficit (Martin, 1987).

Recently there has been increasing evidence that lexical or semantic factors may influence verbal span performance, suggesting that these types of representations also need to be taken into account in the working memory system (Brooks & Watkins, 1990; Friedrich, 1990a; Saffran & Martin, 1990; Shelton, Martin, & Yaffee, 1992). Models now emerging reflect a multiple-representations approach, including buffers for auditory, visual, articulatory, lexical, and semantic representations (e.g., Monsell, 1984; Schneider & Detweiler, 1987). Although less extensively studied, visual and spatial representations may also be dissociable (Farah, Hammond, Levine, & Calvanio, 1988) and thus make separable contributions to selective deficits of the visual–spatial scratchpad (Hanley, Young, & Pearson, 1991).

Overall, therefore, reduction in short-term memory span may result from a variety of impairments; the nature of the deficit in turn provides a link to other systems (i.e., phonological, spatial, semantic) that can shed light on the functional consequences of such a deficit—for example, the way in which the STM deficit will influence sentence processing (e.g., Friedrich, Martin, & Kemper, 1985; Martin, 1990). Standardized assessment devices do not currently provide for such a detailed analysis of the source of reduced STM capacity, although some experimental protocols are now emerging (Shelton et al., 1992).

Long-Term Memory

As in the case of short-term memory, our conceptualization of long-term memory processes has become increasingly complex in recent years, guided to some extent by evidence of dissociations among different measures of memory. Quite a number of frameworks for distinguishing different LTM systems have been proposed, based on data from animal studies, and normal and neurologically impaired human populations. An early distinction based on neuropsychological data concerned modality-specific learning. Patients with left temporal lobe lesions have been shown to have deficits in verbal learning but not maze-learning tasks; conversely, patients with right temporal lobe lesions have shown normal verbal learning performance but impaired spatial learning (Milner, 1971). Modality-specific distinctions remain an important consideration in describing distinct memory stores, as they indicate that information can be stored in memory in a variety of different representations. More recently, however, models have been proposed that suggest distinct memory stores that operate according to different principles and for different purposes.

One of the most influential of these frameworks, and one which has evolved over the course of several years, has come from the work of Tulving (1972, 1985), who proposed separable episodic, semantic, and procedural memory systems. A key distinction among these proposed types of memory is the nature of the information. Episodic memory refers to memory for events that have occurred (generally personally experienced or autobiographical events) within a specific temporal and spatial context; that is, memories of this sort have a particular contextual "tag" that makes that event unique. Semantic information includes facts, concepts, word meanings, and so on, which constitute an individual's knowledge of the world. For example, knowing the meaning of a word would reflect semantic memory, whereas remembering that a given word was on a list that you were asked to recall would be an example of episodic memory. Procedural memory is described as memory for how to perform a task; it is both acquired and measured through performance, and thus may not involve a conscious effort to recall.

According to Tulving (1985), these three systems differ in how information is acquired, represented, expressed, and, in the nature of the conscious experience, associated with it. However, these systems are not completely independent; rather, the relation among them is "monohierarchical," in which each higher level system depends on a lower system, but also has some unique characteristics. According to this framework, procedural memory comprises the lowest or most basic level of the hierarchy, and thus can function without either of the other systems. Semantic memory is now thought to be a "specialized subsystem" within procedural memory and episodic memory a subsystem within semantic memory. Based on this proposed relationship among the different memory stores, only certain dissociations would be expected in neurologically impaired patient populations; therefore, a patient may retain procedural memory with either semantic or episodic memory loss, but a semantic impairment would necessarily have consequences for episodic memory.

The strongest support for distinctions among LTM systems is evidence from both normal and patient populations demonstrating a distinction between procedural and other memory systems. Indeed, a number of alternative frameworks identify only two types of LTM stores, a procedural and a nonprocedural memory, the latter variously referred to as propositional, declarative, explicit, or representational memory (e.g., Graf & Schacter, 1985; Mishkin & Appenzeller, 1987; Squire, 1987). The classic example of the procedural/nonprocedural distinction comes from cases of amnesic patients, such as HM, who demonstrate procedural learning across training sessions in perceptual-motor tasks, such as mirror reading or rotor pursuit, but who have no conscious memory of ever having performed the task before (e.g., Cohen & Squire, 1980; Corkin, 1968; Shimamura, 1986). Considerable evidence now exists that procedural learning—as demonstrated on a variety of tasks—can be quite robust in the face of otherwise dense amnesia. Defining exactly what constitutes procedural memory remains a problem, however. There has been a tendency to assume that any residual learning ability in an amnesic patient must reflect procedural memory, so that highly dissimilar tasks have been lumped into the same category. Squire (1987) has suggested that the category of procedural learning is actually a collection of abilities (e.g., motor skill learning, perceptual learning, classical conditioning, priming, habituation), each of which has a specialized processing system involving particular brain structures. This situation calls into question the utility of the concept of procedural memory, but also suggests that the number of elements or components contributing to long-term memory performance may be even greater than previously imagined.

Although the potential number of procedural memory systems has been expanding, Tulving's original distinction between episodic and semantic memory has faced increasing criticism. The distinction between episodic and semantic memory has heuristic value and is commonly accepted in the field (as reflected in current textbooks); however, McKoon, Ratcliff, and Dell (1986) reviewed evidence questioning the distinction and provide a comprehensive critique of the issue. They argued that the theoretical distinction is not clearly defined and that supporting evidence is weak.

In addition to reviewing evidence from normal populations, McKoon et al. pointed out some problems in interpreting the neuropsychological data. For example, from Tulving's perspective, some forms of amnesia should impair episodic but not semantic information; indeed, cases have been presented demonstrating such a dissociation (e.g., Cermak & O'Connor, 1983; Schacter & Tulving, 1982; Tulving, Hayman, & MacDonald, 1991; Wood, Ebert, & Kinsbourne, 1982). However, the picture is complicated by issues of retrograde versus anterograde amnesia; that is, evaluating whether the memory impairment affects information acquired before or after the brain injury. Squire (1987) has suggested that reports showing a dissociation between episodic and semantic memory in amnesics have tended to evaluate intact semantic knowledge from *before* the injury and contrast it with impaired ability to learn new episodic information presented *after* the injury. Therefore, Squire (1987; Cohen & Squire, 1981) has argued that patients with difficulty acquiring new episodic information also have a deficit in acquiring new semantic information. In response, Tulving et al. (1991) described a patient who does appear to be able to acquire new semantic facts in the face of a severe anterograde amnesia.

This approach of evaluating memory performance in terms of the contributions of isolable elements or components has been extended to another level of analysis: the contents and organization of semantic knowledge. The primary focus of this work has been the study of memory deficits in patients with dementia of the Alzheimer's type (DAT). In addition to a pattern of anterograde amnesia similar to that of patients with bilateral medial temporal damage, DAT patients seem to suffer a progressive loss of previously acquired semantic knowledge (word meanings, categorical knowledge) that is reflected in language as well as memory tasks (e.g., Chertkow & Bub, 1990; Schwartz, Marin, & Saffran, 1979). Recent work in this area has considered the possibility of semantic systems, based on specific modalities or on distinct categories of knowledge (e.g., Chertkow & Bub, 1990; Farah &

McClelland, 1991; Warrington & McCarthy, 1983; Warrington & Shallice, 1984). Many issues in this area have yet to be resolved, but the exciting potential of this work is clearly represented in a computational model developed by Farah and McClelland. The model consists of distributed representations of visual and functional semantic information; when "lesioned," it can produce a pattern of performance consistent with selective impairments of other hypothesized categories of semantic information, such as living and nonliving things. Such an approach may help us understand the basic elements of memory, as well as how these elements and types of representation interact to produce a variety of patterns of performance in different contexts.

The theoretical utility and degree of empirical support for the various proposed components of the memory system(s) described here clearly have yet to be resolved. The direction of recent work in memory holds a number of lessons for us, however. First, it is clear that progress in the development of cognitive models and in neuropsychological analyses of deficits can influence and benefit one another. Ultimately, a successful model must account for both normal and impaired patterns of performance. Moreover, evidence from neuropsychology can provide an independent means of evaluating hypotheses developed based on traditional cognitive tasks, and vice versa (Schacter, 1992). Second, the benefits of using neuropsychological data depend on identifying what is spared as well as what is impaired; this type of information can give us a window on possible components within the system. Third, there is also a danger of abusing the component process approach by assuming a separable system or independent process for every variation of memory deficit that is described. Such distinctions need to be clearly defined so as to be testable and supported by empirical evidence, criteria that some would say have not been met in some proposed multiple-memory systems. Nevertheless, the potential richness and complexity of current conceptions of memory are certainly intriguing.

SPATIAL ATTENTION

The concept of attention has been important to understanding human thought since the earliest writings on cognition (James, 1890), at least in part because it provides a mechanism responsible for choosing important information for further processing. The concept itself is often vaguely defined and seems to acquire a variety of meanings and characteristics depending on the situation. Posner and Boies (1971) discussed three main aspects of attention: alertness, selectivity, and processing capacity. Alertness is a general readiness to process all sources of information or to improve selection of a particular type of stimulus. Selectivity refers to choosing a source of information for further processing. Processing capacity involves limits in processing speed or accuracy when mental operations such as response selection or rehearsal are performed on encoded information. Different tasks are often associated with these features of attention, including vigilance, sustained attention, orienting, and both focused and divided attention tasks. Even within a subtype of attention, such as selective attention, a range of potential functions have been identified: facilitating perception, acquiring skills, response selection, learning, object recognition, and so on. Deficits of attention are similarly varied in their descriptions and presumed consequences.

One of the most detailed models of attention, and one that demonstrates a component process approach, has focused on visual–spatial attention. A number of models have been proposed; those based primarily on work with normal populations differ in terms of how attention is allocated and distributed across space (e.g., Erikson & Yeh, 1985; Juola, Bouwhuis, Cooper, & Warner, 1991; LaBerge & Brown, 1989) and whether attention moves across space in an analog or discrete fashion (e.g., Eriksen & Murphy, 1987; Shulman,

Remington, & McLean, 1979). We begin our discussion by focusing on a specific spatial-orienting model, which accords well with data from both normal and neurological populations. This work has produced a picture of a multicomponent attentional system, linking several brain regions in an interactive system that extends beyond visual orienting and encompasses mechanisms for semantic selection as well.

Components of Spatial Orienting

Consider the following task: You are watching a computer screen that contains a row of three boxes, with a small cross located in the center of the middle box. You are instructed to keep your eyes fixated on the cross at all times, and to expect the appearance of a target, a small bright star, which could appear in either the left or the right box. When it does, you are to press a key as quickly as possible. However, before the target appears, one of the three boxes quickly flashes. The target then appears after a variable interval of time in an outer box. In such studies, the flashing of the box, or the cue, can be valid, when it is in the same location as the target; neutral, when it is in the center and provides no information about the location of the subsequent peripheral target; or invalid, when it is on the opposite side as the target.

This orienting task has proven to be simple yet powerful; the nature of the task allows it to be adapted for use in single-cell recording in animals, in PET scan studies, and with different populations of neurological and psychiatric patients. Based on these types of data, Posner and his colleagues developed a model of the component processes underlying attentional orienting (e.g., Posner, 1980; Posner, Walker, Friedrich, & Rafal, 1984).

Intuitively, the process of orienting spatial attention would seem to involve disengaging it from its present location, moving it to the new location, and engaging it there. Studies of brain-injured patients have indeed supported the existence of these components of orienting. Patients with damage to the posterior parietal lobes show particular difficulty in disengaging attention from the location ipsilateral to the lesion (e.g, Baynes, Holtzman, & Volpe, 1986; Friedrich, Egly, Rafal, & Beck, in preparation; Morrow & Ratcliff, 1988; Posner et al., 1984; Posner, Walker, Friedrich, & Rafal, 1987). If a patient with damage to the right posterior parietal lobe engages attention to a cue in the right (intact) field, response time to a target occurring in the left (impaired) field will be longer than in any other condition. The problem is not in moving attention per se, because valid trials in the left and right fields are often comparable in these patients. Therefore, a distinct disengage mechanism is implicated by such findings.

Patients with damage to the superior colliculus show a markedly different pattern of deficit in the same task. Such damage occurs in progressive supranuclear palsy (PSP), which is marked by deterioration of midbrain structures. PSP patients have difficulty making eye movements, especially in the vertical plane, and, it appears, also show deficits in attentional movements. When performing the aforementioned spatial attention task, patients with PSP show markedly slowed response times regardless of the hemifield in which the stimulus occurs and where attention had been previously engaged (Rafal, Posner, Friedman, Inhoff, & Bernstein, 1988). This finding suggests that the colliculus performs a computation involved in moving attention and that this computation may be closely tied to that which is used for movements of the eyes.

Patients with collicular damage demonstrate an additional deficit. Normal subjects show a reduced probability of returning attention to a previously attended location, a phenomenon termed *inhibition of return* (Posner & Cohen, 1984). Collicular damage results in the loss of this aspect of orienting (Posner, Rafal, Choate, & Vaughan, 1985), which has recently been shown to be closely associated with preparation to make an eye movement (Rafal, Calabresi, Brennan, & Sciolto, 1989).

The engage operation seems to be associated with the pulvinar nucleus of the thalamus (Rafal & Posner, 1987). Patients with thalamic damage show slowed response times for targets on the side contralateral to the lesion whether or not attention had been cued to that location previously, even when attention has had plenty of time to be moved there. This suggests a deficit in engaging attention in contralateral targets. In addition, PET scan studies of intact subjects performing attention tasks suggest activity in the pulvinar region when the task requires the filtering of a target letter from a cluttered visual field (LaBerge, 1991). Engaging attention at the target location would presumably be required for such a filtering operation to occur.

The involvement of posterior areas of the brain in visual attention has been confirmed by other techniques, in addition to the response time and PET scan studies mentioned earlier. For example, recordings of single cells in alert monkeys have confirmed the involvement of the parietal lobes, the pulvinar nucleus of the thalamus, and the superior colliculus in visual attention (Mountcastle, 1978; Petersen, Robinson, & Morris, 1987; Wurtz, Goldberg, & Robinson, 1980). Event-Related Potential (ERP) studies have shown similar results in human subjects, supporting the idea that posterior cortical regions are involved in spatial attention (e.g., Hillyard & Munte, 1984).

One of the benefits of this component process approach is that it can be related to clinical syndromes resulting from brain injury. For example, it is well documented that neglect, or some form of spatial attention deficit, can result from injury to any of several brain regions, including the frontal lobe, thalamic regions, and the posterior parietal lobe, although the right parietal lobe is by far the region most frequently associated with severe spatial attention deficits (De Renzi, 1982; Heilman & Valenstein, 1985). In the case of severe neglect, the patient fails to notice stimuli presented to the contralesional visual field, despite adequate visual acuity. In less severe forms, a patient may show extinction, or failure to detect an item in the contralesional field when a competing item is in the ipsilesional field. What is the relationship between clinical neglect and the components of orienting discussed earlier? Morrow and Ratcliff (1988) compared disengage impairments to clinical neglect in patients with right- or left-parietal damage. Additionally, they studied patients longitudinally to look at changes in neglect and the disengage deficit over time. They found that the size of the disengage impairment correlated significantly with the amount of neglect demonstrated through clinical tests for patients with right-hemisphere lesions but not for patients with left-hemisphere lesions.

Morrow and Ratcliff (1988) found further evidence of a relationship between clinical neglect and disengage difficulties in longitudinal studies of their patients. Two subjects who showed improvement in clinical neglect measures over time also showed reduced disengage difficulties. Two patients who did not show such clinical improvements also failed to improve in the cued-target detection task. It should be noted, however, that response time tasks seem to provide an extraordinarily sensitive measure of possible "subclinical" attentional deficits; chronic parietal patients who no longer have any clinical evidence of neglect or extinction still show visual field asymmetries in this type of orienting task (Posner et al., 1984). Similarly, in a longitudinal case study, a patient with a right subcortical lesion continued to show a visual field asymmetry in the response time task for over a year and a half after all clinical evidence of neglect or extinction had resolved (Friedrich & Margolin, 1993).

Therefore, for the seemingly simple task of orienting to a location in space, it appears that several brain regions are needed to perform all the required operations. However, there are also many different types of tasks in addition to spatial orienting that require attention. For example, categorizing words and orienting in space both require attention, but in different ways. Posner and colleagues (e.g., Posner, Petersen, et al., 1988) have suggested that the posterior attentional system involved in the orienting of spatial attention shares operations with other processes requiring attention, such as language processes, through an anterior attention system, possibly centered in the anterior cingulate gyrus. Evidence of a shared system comes from studies demonstrating delayed orienting effects when the spatial task is performed simultaneously with a language task (Posner, Inhoff, Friedrich, & Cohen, 1987). Moreover, PET studies suggest that the left frontal lobe is associated with semantic language tasks and that the anterior cingulate gyrus is important in selecting activated semantic targets for action (Posner, Petersen, et al., 1988).

Interesting extensions of this work have been made with other patient populations. Several disorders, such as schizophrenia and ADD, have long been thought to involve attentional problems. Recently, the orienting task has been used to investigate attentional processing in both ADD and schizophrenic populations. Swanson et al. (1991) studied cued-target detection in children with ADD and found evidence suggesting an abnormality in the anterior action system. Similarly, Posner, Early, and Reiman (1988) studied attention in individuals with schizophrenia and found abnormalities consistent with a left-hemisphere disorder. Therefore, the analysis of spatial attention has helped us to understand important components of several clinical disorders.

What is emerging from this type of component process analysis is a picture of a complex, multifaceted system, associated with several different brain regions, whose operations can be combined in a variety of ways depending upon the task demands. Even so, the attention systems described here do not tell the entire story. In recent years, there has been some question as to whether attention is allocated on the basis of spatial location or whether allocation is actually object-based (e.g., Duncan, 1984). That is, when an individual orients attention to the cue in the orienting task discussed previously, is attention allocated to a spatial position or to the box that demarcates the cue position? Although it can be demonstrated that attention can be oriented to spatial locations in an otherwise empty field (e.g., Posner, 1980), there is also evidence that performance is better if subjects are asked to judge two properties from the same object compared to the same two properties from different objects (e.g., Duncan, 1984). Moreover, the inhibition of return effect, reflecting a bias against returning to a previously attended location, may actually reflect a bias against reattending to an specific object rather than the location: If the cued box moves to a new location, inhibition of return seems to follow the box (Tipper, Driver, & Weaver, 1991).

Evidence supporting an object-based attention system also comes from studies of patients with right parietal lobe lesions and demonstrated spatial attention deficits. Such patients have more trouble attending to the left side of a object, whether it occurs in the left or right visual field (e.g., Driver, Baylis, & Rafal, 1992; Driver & Halligan, 1991). In fact, recent work with parietal lesions patients suggests that the visual attention system has both a space-based and an object-based component and that the two hemispheres may be differentially specialized for the two components (Egly, Driver, & Rafal, 1992).

The body of literature concerning models of spatial attention is impressive, in particular because there has been a remarkable convergence of methodologies and data from some traditionally disparate areas. A number of questions remain to be pursued, however. For example, some have suggested that separate neural mechanisms underlie orienting initiated by a cue in the periphery, such as a flash of light, and orienting that is internally initiated (e.g., Friedrich et al., in preparation; Rafal & Henik, 1994). The function of attention in different contexts, and thus the consequences of a spatial attention deficit, need to be clarified: Does attention or the absence of it have different consequences for detection and identification tasks? If, as Treisman (e.g., Treisman & Gelade, 1980) has suggested, attention is important for feature integration processes during object recognition, what are the consequences of lesions to different components of the attention system(s)? How would such lesions affect other presumed functions of attention, such as skill acquisition or learning? It is our belief that the component process approach discussed here provides a framework for addressing these issues in a coherent and meaningful way.

MENTAL IMAGERY

Mental imagery is one of the most intriguing areas of research in brain–behavior relationships, at least in part because its subjective and transitory nature would seem to make it nearly impossible to study experimentally. Mental imagery involves the set of internal cognitive processes necessary in order for us to visualize, for example, whether or not we would be able to carry our dining room table directly out through the front door or whether it would need to be angled. Many researchers have shown that in order to answer such questions without looking at the dining room table or the front door, we must retrieve stored images of objects and locations, and process them much as we would visually process an actual object or scene (Shepard & Chipman, 1970).

Universal agreement does not exist concerning the nature and diversity of internal codes or representations; some have argued for a single propositional coding system (e.g., Pylyshyn, 1973), although considerable evidence supporting a multiple representation view has been amassed (e.g., Posner, 1978). In recent years, a good deal of research has been done with normal populations demonstrating similarities in how certain factors (e.g., visual angle, orientation) affect both visual perception and imagery task performance, and suggesting that the two systems may share some mechanisms and some neural substrates. In this section we focus on one of the most explicit and best articulated theories of the mental imagery process (Kosslyn, 1980, 1987), and discuss it in relation to the relevant neuropsychological data.

Components of Mental Imagery

Like other cognitive systems, mental imagery can be seen as a complex set of operations incorporating several processing subsystems. Kosslyn (1980) has identified a number of separate *structures* and *processes*. The structures include (a) long-term visual memories of objects, which are the representations of images, and (b) a visual buffer, which is the medium in which images are held. The processes involve (a) generating the image, which creates activation patterns in the buffer from information in long-term memory, (b) inspecting the image, which converts the activation patterns in the buffer to meaningful percepts, and (c) transforming the image, which rotates or translates the image if necessary. Some of these processes may in turn be described in terms of even more basic operations or computations.

Work with normal populations have helped define some of these component processes. For example, the component theory suggests that in some cases images are constructed one segment at a time during the image generation process, requiring a specific subsystem to locate and arrange the segments appropriately. Subsequent work using response time measures have supported this sequential process and the assumption that some information about the categorical relations of the different parts is required (Kosslyn, 1987). Thus, the data from normal populations suggest separable representational subsystems for shape and spatial relations. Some of the most compelling data supporting this distinction as well as other aspects of the component process approach, however, have come from the neuropsychological literature.

Representational Subsystems. The idea that mental imagery may have dissociable visual and spatial subsystems has its basis in neural evidence for a similar distinction in visual object recognition. Ungerleider and Mishkin (1982), for example, have shown that parietal-lesioned monkeys can perform well in tasks requiring discrimination of objects based on differences in appearance, but are markedly impaired at tasks requiring spatial location discrimination. Animals with damage to the inferior temporal cortex, however, show the opposite pattern of results. These data, as well as much other data, suggest that independent visual systems perform analyses based on these two types of information.

Does the same separation apply for mental imagery? Levine, Warach, and Farah (1985) presented data of brain-damaged humans that support the same distinction in mental imagery. Patients with parietal lesions, who were impaired in the perception of spatial location, were also impaired at describing or drawing the spatial layout of remembered scenes without impairment in imagining the characteristics of objects. Similarly, inferior temporal lobe damaged subjects had difficulty describing the appearance of imagined objects even though they had no trouble with the spatial layouts of imagined objects or scenes.

Farah, Hammond et al. (1988) tested a brain-damaged patient who demonstrated deficits in object recognition but showed intact object localization on various types of mental imagery tasks. This patient, who had bilateral posterior inferior temporal lobe injury, was tested on imagery tasks designed to tap into spatial and visual components of imagery separately. The visual imagery tasks involved using information about objects' visual properties, such as color, size, and shape. The spatial tasks used information regarding relative locations of objects as well as the ability to process transformations of these objects.

The patient's performance was markedly impaired on the visual imagery tasks while being well within the normal range (compared to performance of age-matched controls) on the spatial tasks. Farah, Hammond, et al. argued that the patient's impairment is in long-term visual memory and concluded that imagery involves both spatial and visual representations.

Processing Subsystems. Recall that Kosslyn's theory proposes that mental imagery involves generating, inspecting, and transforming the image. Do neuropsychological data support the existence of these subprocesses of mental imagery in the brain?

Farah (1984) reviewed case descriptions of 37 cases of reported visual imagery deficits found in the literature. The detail of description and the nature of the tasks employed varied widely across the reports: Farah determined that there was sufficient evidence to demonstrate imagery deficits in 27 of the cases. In order to determine the nature of the deficit in these cases, she analyzed the tasks used to test these patients in terms of the component processes needed to perform the task. Therefore, although different patients were evaluated on different tasks, it was possible to narrow down the source of the deficit in most cases. The locus of the damage was also variable across patients; however, several distinct patterns of deficit were apparent.

One group of patients showed evidence of an image-generation deficit, as demonstrated in a variety of tasks. Some patients were unable to describe visualized objects but could describe remembered objects that did not require visualization. For example, a construction worker could not visualize plans but could describe his house. Other cases described patients who could not draw common objects from memory but could copy drawings of objects. In these cases, according Farah's task analysis, the only component involved in the failed tasks that does not occur in the successful tasks is the generation process.

When lesion sites of these patients were considered together, a pattern was apparent. The locus of damage seemed mainly to be the posterior region of the left hemisphere. This association of image generation with the left hemisphere seems quite counterintuitive, as imagery processes have been the domain of the right hemisphere according to many accounts of hemispheric specialization (e.g., Springer & Deutsch, 1985). However, some split-brain patients, whose corpus callosi have been severed rendering the two hemispheres functionally independent, have been evaluated on imagery tasks, and the results tend to support an image-generation process in the left posterior brain regions (Kosslyn, Holtzman, Farah, & Gazzaniga, 1985). More specifically, Kosslyn (1987) argued that both hemispheres can encode shapes, generate images of general shapes, and retain those images. However, the two hemispheres may differ in how location information is represented, with the right hemisphere using spatial coordinates, whereas the left hemisphere uses categorical spatial relations. In Kosslyn's view, the categorical relations are needed in order to construct a complex image one segment at a time. Therefore, even within the category of generation deficits, the exact source of the deficit and pattern of impairment may vary depending on which subsystem is affected and how imagery abilities are evaluated.

A second pattern revealed by Farah's (1984) case study review suggested that several patients had an impairment in the inspection process, as demonstrated through poor performance on imagery question–answer tasks, descriptions of imagined objects, and drawings of objects from memory. The performance of these patients was quite poor across the board, so it is difficult to infer damage specifically to the inspection process. However, the only component that occurs in all of and only the failed tasks is inspection.

Some cases of transformation process deficits have also been reported. This impairment most commonly occurs with right hemisphere lesions. Riddoch and Humphreys (1986) studied object naming in five patients who had suffered strokes. Subjects were asked to name photographs of objects whose sizes or orientations had been changed. Three of these patients, all with lesions of the right hemisphere, named objects that were shown in prototypical views very well, but were markedly disturbed at naming objects that had undergone transformations resulting in feature reduction or enlargement. Further tests revealed that mere depth transformations were not enough to impair the performance of these patients. Although these results imply impaired perception of transformed objects, it is reasonable to suggest that the transformation process in mental imagery would be damaged as well, although this was not explicitly studied by Riddoch and Humphries.

Ratcliffe (1979), however, described the cases of several patients with penetrating right-hemisphere head wounds and found that they were impaired at mental rotation tasks. Cerebral blood flow studies as well as evoked potential studies have indicated greater blood flow to the right parietal lobe as well as greater suppression of evoked potentials over the right hemisphere when patients performed mental rotation versus passively viewing the same stimuli (Papanicolaou, Deutsch, Bourbon, & Will, 1987).

Not all patients have highly selective deficits, of course. Riddoch (1990) studied a patient with a left temporoparietal lesion who showed impaired generation and transformation processes. He was tested on several tasks requiring generation, inspection, and transformation of imagery. The patient was found to be at chance in most of the generation and transformation tests. Riddoch discussed two possible explanations for the pattern of deficits shown in this patient: that generation and transformation are separate processes and both are damaged, and that the processes are related and the patient's performance reflects disruption of a particular form of image representation. She argued that the types of transformations this patient was asked to do require active maintenance of an image in the visual buffer. This patient shows evidence of two separate generation problems: generating from long-term memory to the image buffer, and generating from the visual buffer to the image buffer in order to do the transformation. This is consistent with Farah's (1984) hypothesis that generation and transformation are left- and right-hemisphere functions, respectively.

As mentioned previously, the types of processes that are carried out on images are similar to those done in the perception of actual objects. It seems intuitive, therefore, that they should share neural substrates. Many different types of studies have supported this claim. Studies of ERP (Farah, Peronnet, Gonon, & Giard, 1988) and regional blood flow (Roland &

Friberg, 1985) have suggested that brain activity is similar in visual perception and visual imagery, with active areas being occipital, temporal, and parietal cortices. In addition, as discussed previously, the blood flow and evoked potential studies have supported some lateralization of processes, with generation processes associated with left-hemisphere functions and transformation processes associated with the right hemisphere.

It should be noted, however, that although some mechanisms seemed to be shared in visual perception and imagery tasks, dissociations between the two are also possible. Often patients have the same type of deficit for both perception and imagery tasks, but some cases have been reported of patients with impaired object recognition but intact visual imagery skills (Behrmann, Winocur, & Moscovitch, 1992; Jankowiak, Kinsbourne, Shalev, & Bachman, 1992). New variations of visual perceptual and imagery deficits will undoubtedly be reported with greater frequency. It is likely that until recently, imagery abilities were not systematically evaluated in many patients with potential deficits; the formulation of a component process model of this type makes specific predictions about what type of dissociations should occur and thus may help guide clinical evaluation of these patients.

The nature of the approach to the study of mental imagery and spatial attention has been similar—the cognitive function is decomposed into separable but interacting components. Many different types of evidence, including data from cognitive, neuropsychological, evoked potential, cerebral blood flow, and single unit recording studies, have converged to suggest that these components can be separated out and studied independently. Furthermore, different neural substrates are probably involved in the different components of imagery. The coming years will most likely see research in mental imagery become more sophisticated and precise in terms of separating out the components of imagery processing, whereas advancements in technology will provide ways to chart more accurately the neural areas underlying these processes.

IMPLICATIONS FOR ASSESSMENT AND TREATMENT

We have described three areas in which a component process analysis of cognitive functions has provided a productive interaction between the development of experimental models and the study of clinical syndromes. The same principles can be, and have been, applied in other domains as well. For example, a number of models of language processing have emerged in recent years, including models of speech perception and production (e.g., Caramazza & Berndt, 1978; Saffran, Schwartz, & Marin, 1980), reading (e.g., Coltheart, 1985; Ellis, 1984), writing, and oral spelling (e.g., Margolin, 1984; Patterson & Shewell, 1987). All of these approaches attempt to identify various pathways (i.e., phonological, visual), or types of representations (i.e., abstract letter identities, lexical, semantic, articulatory, syntactic) that will account for the types of dissociations seen. Similarly, models consistent with a component process approach are being developed in the study of agnosia and high-level visual operations (e.g, Coslett & Saffran, 1991; Farah, 1990) and calculation deficits (e.g., McCloskey, Caramazza, & Basili, 1985).

The theoretical distinctions among the various specific operations hypothesized to underlie these cognitive functions may seem irrelevant, at first glance, to more practical concerns of clinical assessment and the development of treatment plans. On the contrary, the incorporation of this type of approach can enhance both assessment and treatment strategies. To support this claim, let us first make explicit three principles that follow from the logic of the component process approach:

1. Even seemingly simple cognitive tasks (e.g., orienting attention, naming an object)

require several elementary operations, and possibly several cognitive systems (e.g., spatial attention, memory, object recognition).

2. Conversely, a given clinical deficit (e.g., neglect, STM deficit, visual agnosia) may be caused by an impairment of any of the operations underlying that function. For example, an impairment in either the engage, move, or disengage operations may result in a spatial orienting deficit. Similarly, STM abilities may be reduced by deficits involving phonological, articulatory, semantic, or attentional (strategic) processes.

3. A given operation or type of representation may play a role in several different cognitive functions. This idea is made most explicit in the imagery literature, where it is assumed that long-term visual representations and operations such as scanning or rotation are shared by the visual perception and imagery systems. This principle may extend to other domains as well, however, such as the role a phonological operation may play in STM, reading, repetition of speech, and sentence comprehension (e.g., Friedrich et al., 1984, 1985).

Following from these principles, it is clear that traditional diagnostic categories and techniques used in assessment may actually mask differences in deficits and contribute to confusions in the localization of functions. Farah (1990) has suggested that the taxonomic categories used to differentiate visual agnosias have in some cases been based on theoretical assumptions about the nature of visual processes rather than on empirical data and clinical observations; as a result, in some analyses patients with distinctly different patterns of deficits have been grouped together. Similarly, Dronkers, Redfern, and Shapiro (1993) demonstrated that patients classified as severe Broca's aphasics by traditional measures can be subdivided into two groups with different clinical profiles and different lesion locations (see also Behrmann & Byng, 1992).

A component process analysis can help address problems of heterogeneity within diagnostic categories by providing guidance regarding which underlying operations need to be evaluated. A critical element is an understanding of what a given task is actually evaluating; therefore, tasks must be logically decomposed to identify presumed cognitive requirements and then selected so that deficits can be isolated as well as possible. Farah's (1984) analysis of imagery tasks provides a useful model of this process.

A number of assessment devices based on these general ideas are emerging. As indicated previously, the Boston Process approach to assessment is explicitly designed to allow the qualitative nature of the deficit to reveal itself (Kaplan, 1988). Errors on the Block Design and other visual construction tasks have long been considered a marker of right-hemisphere damage. Kaplan's description of the strategies and errors of both left- and right-hemisphere patients on the Block Design test accords well with models of attention and spatial processing. The two hemispheres may have different ways of representing spatial information (e.g., Kosslyn, 1987), which could result in different patterns of errors. In addition, the fact that both left- and right-parietal-lobe patients show a disengage deficit on the Posner spatial-orienting task make it less surprising that left-hemisphere patients are likely to make errors on the right side of the design. The Block Design task requires attentional, spatial, visuo–perceptual, sequencing, and motor operations; a number of different deficits may impair performance, but the types of errors and the other types of tasks on which the patient shows impairment should provide converging information regarding the underlying nature of the deficit.

Systematic assessment protocols reflecting this approach are beginning to emerge in several domains, although many are still in development. For example, progress has been made in assessment of STM (e.g., Shelton et al., 1992), LTM (e.g., Feher & Martin, 1992), reading disorders (e.g., Coltheart, 1985), dyscalculia (e.g., Macaruso, Harley, & Mc-

Closkey, 1992), dysgraphia (Goodman & Caramazza, 1985), and acquired language disorders (e.g., Behrmann & Byng, 1992). A number of treatment plans based on this type of analysis have also been reported (e.g., Behrmann & Byng, 1992; Seron & Deloche, 1989). It should be noted, however, that even the most accurate assessment of the deficit does not automatically prescribe the appropriate treatment plan. For example, should the focus be on retraining the deficient process or on teaching compensatory strategies? In any case, a better understanding of the nature of deficits and how they manifest themselves in different contexts will certainly enhance our ability to design and evaluate rehabilitation techniques.

REFERENCES

Atkinson, R. C., & Shiffrin, R. M. (1968). Human memory: A proposed system and its control process. In K. W. Spence & J. T. Spence (Eds.), *The psychology of learning and motivation: Advances in research and theory* (Vol. 2, pp. 89–195). New York: Academic Press.

Baddeley, A. (1986). *Working memory*. New York: Oxford University Press.

Baddeley, A. (1992). Is working memory working? *Quarterly Journal of Experimental Psychology*, *44A*(1), 1–31.

Baddeley, A., & Hitch, G. (1974). Working memory. In G. Bower (Ed.), *Recent advances in learning and motivation* (Vol. 8, pp. 47–89). New York: Academic Press.

Baddeley, A., Lewis, V. J., & Vallar, G. (1984). Exploring the articulatory loop. *Quarterly Journal of Experimental Psychology*, *36*, 233–252.

Baynes, K., Holtzman, J. D., & Volpe, B. (1986). Components of visual attention: Alterations in response patterns to visual stimuli following parietal lobe infarction. *Brain*, *109*, 99–114.

Behrmann, M., & Byng, S. (1992). A cognitive approach to the neurorehabilitation of acquired language disorders. In D. I. Margolin (Ed.), *Cognitive neuropsychology in clinical practice* (pp. 327–353). New York: Oxford University Press.

Behrmann, M., Winocur, G., & Moscovitch, M. (1992). Dissociation between mental imagery and object recognition in a brain-damaged patient. *Nature*, *359*, 636–637.

Brooks, J. O., & Watkins, M. J. (1990). Further evidence on the intricacy of memory span. *Journal of Experimental Psychology: Learning, Memory and Cognition*, *16*, 1134–1141.

Brooks, L. R. (1968). Spatial and verbal components of the act of recall. *Quarterly Journal of Experimental Psychology*, *10*, 12–21.

Caplan, D. (1987). *Neurolinguistics and linguistic aphasiology: An introduction*. Cambridge: Cambridge University Press.

Caramazza, A., & Berndt, R. (1978). Syntactic and semantic processes in aphasia: A review of the literature. *Psychological Review*, *85*, 898–918.

Caramazza, A., & Hillis, A. E. (1991). Lexical organization of nouns and verbs in the brain. *Nature*, *349*, 788.

Cermak, L. S., & O'Connor, M. (1983). The anterograde and retrograde retrieval ability of a patient with amnesia due to encephalitis. *Neuropsychologia*, *21*, 213–234.

Chertkow, H., & Bub, D. (1990). Semantic memory loss in Alzheimer-type dementia. In M. Schwartz (Ed.), *Modular deficits in Alzheimer-type dementia* (pp. 207–244). Cambridge, MA: MIT Press.

Cohen, N. J., & Squire, L. R. (1980). Preserved learning and retention of pattern analyzing skill in amnesia: Dissociation of knowing how and knowing that. *Science*, *210*(10), 207–209.

Cohen, N. J., & Squire, L. R. (1981). Retrograde amnesia and remote memory impairment. *Neuropsychologia*, *19*, 337–356.

Coltheart, M. (1985). Cognitive neuropsychology and the study of reading. In M. I. Posner & O. S. M. Marin (Eds.), *Attention and performance XI* (pp. 3–37). Hillsdale, NJ: Lawrence Erlbaum Associates.

Corkin, S. (1968). Acquisition of motor skill after bilateral medial temporal lobe excision. *Neuropsychologia*, *6*, 225–265.

Coslett, H. B., & Saffran, E. (1991). Simultanagnosia. *Brain*, *114*, 1523–1545.

De Renzi, E. (1982). *Disorders of space exploration and cognition*. New York: Wiley.

De Renzi, E., & Nichelli, P. (1975). Verbal and non-verbal short-term memory impairment following hemispheric damage. *Cortex*, *11*, 341–354.

Driver, J. S., Baylis, G. C., & Rafal, R. D. (1992). Preserved figure-ground segmentation and symmetry in a patient with neglect. *Nature*, *360*, 73–75.

Driver, J. S., & Halligan, P. (1991). Can visual neglect operate in object-centred coordinates? An affirmative case study. *Cognitive Neuropsychology*, *8*(6), 475–496.

Dronkers, N., Redfern, B., & Shapiro, J. K. (1993, February). *Neuroanatomic correlates of production deficits in*

severe Broca's aphasia. Paper presented at the annual meeting of the International Neuropsychological Society, Galveston, TX.
Duncan, J. (1984). Selective attention and the organization of visual information. *Journal of Experimental Psychology: General, 113*, 501–517.
Egly, R., Driver, J., & Rafal, R. D. (1992, November). *Deficits in visual attention following parietal damage: Object based or space based*? Poster presented at the annual meeting of the Psychonomics Society, St. Louis, MO.
Ellis, A. W. (1984). *Reading, writing and dyslexia: A cognitive analysis*. Hove, UK: Lawrence Erlbaum Associates.
Eriksen, C. W., & Murphy, T. D. (1987). Movement of attentional focus across the visual field: A critical look at the evidence. *Perception and Psychophysics, 12*, 201–204.
Eriksen, C. W., & Yeh, Y. (1985). Allocation of attention in the visual field. *Journal of Experimental Psychology: Human Perception and Performance, 11*, 583–597.
Farah, M. J. (1984). The neurological basis of mental imagery: A componential analysis. *Cognition, 18*, 245–272.
Farah, M. J. (1990). *Visual agnosia: Disorders of object recognition and what they tell us about normal vision*. Cambridge, MA: MIT Press.
Farah, M. J., Hammond, K. M., Levine, D. N., & Calvanio, R. (1988). Visual and spatial mental imagery: Dissociable systems of representation. *Cognitive Psychology, 20*, 439–462.
Farah, M. J., Peronnet, F., Gonon, M. A., & Giard, M. H. (1988). Electrophysiological evidence for a shared representational medium for visual images and visual percepts. *Journal of Experimental Psychology: General, 117*(3), 248–257.
Farah, M., & McClelland, J. (1991). A computational model of semantic memory impairment: Modality specificity and emergent category specificity. *Journal of Experimental Psychology: General, 120*(4), 339–357.
Feher, E. P., & Martin, R. C. (1992). Cognitive assessment of long-term memory disorders. In D. I. Margolin (Ed.), *Cognitive neuropsychology in clinical practice* (pp. 168–206). New York: Oxford University Press.
Friedrich, F. J. (1990a). Multiple phonological representations and verbal short-term memory. In G. Vallar & T. Shallice (Eds.), *Neuropsychological impairments of short-term memory*. Cambridge, England: Cambridge University Press.
Friedrich, F. J. (1990b). Frameworks for the study of human spatial impairments. In R. P. Kesner & D. S. Olton (Eds.), *Neurobiology of comparative cognition* (pp. 317–337). Hillsdale, NJ: Lawrence Erlbaum Associates.
Friedrich, F. J., Egly, R., Rafal, R., & Beck, D. (In preparation). *Covert orienting of attention and superior temporal gyrus lesions*.
Friedrich, F. J., Glenn, C., & Marin, O. S. M. (1984). Interruption of phonological coding in conduction aphasia. *Brain and Language, 22*, 253–296.
Friedrich, F. J., & Margolin, D. I. (1993). Response time measures of hemi-inattention: A longitudinal case report. *Neuropsychiatry, Neuropsychology and Behavioral Neurology, 6*(2), 54–59.
Friedrich, F. J., Martin, R. C., & Kemper, S. J. (1985). Consequences of a phonological coding deficit in sentence processing. *Cognitive Neuropsychology, 2*, 385–412.
Goodman, R. A., & Caramazza, A. (1985). *The Johns Hopkins University dysgraphia battery*. Baltimore: Johns Hopkins University Press.
Graf, P., & Schacter, D. L. (1985). Implicit and explicit memory for new associations in normal and amnesic subjects. *Journal of Experimental Psychology: Learning, Memory, and Cognition, 11*, 501–518.
Hanley, J. R., Young, A. W., & Pearson, N. A. (1991). Impairment of the visuo-spatial sketchpad. *Quarterly Journal of Experimental Psychology, 43A*, 101–126.
Heilman, K. M., & Valenstein, E. (1985). *Clinical neuropsychology* (2nd ed.). New York: Oxford University Press.
Hillyard, S. A., & Munte, T. F. (1984). Selective attention to color and location: An analysis with event-related brain potentials. *Perception and Psychophysics, 36*, 185–198.
Jackson, J. H. (1915). On the duality of the brain. *Brain, 38*, 80–103. (Original work published 1874)
James, W. (1890). *Principles of psychology*. New York: Holt.
Jankowiak, J., Kinsbourne, M., Shalev, R. S., & Bachman, D. L. (1992). Preserved visual imagery and categorization in a case of associative visual agnosia. *Journal of Cognitive Neuroscience, 4*(2), 119–131.
Juola, J., Bouwhuis, D. G., Cooper, E. E., & Warner, C. B. (1991). Control of attention around the fovea. *Journal of Experimental Psychology: Human Perception and Performance, 17*, 125–141.
Kaplan, E. (1988). A process approach to neuropsychological assessment. In T. Boll & B. Bryant (Eds.), *Clinical neuropsychology and brain function: Research, measurement and practice* (pp. 129–167). Washington, DC: American Psychological Association.
Kesner, R. P. (1991). Neurobiological views of memory. In J. S. Martinez & R. P. Kesner (Eds.), *Learning and memory: A biological view*, (2nd ed. pp. 499–547). New York: Academic Press.
Kolb, B., & Whishaw, I. (1985). *Fundamentals of human neuropsychology*. San Francisco: Freeman.
Kosslyn, S. M. (1980). *Images and mind*. Cambridge, MA: Harvard University Press.

Kosslyn, S. (1987). Seeing and imagining in the cerebral hemispheres: A computational approach. *Psychological Review, 94*(2), 148–175.

Kosslyn, S., Holtzman, J., Farah, M. J., & Gazzaniga, M. (1985). A computational analysis of mental image generation: Evidence from functional dissociations in split-brain patients. *Journal of Experimental Psychology: General, 114*(3), 311–341.

LaBerge, D. (1991). Thalamic and cortical mechanisms of attention suggested by recent positron emission tomographic experiments. *Journal of Cognitive Neuroscience, 4*(2), 358–372.

LaBerge, D., & Brown, V. (1989). Theory of attentional operations in shape identification. *Psychological Review, 96*, 101–124.

Levine, D. N., Warach, J., & Farah, M. J. (1985). Two visual systems in mental imagery: Dissociation of "what" and "where" in imagery disorders due to bilateral posterior cerebral lesions. *Neurology, 35*, 1010–1018.

Lezak, M. D. (1983). *Neuropsychological assessment* (2nd ed.). New York: Oxford University Press.

Luria, A. R. (1973). *The working brain*. New York: Basic Books.

Macaruso, P., Harley, W., & McCloskey, M. (1992). Assessment of acquired dyscalculia. In D. I. Margolin (Ed.), *Cognitive neuropsychology in clinical practice* (pp. 405–435). New York: Oxford University Press.

Margolin, D. I. (1984). The neuropsychology of writing and spelling: Semantic, phonological, motor, and perceptual processes. *Quarterly Journal of Experimental Psychology, 34a*, 459–489.

Margolin, D. I. (1991). Cognitive neuropsychology: Resolving enigmas about Wernicke's aphasia and other higher cortical disorders. *Archives of Neurology, 48*, 751–765.

Marslen-Wilson, W. D., & Welsh, A. (1978). Processing interactions and lexical access during word recognition in continuous speech. *Cognitive Psychology, 10*, 29–63.

Martin, R. C. (1987). Articulatory and phonological deficits in short-term memory and their relation to syntactic processing. *Brain and Language, 32*, 137–158.

Martin, R. C. (1990). Neuropsychological evidence on the role of short-term memory in sentence processing. In G. Vallar & T. Shallice (Eds.), *Neuropsychological impairments of short-term memory* (pp. 390–427). Cambridge, England: Cambridge University Press.

McClelland, J. L. (1979). On the time-relations of mental processes: An examination of systems of processes in cascade. *Psychological Review, 86*, 287–330.

McClelland, J. L., & Rumelhart, D. E. (1981). An interactive activation model of context effects in letter perception: Part 1. An account of basic findings. *Psychological Review, 88*, 375–407

McClelland, J. L., Rumelhart, D. E., & Hinton, G. E. (1987). The appeal of parallel distributed processing. In D. E. Rumelhart & J. L. McClelland (Eds.), *Parallel distributed processing*, (Vol. 1, pp. 3–44). Cambridge, MA: MIT Press.

McCloskey, M., Caramazza, A., & Basili, A. G. (1985). Cognitive mechanisms in number processing and calculation: Evidence from dyscalculia. *Brain and Cognition, 4*, 171–196.

McKoon, G., Ratcliff, R., & Dell, G. (1986). A critical evaluation of the semantic-episodic distinction. *Journal of Experimental Psychology: Learning, Memory and Cognition, 12*(2), 295–306.

Melton, A. W. (1963). Implications of short-term memory for a general theory of memory. *Journal of Verbal Learning and Verbal Behavior, 2*, 1–21.

Milberg, W. P., Hebben, N., & Kaplan, E. (1986). The Boston process approach. In I. Grant & K. M. Adams (Eds.), *Neuropsychological assessment of neuropsychiatric disorders* (pp. 65–86). New York: Oxford University Press.

Milner, B. (1971). Interhemispheric differences in the localization of psychological processes in man. *British Medical Bulletin, 27*(3), 272–277.

Mishkin, M., & Appenzeller, T. (1987). The anatomy of memory. *Scientific American, 256*, 80–89.

Monsell, S. (1984). Components of working memory underlying verbal skills: A "distributed capacities" view. In H. Bouma & D. G. Bouwhuis (Eds.), *Attention and performance X* (pp. 327–350). Hove, UK: Lawrence Erlbaum Associates.

Morrow, L. A., & Ratcliff, G. (1988). The disengagement of covert attention and the neglect syndrome. *Psychobiology, 16*(3), 261–269.

Mountcastle, V. B. (1978). Brain mechanisms of directed attention. *Journal of the Royal Society of Medicine, 71*, 14–27.

Papanicolaou, A. C., Deutsch, G., Bourbon, W. T., & Will, K. W. (1987). Convergent evoked potential and cerebral blood flow evidence of task-specific hemispheric differences. *Electroencephalography and clinical neurophysiology, 66*(6), 515–520.

Patterson, K., & Shewell, C. (1987). Speak and spell: Dissociations and word class effects. In M. Coltheart, R. Job, & G. Satori (Eds.), *The cognitive neuropsychology of language* (pp. 273–294). Hove, UK: Lawrence Erlbaum Associates.

Petersen, S. E., Robinson, D. L., & Morris, J. D. (1987). Contributions of the pulvinar to visual spatial attention. *Neuropsychologia, 25*(1A), 97–105.

Posner, M. I. (1978). *Chronometric explorations of mind.* Hillsdale, NJ: Lawrence Erlbaum Associates.
Posner, M. I. (1980). Orienting of attention. *Quarterly Journal of Experimental Psychology, 32*, 3–25.
Posner, M. I., & Boies, S. J. (1971). Components of attention. *Psychological Review 78*(5), 391–408.
Posner, M. I., & Cohen, Y. (1984). Components of attention. In H. Buoma & D. Bowhuis (Eds.), *Attention and performance X* (pp. 531–556). Hillsdale, NJ: Lawrence Erlbaum Associates.
Posner, M. I., Early, T. S., & Reiman, E. (1988). Asymmetries in hemispheric control of attention in schizophrenia. *Archives of general psychiatry, 45*(9), 814–821.
Posner, M. I., Inhoff, A., Friedrich, F. J., & Cohen, A. (1987). Isolating attentional systems: A cognitive–anatomical analysis. *Psychobiology, 15*, 107–121.
Posner, M. I., Petersen, S. E., Fox, P. T., & Raichle, M. E. (1988). Localization of cognitive operations in the human brain. *Science, 240*, 1627–1631.
Posner, M. I., Rafal, R. D., Choate, L. S., & Vaughan, J. (1985). Inhibition of return: Neural basis and function. *Cognitive Neuropsychology, 2*(3), 211–228.
Posner, M. I., Walker, J. A., Friedrich, F. J., & Rafal, R. D. (1984). Effects of parietal injury on covert orienting of attention. *The Journal of Neuroscience, 4*(7), 1863–1874.
Posner, M. I., Walker, J. A., Friedrich, F. J., & Rafal, R. D. (1987). How do the parietal lobes direct covert attention? *Neuropsychologia, 25*, 134–145.
Pylyshyn, A. (1973). What the mind's eye tells the mind's brain: A critique of mental imagery. *Psychological Bulletin, 80*, 1–24.
Rafal, R. D., Calabresi, P., Brennan, C., & Sciolto, T. (1989). Saccade preparation inhibits reorienting to recently attended locations. *Journal of Experimental Psychology: Human Perception and Performance, 15*(4), 673–685.
Rafal, R. D., & Henik, A. (1994). Inhibitory neural mechanisms for integrating controlled and automatic processes. In D. Dagenbach & T. Carr (Eds.), *Inhibitory processes in attention, memory and language* (pp. 1–50). New York: Academic Press.
Rafal, R. D., & Posner, M. I. (1987). Deficits in human visual spatial attention following thalamic lesions. *Proceedings of the National Academy of Science, 84*, 7349–7353.
Rafal, R. D., Posner, M. I., Friedman, J. H., Inhoff, A., & Bernstein, E. (1988). Orienting of visual attention in progressive supranuclear palsy. *Brain, 111*, 267–280.
Ratcliffe, G. (1979). Spatial thought, mental rotation and the right cerebral hemisphere. *Neuropsychologia, 17*, 49–54.
Riddoch, M. J. (1990). Loss of visual imagery: A generation deficit. *Cognitive Neuropsychology, 7*(4), 249–273.
Riddoch, M. J., & Humphreys, G. W. (1986). Neurological impairments of object constancy: The effects of orientation and size disparities. *Cognitive Neuropsychology, 3*(2), 207–224.
Roland, P. E., & Friberg, L. (1985). Localization of cortical areas activated by thinking. *Journal of Neurophysiology, 53*, 1219–1243.
Saffran, E., & Marin, O. (1977). Reading without phonology: Evidence from aphasia. *Quarterly Journal of Experimental Psychology, 29*, 515–525.
Saffran, E., & Martin, N. (1990). Neuropsychological evidence for lexical involvement in STM. In G. Vallar & T. Shallice (Eds.), *Neuropsychological impairments of short-term memory* (pp. 428–447). Cambridge, England: Cambridge University Press.
Saffran, E., Schwartz, M., & Marin, O. S. M. (1980). Evidence from aphasia: Isolating the components of a production model. In B. Butterworth (Ed.), *Language production* (pp. 221–241). London: Academic Press.
Salame, P., & Baddeley, A. D. (1982). Disruption of short-term memory by unattended speech: Implications for the structure of working memory. *Journal of Verbal Learning and Verbal Behavior, 21*, 150–164.
Schacter, D. (1992). Understanding implicit memory: A cognitive science approach. *American Psychologist, 47*(4), 559–569.
Schacter, D., & Tulving, E. (1982). Amnesia and memory research. In L. Cermak (Ed.), *Human memory and amnesia* (pp. 1–32). Hillsdale, NJ: Lawrence Erlbaum Associates.
Schneider, W., & Detweiler, M. (1987). A connectionist/control architecture for working memory. In G. Bower (Ed.), *The psychology of learning and motivation: Advances in research and theory* (Vol. 21, pp. 54–119). New York: Academic Press.
Schwartz, M., Marin, O., & Saffran, E. (1979). Dissociation of language function in dementia: A case study. *Brain and Language, 7*, 277–306.
Seron, X., & Deloche, G. (1989). *Cognitive approaches in neuropsychological rehabilitation*. Hillsdale, NJ: Lawrence Erlbaum Associates.
Shallice, T., & Warrington, E. (1970). Independent functioning of the verbal memory stores: A neuropsychological study. *Quarterly Journal of Experimental Psychology, 22*, 261–273.
Shelton, J., Martin, R. C., & Yaffee, L. S. (1992). Investigating a verbal short-term memory deficit and its

consequences for language processing. In D. I. Margolin (Ed.), *Cognitive neuropsychology in clinical practice* (pp. 131–167). New York: Oxford University Press.

Shepard, R. N., & Chipman, S. (1970). Second-order isomorphism of internal representations: Shapes of states. *Cognitive Psychology, 1*, 1–17.

Shimamura, A. (1986). Priming effects in amnesia: Evidence for a dissociable memory function. *Quarterly Journal of Experimental Psychology, 38A*, 619–644.

Shulman, G. L., Remington, R., & McLean, J. P. (1979). Moving attention through visual space. *Journal of Experimental Psychology: Human Perception and Performance, 5*, 522–526.

Springer, S. P., & Deutsch, G. (1985). *Left brain, right brain*. San Francisco: Freeman.

Squire, L. R. (1987). *Memory and brain*. New York: Oxford University Press.

Sternberg, S. (1966). High speed scanning in human memory. *Science, 153*, 652–654.

Sternberg, S. (1969). The discovery of processing stages: Extensions of Donder's method. *Acta Psychologica, 30*, 276–315.

Swanson, J. M., Posner, M. I., Potkin, S., Bonforte, S., Youpa, D., Fiore, C., Cantwell, D., & Crinella, F. (1991). Activating tasks for the study of visual–spatial attention in ADHD children: A cognitive anatomical approach. *Journal of Child Neurology, 6*, 119–127.

Tipper, S. P., Driver, J. S., & Weaver, B. (1991). Object-centered inhibition of return of visual attention. *Quarterly Journal of Experimental Psychology, 43A*, 289–298.

Treisman, A. M., & Gelade, G. (1980). A feature-integration theory of attention. *Cognitive Psychology, 12*, 97–136.

Tulving, E. (1972). Episodic and semantic memory. In E. Tulving & W. Donaldson (Eds.), *Organization of memory* (pp. 381–403). New York: Academic Press.

Tulving, E. (1985). How many memory systems are there? *American Psychologist, 40*(4), 385–398.

Tulving, E., Hayman, C. A., & McDonald, C. A. (1991). Long-lasting perceptual priming and semantic learning in amnesia: A case experiment. *Journal of Experimental Psychology: Learning, Memory and Cognition, 17*(4), 595–617.

Ungerleider, L. G., & Mishkin, M. (1982). Two cortical visual systems. In D. J. Ingle, M. A. Goodale, & R. J. W. Mansfield (Eds.), *Analysis of visual behavior* (pp. 549–586). Cambridge, MA: MIT Press.

Vallar, G., & Baddeley, A. D. (1984). Fractionation of working memory: Neuropsychological evidence for a phonological short-term store. *Journal of Verbal Learning and Verbal Behavior, 23*, 151–161.

Vallar, G., & Shallice, T. (Eds.). (1990). *Neuropsychological impairments of short-term memory*. Cambridge, England: Cambridge University Press.

Warrington, E., & McCarthy, R. (1983). Category specific access dysphasia. *Brain, 106*, 859–878.

Warrington, E., & Shallice, T. (1969). The selective impairment of auditory verbal short-term memory. *Brain, 92*, 885–896.

Warrington, E., & Shallice, T. (1984). Category specific semantic impairments. *Brain, 107*, 829–854.

Waugh, N. C., & Norman, D. A. (1965). Primary memory. *Psychological Review, 72*, 89–104.

Wood, F., Ebert, V., & Kinsbourne, M. (1982). The episodic–semantic distinction in memory and amnesia: Clinical and experimental observations. In L. Cermak (Ed.), *Human memory and amnesia* (pp. 167–194). Hillsdale, NJ: Lawrence Erlbaum Associates.

Wurtz, R. H., Goldberg, M. E., & Robinson, D. L. (1980). Behavioral modulation of visual responses in the monkey: Stimulus selection for attention and movement. *Progress in Psychobiology and Physiological Psychology, 9*, 43–83.

4

Forensic Neuropsychology

David A. Pritchard
Roosevelt Warm Springs Institute for Rehabilitation

Forensic neuropsychology may be defined as the use of neuropsychological knowledge and skills to help answer legal questions. It is not the drama of courtroom battle, the publicity of a celebrated case, "grace under fire" during cross-examination, the validation of one's professional worth through designation as an expert witness, nor the fight for "truth" and "justice." It is instead the sometimes dry and studied application of neuropsychological knowledge to the solution of narrow, sometimes esoteric, legal problems.

Forensic neuropsychology is a subspecialty of clinical neuropsychology and a subspecialty of forensic psychology. It is not, however, subsumed by either of these psychological specialties. It is not "lawyering," although its parameters are defined by existing law and it requires knowledge of legal rules. It is not "doctoring," although its application requires knowledge of neuropathology and neuropsychological assessment. Forensic neuropsychology is less than clinical neuropsychology and less than forensic psychology, but at the same time is more than either one.

This chapter explores the dimensions of forensic neuropsychology in an introductory way. The focus is on the conceptual underpinnings and not on the pragmatics of forensic neuropsychology.[1] First, forensic neuropsychology is distinguished from clinical neuropsychology. The legal aspects of expert witnesses in general are then reviewed, followed by a discussion of the unique aspects of neuropsychologists as expert witnesses. The substantive areas of law in which neuropsychologists are most likely to participate are surveyed and the training of forensic neuropsychologists is examined. A brief review of the issue of malingering is also included, because this issue is pervasive throughout forensic neuropsychology. Unique ethical problems facing forensic neuropsychologists are then discussed. Finally, future directions for the development of forensic neuropsychology as a specialty are suggested.

---

[1]Practical advice to psychologists and attorneys regarding trial testimony is offered by Brodsky (1992), Brown (1987), Faust, Ziskin, and Hiers (1991), and Wellman (1986).

DIFFERENCES BETWEEN CLINICAL AND FORENSIC NEUROPSYCHOLOGY

There are subtle, interrelated differences between clinical and forensic neuropsychology that affect the practice of both specialties. The most important distinctions include differences in goals, clients, referral questions, and decision processes.

The goal of clinical neuropsychology is to diagnose and treat neuropsychological problems in individual cases. The clinical neuropsychologist aims to assist clients in improving their functioning, either through direct rehabilitation or through accurate diagnosis and recommendations, which are in turn used by others to design and implement a plan of rehabilitation. In contrast, the goal of forensic neuropsychology is to provide information that may assist legal fact finders in resolving legal disputes. The forensic neuropsychologist is not involved in making final decisions regarding the client or in providing treatment services to the client; the aim here is not therapeutic or rehabilitative, but educational. This difference in goals leads to differences in diagnostic questions asked, in diagnostic data collected, and in diagnostic decisions made.

The recipient of the clinical neuropsychologist's efforts is the individual client and sometimes, by extension, the client's significant others. In contrast, the recipient of the forensic neuropsychologist's efforts is the attorney who hired the neuropsychologist or the fact finder (judge, jury, or both) who is responsible for resolving the legal dispute. This difference in recipient impacts directly on the evaluation of the relative costs of diagnostic errors that inevitably occur during neuropsychological assessment. When the recipient is the individual client (in clinical neuropsychology), the costs of incorrectly diagnosing or missing a central nervous system (CNS) dysfunction are evaluated from the client's point of view. What is the financial, psychological, and prognostic impact on the client of diagnosing a problem that does not exist or of misclassifying the type of problem? What are the various costs to the client of not receiving an accurate diagnosis or of not receiving beneficial treatment?

When the recipient is a legal fact finder (in forensic neuropsychology), the costs of assessment errors are evaluated from the fact finder's point of view. What are the costs to the adjudication process of communicating inaccurate or misleading neuropsychological information? What is the cost of misleading a judge or jury to deny compensation for an actual injury, compared with the cost of misleading a judge or jury to award damages for a nonexistent injury? These two points of reference usually do not produce identical cost estimates and may produce conflicting estimates. They may lead to differing decision rules (i.e., cut-off scores, inclusion criteria) for test interpretations. The neuropsychologist may tend to give the client the "benefit of the doubt" when test results are marginal, because it may be less costly to the client to treat a nonexistent or minor problem than to ignore it. In contrast, the forensic neuropsychologist may adopt stricter decision rules, because it may be less costly for a judge or jury to deny compensation for an actual injury than to award compensation for a nonexistent injury.

The referral questions in clinical neuropsychology typically involve treatment-related issues like diagnosis, prognosis, response to treatment, and recommendations for rehabilitation, placement, and support services. The answers to these practical questions lead to the development or revision of appropriate individualized service plans, which are implemented in whole or in part by the clinical neuropsychologist or by other professionals. In contrast, the referral questions in forensic neuropsychology focus on legally relevant issues that are not necessarily treatment-related. Some forensic questions are identical to clinical referral questions (e.g., Does the client meet the inclusion criteria for a particular diagnostic category?), whereas many forensic questions are nonclinical in nature (e.g., Did the client have the cognitive capacity at some past point in time to form the "mental intent" necessary to support a verdict of first-degree murder?). Regardless of whether or not the forensic question is similar to a clinical referral question, the purpose of the forensic question is not to improve the functioning of the client, but rather to assist some third party (the fact finder) in answering a legal question.

The differences between clinical and forensic neuropsychology in goals, clients, and referral questions are related to differences in the decision-making processes of clinical and forensic neuropsychologists. Both types of specialists use the same tests, techniques, and procedures to gather the information needed to answer their referral questions, but the conclusions, inferences, arguments, and recommendations based on that information may be decidedly different. It may appear paradoxical that the same set of valid tests and procedures can lead to different—even opposing—conclusions and recommendations, but the paradox is unraveled when validity is considered as a feature of "interpretations" rather than of "test scores" (Kane, 1992). According to this view, the meaning of a test score (or pattern of scores) is an argument (conclusion) with the test score as a premise and several more-or-less-credible assumptions as inferences. The resulting argument or conclusion is "credible" (valid) to the extent that the inferred assumptions are credible.

The reason that forensic conclusions may differ from clinical conclusions is that they frequently require different assumptions in order to be credible. For example, a particular pattern of test scores, demographic characteristics, and historical events may lead a clinical neuropsychologist to conclude that a client has suffered a mild head injury in an automobile accident which could improve with cognitive rehabilitation. A forensic neuropsychologist might conclude, based on the same data, that the evidence does not indicate a mild head injury that can be attributed to the automobile accident. This difference in conclusions is due to the differing assumptions made by the clinical and forensic neuropsychologists in interpreting the relevant data. The forensic neuropsychologist assumes, based on current liability law, that the conclusion that the automobile accident induced cognitive problems requires evidence of a *change* in cognitive functioning after the accident compared with before the accident. If such comparative evidence is lacking, the presumption is that the current cognitive problems preexisted the automobile accident. In contrast, the clinical neuropsychologist requires only that the current cognitive problems be *consistent* with a mild head injury caused by an automobile accident. Both neuropsychologists are "correct," even though their conclusions are diametrically opposed. The conclusion of the forensic neuropsychologist is constrained by the legal rule that a defendant will not be assessed damages for an injury without evidence that an injury (i.e., a change in cognitive functioning) actually occurred. The conclusion of the clinical neuropsychologist is not constrained by this legal rule and therefore is still "credible," even though it appears to be contradictory.

Finally, the conclusions of clinical and forensic neuropsychologists may differ because of the "finality" of their respective arguments. In clinical neuropsychology, assessment is usually an ongoing process in which impressions of a client are revised according to newly developed information. Initial impressions are constantly revised in light of new information; interpretations are modified as the results of evaluations by other specialists become available; treatment recommendations are modified in view of the client's response to current therapies. Both the diagnostic and rehabilitative decisions of the clinical neuropsychologist are generally revisable and reversible until the case is closed. In contrast, the forensic neuropsychologist typically has one opportunity to evaluate a client and must arrive at a final, irreversible judgment of the case, which is then handed over to others for their consideration. Although the forensic neuropsychologist will generally begin an evaluation in the same open-ended, hypothesis-testing, recursive mode as the clinical neuropsychologist, the forensic neuropsychologist must eventually formulate a final judgment of the case, which is presented once and for all to the legal fact finders involved. Once a deposition or testimony has been presented, it is extremely difficult (although not impossible) for the forensic neuropsychologist to amend conclusions, interpretations, and predictions.

In summary, clinical and forensic neuropsychology differ in their respective goals, clients, referral questions, and decision-making processes. These differences establish forensic neuropsychology as a practice specialty separate from clinical neuropsychology. Although the assessment procedures and knowledge base of clinical and forensic neuropsychology are similar, the practice of the two specialties is distinct and unique. The forensic neuropsychologist is more than a clinical neuropsychologist sitting in a courtroom.

THE ROLE OF EXPERT WITNESSES IN GENERAL

The law distinguishes between ordinary witnesses and expert witnesses. Ordinary witnesses are those who testify to things personally heard, seen, or otherwise observed (Cleary et al., 1972). Such witnesses may testify to observed facts and to limited inferences from those facts (e.g., identification of a person previously seen; appearance or apparent condition of a person at the time previously seen; mental condition of a person at the time previously seen; judgments of size, speed, weight, color, etc.; value of personally owned property; handwriting of familiar persons). In contrast, expert witnesses are those who testify to inferences from facts that are beyond the ability of the average layman to draw. Such witnesses need not have personal knowledge of the facts in a case, but must possess special knowledge that permits them to interpret available facts in a case.

The purpose of expert testimony is to assist the trier of fact in understanding complex sets of facts that are relevant to the legal questions in dispute. The opinions of expert witnesses are not intended to instruct the fact finder as to a "correct" verdict, but rather to provide him or her with an interpretation of facts that is not obvious to the average layman and that would assist in resolving the legal questions at hand. For example, expert opinion in a malpractice case regarding the customary procedure for conducting a neuropsychological evaluation would assist the fact finder in deciding whether or not the defendant's evaluation conformed to that standard. Expert testimony that a plaintiff who suffered a head injury could (or could not) benefit from cognitive rehabilitation would assist the judge and jury to assess damages in the case. The distinguishing features of expert opinions are that (a) they may be based on facts provided by others and (b) they are based on knowledge beyond that possessed by the average person.

The clinical/forensic neuropsychologist may serve as both an ordinary witness and an expert witness in the same case. The neuropsychologist may testify about the procedures employed in an evaluation, the scores, and other results of the evaluation and personal impressions developed during the evaluation. These statements are no different from those of an eyewitness to an accident or a crime. However, when the neuropsychologist testifies about the meaning of test scores, integrates test scores with the findings of other specialists, or offers diagnoses, prognoses, and recommendations, such statements are expert opinions that go beyond observed facts and require special knowledge.

Before a person is allowed to offer expert testimony, the witness' competence as an expert must first be established. Both federal and state rules require that the potential witness have sufficient skill, knowledge, or experience in a relevant science, profession, business, trade, or occupation. However, trial judges are provided wide latitude in deciding how much and what kind of training, experience, and knowledge are sufficient to qualify a witness as an expert. Professional credentials, years of experience, stature in the field, and number of research publications are all relevant to establishing one's qualification as an expert witness, but none of these factors alone are determinative. In general, the only formal requirement of a court's acceptance of a witness as an expert is the possession of any statutorily required licensure for the claimed profession. If a potential witness is licensed as a psychologist, then it is not an abuse of discretion for a trial judge to allow that psychologist to testify about neuropsychology regardless of the psychologist's specialization (or lack thereof).[2]

Once a witness has been qualified as an expert, the various opinions offered by the witness in the course of testimony are subject to objection and exclusion. The mere fact that a witness is qualified as an expert does not provide carte blanche to state any opinion on any question. Expert opinions must fall within the jurisdiction's rules of admissibility. For example, the Nebraska Supreme Court ruled in *Sanchez v. Denby* (1989) that a trial court had abused its discretion in excluding a neuropsychologist's opinion about the cause of brain damage: "Any questioning of the basis for the neuropsychologist's opinion should go to its weight and credibility, not to its admissibility."[3] However, the Georgia Supreme Court ruled in *Chandler Exterminators, Inc. v. Morris* (1992) that "a psychologist is not qualified to render an opinion concerning a diagnosis of a mental disorder when such disorder requires a professional opinion as to a physical disorder—here, organic brain damage."[4]

Assuming that a professional has been qualified as an expert witness and the subject matter of the professional's opinions are admissible, the question arises as to the degree of confidence that the professional must have in the opinions before those opinions may be accepted as evidence. The degree of confidence with which ordinary witnesses express their observations or opinions determines how much weight the fact finder should attach to the testimony, but does not determine the admissibility of the testimony. An eyewitness who is only slightly confident in the identification of a perpetrator will generally be allowed to testify, although such testimony will not be very persuasive. In contrast, expert witnesses must generally meet or exceed some minimal level of confidence in their opinions before their testimony is even admissible. This threshold level of confidence is usually defined as a *professional certainty* (Hoge & Grisso, 1992), although this term by itself provides little practical guidance to the professional in evaluating potential opinions. At one extreme is the opinion based on a mere possibility (e.g., "It is possible that exposure to this neurotoxin causes cognitive deficits"), and at the other extreme is the opinion based on certitude (e.g., "I am certain that this type of gunshot wound causes cognitive deficits"). The question is where to draw the line between mere possibility and reasonable probability.

Some professionals confuse this minimal level of confidence with the standard of proof required for resolution of the ultimate legal questions by the judge or jury. Some legal proceedings require the judge and jury to base their verdict on a preponderance of the evidence, some require a finding by clear and convincing evidence, and some require evidence beyond a reasonable doubt. These legal thresholds are the standards that the fact finder must use in evaluating *all* the evidence in a case to resolve the *ultimate* questions in the case. They are not the standards required before an expert's opinions may be admitted as evidence.[5] Some professionals confuse professional certainty with empirical accuracy. They

---

[2]In jurisdictions whose psychology licensing law is a "title protection" rather than a "practice protection" act, nonlicensed professionals may be permitted to testify as experts in psychology or neuropsychology so long as they do not call themselves "psychologists." For example, an art therapist may be allowed to render personality descriptions based on drawings so long as the witness sidesteps the title of psychologist. In addition, the *Ethical Principles of Psychologists and Code of Conduct* of the American Psychological Association (1992) limit psychologists to offering opinions only in those areas in which the psychologist is competent.

[3]Credibility is the weight assigned to any particular witness or statement by the trier of fact. It is the subjective evaluation by the judge/jury of the importance of a piece of evidence when considered in the context of all available evidence.

[4]In 1993, the Georgia Legislature remedied this restriction on neuropsychologists' testimony by revising the state's Psychology Licensing Act to include neuropsychological diagnosis and etiology in the definition of the practice of psychology.

[5]See Grisso and Appelbaum (1992, p. 626 and note 7) for a similar discussion of clinical certainty in making predictions of future violence.

argue that expert opinions are inadmissible unless they are "pretty likely accurate" (Faust & Ziskin, 1988, p. 32). However, no legal rules of evidence require a test of the empirical accuracy of an expert's opinions before those opinions may be accepted as evidence (Black, 1988). Although there must be some empirical foundation for the expert's opinion (mere speculation is inadmissible regardless of the expert's degree of confidence), there is no legal requirement that the expert's conclusions meet some minimal level of accuracy. Even opinions that are "more likely wrong than right" (such as predictions of future dangerousness) may be admissible as evidence (e.g., *Barefoot v. Estelle,* 1983). The empirical accuracy of expert opinions affects the weight given the testimony by the judge and jury but does not affect its admissibility.

Professional certainty is not the standard of proof required for a verdict by a fact finder and is not the degree of empirical accuracy of the expressed opinions. It is "the degree of confidence the clinician places in his or her opinion" (Hoge & Grisso, 1992, p. 70). In general, courts have wide latitude in defining the minimal confidence threshold for admissibility of expert opinions:

> Some courts have required an intermediate standard of "reasonable probability" which has been defined as "that standard of persuasion that is in quality sufficient to generate the belief that the tendered hypothesis is, in all human likelihood, the fact." In admitting testimony of cause–effect relationships, courts may require that the witness state that the alleged events did in fact produce the effect; other courts may permit proof that the alleged events might, could, or would have caused the effect. (Schwitzgebel & Schwitzgebel, 1980, p. 240)

In practical terms, the threshold of professional certainty occurs when the professional believes that the opinion is "more likely correct than not"; that is, the expert is at least 51% confident of the correctness of the opinion. However, in particular jurisdictions or in particular types of cases, courts may require a higher degree of confidence than this minimum.

The end result of any expert's testimony is that it may be totally disregarded by the fact finder in resolving the ultimate legal questions. Expert opinions are merely advisory and never determinative. Even when experts unanimously agreed that a defendant was "legally insane" at the time of the commission of a homicide, the jury was free to ignore their opinions and to return a verdict of guilty beyond a reasonable doubt (e.g., *Davasher v. Arkansas,* 1992; *Ellis v. Alabama,* 1990).

In summary, an expert witness is one who is qualified by a court to render opinions on subjects that are beyond the knowledge of the average layman. Both state and federal courts have wide latitude in deciding the minimum qualifications of expert witnesses. Jurisdictions also vary regarding the subject matter on which opinions may be offered by qualified expert. The expert witness must be at least 51% confident of the opinions expressed, but may be required by particular courts to be more certain than this minimal level. Any expert testimony may be totally disregarded by the fact finder in a case.

THE ROLE OF NEUROPSYCHOLOGISTS AS EXPERT WITNESSES

There is considerable controversy in both legal and psychological circles regarding appropriate rules of admissibility for neuropsychological opinions. Faust et al. (1991; see also Faust, 1991) have argued that current methods and procedures in neuropsychology lack sufficient reliability and validity to assist courts in answering neuropsychologically related legal questions. For example, they cited studies showing that neuropsychological tests are less accurate in detecting brain damage in a sample of "subtle" cases than in samples of "obvious" cases. They contended that current neuropsychological procedures do not permit accurate classification of current everyday functioning or prediction of future functioning, and they alleged that neuropsychological evaluations are subject to undetectable faking or malingering. Neuropsychologists are said to be incapable of the kinds of complex, subjective integration of data that is claimed in their reports and in their testimony. They challenged the reliability, validity, standardization and norms of frequently used neuropsychological tests and procedures. In brief, they claimed that neuropsychological practice is too unscientific to form an acceptable basis for courtroom testimony.

In response, critics point out that Faust and colleagues have selectively reviewed the available research and have ignored that literature that upholds neuropsychological practice (Matarazzo, 1990). Indeed, Faust et al. (1991) themselves stated in the preface to their book that "there is literature which is not contained in this book that is supportive of forensic neuropsychology" (p. xv). Barth, Ryan, and Hawk (1992) have argued that much of the literature cited by Faust et al. is not relevant to questions about the neuropsychologist's ability to use clinical judgment in individual cases. In addition, they cited recent studies that address concerns with norms, actuarial interpretations, and predictions of everyday functioning.

This debate among neuropsychologists regarding the sufficiency of current neuropsychological practice is part of the process of normal science. Criticisms of particular procedures or techniques lead to clarifications and revisions and to the development of new technologies. Such debate is necessary for the ordinary development of the profession. However, it is largely irrelevant to the legal question of the admissibility of neuropsychological opinions in testimony. The fact that clinical neuropsychology is not a fully developed technology does not mean that neuropsychological opinions should be excluded from testimony in court. The weaknesses of current neuropsychological methods, when properly acknowledged by the neuropsychologist-as-witness, are matters of credibility that may affect the weight accorded the neuropsychologist's testimony by the fact finder, but are not matters of admissibility that should preclude the testimony per se.

Confusion regarding the admissibility of neuropsychological testimony arose and has persisted because of the adoption by federal courts of the *Frye* test. The Court ruled in *Frye v. U.S.* (1923) that, in order for an expert opinion to be admissible, the methodology on which the opinion is based "must be sufficiently established to have gained general acceptance in the particular field to which it belongs" (p. 1014). The requirement of "general acceptance" has led some neuropsychologists and some courts to evaluate whether or not particular neuropsychological tests, procedures, or practices meet current scientific standards of reliability and validity. To the extent that techniques and procedures do not meet current standards, opinions based on those methods would be inadmissible. This has had the effect of reducing the legal question of admissibility to the scientific question of acceptability. However, in *Daubert v. Merrell Dow Pharmaceuticals* (1993), the U.S. Supreme Court ruled that the *Frye* test was now superseded by Rule 702 of the Federal Rules of Evidence, which states:

> If scientific, technical, or other specialized knowledge will assist the trier of fact to understand the evidence and to determine a fact in issue, a witness qualified as an expert by knowledge, skill, experience, training or education, may testify thereto in the form of an opinion or otherwise.

In *Daubert:*

> The majority of the Court emphasized that it is the responsibility of federal judges to review expert evidence to insure that it rests on a reliable foundation and is relevant to the case. In performing this function the Court suggested that the following factors should be used in

> considering the admissibility of expert testimony: (a) whether it has been tested using some accepted scientific methodology, (b) whether it has been subject to peer review and publication, (c) whether the known or potential rate of error of the scientific technique justifies its use, (d) whether it has achieved a degree of acceptance within the scientific community. The Court emphasized that these were *factors* to be considered and that the essential question is scientific validity within the context of the issues presented by a particular case. The Court also recognized that this is a "flexible" standard. Finally, the Court expressed its view that "vigorous cross-examination, presentation of contrary evidence, and careful instruction on the burden of proof" are sufficient to deal with bad scientific evidence that is presented to a judge or jury. (Smith, 1993, p. 2)

Under *Daubert* there is no longer any requirement that the methods on which expert opinion is based be "generally accepted" in the field. Under this new rule, federal trial courts will have greater latitude than previously in admitting expert testimony. For forensic neuropsychologists this may mean the admissibility of opinions based on single-case studies, on "less-than-perfect" tests, and, perhaps, on clinical experience.

Rule 702 of the Federal Rules of Evidence, however, applies only to federal courts and tribunals. State courts and tribunals are governed by their own rules of evidence and local case law that probably differ in general and most likely also differ in detail from their federal counterparts. These local rules may be found in the state's code of statutes under the general title of evidence, in the published rules of the state's supreme court, and in case reporters of the state's appellate and supreme courts. In addition, a jurisdiction's criminal law, psychology licensing statute, worker's compensation rules, and Social Security disability rules may contain other restrictions that further define the admissibility of expert opinions in particular forums or on particular questions. Daniell (1987) provided an introduction to the use of law libraries for legal research on local rules, although more detailed treatises may be necessary for thorough research (e.g., Cohen, Berry, & Olson, 1989; Kunz, Schmedemann, Bateson, Downs, & Erlinder, 1992). In addition, the *Mental and Physical Disability Law Reporter,* published by the American Bar Association, provides national coverage of recent state and federal court rulings relevant to neuropsychological cases.

Richardson and Adams (1992; see also Rothke, 1992) presented a recent survey to state rules of admissibility for three neuropsychological questions: (a) the presence/absence of brain damage, (b) the cause of brain damage, and (c) the prognosis for future problems caused by brain damage. Of the 11 states whose courts had considered the question of admissibility of neuropsychologists' opinions on the existence of brain damage and on the cause of brain damage, all had approved their admissibility.[6] Of the three states that had considered the question of prognostic opinions, all three had approved their admissibility. However, it is important to recognize that only one of these states involved a ruling by the state's Supreme Court (see Richardson & Adams, 1992, for details). Therefore, all of the remaining rulings are subject to review and possible reversal by the jurisdiction's highest court. Furthermore, the rulings of a local jurisdiction are not precedents in other jurisdictions and are not necessarily good indicators of how other jurisdictions would rule when presented with their own unique cases.

Although it is tempting to leave questions of admissibility to attorneys and judges, there is

---

[6]Richardson and Adams (1992) cited the case of *Chandler Exterminators, Inc. v. Morris* (1991) as supportive of the admissibility of neuropsychologists' opinions on the cause of brain damage. However, this ruling was reversed by the Georgia Supreme Court (416 S.E.2d 277; Ga. Sup. Ct. 1992). Subsequently, the Georgia Legislature passed amendments to the state's psychology licensing law that specifically authorized psychologists to diagnose the existence and etiology of organic mental disorders. Because this new law did not take effect until July 1, 1993, no Georgia court has yet had the opportunity to rule on the admissibility of expert opinions based on this expanded scope of practice.

no substitute for careful study by the neuropsychologist-as-expert-witness of the jurisdiction's statutory, regulatory, and case law restrictions on neuropsychological testimony. Indeed, it is forensic neuropsychologists' ability to articulate neuropsychological knowledge within the requirements of law that distinguishes them from clinical neuropsychologists. First, knowledge of the applicable rules of evidence (and of substantive law, which is discussed in the next section) in a particular case helps the forensic neuropsychologist to educate the client (attorney or judge and jury) regarding which referral questions can be properly answered through a neuropsychological evaluation and which would require mere speculation. Attorneys and judges or juries have particular questions to answer and particular points to argue. They understandably want the neuropsychologist-as-expert-witness to answer these questions as unequivocally as possible. They also have a layman's understanding of the complexities of brain–behavior relationships and want to simplify these complexities in terms that they can understand.

Only the neuropsychologist is in the position to distinguish professional opinions from mere speculations, and to resist inducements to testify beyond one's professional limits. For example, a young man was injured in an automobile accident and claimed to have suffered both cognitive deficits and damage to his potential career as a professional baseball player. Discussion with his attorney clarified that a neuropsychological evaluation could address the claim of cognitive declines, but that neuropsychologists have no expertise in assessing *potential* success as a professional baseball player. Any opinion on injury to his potential as professional baseball player would be mere speculation and therefore would be inadmissible in any jurisdiction.

Second, knowledge of applicable rules of admissibility helps the forensic neuropsychologist to formulate explicitly the assumptions underlying expert opinions. For example, an actuarial prediction that a person would function best in a sheltered workshop requires, among other things, the assumption that the person is similar in essential respects to the sample of subjects on whom the actuarial method was derived. Is *unpublished* data of this kind admissible as a basis for the expert opinion? If not, one of the essential links between the neuropsychologist's evaluation of the person and the expert opinion is missing.

Third, knowledge of rules of admissibility helps the neuropsychologist to collect properly during the neuropsychological evaluation the data needed to support any expert opinions. For example, do the rules of admissibility permit an expert to base an opinion, even in part, on the work of a third party (e.g., a radiologist, a neuropsychological technician)? If not, the expert would need to gather comparable data from an admissible source.

In summary, although rules of admissibility regarding expert opinions are basically legal-procedural issues, they impact directly on the role that neuropsychologists can play in the legal system. They place limits on the types of referral questions that neuropsychologists can properly address in court and restrict the opinions that may be expressed to those whose implicit assumptions are supported by admissible data. Finally, they define the types of data that may be used as the basis for expert opinions.

COMMON TYPES OF QUESTIONS IN FORENSIC NEUROPSYCHOLOGY

The ultimate issues addressed in legal proceedings are questions of substantive law. Substantive questions ask whether or not the evidence presented is sufficient to find that the required legal elements of the case have been proven. These required legal elements vary according to the specific claims made in each case, but they may be broadly classified into questions of *criminal law,* questions of *civil law,* and questions of *administrative law.* Ultimate questions in criminal law ask whether the prosecution has presented evidence sufficient to prove

TABLE 4.1
Legal Questions Potentially Involving Neuropsychological Testimony

- Criminal law
  - Admissibility of confessions
  - Competence to stand trial
  - Competence to be executed
  - Criminal responsibility
- Civil law
  - Competence to assert a timely claim
  - Competence to make a will
  - Competence to make a contract
  - Competence to manage one's affairs
    - Guardianship
    - Need for involuntary treatment
  - Competence to parent
  - Competence to testify
  - Personal tort
    - Neuropsychological injury
    - Neuropsychological prognosis
  - Professional malpractice
    - Standard of care
    - Neuropsychological injury
- Administrative law
  - Social Security
  - Veterans Administration
  - Vocational rehabilitation
  - Workman's compensation

beyond a reasonable doubt that the required elements of the criminal charges were present at the time of the alleged offense. Ultimate questions in civil law ask whether the plaintiff has presented evidence sufficient to prove by a preponderance of the evidence or by clear and convincing evidence that the required elements of the civil complaint are present. Ultimate questions in administrative law ask whether the appellant has presented evidence to prove by a preponderance of the evidence that the required criteria for administrative benefits are satisfied.

To complicate matters further, however, each of these ultimate questions may involve subsidiary questions that entail different standards of proof and different burdens of persuasion. For example, in all jurisdictions, the prosecution in a criminal case must prove the required elements of the charged crime beyond a reasonable doubt. In some jurisdictions, however, the defense must prove an insanity defense beyond a reasonable doubt, whereas in other jurisdictions the defense must only prove by a preponderance of the evidence that the defendant met the legal criteria for "insanity," at which point the prosecution must prove beyond a reasonable doubt that the defendant was in fact legally sane.

This section does not discuss all the variations of criminal, civil, and administrative questions. Rather, it briefly describes those ultimate or subsidiary questions of substantive law that are most likely to involve the expert testimony of neuropsychologists. Table 4.1 lists these legal questions.

Questions of Criminal Law

In criminal law, almost all questions potentially involving neuropsychological testimony are questions of "competence." Does the person have sufficient cognitive capacity to render a voluntary confession, to testify as an ordinary witness, to participate effectively in one's own defense, to be held responsible for criminal conduct, or to be executed? The question for the neuropsychologist is whether the person has neuropsychological impairment so severe that the usual legal presumption of competence should be suspended and, perhaps, that the usual legal outcomes should not accrue. For example, the "confession" to police given by a stroke victim with severe receptive and expressive aphasia was suppressed by the court and the criminal charge of murder against him was dropped for lack of other evidence. A defendant who shot himself in the head after killing a policeman was found incompetent to stand trial because of his current inability to remember the evidence presented against him during trial. A death-row inmate with severe dementia was found incompetent to be executed because he could not appreciate the reasons for his execution.

A confession to a crime is usually admissible as evidence only if the suspect's waiver of Miranda rights was "voluntarily," "knowingly," and "intelligently" made (e.g., *Miranda v. Arizona,* 1966; *In re Gault,* 1967). Whether or not a confession is admissible is usually determined by the court on the basis of the "totality of the circumstances" surrounding the confession, including (a) the suspect's age, intelligence, education, amount of prior experience with the police, and physical and mental condition; (b) the characteristics of the interrogation by the police; and (c) the availability to the suspect of assistance by counsel, parents, or friends (*Fare v. Michael C.*, 1979). Of particular interest to the neuropsychologist is the suspect's cognitive functioning at the time of the confession. Did the suspect have sufficient language functions to understand the literal meaning of the Miranda warning? Did the suspect have sufficient reasoning ability to appreciate the consequences of waiving the right to silence and to assistance of counsel? Did the suspect have sufficient reasoning ability to evaluate alternative courses of action and to choose rationally among them? Did the suspect have sufficient mnestic ability to recall accurately the essence of the warnings? Neuropsychological deficits that impair these basic communicative, mnestic, and executive functions are relevant circumstances that affect the suspect's ability to "knowingly" and "intelligently" waive Miranda rights. It is unconstitutional for police interrogators to play on a suspect's cognitive deficits in order to obtain a confession (*Blackburn v. Alabama,* 1960).

Neuropsychologists may need to pay special attention to the case in which cognitive deficits increase a suspect's susceptibility to leading questions and negative feedback by police interrogators (e.g., Gudjonsson, 1987). However, the U.S. Supreme Court (*Colorado v. Connelly,* 1986) has limited the requirement that confessions be "voluntary" to questions of whether the police used coercion to obtain the confession. The fact that a suspect is "compelled" by a mental disorder (e.g., a delusion) or a neuropsychological deficit (e.g., confusion) to confess to a crime does not make the confession "involuntary" and therefore inadmissible. Grisso (1986, chapter 6) presented a discussion of issues and techniques in evaluating the circumstances of confessions.

A defendant's competence to stand trial is the most frequently raised question in criminal cases (Steadman, Monahan, Hartstone, Davis, & Robbins, 1982). In some cases the question is raised by legitimate concerns about the defendant's current mental state; in other cases, the question is raised because it may be the only way for the defense to obtain a court-ordered evaluation of the defendant that may be used to raise other legal questions (e.g., admissibility of a confession, legal insanity, mitigating circumstances). The question of competence to stand trial addresses whether the defendant has "sufficient present ability to consult with his lawyer with a reasonable degree of rational understanding," and whether the defendant has a "rational as well as factual understanding of the proceedings against him" (*Dusky v. U.S.*, 1960).[7] The mere existence of a mental disorder is insufficient to find that a defendant is

[7]In *Godinez v. Moran* (1993), the U.S. Supreme Court ruled that this same legal standard defines the minimal level of competence required for pleading guilty or waiving the right to counsel.

incompetent to stand trial. The mental condition must be so severe that it interferes with the defendant's present ability to assist counsel in a defense or to understand the criminal proceedings.

Grisso (1986, chapter 5) discussed court rulings and legislative acts that further specify what is meant by incompetence to stand trial. For the neuropsychologist, competence to stand trial involves questions about the communicative, cognitive, mnestic, and executive functions of the defendant during preparation for trial and during the trial itself. Does the defendant have the capacity to communicate with defense counsel? Can the defendant "track" the evidence presented at trial and compare it to personal recollections of events so as to inform counsel of inconsistencies and inaccuracies? Does the defendant have the ability to testify personally at the trial?[8] Of frequent concern to neuropsychologists is a defendant's inability, due to intoxication or traumatic amnesia, to recall circumstances surrounding the alleged criminal act (e.g., Schacter, 1986). In general, amnesia for the alleged crime is not by itself a basis for finding a defendant incompetent to stand trial (e.g., *United States v. Wilson,* 1966), particularly when there is admissible evidence (e.g., eyewitness testimony, videotape evidence) that the defendant committed the criminal act. Grisso (1986, chapter 5; 1988) presented practical guidelines for conducting evaluations of competence to stand trial.

Whether or not a defendant should be held legally responsible for proven criminal acts is the subject of legal defenses. Among the most controversial available legal defenses to criminal behavior is the "insanity defense," which argues that the defendant was so mentally disordered at the time of the criminal act that no criminal responsibility should be ascribed to the defendant. Jurisdictions differ in the availability of the insanity defense, in their respective definitions of what constitutes insanity, and in their respective burdens of persuasion (American Bar Association, 1983; Brakel, Parry, & Weiner, 1985). However, in all jurisdictions that recognize the insanity defense, the diagnostic question is the same: Did the defendant have a psychological incapacity *at the time of the alleged offense* which produced a condition that falls within the scope of the jurisdiction's definition of legal insanity? The question always involves a postdiction of the diagnostic status of the defendant at the time of the criminal behavior and an argument that this diagnosed condition produced a mental state which is, according to local definition, "legally insane." In federal courts, for example, the definition requires that "at the time of the commission of the acts constituting the offense, the defendant, as a result of a mental disease or defect, was unable to appreciate the nature and quality of the wrongfulness of his acts" (18 U.S.C. 20). The requirement of a "mental disease or defect" calls for a post hoc diagnosis; the requirement that the defendant was "unable to appreciate the nature and quality of the wrongfulness of his acts" calls for an argument that the diagnostic condition produced this required mental state. For neuropsychologists, the question is not simply whether the defendant suffered a diagnosable CNS dysfunction at the time of the criminal act, but also whether this dysfunction was of a type and severity to produce the requisite mental state.

Both the post hoc diagnosis and the argument of its effect on the mental state of the defendant require relevant evidence in order to be valid ("credible"). In a case involving the appeal of a death-row inmate for a new trial, a neuropsychologist argued in an affidavit that the inmate had struck his head on a curb as a child, that his current scores on the Tactual Performance Test (TPT) were impaired, that he was therefore brain damaged, that at the *time of the homicide* this "brain damage" caused him to be unable to judge his degree of alcohol intoxication, that his intoxication was therefore involuntary, and that this "involuntary" intoxication should relieve him of criminal responsibility. It may be questioned whether a

[8]The question here is not whether the defendant *wants* to testify or *should* testify, but whether the defendant has the *capacity* to testify.

mild head injury experienced long before the alleged homicide and impairment on the TPT long after the alleged homicide constitutes evidence that the inmate was "brain damaged" at the time of the homicide. It may be further questioned whether the existence of "brain damage" by itself constitutes evidence of pathological intoxication. Finally, there is no argument by the neuropsychologist that the defendant's intoxication produced the mental state specified in the jurisdiction's definition of insanity. This neuropsychologist's arguments lack supporting data and are therefore untenable.

In jurisdictions that do not recognize the insanity defense, and in some other jurisdictions as well, the defense may still argue that a defendant's mental condition at the time of the alleged offense precluded formulation of the specific mental intent required by the charged offense (Clark, 1987). In most crimes "criminal intent" (*mens rea*) is inferred from the illegal act itself (*actus reus*). For example, if a defendant was discovered inside someone else's house with their jewelry in his pocket, no additional evidence is needed that he intended to steal the property. However, some crimes include in their definitions specific mental elements that must be proved in addition to proof of the criminal act. For example, most jurisdictions distinguish between a premeditated, intentional homicide and an impulsive or negligent homicide. The distinguishing feature is the existence of a mental state of intentionality. If the defense can offer evidence that the defendant, by reason of a mental disorder, lacked the capacity to form this required intentionality, then the defendant can only be found guilty of the less serious offense of negligent homicide or manslaughter. Challenging the capacity of a defendant to form requisite intentionality is called the *mens rea* defense. The diagnostic questions for the neuropsychologist in this type of case are the same as in the case of the insanity defense. Did the defendant have at the time of the offense a diagnosable CNS dysfunction? Did this dysfunction produce a state of mind that rendered the defendant incapable of formulating the requisite mental elements of the charged crime?

Both the insanity defense and the *mens rea* defense exclude voluntary intoxication, regardless of its severity, as a mental disorder that will relieve a defendant of criminal responsibility. The law assumes that because the intoxication was initially voluntary, the defendant intends all the subsequent consequences of the intoxication, even though the intoxication becomes so severe that mental incapacity is obvious. However, "involuntary" intoxication (which is locally defined in case law and statutes) does constitute a mental disorder for purposes of the insanity or *mens rea* defense. It is unsettled in law whether a defendant who voluntarily decides to stop taking prescribed medication is similarly assumed to intend the consequences of this noncompliance. Is the noncompliant defendant responsible for inducing the mental state that would otherwise qualify as an insanity or *mens rea* defense?

Once a person has been convicted of a crime and sentenced to prison, the law requires that the prison system afford the inmate necessary medical care (Cohen & Dvoskin, 1992; *Estelle v. Gamble,* 1976). However, only some jurisdictions have defined medical care to include psychological and neuropsychological treatment, and even fewer jurisdictions have defined medical care to include desirable (as opposed to necessary) treatment (Brakel et al., 1985). Therefore, inmates with neuropsychological deficits may or may not have the right to neuropsychological diagnosis and treatment, depending on where they are incarcerated. However, in all jurisdictions with the death penalty, there is a prohibition against execution of the insane inmate. Neuropsychologists may be asked to evaluate death-row inmates who are suspected of having a mental disorder so severe that the nature and purpose of the punishment cannot be appreciated. A related question is the competence of death-row inmates to waive their right to appeal their death sentence. In *Rees v. Peyton, Penitentiary Superintendent* (1966), the U.S. Supreme Court ruled that an inmate could not withdraw appeal of a death sentence if there existed a mental disorder that substantially affected the inmate's capacity to appreciate his position or to make a rational choice regarding further litigation. Although these issues may seem macabre, they arise with regularity in states where opponents of the death penalty are well organized and intent on blocking further executions.

Questions in Civil Law

In civil law, cases potentially requiring neuropsychological testimony variously involve legal questions of *competence, tort liability,* and *malpractice.* As in criminal law, most civil cases require a diagnosis of a CNS deficit *plus* an argument that this deficit produces a state of affairs which is defined by applicable law. For example, in a case of neurotoxin exposure, the question for the neuropsychologist is whether or not a CNS deficit exists at the time of testing that did not exist before exposure to the toxin. In cases of neuropsychological malpractice, however, the focus is not on alleged neuropsychological damage by a claimant, but on the conduct of the neuropsychologist. A neuropsychological witness may be asked to describe the accepted or customary practice of clinical neuropsychology, which the fact finder may use as a standard against which to evaluate the conduct of the defendant–neuropsychologist. The neuropsychological witness may also be asked to opine whether the defendant–neuropsychologist's behavior "caused" the injury claimed by the plaintiff.

All jurisdictions have defined statutes of limitations which require that legal actions be commenced within a prescribed period of time following the accrual of the cause of action. If the statute of limitations expires without filing of the civil action, then the action is barred. Statutes of limitations may vary within a jurisdiction according to the subject matter of the statute (e.g., product liability, negligence, battery). They also may vary from jurisdiction to jurisdiction for the same subject matter. In addition, there are differences in the definition of the "accrual" of the cause of action. Some jurisdictions define accrual as the actual date of the wrongful conduct; some define it as the date on which the plaintiff discovered or should have discovered the injury resulting from the wrongful conduct; still others use a hybrid definition which specifies accrual from the date of discovery of an injury provided that such discovery occurs within a limited period of time from the date of the injury.

Finally, some jurisdictions have defined exceptions to their usual statutes of limitations that toll (suspend) the statute of limitation in particular circumstances. Of interest to the neuropsychologist is the exception for a plaintiff "of unsound mind." For example, a young man suffered a head injury in a fall and was subsequently administered a major tranquillizer by an emergency room physician who thought he was on drugs. He consequently suffered a stroke and went into a coma. When he emerged from the coma, he was partially paralyzed on the left side and exhibited some cognitive deficits. However, he did not file a malpractice suit against the emergency room physician until well after the expiration of the statute of limitations. The task for the neuropsychologist was the determination of the time when the plaintiff had regained sufficient capacity after emerging from his coma to define "accrual of the cause of action." At what point did the plaintiff regain sufficient cognitive functioning that he should have recognized his wrongful injury, and was the lawsuit filed within the statute of limitations from that date of recovery? This general question in civil law is referred to as "competence to file a timely claim" and arises most often in cases of severe neuropsychological impairment.

Other competencies in civil law include competence to make a will, competence to make a contract, competence to manage one's affairs, and parenting competence. With the increasing mean age of Americans, neuropsychologists can expect to encounter an increase in claims that neuropathological conditions such as dementia render older citizens incapable of issuing a valid will or contract, or incapable of caring for themselves or their dependents. In order for a will to be valid, the testator must generally have sufficient capacity to "understand the nature of the testamentary act, understand and recollect the nature and situation of his or her property, and remember and understand his or her relations to his or her living descendants, spouse, and parents, and those whose interests are affected by the will" (Spar & Garb, 1992, p. 169). In addition, the testamentary act must be free of "undue influence" that subjects the testator's mind to another's, that destroys the testator's free agency, or that overpowers the testator's volition. In order for a contract to be enforceable, the promisor must generally have sufficient cognitive capacity to understand the nature, purpose, and effect of the transaction (95 A.L.R. 4th 1442) or to act in a reasonable manner (Restatement [Second] of Contracts 15). In addition, the contract is voidable if the promisor was vulnerable to the influence of the promisee and the promisee used excessive pressure in overcoming the will of the promisor (Eisenberg, 1986, p. 91). For the neuropsychologist, the question is whether or not the testator/promisor suffered at the time of issuing the legal instrument a neuropsychological deficit sufficiently severe to satisfy the local jurisdiction's definition of incompetence. The mere existence of a severe neuropsychological deficit is usually insufficient to prove incompetence; evidence is normally required that the deficit affected the person in precisely those respects defined by local law.

Questions of incapacity to manage one's own affairs or to care for a dependent (i.e., parenting) are somewhat more amorphous than are questions of testamentary or contractual incapacity. In the past, a mere diagnosis of mental disorder was often sufficient to justify curtailment of a person's right to make personal decisions about one's life, including decisions about "the termination of life-support systems; sterilization; voting; the termination of parental rights; divorce; medical diagnostic procedures; and selecting an attorney" (Parry, 1984, p. 29). More recently, courts and legislatures have tried to balance explicitly the wishes and best interests of mentally disordered persons (Anderer, 1990). Under early guardianship laws incompetent persons were stripped of all personal decision-making rights, but the modern trend is to limit substituted or involuntary decision making to just those areas of functioning that are adversely affected (e.g., Commission on the Mentally Disabled, 1989; Saunders & Simon, 1987). For example, in most jurisdictions, persons who have been involuntarily committed to mental institutions now retain their rights to vote, to consent to medical treatment, to refuse medications, and to make contracts unless they have been explicitly found to be incompetent to exercise one of those rights (e.g., Brakel et al., 1985; Parry & Beck, 1990). The challenge for the forensic neuropsychologist is to keep abreast of the evolving local legal standards of civil incompetence as defined in commitment laws, guardianship statutes, and family law. In general, the forensic neuropsychologist must gather evidence that (a) the person currently suffers from a neuropsychological disorder and (b) the legal criteria are satisfied for involuntary commitment to a mental institution, for involuntary administration of medication or other treatment, for third-party decision making, or for termination of parental rights.

The area of civil law most frequently identified with the practice of forensic neuropsychology is *tort* law. A tort is simply damage suffered through the negligent or intentional act(s) of another person. In forensic neuropsychology, examples include CNS injuries caused by another's negligent operation of a motor vehicle, by another's intentional discharge of a firearm, or by another's negligent handling of a neurotoxin. In order for a plaintiff to prevail in a tort action, three elements must be proved: (a) the defendant owed a legal duty to the plaintiff, (b) the defendant breached that duty, and (c) the plaintiff suffered damage as a proximate result of that breach.[9] These necessary elements, therefore, exclude cases where no duty existed between the defendant and plaintiff (e.g., where a plaintiff was exposed to a neurotoxin after trespassing into a restricted area), or where the plaintiff suffered no damages

[9]Intentional torts, such as battery, defamation, and invasion of privacy, require that additional elements be proved.

as a result of a defendant's negligence (e.g., a child defendant was negligently diagnosed as "brain damaged," but the report was lost and the child was placed in regular school classes anyway). In most cases, however, the existence of each of the three elements is a matter of dispute and is subject to proof by the plaintiff.

Tort cases are further complicated by legal questions about the "foreseeability" of the harm caused by the defendant's behavior (i.e., Could or should the defendant have predicted the harm suffered by plaintiff?), by the existence of intervening causes of the damage over which the defendant had no control, by any behavior of the plaintiff that contributed to either the breach of duty or the damage caused thereby, by the plaintiff's consent to defendant's actions, by any assumption of risk by the plaintiff (i.e., Did the plaintiff knowingly accept the risk of damage?), and by questions about the extent of damages. The task for the forensic neuropsychologist is to address the question of the presence of CNS dysfunction and any one (or more) of the legal questions: (a) legal duty, (b) breach of duty, (c) damage as a proximate result, (d) "foreseeability" of harm, (e) causation, (f) extent of damages, (g) consent, (h) contributory negligence, or (i) assumption of risk.

It is beyond the scope of this chapter to discuss the legal complexities of tort actions, except to emphasize that the forensic neuropsychologist's role in tort cases involves more than testimony about the existence of a neuropsychological deficit that appears to be caused by someone else's behavior. It is critical for the forensic neuropsychologist to understand the legal concepts of duty, breach of duty, causation-in-fact, proximate causation, and damages. What appears reasonable and sensible to one who is not a lawyer is not necessarily what is acceptable under local rules of tort law. Introductory reviews to tort law may be found in various law school textbooks, in West Publishing Company's *Nutshell* series of legal texts and in *Gilbert's Law Summaries*. More detailed information about local rules can be obtained in consultation with knowledgeable attorneys. West and Knowles (1991) also reviewed issues and procedures in estimating the costs of care and loss of earnings for brain-damaged victims.

A special case in civil law is professional liability or malpractice law. Physicians, psychologists, attorneys, and other professionals are generally regarded as owing a duty of care to clients once a professional relationship has been established. This duty of care may give rise to torts when that duty is breached through negligence. However, breach of duty is only one legal basis for claims of "malpractice." "Liability may also result, for example, from intentional misconduct, breaches of contracts guaranteeing a specific therapeutic result, defamation, invasions of privacy . . . and failures to prevent injuries to certain non-patients" (King, 1977, p. 4). Malpractice complaints may therefore involve hybrid claims involving tort law, contract law, mental disability law, and professional regulations.

When a claim is based on tort law, it is necessary to prove that (a) the defendant-professional owed a duty of care to the plaintiff (i.e., a professional relationship existed), (b) the defendant's behavior deviated from the accepted standard of care owed to clients of such professionals, and (c) the defendant suffered damage as a proximate result. The element that distinguishes the professional tort from other torts is the necessity of establishing by evidence a professional standard of care which the fact finder can use to judge the defendant's conduct. In cases where the defendant is a neuropsychologist, forensic neuropsychologists may be called on to testify about accepted or customary practices in clinical neuropsychology, about published professional standards of conduct or about limitations in neuropsychological knowledge and techniques—all to establish a standard of care against which a defendant-neuropsychologist's behavior can be evaluated. In addition, a forensic neuropsychologist may be asked to evaluate the former client of a clinical neuropsychologist in order to establish any damages suffered as a consequence of the latter's malpractice. This task would require the difficult responsibility of distinguishing preexisting neuropsychological deficits from those new deficits that were caused by the malpractice.

Questions of Administrative Law

Administrative law is concerned with resolving disputes over eligibility for special services and benefits. Original dispositions of applications for Social Security disability benefits, for Veterans Administration services and benefits, for vocational rehabilitation services, and for worker's compensation benefits are all subject to appeal to administrative tribunals or special courts. Each program's tribunals employ their own rules for establishing eligibility and for considering evidence. For example, Social Security and some worker's compensation programs restrict eligible disabilities to specified diagnostic categories, whereas rehabilitation and Veterans Administration services do not. In addition, each service imposes differing nondiagnostic restrictions on eligibility. For example, Social Security disability and Veterans Administration pension benefits require a complete inability to engage in gainful employment; rehabilitation services require the potential for gainful employment; Veterans Administration programs require for some services that the disability be service connected; worker's compensation benefits require that the disability be employment connected. Finally, the services differ in the jurisdictional scope of their rulings. Social Security and Veterans Administration services are federally defined and operated; rehabilitation services are defined federally and operated by the states; worker's compensation services are defined and operated by the states.

The existence of these diverse legal rules and regulations transforms clinical neuropsychological evaluations for any of these services into forensic neuropsychological evaluations. The neuropsychologist must conform the evaluation to the procedures and techniques the particular service and must conform conclusions to the legal criteria of that service. To do otherwise is to risk losing any appeal on grounds that the admissible evidence does not support the service's definition of eligibility. The Social Security Administration (1992) provides guidelines for conducting Social Security disability determinations. Decisions regarding veterans' benefits are typically made by Veterans Administration personnel and are appealable to special federal courts established to handle veterans' claims.

MALINGERING/DISSIMULATION

A pervasive issue in forensic psychology in general and forensic neuropsychology in particular is the detection of dissimulation. Whenever there is a personal cost or benefit to a client resulting from a neuropsychological evaluation, the possibility of exaggerated, minimized, or fabricated deficits must be considered. The threat of imprisonment or execution, the prospect of financial compensation, or the chance of rehabilitative, therapeutic, or other services may motivate a person to concoct or magnify a disability. The desire for release from an institution or from other restrictions may induce a person to deny or minimize the severity of personal deficits. In forensic cases, these external inducements to dissimulation are nearly always present and therefore the prevalence of dissimulation in legal contexts has often been assumed to be higher than in clinical evaluations.

In addition to the presence of legal disputes, the *Diagnostic and Statistical Manual* (3rd ed., rev.) (DSM–III–R) (American Psychiatric Association, 1987) supports a diagnosis of malingering whenever there is a medicolegal evaluation involving several of these elements: a discrepancy between a person's claimed distress/disability and objective findings, a client who is not cooperative with the evaluation, or a client who can be diagnosed with antisocial personality disorder. The problem with this definition is that it focuses exclusively on the exaggeration or fabrication of symptoms and ignores the minimization or denial of symptoms. This latter condition may occur in legal contexts where the absence of pathology is beneficial (e.g., parole hearings, hospital release hearings) or where an intermediate severity of pathology is desirable (e.g., eligibility for rehabilitation services). In addition, it focuses exclusively on a single type of personality disorder (antisocial personality), instead of viewing dissimulation as an adaptive response that characterizes all human beings (e.g., Lewis & Saarni, 1993; Rogers & Cavanaugh, 1981).

At present, available neuropsychological tests do not include built-in validity scales or other checks for accurate performance. The *Halstead–Reitan Neuropsychological Battery* (Reitan & Wolfson, 1985), the *Luria–Nebraska Neuropsychological Battery* (Golden, Hammeke, & Purisch, 1980), the Benton Laboratory series of tests (Benton, Hamsher, Varney, & Spreen, 1983), and frequently used individual neuropsychological tests (e.g., *Wechsler Adult Intelligence Scale–Revised,* Wechsler, 1981; *Wechsler Memory Scale–Revised,* Wechsler, 1987) all assume a cooperative, "truthful" subject for their proper interpretation. Therefore, some clinicians and researchers have proposed various internal test signs or patterns that directly suggest dissimulation. Others have developed specialized tests or procedures to collect information regarding performance distortions based on the assumption that suspicious performance on these special tests implies suspicious performance on neuropsychological tests.

Rogers (1988) and Hall and Pritchard (1996) have reviewed the extant literature on detection of dissimulation in both clinical and forensic settings. Both reviews include chapters on detection of neuropsychological dissimulation. Rogers, Harrell, and Liff (1993) identified six strategies for the detection of feigned cognitive and neuropsychological deficits: (a) failure on very simple items, (b) differential performance on easy versus difficult items, (c) higher incidence of approximately correct answers ("near misses") compared to clearly incorrect answers, (d) below chance performance on two-alternative choice tasks (i.e., "symptom validity testing"), (e) inconsistent performance on parallel, repeated, or similar tests, and (f) unexpected presence/absence of psychological or psychometric correlates of neuropsychological deficits. In addition, Hall and Pritchard (1994) emphasized the importance of behavior in day-to-day, nontest situations that is inconsistent with obtained test results. These detection strategies vary in their current frequencies of research validation, but all hold promise for further development.

Most of the recent attention to performance distortion has focused on "malingering," that is, the false production of signs and symptoms of pathology. Little attention has been given to the minimization of signs and symptoms of genuine deficits. In neuropsychology, the assumption is often made that test subjects cannot generate performances of which they are incapable. If a person has a genuine deficit in executive functioning, then it should not be possible to perform well on neuropsychological tests of planning, set shifting, or inhibition of interference. This is probably true in the extreme. However, CNS dysfunction rarely produces all-or-nothing neuropsychological deficits. It therefore may be possible for test subjects to improve their test performances through mobilization of atypical motivation and attention beyond what would be expected based on their "true" level of impairment. This relative improvement in test performance may lead to overestimates of everyday functioning where the increased motivation and attention is either not present or cannot be sustained. For example, some schizophrenic patients are able to improve their performance on the Wisconsin Card Sorting Test when they are provided with feedback and monetary incentives (e.g., Summerfelt, Alphs, Wagman, & Funderburk, 1991), although this improvement typically is not retained after the incentives are withdrawn (Van der Does & Van den Bosch, 1992). This minimization of actual deficits is most likely to occur in contexts where the client is motivated to "appear well" (e.g., qualified for employment, eligible for rehabilitation, ready for institutional release) and on tests that collect small samples of behavior or that have low ceilings. However, there is currently no available research on the detection of denial or minimization during neuropsychological evaluations.

Another problem in forensic neuropsychology is the difficulty of interpreting information about dissimulation. On the one hand, it is not possible to conclude that a client is *not* exaggerating or *not* minimizing neuropsychological deficits. The absence of signs of dissimulation may mean that the client has successfully misled the evaluator. The most that can be said in such cases is that there is *no evidence* that a client is distorting test results. On the other hand, when there is evidence of dissimulation during an evaluation, are any of the evaluation results salvageable? What kind of conclusions are possible when there exists *any* evidence of dissimulation? How does the neuropsychologist distinguish between "true" test results and "distorted" test results?

The risk of dissimulation in forensic neuropsychology is probably greater than in clinical neuropsychology. However, the development of accurate techniques for detecting dissimulation has only recently garnered research attention. A general theory of dissimulation and guidelines for interpreting evidence of dissimulation are currently not available. In spite of these limitations, the neuropsychologist-as-expert-witness can safely assume that questions about dissimulation will be asked during cross-examination.

QUALIFICATIONS AND TRAINING OF FORENSIC NEUROPSYCHOLOGISTS

The unique responsibilities of forensic neuropsychologists obviously require specialized training. Some knowledge of and skill in clinical neuropsychology and forensic psychology is necessary for acceptable performance as a forensic neuropsychologist. The questions are how much knowledge and skill is minimally necessary for professional practice and who should define the minimal standards.

It is clear that each trial court has wide latitude in qualifying professionals as expert witnesses. Although education and training, credentials, relevant experience, membership in professional associations, and publications are all indicia of expertise, trial courts are free to define individually the minimal threshold for any or all of these criteria. In some cases, psychologists with no formal neuropsychological training may be acceptable to the court; in other cases, trained neuropsychologists may be disqualified from testifying. The only limitation on a court's qualification of neuropsychologists as expert witnesses appears to be the requirement of licensure in those jurisdictions that limit the practice of psychology to licensed persons.

The establishment and enforcement of minimal standards for forensic neuropsychology is primarily the responsibility of the profession rather than of the courts. Neuropsychology has offered a definition of the neuropsychologist and recommendations for professional training in neuropsychology, but no formal guidelines have been offered for the practice of neuropsychology. Forensic psychology has offered guidelines for practice but has provided no official recommendations for training. The Division of Clinical Neuropsychology of the American Psychological Association (Division 40, 1989) has defined a *clinical neuropsychologist* as (a) a doctoral-level provider, (b) who has completed both classroom and clinical coursework in neuropsychology and neuroscience at a regionally accredited university, (c) who has successfully completed 2 years of supervised training in clinical neuropsychology, (d) who is licensed to practice psychology in the local jurisdiction, and (e) whose competence has been reviewed by peers. Certification by the American Board of Clinical Neuropsychology or the American Board of Professional Psychology (in clinical neuropsychology) is the clearest evidence that these criteria have been satisfied (Bieliauskas & Matthews, 1987, 1990). The American Psychology–Law Society (Division 41 of the American Psychological Association) has not defined comparable minimal standards for forensic psychologists. However, they have defined specialty guidelines for the practice of forensic psychology (Division 41, 1991). Because these guidelines are useful for all practitioners who practice forensic psychology, not just those who regularly practice as forensic psychologists, they are included in the appendix to this chapter.

The problem with these professional standards is that they are unenforceable. If a licensed psychologist wishes to practice clinical neuropsychology without minimal training or certification, there are no regulatory bodies with the authority to restrict the practice. State psychology licensing laws are typically generic, permitting the practice of psychology without regard for specialty. The only restrictions on specialty practice are (a) *Principle A: Competence of the Ethical Principles of Psychologists and Code of Conduct* (American Psychological Association, 1992), which admonishes psychologists to "provide only those services and use only those techniques for which they are qualified by education, training or experience" (p. 3), and (b) *Ethical Standard 1.04a* of the *Ethical Principles,* which similarly restricts psychologists to providing services "within the boundaries of their competence, based on education, training, supervised experience, or appropriate professional expertise" (p. 4). Even these principles and standards are unenforceable in a particular jurisdiction unless the local psychology licensing law incorporates the *Ethical Principles* into its statutory language and the licensing board is willing to promulgate minimal standards of education, training, and experience for various specialties. In actual practice, the only method of enforcing minimal standards for clinical neuropsychology or forensic neuropsychology is the malpractice suit brought against practitioners who violate professional "standards of care."

In spite of the lack of enforceable minimal standards for the practice of clinical neuropsychology or forensic neuropsychology, these two specialties have defined recommended standards for education and training. The International Neuropsychological Society and Division 40 of the American Psychological Association have jointly published recommended curricula and training for clinical neuropsychologists at the predoctoral, internship, and postdoctoral levels (INS–Division 40, 1987). The American Psychology–Law Society (Division 41 of the American Psychological Association) has not adopted a similar "official" set of guidelines for training and education in forensic psychology. However, Poythress (1982) offered a model curriculum for such training and Melton (1987) provided recommendations for current training programs in forensic psychology.

Because forensic neuropsychology is a hybrid of clinical neuropsychology and forensic psychology, neither specialty has recommended standards for their members who wish to practice in both areas. It appears that most psychologists who wish to practice in a specialty area different from their original training obtain their training from workshops and personal study—a practice that has been decried by both neuropsychological and forensic specialists (INS–Division 40, 1987; Melton, 1987). However, because forensic neuropsychology is practiced in the courtroom, it will be the courts and not the profession that effectively sets minimal standards for the practice of forensic neuropsychology. Of course, forensic neuropsychologists who have been qualified by a court as an expert witness may have their credibility challenged to the extent that they do not meet both the prevailing standards of clinical neuropsychology and forensic psychology.

ETHICAL CONSIDERATIONS IN FORENSIC NEUROPSYCHOLOGY

Beyond the minimal standards needed for legal qualification as an expert witness and the variable standards affecting their credibility as witnesses, responsible psychologists subscribe to the ethical standards of the profession (American Psychological Association, 1992) and to various special standards adopted by the American Psychological Association or its subdivisions (e.g., the *General Guidelines for Providers of Psychological Services,* American Psychological Association, 1987; the *Specialty Guidelines for the Delivery of Services,* American Psychological Association, 1981; the *Guidelines for Providers of Psychological Services to Ethnic, Linguistic and Culturally Diverse Populations,* American Psychological

Association, 1990; the *Record Keeping Guidelines*, American Psychological Association, 1993; the *Standards for Educational and Psychological Tests and Measurements*, American Psychological Association, 1985), and the *Specialty Guidelines for Forensic Psychologists* (Division 41, 1991).[10] These standards and guidelines represent the profession's efforts to deal with ethical concerns and dilemmas that arise in the practice of psychology.

Forensic neuropsychology is faced with several unique ethical problems that are not shared by other specialties in psychology. This section discusses three of these problems: (a) limitations of competence and practice, (b) role conflicts, and (c) truthfulness of testimony.

Limitations of Competence and Practice

The *Specialty Guidelines for Forensic Psychologists* (Division 41, 1991) states:

> III. Competence
>
> A. Forensic psychologists provide services only in areas of psychology in which they have specialized knowledge, skill, experience, and education.
>
> B. Forensic psychologists have an obligation to present to the court, regarding the specific matters to which they will testify, the boundaries of their competence. (p. 659)

In order to practice forensic neuropsychology ethically, how knowledgeable and skilled in neuropsychology should the forensic psychologist be? How experienced and educated in forensic psychology should the neuropsychologist be? Should forensic neuropsychologists be held to the educational standards of clinical neuropsychology and to the practice guidelines of forensic psychology? Clinical neuropsychologists and forensic psychologists are unlikely to agree on general answers to these questions. However, Guideline III.B. may provide a case-by-case standard for evaluating the ethical practice of forensic neuropsychology. The key phrase is ". . .regarding the specific matters to which they will testify. . . ." In some cases the legal questions are framed in such a way that broad expertise in clinical neuropsychology may not be required. For example, because amnesia for a criminal act is insufficient by itself to find a defendant incompetent to stand trial, extensive knowledge and skill in assessing mnestic difficulties may not be necessary to answer this legal question.

Similarly, questions of criminal responsibility, competence to confess, competence to testify, competence to make a will or enter a contract, and competence to manage one's affairs or the need for involuntary treatment may be so defined as to require a functional impairment that does not need a clinical neuropsychologist to detect. For example, functional illiteracy—whether due to cerebral dysfunction, poor schooling or poor motivation—may be the critical factor in challenging a person's competence to contract. Even if a forensic psychologist "misses" the correct diagnosis of more subtle deficits that a clinical neuropsychologist could detect, the legal conclusion remains the same. In other cases, a client may be manifesting such a severe degree of impairment that knowledge of legal subtleties is unnecessary for a legal conclusion. For example, a clinical neuropsychologist may diagnose a dementia of such severity that it would undoubtedly meet any legal definition of contractual capacity. Both the forensic psychologist and the clinical neuropsychologist may be ethically

[10]Note that the *Guidelines for Computer-Based Tests and Interpretation*, as modified by Division 40 (1986) of the American Psychological Association, (APA) has been withdrawn recently by APA and will be reissued in the future. At the present time, APA has no guidelines regarding the use of computers in psychological practice. However, Division 40 of APA has issued guidelines for the use of computer-assisted neuropsychological rehabilitation and cognitive remediation that are independent of APA's original guidelines and that presumably remain in effect today (Matthews, Harley, & Malec, 1991).

practicing within their respective areas of competence when addressing extreme questions in forensic neuropsychology.

However, is it likely that the practitioner will not know the clinical and legal parameters of a forensic case until after the referral has been accepted? What should happen if the legal questions asked of a clinical neuropsychologist exceed knowledge, skill, and experience? What should a forensic neuropsychologist do when confronted with legal questions that require subtle, refined neuropsychological assessment? In the long run, the appropriate course of action would involve acquiring the necessary forensic or neuropsychological knowledge, skills, and experience. In the instant case, however, the practitioner could consult with an appropriate expert, request a second opinion from an expert, or refer the case to an expert in both forensic and clinical neuropsychology. Sometimes consultation with an attorney or a forensic psychologist is all that is needed to supply lacking information about legal rules and practices. In other cases, a forensic psychologist may want to ask a clinical neuropsychologist to review a case or even to conduct a separate evaluation and then (local rules of evidence permitting) to base legal opinions and testimony on their collaborative findings. Finally, the practitioner could refer the case to a colleague who is knowledgeable and skilled in both forensic and clinical neuropsychology. The keys to handling these ethical problems are (a) knowledge of one's own limitations and (b) collaboration on a case-by-case basis with colleagues who complement those limitations.

Role Conflicts

The *Guidelines* (Division 41, 1991) state:

> IV. Relationships
>
> D. Forensic psychologists recognize potential conflicts of interest in dual relationships with parties to a legal proceeding, and they seek to minimize their effects.
>
> 1. Forensic psychologists avoid providing professional services to parties in a legal proceeding with whom they have personal or professional relationships that are inconsistent with the anticipated relationship. (p. 659)

For the neuropsychologist who evaluates or treats a client in the course of clinical practice, a conflict of interest may arise if the practitioner is subsequently asked or compelled to testify as an expert witness regarding that client. If the clinical relationship is ongoing, the neuropsychologist may be hesitant to testify about data or impressions that might undermine the client's motivation for treatment or relationship with the clinician. If the case is closed, the neuropsychologist may not have collected data relevant to the current legal questions or to questions about malingering. In either case, the neuropsychologist's role shifts from clinician to expert witness and the attendant decision rules and processes should change from "client-centered" to "court-centered." The clinician's duty and allegiance to the client may conflict with the new duty to the court. In such cases, the *Guidelines* clearly state that the dual relationship should be avoided.

This type of dilemma may be avoided if the clinician clearly defines the limits of the professional relationship at the outset. If the client (or representative) originally enlists the neuropsychologist's services as a potential expert witness or if the clinician reasonably anticipates that litigation may occur in the case, the neuropsychologist should clarify the relationship as "forensic" and should inform the client that the purpose of the evaluation is to perform an objective assessment that may or may not be helpful to client's case. If the practitioner's services were originally secured for clinical purposes, the client should be informed that any subsequent litigation would necessitate a referral to another professional for a forensic evaluation. If the neuropsychologist is compelled by subpoena to testify regarding a clinical case, the neuropsychologist-as-witness should clarify for the court that the relationship is clinical and that a forensic evaluation was not conducted. Testimony should be limited to clinical findings, clinical diagnosis, clinical prognosis, and treatment recommendations. Opinions on disputed legal questions (e.g., future employability, past mental state, causation) should be avoided.[11] The key to handling this ethical problem is clearly defining for all concerned the nature and limitations of the professional relationship.

Truthfulness of Testimony

The Guidelines (Division 41, 1991) state:

> VII. Public and Professional Communications
>
> D. When testifying, forensic psychologists have an obligation to all parties to a legal proceeding to present their findings, conclusions, evidence, or other professional products in a fair manner. This principle does not preclude forceful representation of the data and reasoning upon which a conclusion or professional product is based. It does, however, preclude an attempt, *whether active or passive,* to engage in partisan distortion or misrepresentation. Forensic psychologists do not, *by either commission or omission,* participate in a misrepresentation of their evidence, nor do they participate in partisan attempts to avoid, deny, or subvert the presentation of evidence contrary to their own position. (p. 664, emphasis added)

Some expert witnesses get caught up in the adversarial nature of litigation. They believe that they have been hired by one party to a controversy and that they are expected to "fight" for their side. This partisanship is dictated in part by the procedures involved in litigation. First, the expert is cautioned not to talk to the opposing side unless counsel is present. Second, the expert's written report is kept hidden until compelled to be shared. Finally, at trial the witness is first directly examined by "compatriots," then cross-examined by the "enemy," then redirected by "compatriots," and finally recrossed by the "enemy." The nature of litigation emphasizes secrecy, "surprise attacks," "stealth," "tactics," "sparring," and other adversarial practices. In part, this bias is dictated by the all-or-none, winner-take-all nature of many legal decisions. The role of the fact finder is to resolve legal questions one way or the other, not to wallow in the "shades of grey" that characterize real life.

This adversarial system leads some expert witnesses to believe that they, too, are partisans who must use concealment, disguise, and distortion to help their side "win." There exists a small group of unethical expert witnesses who will testify in any case for either side on any question. They are able to find some evidence that is supportive of their position; they are willing to present that evidence as if it were complete and objective; they are willing to conceal contrary evidence unless specifically asked by opposing counsel. They justify their partisanship on the grounds that they are not lying and that they are obligated only to answer the questions asked of them.

The proper role for the expert witness, however, is not that of advocate but of educator. Even when the witness has been hired by one party to the legal dispute, the job of the witness is to educate the fact finder regarding findings and conclusions that bear on the legal questions at hand. This means acknowledging that those findings and conclusions are not nearly so clear-cut as the adversaries would like. It means admitting the limitations of one's knowledge and skills and of available techniques and methods. It also means conceding that some facts in the case are supportive of opposing arguments and conclusions. The key to

[11] It is always acceptable for an expert witness to state that no opinion has been formed on a particular question. Although a practitioner may be compelled to testify, no expert witness can be compelled to express a professional opinion.

avoiding unethical partisanship is complete truthfulness that eschews both lies of omission and lies of commission.

A more subtle question than partisanship is the adequacy of the scientific basis for an expert opinion. What is the minimal scientific/professional basis needed ethically to render an expert opinion? Is it sufficient to have seen a few clients in private practice all of whom shared a common characteristic that forms the basis for an expert opinion? Is reliance on the unpublished data or reports of other professionals an ethically acceptable basis for an expert opinion? Is the unreplicated published report of a single case study adequate to support an expert opinion? How does one evaluate the conflicting results of published group studies in order to find the scientific basis for an expert opinion?

These are not easily answered questions in forensic neuropsychology where controversy abounds regarding the proper methods of study in neuropsychology and the best techniques for assessment in clinical neuropsychology. In neuropsychology, debate continues whether the study of brain–behavior relationships is best pursued in single case studies or in group comparisons (e.g., Marshall & Newcombe, 1984; McCloskey, 1993; Robertson, Knight, Rafal, & Shimamura, 1993; Shallice, 1979). In clinical neuropsychology, assessment methods include empirical–normative (e.g., Halstead–Reitan Neuropsychological Battery; Benton Laboratory tests), theoretical–normative (e.g., Luria–Nebraska Neuropsychological Battery), theoretical–clinical (e.g., Kaplan, Fein, Morris, & Delis, 1991), and clinical–process (e.g., Luria) approaches. This variety hardly provides sure footing for the forensic neuropsychologist who must defend the choice of assessment methods and the soundness of conclusions.

It is important, however, in considering the ethics of expert opinions based on various clinical and research methods, to distinguish between scientific debate over proper methods and ethical condemnation of particular methods. It is possible to disagree vigorously over the proper methods of study in neuropsychology and the optimal methods of assessment in clinical neuropsychology without accusing opponents of unethical practice. Perhaps the best approach is similar to that adopted by some courts in regard to the admissibility of expert opinion: It is ethically permissible for a forensic neuropsychologist to base an expert opinion on a disputed fact or controversial method provided that the limitations are made public. As the U.S. Supreme Court stated in *Daubert* (1993), "vigorous cross-examination, presentation of contrary evidence, and careful instruction on the burden of proof" (p. 4805) will illuminate the strengths and weaknesses of an expert's methods and conclusions.

SUMMARY AND FUTURE DEVELOPMENTS IN FORENSIC NEUROPSYCHOLOGY

Forensic neuropsychology is a hybrid specialty whose parameters are defined in part by local law and in part by current neuropsychological knowledge and methods. Although both forensic psychology and clinical neuropsychology may lay claim to forensic neuropsychology, it is synonymous with neither. The practicing forensic neuropsychologist must be knowledgeable of applicable law and legal procedure, as must the forensic psychologist, and must be knowledgeable of neuropsychology and clinical methods, as must the clinical neuropsychologist. Whether or not a professional is recognized as an expert in forensic neuropsychology is ultimately a question for the courts to decide; whether or not an expert's testimony is persuasive is ultimately a question for the fact finder to decide. Forensic neuropsychology's responsibility is to prepare practitioners to serve as knowledgeable, skilled, and unbiased practitioners.

Unfortunately, neither forensic psychology nor clinical neuropsychology has met this responsibility. Training programs and continuing education in forensic psychology do not typically prepare their students to conduct adequate neuropsychological evaluations. Although knowledgeable in law and general clinical practice, most forensic psychologists lack sufficient education in clinical neuropsychology. Training programs and continuing education in clinical neuropsychology have typically focused on the appearances of forensic neuropsychology to the exclusion of its substance. Clinical neuropsychologists are frequently advised about courtroom demeanor and cross-examination tactics, but are rarely taught how to do legal research, how to evaluate a court ruling, or how to translate legal concepts into clinical terms. Both specialties bring to the courtroom their own strengths which are, by themselves, inadequate to the task.

The usefulness and viability of forensic neuropsychology depends entirely on the link between clinical neuropsychology and law. Forensic neuropsychology will develop and prosper only to the extent that it provides valid and meaningful answers to legal questions. Valid answers are those that are "highly plausible, given all available evidence" (Kane, 1992, p. 527). In this sense, validity is equivalent to the legal concept of "probative value," which is that aspect of evidence that "tends to prove an issue" (Black, 1981, p. 1160). Meaningful answers are those that are related to a legally contested matter. In this sense, meaningfulness is equivalent to the legal concept of "relevancy," which is that aspect of evidence that makes it "applicable in determining the truth and falsity of the matters in issue" between litigants (Black, 1981, p. 1160).

The relevancy of neuropsychological testimony in legal forums is beyond question. This chapter has outlined in broad terms the variety of legal questions to which forensic neuropsychology may contribute meaningful answers. The current controversy involves the extent to which such answers are valid or plausible. Do the answers offered by forensic neuropsychologists point to singular interpretations of available facts to the relative exclusion of competing interpretations?

The greatest threat to the validity of forensic neuropsychological testimony is the current gap between neuropsychological data and conclusions regarding impairment, disability, or incompetence. A proper neuropsychological evaluation and a correct neuropsychological diagnosis are usually insufficient for forensic purposes. Abnormal test scores, pathognomonic signs, neurological diagnoses, and even tangible lesions do not, by themselves, imply the functional impairment, handicap, or incapacity that is usually the ultimate concern of the courts.

Several developments in clinical neuropsychology would help to bridge this threatening gap. First, many current neuropsychological tests are inadequately scaled to permit cross-test comparisons and consensual interpretation. Some published test norms are based on too small or unrepresentative samples to justify statements about the relative probability of various test scores in the general population.[12] Extreme test scores on such tests are subject to the rival interpretations of "abnormality" versus "unrepresentativeness." Some derived test scores (e.g., *T* scores) are linear transformations of skewed raw score distributions and comparisons of extreme test scores are therefore distorted by unequal test score variances. A *T* score of 90 on a scale may represent a ceiling effect or a low difficulty level in the particular test rather than a "true" abnormality in the neuropsychological function being measured (e.g., Mortensen & Gade, 1992). Finally, most neuropsychological test scores contain no information regarding the relative severity of abnormal test scores. A score at the 99th percentile of the general population is interpretable as either extreme normal variation or severe impairment.

Russell (1987) advocated construction of a reference scale that is based on the combined distributions of normal and brain-damaged subjects, but is anchored in the normal sample. First, brain-damaged subjects' test scores are converted to *z* scores based on the mean and

[12]Such reference-group norms still have limited utility in permitting comparisons across tests, because scores on the subtests can all be interpreted in reference to a common scale derived on the same sample. Such comparisons may provide the basis for "profile analysis" without providing information about the abnormality of the profiles.

standard deviation of normal subjects' test scores; each subject's *z* scores are then averaged across all the administered tests to produce a distribution of average *z* scores (the reference scale); finally, the reference scale scores are used to predict the raw scores of each administered test. This procedure has the effect of producing equal-interval score distributions for each of the tests in which low scores represent the performance of normal subjects and higher scores represent the increasingly abnormal scores of brain-damaged subjects. In forensic neuropsychology, this is precisely the type of information which is needed to argue that abnormal test scores actually represent impairment.

Another approach to increasing the validity of neuropsychological testimony is the development of regression equations to predict "everyday functioning" from neuropsychological test results (Heaton & Pendleton, 1981). For example, McCarron and Dial (1986) developed a battery of neuropsychological tests that were subsequently used to predict residential placement (e.g., institutional vs. group vs. independent living) and vocational outcomes (e.g., sheltered vs. supported vs. competitive employment) of mentally retarded persons (Dial, Freeman, McCarron, & Swearington, 1979; Dial & Swearington, 1976; McCarron & Dial, 1972; Rubinsky, 1991). Dial, Chan, Parker, Carter, and Pomeroy (1985) used one test from this battery to predict independent living skills. Fortune and Eldredge (1982) extended the predictive system to psychiatric patients. This type of system would be useful in legal cases involving questions about eligibility for rehabilitation services and about the future cost of care and loss of income. The problem with this approach is that the selection of the best neuropsychological test scores to include in a prediction equation must be replicated and the regression weights must be locally developed for each criterion to be predicted. Regression equations are not "portable" across populations or across criteria.

A third approach to dealing with this problem is the development of new neuropsychological tests that directly assess everyday functioning (Heinrichs, 1990). Crook, Youngjohn, and Larrabee (1992), for example, developed computerized batteries of memory tasks that parallel everyday memory tasks (e.g., remembering phone numbers and shopping lists, associating names with faces). This approach has high face validity and therefore may be persuasive to legal fact finders; it may also be as accurate in detecting functional incapacities in everyday life as more traditional memory tests (Larrabee & Crook, 1989; Youngjohn, Larrabee, & Crook, 1992). The problem with this approach is that it is task-oriented rather than process-oriented. Remembering phone numbers and stranger's faces says nothing about the underlying mnestic processes that might be impaired, and therefore it does not permit clear predictions about performance on other tasks (e.g., recollection of one's estate and relatives) (cf. Loftus, 1991). This approach is most likely to be useful in forensic neuropsychology if the tasks contain legally relevant content rather than "everyday" content.

Notably lacking in the neuropsychological literature are studies of the temporal stability of various neuropsychological measures. In forensic neuropsychology, predictions and postdictions are sometimes required from test scores obtained at one point in time. The validity of these conclusions about past or future functioning is threatened by plausible arguments that little is known about the temporal stability of the test scores. Most test–retest studies in neuropsychology have investigated the reliability of neuropsychological tests or the effects of practice on such tests rather than the natural time course of neuropsychological test scores. What is the predictive horizon of various neuropsychological tests; that is, at what point in the future (or past) do tests lose their ability to forecast accurately? What is the effect of progressive conditions such as alcoholism or dementia of the Alzheimer's type on this time horizon? How frequently should neuropsychological tests be readministered during recovery from head injury in order to make accurate estimates of future functioning? The answers to these fundamental questions are essential for forensic neuropsychologists to present valid conclusions regarding premorbid functioning or permanent loss.

Finally, forensic neuropsychology would benefit from more publication of meta-analyses (e.g., Hunter & Schmidt, 1990; Rosenthal, 1991) of extant data regarding the psychometric characteristics of neuropsychological tests (e.g., reliability, criterion-related validity), the life expectancies, cost of care, or future earnings of various types of neurological patients, the accuracy of tests of malingering, and other empirical questions. Such studies objectively separate methodological variance (e.g., differences in sample size or composition) from substantive differences and thus provide clear summaries of multiple studies. Furthermore, they focus on effect size rather than statistical significance and thus emphasize the practical importance of research results. These analyses would serve to highlight both areas of agreement among opposing expert witnesses and areas where data are too sparse or conflicting to serve as a basis for firm conclusions. Such reports also would promote the role of forensic neuropsychologist as educator rather than as advocate.

Forensic neuropsychology as a distinct specialty has considerable progress to make to validate procedures for making objective, legally relevant conclusions that are based on objective, standardized neuropsychological evaluations. There is an obvious need for better training and continuing education of both clinical neuropsychologists and forensic psychologists in this hybrid specialty. However, forensic neuropsychology serves such a useful role in America's courts and tribunals that the legal system will not wait until all these problems have been resolved. Although practitioners of this specialty are ultimately responsible collectively for solving these problems, the individual practitioner, in the meantime, must assume the personal responsibilities of carefully defining the boundaries of the specialty, of recognizing limitations of competence, and of always telling the truth.

REFERENCES

American Bar Association. (1983). The insanity defense: ABA and APA proposals for change. *Mental and Physical Disability Law Reporter, 7*(2), 136–147.

American Psychiatric Association. (1987). *Diagnostic and statistical manual of mental disorders* (3rd. ed., rev.). Washington, DC: Author.

American Psychological Association. (1981). Specialty guidelines for the delivery of services. *American Psychologist, 36*(6), 640–681.

American Psychological Association. (1985). *Standards for educational and psychological testing*. Washington, DC: Author.

American Psychological Association. (1987). *General guidelines for providers of psychological services*. Washington, DC: Author.

American Psychological Association. (1990). *Guidelines for providers of psychological services to ethnic, linguistic and culturally diverse populations*. Washington, DC: Author.

American Psychological Association. (1992). *Ethical principles of psychologists and code of conduct*. Washington, DC: Author.

American Psychological Association. (1993). *Record keeping guidelines*. Washington, DC: Author.

Anderer, S. (1990). A model for determining competence in guardianship proceedings. *Mental and Physical Disability Reporter, 14*(2), 107–114.

Barefoot v. Estelle, 103 S. Ct. 3383 (U.S. Sup. Ct. 1983).

Barth, J., Ryan, T., & Hawk, G. (1992). Forensic neuropsychology: A reply to the method skeptics. *Neuropsychology Review, 2*(3), 251–261.

Benton, A., Hamsher, K., Varney, N., & Spreen, O. (1983). *Contributions to neuropsychological assessment*. New York: Oxford University Press.

Bieliauskas, L., & Matthews, C. (1987). American Board of Clinical Neuropsychology: Policies and procedures. *The Clinical Neuropsychologist, 1*(1), 21–28.

Bieliauskas, L., & Matthews, C. (1987). American Board of Clinical Neuropsychology: Update 1990. *The Clinical Neuropsychologist, 4*(4), 337–343.

Black, B. (1988). Evolving legal standards for the admissibility of scientific evidence, *Science, 39*, 1508–1512.

Black, H. (1981). *Black's law dictionary* (5th ed.). St. Paul, MN: West.

Blackburn v. Alabama, 361 U.S. 199 (U.S. Sup. Ct. 1960).

Brakel, S., Parry, J., & Weiner, B. (1985). *The mentally disabled and the law* (3rd ed.). Chicago: American Bar Association.

Brodsky, S. (1992). *Testifying in court.* Washington, DC: American Psychological Association.

Brown, P. (1987). *The art of questioning: Thirty maxims of cross-examination.* New York: MacMillan.

Chandler Exterminators, Inc. v. Morris, 409 S.E. 2d 49 (Ga. App. 1991).

Chandler Exterminators, Inc. v. Morris, 416 S.E. 2d 277 (Ga. Sup. Ct. 1992).

Clark, C. (1987). Specific intent and diminished capacity. In I. Weiner and A. Hess (Eds.), *Handbook of forensic psychology* (pp. 352–377). New York: Wiley.

Cleary, E., Ball, V., Barnhart, R., Brown, K., Dix, G., Gellhorn, E., Meisenholder, R., Roberts, E., & Strong, J. (1972). *McCormack's handbook of the law of evidence* (2nd ed.). St. Paul, MN: West.

Cohen, M., Berring, R., & Olson, K. (1989). *How to find the law* (9th ed.). St. Paul, MN: West.

Cohen, F., & Dvoskin, J. (1992). Inmates with mental disorders: A guide to law and practice. *Mental and Physical Disability Law Reporter, 16*(3), 339–346.

Colorado v. Connelly, 107 S. Ct. 515 (U.S. Sup. Ct., 1986).

Commission on the Mentally Disabled (1989). Guardianship: An agenda for reform: Recommendations of the National Guardianship Symposium and policy of the American Bar Association. *Mental and Physical Disability Law Reporter, 13*(3), 271–313.

Crook, T., Youngjohn, J., & Larrabee, G. (1992). Multiple equivalent test forms in a computerized, everyday memory battery. *Archives of Clinical Neuropsychology, 7*(3), 221–232.

Daniell, D. (1987). Accessing legal literature. In I. Weiner & A. Hess (Eds.), *Handbook of forensic psychology* (pp. 50–60). New York: Wiley.

Daubert v. Merrell Dow Pharmaceuticals, 61 L.W. 4805 (U.S. Sup. Ct. 1993).

Davasher v. Arkansas, 823 S.W. 2d 863 (Ark. Sup. Ct. 1992).

Dial, J., Chan, F., Parker, H., Carter, S., & Pomeroy, V. (1985). SSSQ predictors of independent living skills: A criterion validity study. *Vocational Evaluation and Work Adjustment Bulletin, 18*(4), 141–145.

Dial, J., Freeman, L., McCarron, L., & Swearington, S. (1979). Predictive validation of the McCarron–Dial Evaluation System. *Vocational Evaluation and Work Adjustment Bulletin, 12*(1), 11–18.

Dial, J., & Swearington, S. (1976). The prediction of sheltered workshop performance: Special applications of the McCarron–Dial Work Evaluation System. *Vocational Evaluation and Work Adjustment Bulletin, 9,* 24–33.

Division 40. (1986). Division 40: Task force report on computer assisted neuropsychological evaluation. *The Clinical Neuropsychologist, 1*(2), 161–184.

Division 40. (1989). Definition of a clinical neuropsychologist. *The Clinical Neuropsychologist, 3*(1), 22.

Division 41. (1991). *Specialty guidelines for forensic psychologists.* Washington, DC: American Psychological Association.

Dusky v. U.S., 362 U.S. 402 (U.S. Sup. Ct. 1960).

Eisenberg, M. (1986). *Contracts.* Chicago: Harcourt Brace Jovanovich Legal and Professional.

Ellis v. Alabama, 570 So. 2d 744 (Ala. Crim. App. 1990).

Estelle v. Gamble, 429 U.S. 97 (U.S. Sup. Ct. 1976).

Faust, D. (1991). Forensic neuropsychology: The art of practicing a science that does not yet exist. *Neuropsychology Review, 2*(3), 205–231.

Faust, D., & Ziskin, J. (1988). The expert witness in psychology and science. *Science, 241,* 31–35.

Faust, D., Ziskin, J., & Hiers, J. (1991). *Brain damage claims: Coping with neuropsychological evidence.* Los Angeles: Law and Psychology Press.

Fare v. Michael C., 442 U.S. 707 (U.S. Sup. Ct. 1979).

Fortune, J., & Eldredge, G. (1982). Predictive validation of the McCarron–Dial Evaluation System for psychiatrically disabled sheltered workshop workers. *International Journal of Rehabilitation Research, 5*(4), 540–541.

Frye v. U.S., 54 U.S. App. 46 (D.C. App., 1923).

Godinez v. Moran, 113 S. Ct. 2680 (U.S. 1993).

Golden, C., Hammeke, T., & Purisch, A. (1980). *The Luria–Nebraska Neuropsychological Battery manual.* Los Angeles: Western Psychological Services.

Grisso, T. (1986). *Evaluating competencies: Forensic assessments and instruments.* New York: Plenum.

Grisso, T. (1988). *Competence to stand trial evaluations: A manual for practice.* Sarasota, FL: Professional Resource Exchange.

Grisso, T., & Appelbaum, P. (1992). Is it unethical to offer predictions of future violence? *Law and Human Behavior, 16*(6), 621–633.

Gudjonsson, G. (1987). A parallel form of the Gudjonsson Suggestibility Scale. *British Journal of Clinical Psychology, 26,* 215–221.

Hall, H., & Pritchard, D. (1996). *Detecting malingering and deception: Forensic distortion analysis.* DelRay Beach, FL: St. Lucie Press.

Heaton, R., & Pendleton, M. (1981). Use of neuropsychological tests to predict adult patients' everyday functioning. *Journal of Consulting and Clinical Psychology, 49*(6), 807–821.
Heinrichs, R. (1990). Current and emergent applications of neuropsychological assessment: Problems of validity and utility. *Professional Psychology: Research and Practice, 21*(3), 171–176.
Hoge, S., & Grisso, T. (1992). Accuracy and expert testimony. *Bulletin of the American Academy of Psychiatry and Law, 20*(1), 67–76.
Hunter, J., & Schmidt, F. (1990). *Methods of meta-analysis.* Newbury Park, CA: Sage.
In re Gault, 387 (U.S. Sup. Ct. 1967).
INS–Division 40. (1987). Reports of the INS–Division 40 Task Force on education, accreditation and credentialing. *The Clinical Neuropsychologist, 1*(1), 29–34.
Kane, M. (1992). An argument-based approach to validity. *Psychological Bulletin, 112*(3), 527–535.
Kaplan, E., Fein, D., Morris, R., & Delis, D. (1991). *WAIS–R as a neuropsychological instrument.* San Antonio, TX: The Psychological Corporation.
King, J. (1977). *The law of medical malpractice.* Minneapolis, MN: West.
Kunz, C., Schmedemann, D., Bateson, A., Downs, M., & Erlinder, C. (1992). *The process of legal research: Successful strategies* (3rd ed.). Boston: Little, Brown.
Larrabee, G., & Crook, T. (1989). Dimensions of everyday memory in age-associated memory impairment. *Psychological Assessment, 1*(2), 92–97.
Lewis, M., & Saarni, C. (Eds.). (1993). *Living and deception in everyday life.* New York: Guilford.
Loftus, E. (1991). The glitter of everyday memory . . . and the gold. *American Psychologist, 46*(1), 16 et seq.
Marshall, J., & Newcombe, F. (1984). Putative problems and pure progress in neuropsychological single-case studies. *Journal of Clinical Neuropsychology, 6*(1), 65–70.
Matarazzo, J. (1990). Psychological assessment versus psychological testing: Validation from Binet to the school, clinic and courtroom. *American Psychologist, 45*(9), 999–1017.
Matthews, C., Harley, J., & Malec, J. (1991). Guidelines for computer-assisted neuropsychological rehabilitation and cognitive remediation. *The Clinical Neuropsychologist, 5*(1), 3–19.
McCarron, L., & Dial, J. (1986). *McCarron–Dial Evaluation System.* Dallas, TX: McCarron–Dial Systems.
McCarron, L., & Dial, J. (1972). Neuropsychological predictors of sheltered workshop performance. *American Journal of Mental Deficiency, 77,* 244–250.
McCloskey, M. (1993). Theory and evidence in cognitive neuropsychology: A "radical" response to Robertson, Knight, Rafal, and Shimamura (1993). *Journal of Experimental Psychology: Learning, Theory and Cognition, 19*(3), 718–734.
Melton, G. (1987). Training in psychology and law. In I. Weiner & A. Hess (Eds.), *Handbook of forensic psychology* (pp. 681–697). New York: Wiley.
Miranda v. Arizona, 384 U.S. 436 (U.S. Sup. Ct. 1966).
Mortensen, E., & Gade, A. (1992). Linear versus normalized *T* scores as standardized neuropsychological test scores. *Scandanavian Journal of Psychology, 33*(3), 230–237.
Parry, J. (1984). *Mental disability law: A primer.* Washington, DC: American Bar Association.
Parry, J., & Beck, J. (1990). Revisiting the civil commitment/involuntary treatment stalemate using limited guardianship, substituted judgment and different due process considerations: A work in progress, *Mental and Physical Disability Law Reporter, 14*(2), 102–107.
Poythress, N. (1982). A proposal for training in forensic psychology. *American Psychologist, 34,* 612–621.
Rees v. Peyton, Penitentiary Superintendent, 384 U.S. 312 (U.S. Sup. Ct. 1966).
Reitan, R., & Wolfson, D. (1985). *The Halstead–Reitan Neuropsychological Test Battery: Theory and clinical interpretation.* Tuscon, AZ: Neuropsychology Press.
Richardson, R., & Adams, R. (1992). Neuropsychologists as expert witnesses: Issues of admissibility. *The Clinical Neuropsychologist, 6*(3), 295–308.
Robertson, L., Knight, R., Rafal, R., & Shimamura, A. (1993). Cognitive neuropsychology is more than single-case studies. *Journal of Experimental Psychology: Learning, Memory and Cognition, 19*(3), 710–717.
Rogers, R. (Ed.). (1988). *Clinical assessment of malingering and deception.* New York: Guilford.
Rogers, R., & Cavanaugh, J. (1981). "Nothing but the truth" . . . A re-examination of malingering. *Journal of Psychiatry and Law, 11,* 443–460.
Rogers, R., Harrell, E., & Liff, C. (1993). Feigning neuropsychological impairment: A critical review of methodological and clinical considerations. *Clinical Psychology Review, 13,* 255–274.
Rosenthal, R. (1991). *Meta-analytic procedures for social research.* Newbury Park, CA: Sage.
Rothke, S. (1992). Expert testimony by neuropsychologists: Addendum to Schwartz and Satz. *The Clinical Neuropsychologist, 6*(1), 85–91.
Rubinsky, S. (1991). The use of the McCarron–Dial Work Evaluation System to predict success in sheltered, supported and competitive employment settings. *Vocational Evaluation and Work Adjustment Bulletin, 24*(4), 129–135.

Russell, E. (1987). A reference scale method for constructing neuropsychological test batteries. *Journal of Clinical and Experimental Neuropsychology, 9*(4), 376–392.
Sanchez v. Denby, 433 N.W. 2d 523 (Neb. Sup. Ct. 1989).
Saunders, A., & Simon, M. (1987). Individual functional assessment: An instruction manual. *Mental and Physical Disability Law Reporter, 11*(1), 60–70.
Schacter, D. (1986). Amnesia and crime. *American Psychologist, 41*(3), 265–295.
Schwitzgebel, R., & Schwitzgebel, R. (1980). *Law and psychological practice.* New York: Wiley.
Shallice, T. (1979). Case study approach in neuropsychological research. *Journal of Clinical Neuropsychology, 1*(3), 183–211.
Smith, S. (1993). The 1992–1993 Supreme Court and psychologists. *Bulletin of the American Academy of Forensic Psychology, 14*(1), 1–8.
Social Security Administration. (1992). *Disability evaluation under Social Security.* Washington, DC: U.S. Government Printing Office.
Spar, J., & Garb, A. (1992). Assessing competency to make a will. *American Journal of Psychiatry, 149*(2), 169–174.
Steadman, H., Monahan, J., Hartstone, E., Davis, S., & Robbins, P. (1982). Mentally disordered offenders: A national survey of patients and facilities. *Law and Human Behavior, 6,* 31–38.
Summerfelt, A., Alphs, L., Wagman, A., & Funderburk, F. (1991). Reduction of perseverative error in patients with schizophrenia using monetary feedback. *Journal of Abnormal Psychology, 100*(4), 613–616.
United States v. Wilson, 391 F. 2d 460 (1966).
Van der Does, A., & Van den Bosch, R. (1992). What determines Wisconsin Card Sorting performance in schizophrenia? *Clinical Psychology Review, 12*(6), 567–583.
Wechsler, D. (1981). *WAIS–R manual: Wechsler Adult Intelligence Scale–Revised.* New York: The Psychological Corporation.
Wechsler, D. (1987). *WMS–R manual: Wechsler Memory Scale–Revised.* New York: The Psychological Corporation.
Wellman, F. (1986). *The art of cross-examination* (4th ed.). New York: Dorsey.
West, M., & Knowles, D. (1991). Estimating cost of care and economic loss in brain injury. In H. Doerr & A. Carln (Eds.), *Forensic neuropsychology* (pp. 214–228). New York: Guilford.
Youngjohn, J., Larrabee, G., & Crook, T. (1992). Discriminating age-associated memory impairment from Alzheimer's disease. *Psychological Assessment, 4*(1), 54–59.

APPENDIX

SPECIALTY GUIDELINES FOR FORENSIC PSYCHOLOGISTS:[13] COMMITTEE ON ETHICAL GUIDELINES FOR FORENSIC PSYCHOLOGISTS[14]

The Specialty Guidelines for Forensic Psychologists, while informed by the Ethical Principles of Psychologists (APA, 1990) and meant to be consistent with them, are designed to provide more specific guidance to forensic psychologists in monitoring their professional

[13]The Specialty Guidelines for Forensic Psychologists were adopted by majority vote of the members of Division 41 and the American Psychology–Law Society. They have also been endorsed by majority vote by the American Academy of Forensic Psychology. The Executive Committee of Division 41 and the American Psychology–Law Society formally approved these Guidelines on March 9, 1991. The Executive Committee also voted to continue the Committee on Ethical Guidelines in order to disseminate the *Guidelines* and to monitor their implementation and suggestions for revision.

[14]These *Guidelines* were prepared and principally authorized by a joint Committee on Ethical Guidelines of Division 41 and the American Academy of Forensic Psychology (Stephen L. Golding, Chair; Thomas Grisso, David Shapiro, and Herbert Weissman, Co-chairs). Other members of the Committee included Robert Fein, Kirk Heilbrun, Judith McKenna, Norman Poythress, and Daniel Schuman. Their hard work and willingness to tackle difficult conceptual and pragmatic issues is gratefully acknowledged. The Committee would also like to acknowledge specifically the assistance and guidance provided by Dort Bigg, Larry Cowan, Eric Harris, Arthur Lerner, Michael Miller, Russell Newman, Melvin Rudov, and Ray Fowler. Many other individuals also contributed by their thoughtful critique and suggestions for improvement of earlier drafts, which were widely circulated.

conduct when acting in assistance to courts, parties to legal proceedings, correctional and forensic mental health facilities, and legislative agencies. The primary goal of the Guidelines is to improve the quality of forensic psychological services offered to individual clients and the legal system and thereby to enhance forensic psychology as a discipline and profession. The Specialty Guidelines for Forensic Psychologists represent a joint statement of the American Psychology-Law Society and Division 41 of the American Psychological Association and are endorsed by the American Academy of Forensic Psychology. The Guidelines do not represent an official statement of the American Psychological Association.

The Guidelines provide an aspirational model of desirable professional practice by psychologists, within any subdiscipline of psychology (e.g., clinical, developmental, social, experimental), when they are engaged regularly as experts and represent themselves as such, in an activity primarily intended to provide professional psychological expertise to the judicial system. This would include, for example, clinical forensic examiners; psychologists employed by correctional or forensic mental health systems; researchers who offer direct testimony about the relevance of scientific data to a psycholegal issue; trial behavior consultants; psychologists engaged in preparation of amicus briefs; or psychologists, appearing as forensic experts, who consult with, or testify before, judicial, legislative, or administrative agencies acting in an adjudicative capacity. Individuals who provide only occasional service to the legal system and who do so without representing themselves as forensic experts may find these Guidelines helpful, particularly in conjunction with consultation with colleagues who are forensic experts.

While the Guidelines are concerned with a model of desirable professionals practice, to the extent that they may be construed as being applicable to the advertisement of services or the solicitation of clients, they are intended to prevent false or deceptive advertisement or solicitation, and should be construed in a manner consistent with that intent.

I. PURPOSE AND SCOPE

A. Purpose
   1. While the professional standards for the ethical practice of psychology, as a general discipline, are addressed in the American Psychological Association's Ethical Principles of Psychologists, these ethical principles do not relate, in sufficient detail, to current aspirations of desirable professional conduct for forensic psychologists. By design, none of the Guidelines contradicts any of the Ethical Principles of Psychologists; rather, they amplify those Principles in the context of the practice of forensic psychology, as herein defined.
   2. The Guidelines have been designed to be national in scope and are intended to conform with state and Federal law. In situations where the forensic psychologist believes that the requirements of law are in conflict with the Guidelines, attempts to resolve the conflict should be made in accordance with the procedures set forth in these Guidelines [IV(G)] and in the Ethical Principles of Psychologists.

B. Scope
   1. The Guidelines specify the nature of desirable professional practice by forensic psychologists, within any subdiscipline of psychology (i.e., clinical, developmental, social, experimental), when engaged regularly as forensic psychologists.
      a. "Psychologist" means any individual whose professional activities are defined by the American Psychological Association or by regulation of title by state registration or licensure, as the practice of psychology.
      b. "Forensic psychology" means all forms of professional psychological conduct

when acting, with definable foreknowledge, as a psychological expert on explicitly psycholegal issues, in direct assistance to courts, parties to legal proceedings, correctional and forensic mental health facilities, and administrative, judicial, and legislative agencies acting in an adjudicative capacity.

c. "Forensic psychologist" means psychologists who regularly engage in the practice of forensic psychology as defined in I(B)(1)(b).

2. The Guidelines do not apply to a psychologist who is asked to provide professional psychological services when the psychologist was not informed at the time of delivery of the services that they were to be used as forensic psychological services as defined above. The Guidelines may be helpful, however, in preparing the psychologist for the experience of communicating psychological data in a forensic context.
3. Psychologists who are not forensic psychologists as defined in I(B)(1)(c), but occasionally provide limited forensic psychological services, may find the Guidelines useful in the preparation and presentation of their professional service.

C. Related Standards

1. Forensic psychologists also conduct their professional activities in accord with the Ethical Principles of Psychologists and the various other statements of the American Psychological Association that may apply to particular subdisciplines or areas of practice that are relevant to their professional activities.
2. The standards of practice and ethical guidelines of other relevant "expert professional organizations" contain useful guidance and should be consulted even though the present Guidelines take precedence for forensic psychologists.

II. RESPONSIBILITY

A. Forensic psychologists have an obligation to provide services in a manner consistent with the highest standards of their profession. They are responsible for their own conduct and the conduct of those individuals under their direct supervision.

B. Forensic psychologists make a reasonable effort to ensure that their services and the products of their services are used in a forthright and responsible manner.

III. COMPETENCE

A. Forensic psychologists provide services only in areas of psychology in which they specialized knowledge, skill, experience, and education.

B. Forensic psychologists have an obligation to present to the court, regarding the specific matters to which they will testify, the boundaries of their competence, the factual bases (knowledge, skill, experience, training, and education) for their qualification as an expert, and the relevance of those factual bases to their qualification as an expert on the specific matters at issue.

C. Forensic psychologists are responsible for a fundamental and reasonable level of knowledge and understanding of the legal and professional standards that govern their participation as experts in legal proceedings.

D. Forensic psychologists have an obligation to understand the civil rights of parties in legal proceedings in which they participate, and manage their professional conduct in a manner that does not diminish or threaten those rights.

E. Forensic psychologists recognize that their own personal values, moral beliefs, or personal and professional relationships with parties to a legal proceeding may interfere with their ability to practice competently. Under such circumstances, forensic psychologists are obligated to decline participation or to limit their assistance in a manner consistent with professional obligations.

IV. RELATIONSHIPS

A. During initial consultation with the legal representative of the party seeking services, forensic psychologists have an obligation to inform the party of factors that might reasonably affect the decision to contract with the forensic psychologist. These factors include, but are not limited to:
   1. the fee structure for anticipated professional services;
   2. prior and current personal or professional activities, obligations, and relationships that might produce a conflict of interests;
   3. their areas of competence and the limits of their competence; and
   4. the known scientific bases and limitations of the methods and procedures that they employ and their qualifications to employ such methods and procedures.

B. Forensic psychologists do not provide professional services to parties to a legal proceeding on the basis of "contingent fees," when those services involve the offering of expert testimony to a court or administrative body, or when they call upon the psychologist to make affirmations or representations intended to be relied upon by third parties.

C. Forensic psychologists who derive a substantial portion of their income from fee-for-service arrangements should offer some portion of their professional service on a pro bono or reduced fee basis where the public interest or the welfare of clients may be inhibited by insufficient financial resources.

D. Forensic psychologists recognize potential conflicts of interest in dual relationships with parties to a legal proceeding, and they seek to minimize their effects.
   1. Forensic psychologists avoid providing professional services to parties in a legal proceeding with whom they have personal or professional relationships that are inconsistent with the anticipated relationship.
   2. When it is necessary to provide both evaluation and treatment services to a party in a legal proceeding (as may be the case in small forensic hospital settings or small communities), the forensic psychologist takes reasonable steps to minimize the potential negative effects of these circumstances on the rights of the party, confidentiality, and the process of treatment and evaluation.

E. Forensic psychologists have an obligation to ensure that prospective clients are informed of their legal rights with respect to the anticipated forensic service, of the purposes of any evaluation, of the nature of procedures to be employed, the intended uses of any product of their services, and of the party who has employed the forensic psychologist.
   1. Unless court ordered, forensic psychologists obtain the informed consent of the client or party, or their legal representative, before proceeding with such evaluations and procedures. If the client appears unwilling to proceed after receiving a thorough notification of the purposes, methods, and intended uses of the forensic evaluation, the evaluation should be postponed and the psychologist should take steps to place the client in contact with his/her attorney for the purpose of legal advice on the issue of participation.
   2. In situations where the client or party may not have the capacity to provide informed consent to services or the evaluation is pursuant to court order, the forensic psychologist provides reasonable notice to the client's legal representative of the nature of the anticipated forensic service before proceeding. If the client's legal

representative objects to the evaluation, the forensic psychologist notifies the court issuing the order and responds as directed.

3. After a psychologist has advised the subject of a clinical forensic evaluation of the intended uses of the evaluation and its work product, the psychologist may not use the evaluation work product for other purposes without explicit waiver to do so by the client or the client's legal representative.

F. When forensic psychologists engage in research or scholarly activities that are compensated financially by a client or party to a legal proceeding, or when the psychologist provides those services on a pro bono basis, the psychologist clarifies any anticipated further use of such research or scholarly product, discloses the psychologist's role in the resulting research or scholarly products, and obtains whatever consent or agreement is required by law or professional standards.

G. When conflicts arise between the forensic psychologist's professional standards and the requirements of legal standards, a particular court, or a directive by an officer of the court or legal authorities, the forensic psychologist has an obligation to make those legal authorities aware of the source of the conflict and to take reasonable steps to resolve it. Such steps may include, but are not limited to, obtaining the consultation of fellow forensic professionals, obtaining the advice of independent counsel, and conferring directly with the legal representatives involved.

V. CONFIDENTIALITY AND PRIVILEGE

A. Forensic psychologists have an obligation to be aware of the legal standards that may affect or limit the confidentiality or privilege that may attach to their services or their products, and they conduct their professional activities in a manner that respects those known rights and privileges.

1. Forensic psychologists establish and maintain a system of record keeping and professional communication that safeguards a client's privilege.
2. Forensic psychologists maintain active control over records and information. They only release information pursuant to statutory requirements, court order, or the consent of the client.

B. Forensic psychologists inform their clients of the limitations to the confidentiality of their services and the products (see also Guideline IV E) by providing them with an understandable statement of their rights, privileges, and the limitations of confidentiality.

C. In situations where the right of the client or party to confidentiality is limited, the forensic psychologist makes every effort to maintain confidentiality with regard to any information that docs not bear directly upon the legal purpose of the evaluation.

D. Forensic psychologists provide clients or their authorized legal representatives with access to the information in their records and a meaningful explanation of that information, consistent with existing federal and state statutes, the Ethical Principles of Psychologists, the Standards for Educational and Psychological Testing, and institutional rules and regulations.

V. METHODS AND PROCEDURES

A. Because of their special status as persons qualified as experts to the court, forensic psychologists have an obligation to maintain current knowledge of scientific, professional and legal developments within their area of claimed competence. They are obligated also to use that knowledge, consistent with accepted clinical and scientific standards, in selecting data collection methods and procedures for an evaluation, treatment, consultation or scholarly/empirical investigation.

B. Forensic psychologists have an obligation to document and be prepared to make available, subject to court order or the rules of evidence, all data that form the basis for their evidence or services. The standard to be applied to such documentation or recording anticipates that the detail and quality of such documentation will be subject to reasonable judicial scrutiny; this standard is higher than the normative standard for general clinical practice. When forensic psychologists conduct an examination or engage in the treatment of a party to a legal proceeding, with foreknowledge that their professional services will be used in adjudicative forum, they incur a special responsibility to provide the best documentation possible under the circumstances.
   1. Documentation of the data upon which one's evidence is based is subject to the normal rules of discovery, disclosure, confidentiality, and privilege that operate in the jurisdiction in which the data were obtained. Forensic psychologists have an obligation to be aware of those rules and regulate their conduct in accordance with them.
   2. The duties and obligations of forensic psychologists with respect to documentation of data that form the basis for their evidence apply from the moment they know or have a reasonable basis for knowing that their data and evidence derived from it are likely to enter into legally relevant decisions.

C. In providing forensic psychological services, forensic psychologists take special care to avoid undue influence upon their methods, procedures, and products, such as might emanate from the party to a legal proceeding by financial compensation or other gains. As an expert conducting an evaluation, treatment, consultation, or scholarly/empirical investigation, the forensic psychologist maintains professional integrity by examining the issue at hand from all reasonable perspectives, actively seeking information that will differentially test plausible rival hypotheses.

D. Forensic psychologists do not provide professional forensic services to a defendant or to any party in, or in contemplation of, a legal proceeding prior to that individual's representation by counsel, except for persons judicially determined, where appropriate, to be handling their representation *pro se*. When the forensic services are pursuant to court order and the client is not represented by counsel, the forensic psychologist makes reasonable efforts to inform the court prior to providing the services.
   1. A forensic psychologist may provide emergency mental health services to a pretrial defendant prior to court order or the appointment of counsel where there are reasonable grounds to believe that such emergency services are needed for the protection and improvement of the defendant's mental health and where failure to provide such mental health services would constitute a substantial risk of imminent harm to the defendant or to others. In providing such services the forensic psychologist nevertheless seeks to inform the defendant's counsel in a manner consistent with the requirements of the emergency situation.
   2. Forensic psychologists who provide such emergency mental health services should attempt to avoid providing further professional forensic services to that defendant unless that relationship is reasonably unavoidable [see IV(D)(2)].

E. When forensic psychologists seek data from third parties, prior records, or other sources, they do so only with the prior approval of the relevant legal party or as a consequence of an order of a court to conduct the forensic evaluation.

F. Forensic psychologists are aware that hearsay exceptions and other rules governing expert testimony place a special ethical burden upon them. When hearsay or otherwise inadmissible evidence forms the basis of their opinion, evidence, or professional product, they seek to minimize sole reliance upon such evidence. Where circumstances reasonably permit, forensic psychologists seek to obtain independent and personal verification of data relied upon as part of their professional services to the court or to a party to a legal proceeding.

1. While many forms of data used by forensic psychologists are hearsay, forensic psychologists attempt to corroborate critical data that form the basis for their professional product. When using hearsay data that have not been corroborated, but are nevertheless utilized, forensic psychologists have an affirmative responsibility to acknowledge the uncorroborated status of those data and the reasons for relying upon such data.
2. With respect to evidence of any type, forensic psychologists avoid offering information from their investigations or evaluations that does not bear directly upon the legal purpose of their professional services and that is not critical as support for their product, evidence or testimony, except where such disclosure is required by law.
3. When a forensic psychologist relies upon data or information gathered by others, the origins of those data are clarified in any professional product. In addition, the forensic psychologist bears a special responsibility to ensure that such data, if relied upon, were gathered in a manner standard for the profession.

G. Unless otherwise stipulated by the parties, forensic psychologists are aware that no statements made by a defendant, in the course of any (forensic) examination, no testimony by the expert based upon such statements, nor any other fruits of the statements can be admitted into evidence against the defendant in any criminal proceeding, except on an issue respecting mental condition on which the defendant has introduced testimony. Forensic psychologists have an affirmative duty to ensure that their written products and oral testimony conform to this Federal Rule of Procedure (12.2[c], or its state equivalent.

1. Because forensic psychologists are often not in a position to know what evidence, documentation, or element of a written product may be or may lend to a "fruit of the statement," they exercise extreme caution in preparing reports or offering testimony prior to the defendant's assertion of a mental state claim or the defendant's introduction of testimony regarding a mental condition. Consistent with the reporting requirements of state or federal law, forensic psychologists avoid including statements from the defendant relating to the time period of the alleged offense.
2. Once a defendant has proceeded to the trial state, and all pretrial mental health issues such as competency have been resolved, forensic psychologists may include in their reports or testimony any statements made by the defendant that are directly relevant to supporting their expert evidence, providing that the defendant has "introduced" mental state evidence or testimony within the meaning of Federal Rule of Procedure 12.2(c), or its state equivalent.

H. Forensic psychologists avoid giving written or oral evidence about the psychological characteristics of particular individuals when they have not had an opportunity to conduct an examination of the individual adequate to the scope of the statements, opinions, or conclusions to be issued. Forensic psychologists make every reasonable effort to conduct such examinations. When it is not possible or feasible to do so, they make clear the impact of such limitations on the reliability and validity of their professional products, evidence, or testimony.

VII. PUBLIC AND PROFESSIONAL COMMUNICATIONS

A. Forensic psychologists make reasonable efforts to ensure that the products of their services, as well as their own public statements and professional testimony, are communicated in ways that will promote understanding and avoid deception, given the particular characteristics, roles, and abilities of various recipients of the communications.

1. Forensic psychologists take reasonable steps to correct misuse or misrepresentation of their professional products, evidence, and testimony.
2. Forensic psychologists provide information about professional work to clients in a manner consistent with professional and legal standards for the disclosure of test results, interpretations of data, and the factual bases for conclusions. A full explanation of the results of tests and the bases for conclusions should be given in language that the client can understand.
   a. When disclosing information about a client to third parties who are not qualified to interpret test results and date, the forensic psychologist complies with Principle 16 of the *Standards for Educational and Psychological Testing*. When required to disclose results to a nonpsychologist, every attempt is made to ensure that test security is maintained and access to information is restricted to individuals with a legitimate and professional interest in the data. Other qualified mental health professionals who make a request for information pursuant to a lawful order are, by definition, "individuals with a legitimate and professional interest."
   b. In providing records and raw data, the forensic psychologist takes reasonable steps to ensure that the receiving party is informed that raw scores must be interpreted by a qualified professional in order to provide reliable and valid information

B. Forensic psychologists realize that their public role as "expert to the court" or as "expert representing the profession" confers upon them a special responsibility for fairness and accuracy in their public statements. When evaluating or commenting upon the professional work product or qualifications of another expert or party to a legal proceeding, forensic psychologists represent their professional disagreements with reference to a fair and accurate evaluation of the data, theories, standards, and opinions of the other expert or party.

C. Ordinarily, forensic psychologists avoid making detailed public (out-of-court) statements about particular legal proceedings in which they have been involved. When there is a strong justification to do so, such public statements are designed to assure accurate representation of their role or their evidence, not to advocate the positions of parties in the legal proceedings. Forensic psychologists address particular legal proceedings in publications or communications only to the extent that the information relied upon is part of a public record, or consent for that use has been properly obtained from the party holding any privilege.

D. When testifying, forensic psychologists have an obligation to all parties to a legal proceeding to present their findings, conclusions, evidence, or other professional products in a fair manner. This principle does not preclude forceful representation of the data and reasoning upon which a conclusion of professional product is based. It does, however, preclude an attempt, whether active or passive, to engage in partisan distortion or misrepresentation. Forensic psychologists do not, by either commission or omission, participate in a misrepresentation of their evidence, nor do they participate in partisan attempts to avoid, deny, or subvert the presentation of evidence contrary to their own position.

E. Forensic psychologists, by virtue of their competence and rules of discovery, actively disclose all sources of information obtained in the course of their professional services; they actively disclose which information from which sources was used in formulating a particular written product or oral testimony.

F. Forensic psychologists are aware that their essential role as expert to the court is to assist the trier of fact to understand the evidence or to determine a fact in issue. In offering expert evidence, they are aware that their own professional observations, inferences, and conclusions must be distinguished from legal facts, opinions, and conclusions. Forensic psychologists are prepared to explain the relationship between their expert testimony and the legal issues and facts of an instant case.

5

Personality Assessment of Brain-Impaired Patients

Lloyd I. Cripe
Private practice, Seattle, WA

It is faulty in principle to try to make a distinction between so-called organic and functional diseases, as far as symptomatology and therapy are concerned. In both conditions, one is dealing with abnormal functioning of the same psychophysical apparatus and with the attempts of the organism to come to terms with that . . . Our task is to help the patients in this adjustment by physical and psychological means; the procedure and goal of the therapy in both conditions is, in principle, the same.

—Kurt Goldstein (1952)

Persons who are close to brain-impaired patients often report changes in the patients' personalities. They emphatically state: "It is like I am living with a new person!" A quote from the wife of a 42-year-old man recovering from a right hemisphere vascular accident due to carotid artery occlusion and mild neurocognitive findings illustrates such a concern:

> He's changed and it has been a long 10 months. It is like being married to a stranger. He seems to have problems initiating activities. He has no ambition. This is a decided change, because he used to be so energetic and on the go. It's like he has no importance to anything. If he is left to his own, he doesn't do much. If I ask him if anything is wrong, he simply says "No." He doesn't like to be around people. He behaves strangely and inappropriately in social situations. He is either too calm or too mad. He cannot function sexually. He needs structure to get anything done. I don't know what to do. It is like I am living with a different person. His personality has changed. What am I going to do?

Although the form and intensity of these complaints vary, the theme is always the same—personality has changed since the brain damage.

These subjective complaints raise many questions: What are they seeing that leads to this conclusion? What is their definition of personality? How do they know the personality has changed? What was the personality like before the insult? How much of this is a pre-illness versus post-illness issue?

The assessment of personality is one of the most important and challenging aspects of clinical neuropsychological practice. We constantly make judgments about the personality of our patients, and our diagnoses are affected by these decisions. The treatment and management of the patient are affected by our judgments regarding their personalities. Despite the importance of this issue, there is unfortunately little research or writing on it.

Our focus in clinical neuropsychology is usually riveted on the neuropsychological assessment of brain functions as they relate to cognitive and sensorimotor abilities. This focus often interferes with seeing larger issues such as personality. Our training has often emphasized neuropsychology rather than psychology. Assumptions about personality are poorly conceived; we assume we know how to assess this complicated matter without clearly thinking through our assumptions. We frequently rely on poorly validated single-test measures to make our decisions and think we are assessing personality, when in fact we are only looking at very limited data.

The primary goal of this chapter is to stimulate and challenge the reader's thinking regarding the assessment of personality in brain-impaired persons and to spur more creative thinking and research in this important, neglected area. Perhaps it will also lead to a deeper understanding of the existential dilemmas faced by persons suffering from brain damage.

This chapter is written from the perspective of a practicing clinician rather than a specialized authority in personality research. I am a thinking, caring, dedicated clinician who carefully studies, experiences, and understands each patient as an individual. Despite their limitations, I use all the tools available to observe the behavioral effects of brain disease. I observe how the *person* has been affected by the disease. I recognize the limitations of this endeavor, but have a firm belief that it is a worthy and honorable one. Based on clinical experience, I share with you some of my thinking and concerns regarding personality and brain disorder.

This chapter addresses a variety of questions relative to the personality assessment of brain-injured patients: What is personality? What do we know about the neuroanatomy and neurophysiology of personality? How is personality affected by brain functioning and brain impairment? How does premorbid personality affect adjustment to brain impairment? How do we study and measure personality? What methods do we have available to study personality? How good are these methods? How can we improve our assessment of personality factors in brain-impaired persons? What should be the future direction of research in this area?

WHAT IS PERSONALITY?

Concepts are not reality. They are not inevitable and "true" representations of the objective world. The conceptual language of a theory is an optional tool utilized to organize observable experience in a logical manner.

—Millon (1981)

Reber (1985) made the following comment regarding the term *personality* in his *Dictionary of Psychology*:

> Personality: One of the classic "chapter heading" words in psychology. That is, a term so resistant to definition and so broad in usage that no coherent simple statement about it can be made—hence, the wise author uses it as the title of a chapter and then writes freely about it without incurring any of the definitional responsibilities incurred were it introduced in the text. Rather than repeat here the folly of several score unwise authors . . . we shall not characterize the term definitionally but rather according to its role in personality theory. This approach seems best, since each author's meaning of the term tends to be colored by his or her theoretical biases and by the empirical tools used in evaluation and test of the theory. (p. 533)

Personality is very difficult to define. We use the term freely, we each have one, we think we understand it, but we are hard-pressed to carefully define it. Before you read further, reflect and write down your definition of personality. It is not easy, is it? As Reber (1985) noted, any definition is the product of the biases and theoretical bent of the author. Your definition will be based on numerous factors unique to your experience. Regardless of the difficulty in trying to define personality, before we can talk intelligently about it, and certainly before we can measure it, we must define what it is.

We begin with a definition from *Webster's* (Guralnik, 1992):

> The quality or fact of being a person . . . the quality or fact of being a particular person; personal identity; individuality . . . habitual patterns and qualities of behavior of any individual as expressed by physical and mental activities and attitudes: distinctive individual qualities of a person considered collectively. (p. 1062)

Next we turn to Wolman (1973), a noted clinical psychologist who offered the following definition of personality:

> The pattern of traits characterizing an individual person, trait here meaning any psychological characteristic of a person, including dispositions to perceive different situations similarly and to react consistently despite changing stimulus conditions, values, abilities, motives, defenses, and aspects of temperament, identity, and personal style. (p. 275)

An earlier definition given by Drever (1965) incorporated a social dimension:

> A term used in various senses, both popularly and psychologically, the most comprehensive and satisfactory being the integrated and dynamic organization of the physical, mental, moral, and social qualities of the individual, as that manifests itself to other people, in the give and take of social life; on further analysis it would appear in the main to comprise the natural and acquired impulses, and habits, interests, and complexes, the sentiments and ideals, the opinions and beliefs, as manifested in his relations with his social milieu. (p. 208)

Psychiatrists Kaplan and Sadock (1991) provided a terse but understandable definition: "Personality can be defined as the totality of emotional and behavioral traits that characterize the person in day-to-day living under ordinary conditions; it is relatively stable and predictable" (p. 525).

The *Diagnostic and Statistical Manual of Mental Disorders Revised (DSM–III–R)* (American Psychiatric Association, 1987) states: "Personality *traits* are enduring patterns of perceiving, relating to, and thinking about the environment and oneself, and are exhibited in a wide range of important social and personal contexts" (p. 335).

Discussing "What is personality?," Millon (1981), a leading scholar and creative thinker in personality theory and measurement, concluded:

> Personality is seen today as a complex pattern of deeply embedded psychological characteristics that are largely unconscious, cannot be eradicated easily, and express themselves automatically in almost every facet of functioning. Intrinsic and pervasive, these traits emerge from a complicated matrix of biological dispositions and experiential learning and now comprise the individual's distinctive pattern of perceiving, feeling, thinking, and coping. (p. 8)

I have asked many patients and their significant others what they mean by the statement that "personality has changed." Although they are never able to provide a very precise definition of personality, they can specify the changes in functioning that lead them to conclude that the personality has changed. Their idea of personality stems from a global gestalt of the person. This perceived gestalt is predictable and they expect this presentation from the person. This perception includes the person's predictable abilities, perception, habits of thought and emotion, and actions. Both the onlooker and the person is accustomed to this predictable pattern of abilities, perceptions, thoughts, emotions, and actions. They sense this expected constellation of behaviors as "the normal person" or "personality."

When *any* of this changes, there is a perception that "the person has changed." Therefore, they conclude that the "personality has changed." Changes in emotions (especially the control and expression of emotion) are particularly important in making the inference that personality has changed.

Borrowing from all of these definitions and my experience, the following definition of personality is used in this chapter: *Personality is an abstract concept that refers to a person's characteristic habitual and predictable manner of perceiving, thinking, emoting, and acting under similar situations*. The major components of personality are the perception, cognition, emotion, motivation, and action of the person as they interact with various environmental situations.

The person's predictable manner of perceiving, thinking, emoting, and acting results in a global gestalt to onlookers that is labeled "personality." Those who are close to a person expect him or her to behave in the manner of this gestalt. When the person does not behave in this expected manner, he or she is perceived by others as having a changed personality.

Potentially, any perceived change in perception, thinking, emotion, or action that deviates from the expected gestalt will be seen as a change in personality. Even changes in cognition (e.g., memory) are often seen by others as a change in the personality.

WHAT CAUSES PERSONALITY?

The origin of all science is the desire to know causes. *And the origin of all false science and imposture is in the desire to accept false causes rather than none; or, which is the same thing, in the unwillingness to acknowledge our own ignorance.*

—William Hazlitt

In exploring the causes of personality, we can ask the question, "What causes perception, cognition, emotion, motivation and action in various situations?" The matrix of causes that produce a particular individual's perception, cognition, emotion, motivation and action is extremely complicated. The causes are multiple, complex, and interrelated. *Personality is always the joint product of the person's biology, learned habits, and situation*. To understand an individual's personality, we must study all of these contributing factors. The factors are never exactly the same for any two persons; that is why there are as many personalities as there are faces.

The biology of the person includes inherited genetics and constitution, the current physiology, and the health of the system. A part of this biology is brain structure, chemistry and physiology. The learned habits of the person include habits of perceiving, thinking, emoting, and acting. This learning is strongly affected by the person's socialization history, especially the early social interactions when enduring habits are formed. Learning is also affected by the person's inherited biological capacity to learn. Current situations affect behavior. The environment in which the person operates has a strong influence on action. The current situation often includes a social milieu that affects the person. A situational factor is the person's place in the life process. Life stages provide situations that influence personality.

Thompson (1988) discussed emotions, a particularly prominent aspect of personality. He reviewed various models from the time of William James to the present and concluded that an "interactionistic model" best explains the causes:

> The emerging picture of human emotions is clearly interactionistic. Yet we must avoid the simplistic conclusion that "mind and body are inseparable." The relative contribution of our

biological states and our cognitions in determining our emotions varies with cultural, dispositional, and situational factors. In some instances, our biology dominates our cognitions. . . . In other instances, our cognitions dominate our biology. We often can think ourselves in and out of anger, depression, or other emotional states. To further complicate matters, our biological states and psychological states may covary or display marked dissociation.

Given the complexity of mind–body interactions, we should be leery of simple explanations such as "repressed anger causes ulcers" . . . researchers have repeatedly tested such simple explanations and found them inadequate. If we wish to comprehend the full richness and variety of human emotions, we must develop a greater appreciation of biological, psychological, and cultural variability. (pp. 343–344)

All of the factors of genetics, biology, socialization, and situation interact in complicated ways to produce personality. For deeper insights into this complicated interaction, I recommend a careful reading of Millon (1981).

WHAT DO WE KNOW ABOUT PERSONALITY AND THE BRAIN?

Virtually any alteration of central nervous system activity can change an individual's personality; impairments of movement, perception, language, or memory affect how an individual behaves and is perceived by others. Nevertheless, the scientific study of changes in personality, emotion, and social behavior following brain injury lags far behind the study of cognitive functions, in large part due to the difficulties in defining, recording, and evaluating these behaviors.

—Kolb & Whishaw (1990)

The general study of personality has a long history in both academic and clinical settings (see, for example, Hall & Lindzey, 1978; Kaplan & Sadock, 1991; Millon, 1981). The more specific study of the relationship between the brain and personality comes from both clinical and laboratory observations (Kolb & Whishaw, 1990).

Because personality is a global concept and the causes are complex, researching the relationship between personality and the brain is very difficult. It involves the study of the relationship of the brain to perception, cognition, emotion, motivation, and action. Where does one start to study such a complex phenomenon? Science typically tackles global complex realities by a reductionistic focus on some detail, hoping that eventually enough details will be known to understand the larger issue.

To reduce the problem of the personality–brain relationship to a more manageable size, most of the research focuses on one aspect of personality—the study of emotions. Although this is understandable, it is important that we do not see emotions as equivalent to personality, because emotions are but one aspect of it.

This section briefly discusses the findings regarding personality and the brain from laboratory and clinical research, and observations from my clinical experience.

Research Knowledge

One of the consistent principles of neural organization is that there are multiple systems controlling virtually every behavior.

—Kolb & Whishaw (1990)

Historically, the well-known case of Phineas Gage (Harlow, 1868) marked the beginning of reported interest in personality change following brain damage. From this and other frontal-brain-damage cases, the idea developed that personality can be dramatically affected by brain damage (Stuss & Benson, 1986). The concept of "frontal brain syndrome" was born.

A recent review of the frontal brain and personality disorder by Stuss, Gow, and Hetherington (1992) challenges the concept of a unitary frontal brain syndrome. The matter is not so simple. They emphasized the complexity of changes in personality associated with frontal brain disorder and argued for a new conceptualization, *frontal personality disturbance*:

> Rather than using the term *frontal syndrome* to describe the overall complex of emotional/social changes after frontal system damage, it is more appropriate to use the term *frontal personality disturbance*; that is, a change in the behavioral response patterns that define an individual as a unique self. Although these personality changes may include disturbances in drive, mood and affect, it is proposed that multiple factors are involved, particularly other cognitive functions related to the frontal lobes, such as vulnerability to interference, impoverished judgment, and an inability to self-correct and self-monitor. Quantitative methods of assessing frontal social disturbances are not readily available. . . . Multiple neurological causes can result in frontal dysfunction. Certain symptoms exhibited by patients with frontal dysfunction are at risk for misdiagnosis as idiopathic psychiatric disorders. . . . Several functional disorders are related to frontal dysfunction. The association of frontal deficit and so many functional disorders suggests caution in interpretation and the necessary establishment of criteria for association. Our understanding of the biological bases of functional disorders remains at an elementary level. (p. 355)

Physiological psychology has long studied brain–emotion and brain–behavior relationships in animals and humans (Cacioppo, Klein, Berntson, & Hatfield, 1993). The major portion of personality–brain research has been in the area of the psychology and neuropsychology of emotion. The study of the psychology of emotion began with William James' (1884) famous article, "What is an emotion?" and continues to the present. This study includes the biology of emotions, which of course involves the brain. This extensive literature is not reviewed here, but the reader is encouraged to become aware of its existence and its major findings (see Birbaumer & Ohman, 1993; Lazarus, 1991; LeDoux & Hirst, 1986; Lewis & Haviland, 1993; Thompson, 1988).

An appreciation for the various complex topics addressed by researchers in this area is quickly obtained by looking at the chapters related to biological aspects of emotion from a recent major publication by Lewis and Haviland (1993). Their book devotes 9 out of 44 chapters (21% of the book) to "Biological and Neurophysiological Approaches to Emotion." The chapter titles are: "Neurochemical Control of Moods and Emotions: Amino Acids to Neuropeptides," "Emotional Networks in the Brain," "The Psychophysiology of Emotion," "The Neuropsychology of Emotion and Affective Style," "Emotion and Behavior Genetics in Vertebrates and Invertebrates," "Multiple-Measure Approaches to the Study of Infant Emotion," "Vocal Expression and Communication of Emotion," "Facial Expression," and "Brain Temperature and Subjective Emotional Experience." This is an impressive display of research, strongly supporting the notion that emotion has an underlying biology which includes the brain. The fact that emotion is just one component of personality suggests that we are only seeing the tip of the knowledge iceberg in this study.

Borod (1993) recently edited a special section in *Neuropsychology* entitled "Neuropsychological Perspectives on Components of Emotion." Borod's basic premise is that emotion consists of processing modes utilizing different brain systems. The modes include cognitive appraisal or perception, expressive behavior, physiological arousal, and subjective experience. The model presented provides a useful organization of the current knowledge of emotion and illustrates the complexity of emotion–brain relationships. The components of this model are discussed in the seven articles composing this special section. The articles provide an understanding of current theory, methods, and knowledge regarding the neuropsychology of emotion.

Kolb and Whishaw (1990) provided a useful summary of the animal and human research regarding emotional process. They summarized the studies of primates with prefrontal and paralimbic lesions and noted the following symptoms: reduced and inappropriate social interaction, loss of social dominance, altered social preference, reduced facial expression and body gestures, and reduced vocalization. They summarized the research with neurologic patients indicating problems with the production and interpretation of affective behavior. They also pointed out the neurobiological aspects of schizophrenia and depression, and the effects of psychosurgery to further develop the evidence for brain mechanisms underlying emotions and personality. They concluded with this summary:

> It does not seem possible to provide a theory of the anatomical circuit of emotions at present. Although it is likely that the right hemisphere plays a different role from that of the left in certain emotional processes, especially cognitive processes, the nature of this difference is unclear. The left–right distinction is certainly not as distinct as it is for language, and it would be a naive mistake to suggest that the right hemisphere is emotional and the left verbal. Furthermore, one of the principles of cortical organization is that functions are localized. Thus, even if the right hemisphere plays a special role in some emotional processes, we must specify the anatomical focus and the precise nature of this function. This will require not only better behavioral–pathological correlations on large samples of subjects, but it will require a better identification of the components of emotional processing that are being effected. This is a tall order and represents a significant challenge for future studies. (pp. 636–637)

Haaland (1992) recently edited a collection of well-thought-out articles regarding "The Emotional Concomitants of Brain Damage." This highly recommended collection of seven articles spans many topics relevant to understanding the complexities of the brain and its relationship to personality and emotion. In this series, Derryberry and Tucker (1992) discussed the neural mechanisms of emotion. After discussing emotional functions of the brainstem (descending effector and ascending regulatory systems), the limbic system (hippocampal system, amygdala, descending and ascending limbic influences), and paralimbic cortices (cingulate, retrosplenial, parahippocampal, orbital frontal, insular, temporal polar, descending and ascending paralimbic influences, posterior and anterior cortex), they commented: "Although our review of the neural systems of emotion has been fairly cursory, it should show that the brain's workings are formidably complex" (p. 336). This statement emphasizes the complicated nature of brain–personality anatomy and physiology. It underscores how this single aspect of personality (emotion) involves multiple brain parts and systems.

The relationship of emotion to the right and left cerebral hemispheres has been the focus of much discussion and research (Borod, 1992; Robinson & Chait, 1985; Ruckdeschel-Hubbard, Gordon, & Diller, 1986). Borod (1992) reviewed the research regarding "Interhemispheric and intrahemispheric control of emotion," the current neuropsychological theories of emotions, and the literature of normal and brain-damaged subjects regarding *perception* and *expression* of emotion. She concluded that the findings support the idea that the right cerebral hemisphere is more dominant for emotion than the left. This is especially true for the perception of emotion.

Another approach to the investigation of the relationship of personality factors and the brain has been to study groups of persons suffering from the same neuropathology and to draw conclusions regarding "emotional and personality" problems (e.g., Dodrill, 1986; Dodrill, Batzel, Queisser, & Temkin, 1980; Rao, Huber, & Bornstein, 1992; Teri & Wagner,1992). This type of research is generally poorly conceptualized: Personality is not well defined, concepts of emotion and personality are fused, and two important realities are ignored. First, neuropathology is not a homogeneous entity. A similar neuropathology in different individuals often involves different specific brain areas and results in different effects. One cannot safely assume that two patients suffering from any similar neuropathology are comparable as to locus of insult or neuropsychological effect. Lumping all of these patients together for group study is an unsafe generalization.

Second, as is discussed in more detail later, the methods used to measure "personality and emotional factors" are significantly limited (Borod et al., 1990) and may not be measuring what is intended. The methods used to measure emotions and personality often rely on very subjective data (i.e., self-reports) and cannot be assumed to be directly measuring personality or emotions.

A recent review of the "emotional" changes of multiple sclerosis and Parkinson's disease by Rao et al. (1992) discusses some of these conceptual and methodological problems and avoids the pitfalls of overgeneralizing a neuropathology and the measurement of personality by realistically limiting conclusions and making constructive recommendations for further research regarding the emotional changes.

Prigatano (1992) discussed personality-change issues associated with traumatic brain injury. He reviewed numerous studies reporting emotional and motivational disturbances in traumatically brain-injured patients and divided 25 commonly reported affective problems into three categories: active, passive, and syndromic. He pointed out that we do not really know what brain mechanisms underlie these problems and emphasized that our methods of assessment are very limited while urging further research for both clinical and scientific reasons.

There are attempts to review and integrate the myriad of details of neuroanatomy and neuropsychology into an understanding of brain–emotion relationships (Heilman, Bowers, & Valenstein, 1985; Heilman & Satz, 1983; Joseph, 1990; Kolb & Whishaw, 1990; Mesulam, 1985; Ross, 1985). Miller (1991, 1992, 1993) postulated a relationship of the brain with psychodynamics and personality types. His work is creative, thought provoking, and deserving of consideration. Sherman, Shaw, and Glidden (1994) have recently proposed a reciprocal inhibition of lateralized emotional functioning model to explain *functional versus organic* emotional behavior in neurologic and psychiatric disorders. All of these attempts to develop a "grand unified field theory" of personality and the brain are impressive, but they are mainly based on limited facts, excessive interpretation, and theorizing far beyond our

TABLE 5.1
Probable Brain Systems Associated With Emotion

Subjective experience
Deep brain structures
Limbic system
Memory system
Physiological reactions
Deep brain structures
Endocrine systems
Autonomic nervous system
Control and management
Frontal brain structures
Frontal brain systems
Verbal coding & decoding
Left hemisphere systems
Nonverbal coding & decoding
Right hemisphere systems

scientific knowledge base. These attempts are premature but are not to be discouraged. They help to punctuate the complexity of brain–emotion relationships, the limits of our knowledge, and the need for much more research.

Based on a review of the literature, I conclude that there is growing evidence for probable brain structures and systems associated with various aspects of emotion. Table 5.1 summarizes the major brain systems that are likely associated with emotion. There are bits and pieces starting to fit together in this complex puzzle, but there are too many missing parts to be confident of its true nature. It is safe to conclude that there are multiple brain mechanisms and systems underlying personality, but the details of this brain–personality relationship are obscure and yet to be discovered. *Part* of the cause of personality is accounted for by brain mechanisms and systems, but the size and form of this contribution is not known.

Clinical Experience

We know what a person thinks not when he tells us what he thinks but by his actions.
—Issach Bashevis Singer

There are three distinct but related issues to consider in the clinical neuropsychological study of personality factors in patients: (a) personality changes directly related to the brain damage; (b) reactions to the situation of being brain damaged; and (c) the interaction of brain damage with individual personalities.

Some changes in emotion and personality seem to be clearly linked to brain pathology. One example is the reflexive laughing and crying (pseudo-bulbar affect) seen most often with stroke patients having bilateral brain lesions who display sudden bursts of laughing and crying with either minimal positive or negative emotional stimulation. Another example is the patient with deep frontal–thalamic disruption who lacks initiative and becomes "adynamic" with emotions and other behaviors. There are those patients with extensive bilateral medial–sagittal frontal damage that results from bilateral anterior infarcts who never again experience a subjective sense of emotion, although they can often perceive emotion in others. Finally, consider the postcoma agitated and uncontrolled patient or the dysinhibited sexual behavior of the Klüver–Bucy syndrome patient. Patients with behavioral manifestations of these types following brain damage present compelling evidence that personality can be dramatically altered with brain disease. They have *obvious* changes of personality as a result of the brain conditions.

There are other patients who present a more *subtle* neurobehavioral disruption. Their problems raise suspicion of brain-based personality changes because of the frequency of presentation even in persons with good preinjury adjustment. Examples of these problems include decreased energy, lack of initiative, sleep disturbance, lability of emotion, irritability and impatience, reduced tolerance for stress, tension, anxiety, and depression, and a lack of confidence.

The most common problems reported to me by neurologic patients following their disorders is decreased energy and emotional reactivity. These patients often have a decreased tolerance for stress and over react to stimuli that did not previously bother them. Although such problems are less clearly linked to the brain disorder, these symptoms occur so frequently that it seems probable that they are linked to changes in brain mechanisms.

Another common presentation is the patient-specific manifestation of the interaction of the personality makeup and the injury. All patients come to a neurologic disorder with an established personality—habits of perceiving, thinking, emoting, and acting. The neurologic disorder is a significant life event creating a unique challenging situation for the person. Erosion of fundamental abilities of the mind and body pose an existential dilemma like no other. This event interacts with each individual's personality to produce an idiosyncratic response. Some persons appear to have excessive or unusual reactions to their neurologic disorders and a poor adjustment that seems more related to their well-established adaptive styles than to the actual brain-based problem.

Drawing from clinical experience, the following hypotheses regarding the brain and personality seem merited:

- There is some relationship between the condition of the brain and personality.
- Some brain disorders seriously disrupt and change the personality.
- Some aspects of personality are related to factors other than the brain.
- Some personality problems following neurologic disease are very obviously linked to brain mechanisms and systems.
- There are personality problems following neurologic disease that are more subtly linked to brain mechanisms and systems.
- A neurologic disorder and its effects on the person is often a very significant existential event.
- The person's well-established personality (habits of perceiving, thinking, emoting, and acting) always interacts with the neurologic event in some manner to produce a unique reaction.
- The unique reaction can be best understood by studying both the brain condition and the established personality.
- Some persons have what appear to be extreme reactions, but they are understandable in the context of the personality and situations of the person.
- The reaction can exceed and complicate the effects of the brain-based problem.
- It is not always clear how much of the reaction is due to the brain, the established personality habits, or an interaction of the two.
- Our technology for objectively evaluating all of this is limited.

In summary, this section has briefly reviewed some of what we know about personality through research and clinical experience. Emotion is only one aspect of personality, but it is often the focus of brain–personality research. Personality is a concept referring to a very complex constellation of factors (perception, cognition, emotion, motivation, and action). Although emotion is only one aspect of personality, it is also very complicated. We know through both research and clinical experience that there is a relationship between the brain and personality, but the exact nature of this relationship is yet to be discovered. Clinical experience reveals a variety of hypotheses that are useful in understanding the relationship of the brain and personality.

WHAT ARE THE METHODS TO STUDY PERSONALITY FACTORS?

The only sensible person I know is my tailor. He measures me anew each time he sees me. The others go on with the same old measures.

—George Bernard Shaw

Neuropsychologists are interested in assessing personality because brain mechanisms are related to personality, changes in the brain can affect personality, and personality issues always interact with the neurologic event to produce some type of reaction. The differential diagnosis of psychiatric and neurologic disorders also motivates the neuropsychologist to study personality issues.

How do we make inferences about someone's personality? Stop for a moment and identify in your mind the person that you know best, then ask yourself, "How did I get to know this person? What methods did I use?" You probably spent considerable time with this person, listened to them, discussed many things, watched their verbal and nonverbal reactions in many situations, and took risks with them by sharing your more private thoughts. You collected many samples of their verbal and nonverbal behavior and formed a belief about who they are, how they perceive, think, feel, and act in various situations. These were your methods. Did your methods include psychological tests?

Personality is inferred from a variety of observable behaviors. No one sees "personality" or "emotions." They see behavioral manifestations and deduce from the manifestations a constellation of actions to infer the existence of personality. Basically, there are no direct measures of personality.

What are the behaviors observed by onlookers to make inferences about the habits of perception, cognition, emotion, motivation, and action of other persons? The behaviors are both *nonverbal* and *verbal* displays observed over varying spans of time. Facial gestures, actions of the eyes (movement, focus, moisture), body gestures (movement and position), breathing, vocalizations, verbal content, tone of voice, speed of speech, verbal inflection, timing of verbalizations, and many other factors all combine to provide the raw data from which the observer interprets and forms the concept of personality. Interpretation of many points of observed information is always a part of this process.

What methods do neuropsychologists use to assess "personality factors"? They rely on a combination of formal and informal direct and indirect observations that usually include direct observations of the patient, the reports of the patient and others, and test instruments. All of the information collected by these methods is analyzed and interpreted to form an opinion regarding personality. The interpretations are of course always subjected to the filters of the examiner's knowledge, experience, and personality.

There are a number of test instruments used by neuropsychologists to aid in the study of personality. Table 5.2 lists the major tests used. These tests can be grouped into four major categories: self-report inventories administered to patients, self-report inventories administered to others who know the patient, examiner-completed ratings, and examiner-adminis-

TABLE 5.2
Test Instruments Commonly Used to Assess Personality Factors in Neurologic Patients

Patient-reported inventories & ratings:
Beck Depression Inventory (Beck et al., 1961)
Geriatric Depression Scale (Yesavage et al., 1983)
Millon Clinical Multiaxial Inventory (Millon, 1983)
Millon Clinical Multiaxial Inventory–II (Millon, 1987)
Minnesota Multiphasic Personality Inventory (Butcher et al., 1989; Hathaway & McKinley, 1951)
Sickness Impact Profile (Berger et al., 1981)
Symptom Checklist 90–Revised (Derogatis, 1977, 1983)
Washington Psychosocial Seizure Inventory (Dodrill et al., 1980)
Other-reported inventories & ratings:
Brief Psychiatric Rating Scale (Overall & Gorham, 1962)[E]
Hamilton Rating Scale for Depression (Hamilton, 1967)[E]
Katz Adjustment Scales (Katz & Lyerly, 1963)[S,P]
Neurobehavioral Rating Scale (Levin et al., 19867)[E]
Examiner-administered tests:
Rorschach Inkblot Test (Exner, 1986)

[E]Completed by the examiner; [P]Completed by the patient; [S]Completed by significant others

tered tests. Most of these instruments are borrowed from clinical psychology and not specifically developed to study personality issues in neurologic patients. Most of them are discussed in a recent book that was written primarily for clinical psychologists but that also is useful to neuropsychologists (see Maruish, 1994).

The most common practice in North America is to use one of two versions of the same personality assessment instrument, the Minnesota Multiphasic Personality Inventory (MMPI or MMPI–2). Along with a battery of "brain-sensitive tests" (neuropsychological tests), a "personality test," usually the MMPI, is administered. Clinicians hope that this easily administered test will aid in identifying the various personality issues in brain-impaired persons. Additionally, the hope is that it will help with differential diagnosis (neurologic vs. psychiatric, depression vs. dementia, etc.). Some examiners spend little or no time with the person and make their inferences about personality primarily from the "test data."

The only direct examiner-administered test on the list in Table 5.2 is the Rorschach Inkblot test. This test has a long history of use in clinical psychology, but is only occasionally used in clinical neuropsychology. Weiner (1994) reviewed the history of this perceptual–cognitive task and provides a useful summary of many Rorschach variables and their "maladaptive corollaries." Erdberg (1990) presented a very useful conceptualization of Rorschach test variables that provides practical clinical information regarding the person's perception, cognition, and emotion.

The use of the Rorschach with neurologic patients has a long history. Frank (1991) reviewed the literature regarding the assessment of cerebral dysfunction with the Rorschach and concluded that although a sign approach is not merited, there is usefulness with the instrument in understanding the quality of thought process. Robbins (1989) discussed validity and reliability issues with neurologic patients. He concluded that there have been significant methodological problems in researching this instrument with neurologic patients because of the use of "organicity" as a unitary concept. He recommended further research with better definitions of the issues.

HOW GOOD ARE THE TESTS?

When science starts to be interpretive, it is more unscientific even than mysticism.
—D. H. Lawrence

General Limitations

Although the test instruments used by neuropsychologists to study personality issues in neurologic patients deliver some information, they are limited: The measures are indirect, they rely heavily on self-report of the patient, and are dependent on the interpretation of the examiner. They also lack solid investigation of their validity and reliability with neurologic patients. The most significant problem is the limited indirect sampling of a very complex phenomenon. As discussed earlier, personality encompasses multiple aspects of the person (perception, thought, emotion, action, etc.). The data available to make inferences about personality include a myriad of verbal and nonverbal behaviors. Tests sample very little of this behavioral repertoire.

A careful analysis of the process that occurs when a patient is given a psychological inventory illustrates how *indirect* and limited observations are when the only method used is an inventory. Figure 5.1 demonstrates the process of inferring personality variables from indirect inventories as compared with a more direct observation through an interview. Although some information is gathered from the inventory, it is a limited and constricted

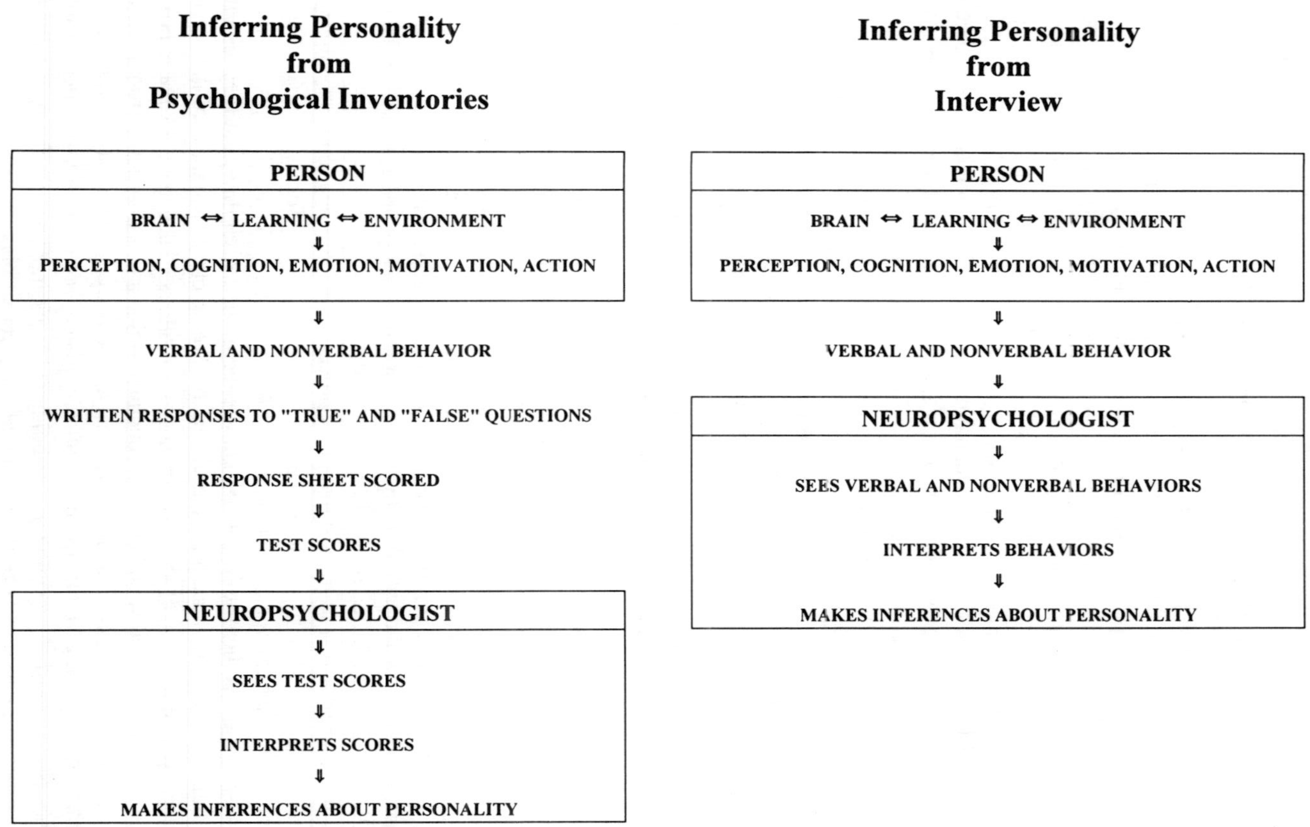

FIG. 5.1. A comparison of the process of observing and inferring personality from test or interview situations.

sampling of the person's "personality behaviors." No direct cues are observed. The test scores are the focus of observation by the examiner. The examiner does not directly see the actual behavior of the person. The examiner is given test scores that are far removed from the actual object of study—the person. It is possible that a person responding to a psychological questionnaire could be displaying many extreme behavioral cues that would not manifest at all on the test response sheet.

In contrast, the interview provides a direct observation of the personality. Many verbal and nonverbal ques become the raw data for inferring personality. Although the interview is but a small sampling of a person's repertoire of behavior, an in vivo observation provides much more data. The interview clearly provides more direct sources of information about the "personality" than a test score. It is highly improbable that an examiner would miss emotional displays during an interview that would be undetected on a test inventory. In sum, *if you want to see all of the raw data it is important to see the person in the flesh.*

Another significant limitation of the psychological inventory test method is its reliance on self-report. Although self-report delivers some information about a person, it is fragile information that may or may not be correlated to the reality of the person. Self-report is particularly problematic with some neurologic patients because their capacity for self-appraisal can be impaired (Prigatano & Schacter, 1991). Neurologic patients often have attention and language problems (receptive or expressive) that make it difficult for them to understand written communications or to express themselves adequately on test instruments. With some patients it is very laborious to try to answer hundreds of items on a questionnaire when their attention is compromised by brain dysfunction. Due to slowed mentation and difficulty in processing complex information, they can spend hours trying to make judgments about the test items and their relevance to their situation. In some cases, such demands are inhumane.

Another weakness with the use of inventory tests in understanding complex personality factors in neurologic patients is the reliance on interpretation. The test scores, several times removed from the reality of the person, are subjected to the "personality factors" of the examiner. The perceptions, thoughts, beliefs, biases, emotions, motivations, and so on of the examiner come into play and affect whatever judgments and opinions are made. The reliance on such limited data subjected to the examiner's personality and bias can be a precarious process as emphasized by the biased interpretations of our critics (Faust et al., 1988; Faust & Ziskin, 1988; Faust, Ziskin, & Hiers, 1991a, 1991b).

Due to the indirect nature of the test inventory process, the interpretation of psychological test scores can be as much a psychological test for examiners as it is for patients. This is why it is so important that examiners have keen insight into their own psychology. Examiners need training that gives them solid general knowledge in their discipline, but they also need specialty training that provides close supervision to develop clear awareness of the personal biases which potentially effect their observations of others. They have to learn how to observe openly, think logically, and come to conclusions that are as unfettered from their own cauldron of psychological issues as possible. Just as good psychotherapists need the experience of training and their own therapy to adequately manage complex transference–countertransference issues, persons engaging in psychological assessment need a sharp awareness of their own psychology to minimize the pitfalls of interpretive bias.

There are problems with the validity and reliability of inventory test measures as they relate to neurologic patients (Franzen, 1989). Most of the measures were not developed specifically for neurologic patients. They have been adapted from general clinical psychological measures with the assumption that if they are measuring personality in psychiatric patients, they will measure personality in neurologic patients.

Whether or not these instruments actually measure personality and emotions is doubtful when we consider the complex nature of personality and emotions. Whether or not they will discriminate the presence or absence of problems with personality and emotions in heterogeneous neurologic populations and discriminate them from psychiatric patients is also questionable. The ability of these measures to do all of this has not been clearly validated. Assumptions are made that the instruments measure personality or emotions, discriminate abnormality of personality in neurologic patients, and discriminate between psychiatric and neurologic diagnoses with limited or absent systematic investigation of the validity of the assumptions.

There are arguments that computer-generated interpretations are more reliable than clinician-dependent interpretations. Computer-generated interpretive statements also are far removed from the real behavioral demonstrations of personality. They are the product of the particular psychological theories that have created them. Regardless of their mechanized scientific appearance, they represent the thinking and biases of their creators. Consistent statements do not necessarily equal accurate or useful information. As Emerson said, "Consistency is the hobgoblin of little minds." This seems especially true when interpreting very complicated dynamic phenomenon. A parrot can be incredibly consistent (reliable) with its verbalizations, but horribly mismatched to the situation (invalid)! To make accurate, consistent, individualized, "canned" statements about the very dynamic, complex phenomenon of personality is highly suspect (Matarazzo, 1986).

Several basic observational facts (Sheehan, 1988) are relevant to the process of trying to observe personality from indirect observations:

- The greater the distance between an object and the observer, the more difficult it becomes to see the object.
- When objects become very difficult to see, interpretation of their meaning becomes more difficult.
- Interpretations of ambiguous objects (stimuli) often tell you more about the interpreter than the objects.

MMPI Limitations

Given the popularity of using the MMPI in neuropsychological assessment, its limitations merit specific discussion. The MMPI is subject to all of the general limitations discussed earlier plus additional flaws. Its item pool and scale construction create special problems when used as part of a neuropsychological assessment.

Many of the items in the MMPI include symptoms and problems experienced by neurologic patients because of their neurologic disorder (Alfano, Finlayson, Stearns, & Nielson, 1990; Cripe, 1988, 1989; Gass, 1991a, 1991b). When the patient endorses these items the profile is elevated for reasons other than the presence of psychiatric disorder or traits. The scales most commonly affected are 1 (Hypochondriasis), 2 (Depression), 3 (Hysteria), 7 (Psychasthenia), and 8 (Schizophrenia). Consequently, group studies of neurologic patients using the MMPI as a measure of "emotion or personality" typically demonstrate profiles with these scales elevated (Mack, 1979).

Because of item overlap, the same item endorsed by a neurologic patient can affect more than one scale. This can have multiple effects on the profile, not because of the presence of some psychiatric or personality problem, but simply because the person has honestly reported their neurobehavioral symptoms.

Because different patients can endorse the same items for different reasons, it is not possible to infer the same meaning from scale elevations across patients. For example, three different patients may have elevated scores on scale 2 (Depression) at the same level, but for distinctly different reasons (one person is very depressed due to an affective disorder; one person is not depressed but has endorsed items on that scale because of neurologic symptoms; and one person is malingering). It is not possible to discriminate on the basis of the profile alone which person belongs in which patient group. They all have elevated scores on scale 2, but for very different reasons. There is no way a clinician could determine the group membership on the basis of the summary test profile alone (Cripe, Maxwell, & Hill, 1995). It is not accurate to conclude that these patients are all suffering from depression.

Because so many items are potentially endorsed by neurologic patients for reasons other than personality or psychiatric dysfunction and the endorsement effects scale and profile elevations (especially scales 1, 2, 3, 7, and 8), the use of traditional cookbook clinical interpretations with neurologic patients is inappropriate.

Some have suggested correction strategies that eliminate the most vulnerable items (Alfano et al., 1990; Gass, 1991a, 1991b). This practice is suspect because the elimination of key items from the test results in a different instrument. Validation research is required to justify such changes.

The MMPI was never developed for the purpose of studying neurologic patients. It was designed to be a tool to help to discriminate the presence or absence of psychiatric pathology according to the nomenclature of the time (Colligan, 1985). It was not and is not a measure of personality. It did not grow out of personality research; it grew out of clinical psychopathology research. If the MMPI is a measure of personality, does a flat profile mean that you have no personality?

The popular habit of tacking an MMPI onto a neuropsychological battery with the hope of unmasking personality factors in neurologic patients has been driven by a number of deeply rooted beliefs that:

- The test measures emotions and personality.
- The MMPI measures emotions and personality and the other neuropsychological tests measure brain functioning.
- The MMPI can discriminate psychiatric from neurologic patients.
- Elevations on the scales mean the same for all patient groups.

All of these beliefs are misconceptions based on scant or nonexistent evidence (Cripe, 1988).

Given the complexity of personality, its interaction with the brain and neuropathology, the multiple behaviors involved in the process of inferring personality, the general limitations of indirect observations, and the inherent limitations of the instrument, reliance on the MMPI for the assessment of personality factors in brain-injured persons is unmerited. This reliance often confuses more than it clarifies.

WHAT IS THE BEST ALTERNATIVE?

You can observe a lot by just watching.
—Yogi Berra

The best alternative to reliance on a single limited instrument like the MMPI is to use multiple methods and data sources to make inferences about these complicated matters called personality. Reliance on a single method, such as test scores, is too limiting. It shrinks the aperture of observation, excludes and obscures information in a situation where we need all the enlightenment that is possible.

There are multiple qualitative and quantitative methods available to observe and study personality: the report of the patient, reports of persons who know the patient, history of the person, reports of medical records, direct observations of the patient's verbal and nonverbal behavior, observations during structured and unstructured problem solving tasks (tests), test scores and profiles, the relationship with the patient (transference and countertransference), reason and logic, knowledge, and intuition. These are all valuable observational tools that provide the raw material (data) for understanding and making inferences about personality.

The evaluation of personality issues in neurologic patients should include consideration of the brain-based dysfunction, the habitual personality style, the psychological reaction to the situation of neurologic disease, and all its repercussions. First, consider the patient's habitual style. Every person comes to the neurologic disorder with a personality makeup or style. This style interacts with the neurologic event and results in some type of reaction. There are some generalizations about personality styles that should be studied (Millon, 1981; Shapiro, 1965, 1981), but because every person is unique, each person will have a unique reaction. We should not become so locked into our stereotypes of what styles exist that we impose this frame of reference on the observation and miss seeing the uniqueness of each person.

Clinical neuropsychologists have not discussed or published much about the interaction of personality style with brain injury although they are prone to very quickly blame "premorbid factors" for complicated reactions. Kay (1992), Kay, Newman, Cavallo, Ezrachi, and Resnick (1992), Prigatano (1992), and Miller (1993) are refreshing exceptions who have researched and written about this complicated matter.

Emotional reactions to the neurologic event need to be carefully considered. The reaction will often include very deep grief. There is no other injury that threatens a person like brain injury, which attacks the essence of self. We should be very sensitive to this in our assessments and not close the door to its manifestation. Attentive empathetic listening can facilitate the patient's awareness and resolution of these emotional issues and provide deep insights into the person's personality.

Given the current state of the art–science of assessing personality issues in neurologic patients, the following clinical guidelines are suggested:

- Be fully aware of how complicated the phenomenon of personality is. Do not oversimplify the matter by artificially separating personality from brain functioning.
- Appreciate the long history of personality assessment in clinical psychology and become a student of it (Goldstein & Hersen, 1990; Hersen, Kazdin, & Bellack, 1983; Rapaport, Gill, & Schafer, 1968).
- Be aware of your own limitations. Consider obtaining additional training or supervision if your formal training did not provide adequate training in the clinical assessment of personality. It is not unusual that a neuropsychologist lacks good training in this area. Neuropsychological training is often very focused on neurobehavioral knowledge and assessment with little training provided in understanding and assessing personality. If this happened to you, find a mentor supervisor and expand your experience.
- Recognize the limitations of psychological tests in assessing personality factors in neurologic patients.
- Do not think that something as complicated as personality can be easily or quickly assessed.
- Do not rely on any one method such as a single test and the limited data it provides to make decisions regarding personality habits, brain-based personality changes, or brain–personality reactions to brain disease.
- Use a comprehensive assessment approach that uses as many methods as possible to *directly and indirectly observe* the manifestations of personality.
- When using psychological tests, use only those meeting the criteria of good tests:

standardized materials and procedures, optimal motivation, immediate recording, objective scoring, appropriate norms, and established validity (Dahlstrom, 1993; Matarazzo, 1990; for a reminder and a deeper appreciation of these criteria, carefully read these excellent articles).

- Keep a constant lookout for tests specifically developed to study personality factors in neurologic patients. Review the research behind them and adopt them when indicated (Borod et al., 1990; Nelson, Mitrushina, Satz, Sowa, & Cohen, 1993; Nelson et al., 1989). Better tests will more directly assess the object of study and not rely solely on self-report. Inventories will ideally incorporate the reports of others as well as those of the patient, and will allow judgments about the person's behavior both before and after the onset of neurologic disorder. The Neuropsychology Behavior and Affect Profile of Nelson et al. (1989) is a good example of implementing before and after ratings by both the patient and significant others.
- Review some of the more recently developed tests in clinical psychology. Although they will have the limitations inherent in inventories, they may have built on the past and represent an improved technology. Morey's (1991; Morey & Henry, 1994) *Personality Assessment Inventory* shows promise but there is currently no research regarding neurologic patients. The test must be used cautiously because the test has items that may be endorsed by neurologic patients because of their neurologic disorders and elevate scales for reasons other than psychiatric disorder. Another promising measure is the NEO Personality Inventory–Revised (NEO PI–R; Costa & McCrae, 1991, 1992), but again there is no current research on it with neurologic patients. It is conceptually rooted in well-established personality theory referred to as the "Big Five." The model derives from factor analytic personality psychology research which concludes that personality traits can be summarized into five basic dimensions: Neuroticism (N) versus Emotional Stability; Extraversion (E) or Surgency; Openness to Experience (O) or Intellect; Agreeableness (A) versus Antagonism; and Conscientiousness (C) or Will to Achieve. An effort is in process to apply this Five-Factor Model to clinical settings (Costa & Widiger, 1994). There is an interesting recent review and debate of conceptual issues regarding the MMPI and the NEO PI–R which should be of general interest (Butcher, 1992). Where all of this theorizing will lead and how it will affect the practical neuropsychological assessment of personality is unknown, but it merits close attention.
- When analyzing all of the information/data collected in the study of a patient, specifically consider how *perception, cognition, emotion, motivation*, and *action* are currently functioning for the person. Try to imagine how these components of personality probably functioned prior to onset of the neurologic disorder. It might help to write the five words down a column to the left side of a page and then create two columns labeled "Before" and "Now" with rows from each of the major components of personality crossing the "Before" and "Now" columns. Try filling in the cells of this chart. If you cannot do it, you probably need more information.
- Be open and creative. There are many useful methods for observing the person that we often ignore or consider to be trivial. The relationship with the person is rich with information regarding their personality. The "interpersonal pull" as suggested by Sullivan (1953) provides useful information. *In vivo* real-life observations often reveal more than those based on office contacts (Lhermitte, 1986; Lhermitte, Pillon, & Serdaru, 1986). Photographs (Weiser, 1993) of the person before the disorder are a potential source of understanding the person, the family, and what has happened to them.
- Spend time directly observing the patient. Look at the patient and study their face. Think about that image when you write your report. Thich Nhat Hanh (1991), a

Vietnamese Zen master, poet, and peace advocate who was nominated for the Nobel Peace Prize in 1967, lent insight regarding useful methods to study the personality:

> When we want to understand something, we cannot just stand outside and observe it. We have to enter deeply into it and be one with it in order to really understand. If we want to understand a person, we have to feel his feelings, suffer his sufferings, and enjoy his joy. The word "comprehend" is made up of the Latin roots *cum*, which means "with," and *prehendere*, which means "to grasp it or pick it up." To comprehend something means to pick it up and be one with it. There is no other way to understand something. In Buddhism, we call this kind of understanding "non-duality." Not two.
>
> Fifteen years ago, I helped a committee for orphans who were victims of the war in Vietnam. From Vietnam, the social workers sent out applications, one sheet of paper with a small picture of a child in the corner, telling the name, age, and conditions of the orphan. My job was to translate the application from Vietnamese into French in order to seek a sponsor, so that the child would have food to eat and books for school, and be put into the family of an aunt, an uncle, or a grandparent. Then the committee in France could send money to the family member to help take care of the child.
>
> Each day I helped translate about 30 applications. The way I did it was to look at the picture of the child. I did not read the application, I just took time to look at the picture of the child. Usually after only 30 or 40 seconds, I became one with the child. Then I would pick up the pen and translate the words from the application onto another sheet. Afterwards I realized that it was not me who had translated the application; it was the child and me, who had become one. Looking at his or her face, I felt inspired, and I became the child and he or she became me, and together we did the translation. It is very natural. You don't have to practice a lot of meditation to be able to do that. You just look, allowing yourself to be, and you lose yourself in the child, and the child in you. (pp. 100–101)

SUMMARY AND CONCLUSIONS

The scientist has marched in and taken the place of the poet. But one day somebody will find the solution to the problems of the world and remember, it will be a poet, not a scientist.
—Frank Lloyd Wright

In summary, we briefly discussed a definition of personality, the relationship between brain and personality, the methods onlookers use to infer personality, the methods commonly used by neuropsychologists, the limits of so-called personality tests, the best observational alternatives, and some clinical guidelines. More specifically, the discussion revealed several important points. The concept of personality is a very complicated abstraction referring to a person's characteristic habitual and predictable manner of perceiving, thinking, emoting, and acting under similar situations with the major components of personality being perception, cognition, emotion, motivation, and action. The underlying causes of these actions include many interacting biological, sociological, and environmental factors. There are many interacting brain systems contributing to these processes that can be disrupted in obvious and subtle ways by brain disorder—the exact mechanisms are poorly understood and yet to be discovered. Personality is inferred by onlookers from multiple verbal and nonverbal manifestations. A variety of methods provide the raw data from which to make inferences regarding personality. One of the methods used by neuropsychologists is the psychological test that yields some information but has a number of limitations when used as part of a neuropsychological assessment. The best approach to the assessment of personality in neurologic patients avoids reliance on single measures and uses all available methods of observation to collect as much data as possible from which to make inferences regarding someone's personality.

Future research into this complicated area should be based on clearer conceptualizations. An appreciation for the complexity of personality is fundamental to designing relevant studies. We should no longer assume that a particular test is an adequate measure of personality. Also, we should no longer assume homogeneity of neuropathologies and think that we can artificially lump groups together while ignoring the obvious variabilities. For example, a study of emotional and personality factors in Parkinson's disease using the MMPI (or any other similar inventory) as the measure of "emotion and personality" denies the reality of the phenomenon under study. Such studies represent a gross violation of what we know, they are poorly conceived and reveal virtually nothing. We can do better.

We can develop more direct measures of the behaviors of personality. We can also develop inventories and rating scales designed to obtain relevant information from patients and significant others, as well as instruments specific to various neuropathologies. Finally, we can study how personality style interacts with the neurologic disorder and investigate other aspects of the inferential process, such as diagnostic decision making and the use of qualitative data.

We can design methods that more directly measure the effects of the brain on personality than is measured by symptom inventories. These measures would focus on the many verbal and nonverbal behaviors from which we make the inferences of personality. Borod's work in this area is an inspiration (see Borod et al., 1990).

Inventories and rating scales can be developed that are more sensitive to the problems of neurologic patients and less confused with the symptoms of psychiatric disorder. Inventories should allow pre- and post-neurologic disorder ratings. They should allow both the patient and significant others to respond. Items can be eliminated that have confusing symptom overlap with psychiatric disorders. Scales can be incorporated in the test that specifically identify psychiatric symptoms. The language used should be simple and understandable. Large print with nonconfusing response sheets should be used. The work of Nelson et al. (1989, 1993) in developing *The Neuropsychology Behavior and Affect Profile* exemplifies a number of these improvements.

Rather than assuming that neurologic patients are a unitary group, specific measures for particular neuropathologies can be developed. This approach recognizes the specific issues to be explored within subgroups of neurologic patients without homogenizing their variability. For example, it is clinically apparent that facial expression of emotion is limited in some persons with Parkinson's disease. This limitation can have some impact on onlookers that affect their perceptions of the patient's personality. Instruments can be developed to better understand this problem among this group of patients. The same instruments might not be relevant to other patient groups.

How personality styles or types interact with brain disorders is clinically recognized as significant but there has been no research in this direction. Kay (1992) discussed how various personality types seem to interact with mild closed head injury and may be related to the functional outcome of the injury. We need research to explore how the premorbid personality affects neurologic adjustment and recovery. A starting point might be to study the adjustment to injury according to Kay's classification. Another approach could look at adjustment to injury with the more obvious problematic personality styles (Shapiro, 1965).

Research of the general neuropsychological evaluation process and methods of collecting data and making inferences about personality also is needed. We have not studied the gamut of available methods; instead, our focus has primarily been on tests and test scores. The reason for this focus on tests and the neglect of other methods has been the belief that the tests we are using are doing the job, and doing it "objectively." We have confused the terms "objective" and "subjective" with "qualitative" and "quantitative." We have mistakenly believed that qualitative methods cannot be objective when, in fact, the very opposite is true

(Cripe, 1995; Taylor & Bogdan, 1984). We need to learn more about qualitative methods and how to effectively use them to directly assess personality.

The interview, direct observations, reports of others, examiner's thought process, and so on are all methods of observation we employ. Because these methods deliver considerable data from which we make inferences regarding personality, we need to study and develop them rather than ignore their existence or deny their important and useful influence on our assessments.

This chapter has argued that the concept of personality and its real world referents are very complicated and that our technology and methods are limited. Does this mean that the challenges for systematic study and measurement are so great and hopelessly limited that we should despair? I think not. The limitations we encounter in this endeavor are not peculiar to the study of humans by humans, as is often portrayed by our critics. Any area of study is complicated and the observational methods are always subjected to our interpretations. It is inherent in the human condition that when we try to study complicated external realities we are challenged and may never know the complete reality. Although the study of ourselves is somewhat of a bootstrap operation and may have limits, we are potentially limitless in our capacity to apply scientific methodology to complicated subjects and to know more.

One of the most honorable things a human can do is to study and understand their fellow human beings and to attempt to alleviate their suffering. At present, the best we can do is to be keenly aware of our limitations, to use all the tools at our disposal, to open-mindedly study each patient appreciating their uniqueness, and to vigilantly research the assessment problem.

We should confront the challenges of assessing personality in brain injury by using all our avenues of knowing to achieve a deeper understanding of the persons who are experiencing fundamental changes in self because of the ravages of brain damage. They need and deserve our dedicated efforts to help find the best possible adaptation to a most unfortunate existential dilemma.

REFERENCES

Alfano, D. P., Finlayson, M. A .J., Stearns, G. M., & Nielson, P. M. (1990). The MMPI and neurologic dysfunction: Profile configuration and analysis. *The Clinical Neuropsychologist, 4*, 69–79.

American Psychiatric Association (1987). *Diagnostic and statistical manual of mental disorders* (3rd ed., rev.). Washington DC: Author.

Beck, A. T., Ward, C. H., Mendelson, M., Mock, J., & Erbaugh, J. (1961). An inventory for measuring depression. *Archives of General Psychiatry, 4*, 561–571.

Berger, M., Bobbit, R. A., Carter, W. B., & Gilson, B. S. (1981). The Sickness Impact Profile: Development and final revision of a health status measure. *Medical Care, 19*, 787–805.

Birbaumer, N., & Ohman, A. (1993). *The structure of emotion*. Seattle: Hogrefe & Huber.

Borod, J. C. (1992). Interhemispheric and intrahemispheric control of emotion: A focus on unilateral brain damage. *Journal of Consulting and Clinical Psychology, 60*, 339–348.

Borod, J. C. (Ed.). (1993). Neuropsychological perspectives on components of emotion (special section). *Neuropsychology, 7*, 427–509.

Borod, J. C., Welkowitz, J., Alpert, M. Brozgold, A. Z., Martin, C. Peselow, E., & Diller, L. (1990). Parameters of emotional processing in neuropsychiatric disorders: Conceptual issues and a battery of tests. *Journal of Communication Disorders, 23*, 247–271.

Butcher, J. N. (Section Ed.). (1992). Special section: Assessing personality characteristics in clinical settings. *Psychological Assessment, 4*, 3–25.

Butcher, J. N., Dahlstrom, W. G., Grahma, J. R., Tellegen, A. M., & Kaemmer, B. (1989). *MMPI–2 manual for administration and scoring*. Minneapolis: University of Minnesota Press.

Cacioppo, J. T., Klein, D. J., Berntson, G. G., & Hatfield, E. (1993). The psychophysiology of emotion. In L. Lewis & J. M. Haviland (Eds.), *Handbook of emotions* (pp. 119–142). New York: Guilford.

Colligan, R. C. (1985). In the beginning: History and development of the MMPI. *Psychiatric Annals, 15*, 524–533.

Costa, P. T., Jr., & McCrae, R. R. (1991). *Manual for the Revised NEO Personality Inventory (NEO PI–R) and NEO Five-Factor Inventory (NEO–FFI)*. Odessa, FL: Psychological Assessment Resources.
Costa, P. T., Jr., & McCrae, R. R. (1992). Normal personality assessment in clinical practice: The NEO Personality Inventory. *Psychological Assessment, 4*, 5–13.
Costa, P. T., Jr., & Widiger, T. A. (Eds.). (1994). *Personality disorders and the Five-Factor model*. Washington, DC: American Psychological Association.
Cripe, L. I. (1988). *The clinical use of the MMPI with neurologic patients: A new perspective*. Paper presented at the Army Medical Department annual psychology conference, Seattle, WA.
Cripe, L. I. (1989). Neuropsychological and psychosocial assessment of the brain-injured person: Clinical concepts and guidelines. *Rehabilitation Psychology, 34*, 93–100.
Cripe, L. I. (1995). The ecological validity of executive function testing. In R. J. Sbordone & C. J. Long (Eds.), *Ecological validity of neuropsychological testing*. Delray Beach, FL: St. Lucie Press.
Cripe, L. I., Maxwell, J. K., & Hill, E. L. (1995). Multivariate discriminate function analysis of neurologic, pain, and psychiatric patients with MMPI. *Journal of Clinical Psychology 51*, (2), 258–268.
Dahlstrom, W. G. (1993). Small samples, large consequences. *American Psychologist, 48*, 393–399.
Derogatis, L. R. (1977). *SCL–90–R: Administration, scoring and procedures manual I*. Baltimore: Clinical Psychometric Research.
Derogatis, L. R. (1983). *SCL–90–R: Administration, scoring and procedures manual II*. Baltimore: Clinical Psychometric Research.
Derryberry, D., & Tucker, D. M. (1992). Neural mechanisms of emotion. *Journal of Consulting and Clinical Psychology, 60*, 329–338.
Dodrill, C. B. (1986). Psychosocial consequences of epilepsy. In S. B. Filskov & T. J. Boll (Eds.), *Handbook of clinical neuropsychology* (Vol. 2, pp. 338–363). New York: Wiley.
Dodrill, C. B., Batzel, L. W., Queisser, H. R., & Temkin, N. R. (1980). An objective method for the assessment of psychological and social difficulties among epileptics. *Epilepsia, 21*, 123–135.
Drever, J. (1965). *A dictionary of psychology* (rev. ed.). New York: Penguin.
Erdberg, P. (1990). Rorschach assessment. In G. Goldstein & M. Hersen (Eds.), *Handbook of psychological assessment* (2nd ed.) (pp. 387–399). New York: Pergamon.
Exner, J. E., Jr. (1986). *The Rorschach: A comprehensive system. Vol. 1: Basic foundations* (2nd ed.). New York: Wiley.
Faust, D., Guilmette, T. J., Hart, K., Arkes, H. R., Fishburne, F. J., & Davey, L. (1988). Neuropsychologist's training, experience, and judgment accuracy. *Archives of Clinical Neuropsychology, 3*, 145–163.
Faust, D., & Ziskin, J. (1988). The expert witness in psychology and psychiatry. *Science*, 241, 31–35.
Faust, D., Ziskin, J., & Hiers, J. B. (1991a). *Brain damage claims: Coping with neuropsychological evidence: Volume I. The scientific and professional literature*. Los Angeles: Law and Psychology Press.
Faust, D., Ziskin, J., & Hiers, J. B. (1991b). *Brain damage claims: Coping with neuropsychological evidence: Volume II. Practical guidelines, cross-examination and case illustration*. Los Angeles: Law and Psychology Press.
Frank, G. (1991). Research on the clinical usefulness of the Rorschach: 2. The assessment of cerebral dysfunction. *Perceptual and Motor Skills, 72*, 103–111.
Franzen, M. D. (Ed.). (1989). *Reliability and validity in neuropsychological assessment*. New York: Plenum.
Gass, C. S. (1991a). Emotional variables and neuropsychological test performance. *Journal of Clinical Psychology, 47*, 153–157.
Gass, C. S. (1991b). MMPI–2 interpretation and closed head injury: A correction factor. *Psychological Assessment: A Journal of Consulting and Clinical Psychology, 3*, 27–31.
Goldstein, G., & Hersen, M. (Eds.). (1990). *Handbook of psychological assessment* (2nd ed.). New York: Pergamon.
Goldstein, K. (1952). The effect of brain damage on the personality. *Psychiatry, 15*, 245–260.
Guralnik, D. B. (Ed.). (1992). *Webster's new world dictionary of the American language* (2nd college ed.). New York: Simon & Schuster.
Haaland, K. Y. (Ed.). (1992). The emotional concomitants of brain damage. *Journal of Consulting and Clinical Psychology, 60*, 327–391.
Hall, C. S., & Lindzey, G. (1978). *Theories of personality* (3rd ed.). New York: Wiley.
Hamilton, M. (1967). Development of a rating scale for primary depressive illness. *British Journal of Social and Clinical Psychology, 6*, 278–296.
Hanh, T. N. (1991). *Peace is every step: The path of mindfulness in everyday life*. New York: Bantam.
Harlow, J. M. (1868). Recovery after severe injury to the head. *Publication of the Massachusetts Medical Society, 2*, 327–346.

Hathaway, S. R., & McKinley, J. C. (1951). *MMPI manual*. New York: Psychological Corporation.
Heilman, K. M., Bowers, D., & Valenstein, E. (1985). Emotional disorders associated with neurological diseases. In K. M. Heilman & E. Valenstein (Eds.), *Clinical neuropsychology* (pp. 461–497). New York: Oxford University Press.
Heilman, K. M., & Satz, P. (Eds.). (1983). *Neuropsychology of human emotion* (3rd ed.). New York: Guilford.
Hersen, M., Kazdin, A. E., & Bellack, A. S. (Eds.). (1983). *The clinical psychology handbook*. New York: Pergamon.
James, W. (1884). What is an emotion? *Mind, 9*, 188–205.
Jennett, B., & Teasdale, G. (1981). *Management of head injuries*. Philadelphia: Davis.
Joseph, R. (1990). *Neuropsychology, neuropsychiatry, and behavioral neurology*. New York: Plenum.
Kaplan, H. I., & Sadock, B. J. (1991). *Synopsis of psychiatry: Behavioral sciences, clinical psychiatry* (6th ed.). Baltimore: Williams & Wilkins.
Katz, M. M., & Lyerly, S. B. (1963). Methods for measuring adjustment and social behavior in the community: I. Rationale, description, discriminative validity and scale development. *Psychological Reports, 13*, 503–535.
Kay, T. (1992). Neuropsychological diagnosis: Disentangling the multiple determinants of functional disability after mild traumatic brain injury. In L. Horn & N. Zasler (Eds.), *Rehabilitation of post-concussive disorders (Physical medicine and rehabilitation: State of the art reviews)* (pp. 109–127). Philadelphia: Hanley & Belfus.
Kay, T., Newman, B., Cavallo, M., Ezrachi, O., & Resnick, M. (1992). Toward a neuropsychological model of functional disability after mild traumatic brain injury. *Neuropsychology, 6*, 371–384.
Kolb, B., & Whishaw, I. (1990). *Fundamentals of human neuropsychology*. New York: Freeman.
Lazarus, R. S. (1991). *Emotion and adaptation*. New York: Oxford University Press.
LeDoux, J. E., & Hirst, W. (Eds.). (1986). *Mind and brain: Dialogues in cognitive neuroscience*. New York: Cambridge University Press.
Levin, H. S., High, W. M., Goethe, K. E., Sisson, R. A., Overall, J. E., Rhoades, H. M., Eisenberg, H. M., Kalisky, Z., & Gray, H. E. (1986). The neurobehavioural rating scale: Assessment of the behavioural sequelae of head injury by the clinician. *Journal of Neurology, Neurosurgery, and Psychiatry, 50*, 183–193.
Lewis, L., & Haviland, J. M. (Eds.). (1993). *Handbook of emotions*. New York: Guilford.
Lhermitte, F. (1986). Human autonomy and the frontal lobes. Part II: Patient behavior in complex and social situations: The "Environmental dependency syndrome." *Annals of Neurology, 19*, 335–343.
Lhermitte, F., Pillon, B., & Serdaru, M. (1986). Human autonomy and the frontal lobes. Part I: Imitation and utilization behavior: A neuropsychological study of 75 patients. *Annals of Neurology, 19*, 326–334.
Mack, J. L. (1979). The MMPI and neurological dysfunction. In C. S. Newmark (Ed.), *MMPI clinical and research trends* (pp. 53–79). New York: Praeger.
Maruish, M. E. (Ed.). (1994). *The use of psychological testing for treatment planning and outcome assessment*. Hillsdale, NJ: Lawrence Erlbaum Associates.
Matarazzo, J. D. (1986). Computerized clinical psychological test interpretations: Unvalidated plus all mean and no sigma. *American Psychologist, 41*, 14–24.
Matarazzo, J. D. (1990). Psychological assessment versus psychological testing: Validation from Binet to the school, clinic, and courtroom. *American Psychologist, 45*, 999–1017.
Mesulam, M. M. (Ed.). (1985). *Principles of behavioral neurology*. Philadelphia: Davis.
Miller, L. (1991). Brain and self: Toward a neuropsychodynamic model of ego autonomy and personality. *Journal of the American Academy of Psychoanalysis, 19*, 213–234.
Miller, L. (1992). Freud's brain: Toward a unified neuropsychodynamic model of personality and psychotherapy. *Journal of the American Academy of Psychoanalysis, 21*, 183–212.
Miller, L. (1993). *Psychotherapy of the brain-injured patient: Reclaiming the shattered self*. New York: Norton.
Millon, T. (1981). *Disorders of personality: DSM–III: Axis II*. New York: Wiley.
Millon, T. (1983). *Millon Clinical Multiaxial Inventory manual* (3rd ed.). Minneapolis, MN: National Computer Systems.
Millon, T. (1987). *Manual for the MCMI–II* (2nd ed.). Minneapolis, MN: National Computer Systems.
Morey, L. C. (1991). *The Personality Assessment Inventory professional manual*. Odessa, FL: Psychological Assessment Resources.
Morey, L. C., & Henry, W. (1994). Personality Assessment Inventory. In M. E. Maruish (Ed.), *The use of psychological testing for treatment planning and outcome assessment* (pp. 185–216). Hillsdale, NJ: Lawrence Erlbaum Associates.
Nelson, L. D., Mitrushina, M., Satz, P., Sowa, M., & Cohen, S. (1993). Cross-validation of the neuropsychology behavior and affect profile in stroke patients. *Psychological Assessment, 5*, 374–376.
Nelson, L. D., Satz, P., Mitrushina, M., Van Gorp, W., Cicchetti, D., Lewis, R., & Van Lanker, D. (1989). Development and validation of the neuropsychology behavior and affect profile. *Psychological Assessment, 1*, 266–272.

Overall, J. E., & Gorham, D. R. (1962). The Brief Psychiatric Rating Scale. *Psychological Reports, 10*, 799–812.
Prigatano, G. P. (1992). Personality disturbances associated with traumatic brain injury. *Journal of Consulting and Clinical Psychology, 60*, 360–368.
Prigatano, G. P., & Schacter, D. (Eds.). (1991). *Awareness of deficit after brain injury: Theoretical and clinical implications*. New York: Oxford University Press.
Rao, S. M., Huber, S. J., & Bornstein, R. A. (1992). Emotional changes with multiple sclerosis and Parkinson's disease. *Journal of Consulting and Clinical Psychology, 60*, 369–378.
Rapaport, D., Gill, M. M., & Schafer, R. (1968). *Diagnostic psychological testing* (rev. ed.). New York: International Universities Press.
Reber, A. S. (1985). *The Penguin dictionary of psychology*. New York: Penguin.
Robbins, D. E. (1989). The Rorschach Inkblots. In M. D. Franzen (Ed.), *Reliability and validity in neuropsychological assessment* (pp. 153–163). New York: Plenum.
Robinson, R. G., & Chait, R. M. (1985). Emotional correlates of structural brain injury with particular emphasis on post- stroke mood disorders. *CRC Critical Reviews in Clinical Neurobiology, 1*, 285–318.
Ross, E. D. (1985). Modulation of affect and nonverbal communication by the right hemisphere. In M. M. Mesulam (Ed.), *Principles of behavioral neurology* (pp. 239–257). Philadelphia: Davis.
Ruckdeschel-Hibbard, M., Gordon, W. A., & Diller, L. (1986). Affective disturbances associated with brain damage. In S. B. Filskov & T. J. Boll (Eds.), *Handbook of clinical neuropsychology* (Vol. 2, pp. 305–337). New York: Wiley.
Shapiro, D. (1965). *Neurotic styles*. New York: Basic Books.
Shapiro, D. (1981). *Autonomy and rigid character*. New York: Basic Books.
Sheehan, W. (1988). *Planets & perception*. Tucson: University of Arizona Press.
Sherman, A. G., Shaw, T. G., & Glidden, H. (1994). Emotional behavior as an agenda in neuropsychological evaluation. *Neuropsychology Review, 4*, 45–69.
Stuss, D. T., & Benson, D. F. (1986). *The frontal lobes*. New York: Raven.
Stuss, D. T., Gow, C. A., & Hetherington, C. R. (1992). "No longer Gage": Frontal lobe dysfunction and emotional changes. *Journal of Consulting and Clinical Psychology, 60*, 349–359.
Sullivan, H. S. (1953). *The interpersonal theory of psychiatry*. New York: Norton.
Taylor, S. J., & Bogdan, R. (1984). *Introduction to qualitative research methods: The search for meanings* (2nd ed.). New York: Wiley.
Teri, L., & Wagner, A. (1992). Alzheimer's disease and depression. *Journal of Consulting and Clinical Psychology, 60*, 379–391.
Thompson, J. G. (1988). *The psychobiology of emotions*. New York: Plenum.
Weiner, I. B. (1994). Rorschach assessment. In M. E. Maruish (Ed.), *The use of psychological testing for treatment planning and outcome assessment* (pp. 249–278). Hillsdale, NJ: Lawrence Erlbaum Associates.
Weiser, J. (1993). *PhotoTherapy techniques: Exploring the secrets of personal snapshots and family albums*. San Francisco: Jossey-Bass.
Wolman, B. B. (Ed.). (1973). *Dictionary of behavioral science*. New York: Van Nostrand Reinhold.
Yesavage, J., Brink, T., Rose, T., Lum, O., Huang, V., Adey, M., & Leirer, V. (1983). Development and validation of a geriatric depression screening scale: A preliminary report. *Journal of Psychiatric Research, 17*, 37–49.

6

Computerized Neuropsychological Assessment

Gary G. Kay
Victoria N. Starbuck
Georgetown University School of Medicine

Computers are playing an increasing role in neuropsychological assessment. Most often, computers are used to assist in the scoring of tests. However, it is becoming increasingly more common to have one or more tests administered on a computer. Some of these tests are likely to be computer versions of conventional neuropsychological tests (e.g., the Wisconsin Card Sorting Test or Halstead Category Test). Others are likely to be tests that were developed specifically for administration on computers (e.g., continuous performance tests). This shift from paper-and-pencil testing to computerized test administration and scoring may be seen as a byproduct of the ubiquitous nature of the desktop personal computer. Has this computerization made a truly significant contribution to neuropsychological assessment, or is this simply new wine in old bottles? What are the benefits of computer applications in neuropsychological assessment? The present chapter offers answers to these questions and provides an overview of computer applications in neuropsychological assessment. The chapter also provides a discussion of many of the issues surrounding the use of computers in neuropsychological test administration.

HISTORICAL PERSPECTIVE

The relatively low cost of personal computers and the potential of having computers perform labor-intensive scoring and test administration procedures may explain the popularity of computer applications in neuropsychological assessment. Computerized testing has promised to be an inexpensive way to routinely administer paper-and-pencil tests. The computer is capable of administering and storing a nearly unlimited number of psychological test forms (i.e., questionnaires, inventories, and tests). The only limitations are media storage, program costs, and copyright considerations.

The computerized scoring programs for the Minnesota Multiphasic Personality Inventory were probably the first computer testing applications to gain wide acceptance. The computer was capable of presenting test items, storing responses, scoring the protocol, generating the profile, interpreting the results, and saving the scores in a database. Computer programs for personality testing have continued to flourish. The development and popularity of computerized neuropsychological tests have lagged somewhat behind developments in personality testing.

Early computer programs (and early computers) were anything but "user-friendly." Fifteen years ago, when computerized test applications were just beginning to enter the mainstream, most psychologists were unwilling, or simply not interested enough, to invest a great deal of their time, money, or both to run computer versions of conventional neuropsychological tests. The computers were slow, the graphics quality was poor, and there was a (well-deserved) feeling that one needed to be either an engineer or a computer scientist in order to get the software working. As a result, early attempts at computerization of cognitive tests were not particularly successful.

Today's computers are far less expensive and far more efficient. It is not unusual for today's computers to be 15 times faster than the computers of 10 years ago. The computers have much greater storage capacity, and the video graphics can present full-motion video and photographic quality color images. Just as important, there has been a dramatic improvement in the "usability" of the software. It is much easier to install and run computer programs. Common software platforms, such as Windows, are used to run large numbers of programs and make it very easy for users to learn new ones. The improvements in graphics and program design are also evident in improved instructions provided to test takers. Computer novices are now able to operate most of the recently developed programs. The nature of the developers has also changed. Ten to 15 years ago software was largely developed in U.S. Department of Defense (DOD) laboratories and in the garages of creative programmers. Now, most of the assessment software is developed and published by major test publishers who can provide the support and maintenance that is essential for commercial applications.

Clearly, the past 10 years have brought us better computers and better (running) software programs. Nevertheless, the question remains as to whether these developments have resulted in any meaningful contribution to the field of neuropsychology. There is a possibility that we have simply created technologically sophisticated workbooks which present tests designed long before the computer age. The challenging question remains: What does computerized testing offer over and above paper-and-pencil testing?

LIMITATIONS OF PAPER-AND-PENCIL TESTS

One way to address these concerns is to review some of the limitations of paper-and-pencil testing. One overriding issue is the lack of standardization in the administration of conventional neuropsychological tests. Although published test instructions are readily available, many neuropsychologists, and their technicians, develop their own style of test administration that may differ somewhat from the standard. For example, the presentation of cues for items on WAIS–R Vocabulary is frequently non-standard and can influence a patient's performance and his or her test score. We have seen a great deal of variability in how a test as simple as the Trail Making Test is administered. It is not unusual to find an examiner incorrectly instructing the subject not to lift his or her pencil when completing this task.

Perhaps the most significant limitation of paper-and-pencil testing, especially in the field of neuropsychology, relates to timing. Timing is an important feature of stimulus presentation, control of interstimulus intervals, and in the measurement of subjects' test responses. Timing provides an important measure of a subject's mental processing. Test administrators often find it difficult to present items at a fixed rate (i.e., at a fixed interstimulus interval). For example, it is quite challenging to present word list items at the rate of one word per second. To do this, the examiner needs to simultaneously attend to both the word list and a stopwatch. Unless word lists and stories are presented on audio tape, there is likely to be considerable variability in the rate of stimulus presentation. Furthermore, timing accuracy can also be adversely affected by the speed of the examiner (in starting the timing interval) and by the type of device used to measure the latency of response or the time to complete a response. Stopwatches are far more accurate than the second hand of a wristwatch; however, the patient's performance anxiety is likely to be raised by the presence of a stopwatch. Furthermore, even if a stopwatch is used, it is still impossible for the administrator to reliably measure reaction times or other events that occur in times less than 1 second.

In addition to these technical limitations of conventional, non-computerized neuropsychological tests, there is also a great deal of cost associated with this approach. First of all, the administration and scoring of these instruments requires a highly trained and skilled individual. It is not only costly to train and employ such individuals, it is difficult to monitor the quality of their test administration skills over time. Furthermore, while administering these measures the clinician is unavailable to perform other clinical or administrative activities.

Conventional tests are also limited in their suitability for repeated administration. For most of these tests there is only a single form; as a result, there tend to be large practice effects associated with repeated administration of the tests. This prevents their being administered to the same subject for serial testing.

Assessment of the cognitive processes underlying an individual's test response requires more than simply noting the accuracy of the response. The "process approach" to neuropsychological assessment (Kaplan, Fein, Morris, & Delis, 1991) is dependent on the examiner recording multiple aspects of the patient's performance. This is particularly difficult using conventional testing methods. The examiner is usually occupied with presenting stimuli, timing response latencies, and recording accuracy of responses. Recording the means by which the examinee arrived at a response is generally beyond the capability of the human examiner.

Finally, conventional paper-and-pencil tests are not well suited for the assessment of certain domains of neuro-cognitive functioning. There are few conventional tests that assess an individual's ability to perform simultaneous tasks. First of all, it would be difficult for the administrator to handle two sets of materials simultaneously. In addition, the administrator would find it very taxing to record the subject's performance on the two different tasks. Although there are some paper-and-pencil tasks that involve simultaneous mental operations (e.g., Auditory Consonant Trigrams, the Paced Serial Auditory Addition Test), these tests do not involve switching or shifting attention between tasks or prioritizing cognitive tasks to maintain an efficient level of performance. Conventional tests are also limited to the presentation of fairly static materials and problems. Therefore, measurement of more dynamic cognitive and perceptual processes is typically omitted in non-computerized neuropsychological assessment. In addition, assessment of sustained attention and vigilance, which are best measured by continuous performance techniques, are simply not possible using paper-and-pencil methods.

FEATURES OF COMPUTERIZED NEUROPSYCHOLOGICAL TESTING

Precise control over timing of stimulus and response characteristics is a common feature of computer-administered tests. This allows for control over stimulus presentation time, interstimulus intervals, and measurement of both response latency and response duration, both of which may be critical elements in assessing aspects of brain functioning.

The extent to which software can provide the timing precision or resolution needed for a particular test application is a function of the software's method of recording time. The least desireable approach to timing uses "delay loops" in the software code. This is a programming technique in which the computer is instructed to repeatedly follow a set of instructions that require a fixed amount of time. However, different computers execute these loops at different rates. A computerized test developed in this fashion can be run reliably only on the model of computer for which it was programmed. This method is not adequate for recording response latencies or for presenting stimuli at the same time a subject is responding. Another approach to timing is accomplished by using the computer's "Time of Day clock" (TODc). On computers following the IBM standard, this approach indirectly generates a 55 msec "tick" rate. When this timing method is used on an IBM-compatible machine one can expect to achieve absolute timing resolution of no greater than one tenth of a second (Thorne, Grenser, Sing, & Hegge, 1985). Although this level of accuracy may be sufficient for controlling stimulus presentation and for obtaining gross estimates of response latency, it is not suitable for reaction times or for some other response latency estimates.

A superior approach to timing uses sophisticated software routines that modify and interact with the computer's basic input and output system (BIOS). By programming at the BIOS level it is possible to attain millisecond or better accuracy (Graves & Bradley, 1991). Similarly, millisecond timing can be attained on the Macintosh using special public domain software timing routines (Westall, Perkey, & Chute, 1986, 1989). This particular approach to timing is becoming increasingly popular among test developers.

A less common method of controlling timing involves the use of hardware timing cards. This method is accurate and effective, but requires programming for the specific hardware timing card being used. The disadvantages of add-in boards include increased equipment costs, more complex installation, and incompatibility with most laptop, notebook, and notepad computers.

Psychologists need to be aware of the method of timing and the degree of accuracy afforded by the technique being employed by their software. They must be sure that the timing resolution is sufficient for the testing application. In reviewing computerized neuropsychological tests we have frequently found tests that report times in the milliseconds (or even the tenths of milliseconds), but which utilize software that could provide only one-tenth-of-a-second resolution at best. Other tests that provide response speed scores compound their software timing resolution problems by requiring subjects to first choose among several response keys and then press the <Enter> key to record their response. This approach does not provide a direct measure of response speed. Another disconcerting observation is the variability in the interstimulus intervals on a number of the Windows-based testing programs. In Windows and other multitasking environments, the timing routines do not necessarily have priority, and events (such as presentation of a test stimulus) can be delayed by other computer operations.

Computer applications utilize a wide range of response input devices: keyboards and keypads, joysticks, touchscreens, mice, and light pens. The impact of response mode on test performance can be significant. For example, lack of keyboard familiarity can affect response time and the stability of a test. Banderet et al. (1988) compared two versions of a computerized addition task with standard paper-and-pencil administration. The initial computerized version required subjects to enter their answers from the keyboard. Although the authors provided subjects with typing lessons, subjects were 35% slower with the keyboard than with the paper-and-pencil version. Scores obtained from the computer version of the task were less stable with repeated administrations than those obtained with the paper-and-pencil version. The second computer version of the addition task provided subjects with a possible sum of the numbers. For this version, subjects simply responded by pressing one of two adjacent keys to indicate if the provided answer was correct or incorrect. This revision, using a simplified method of responding, produced greater stability of scores with repeated administration. It was also more sensitive than either the paper-and-pencil or original computer version of the task to degradations in performance in a study of the effects of altitude.

In retrospect, it appears that over the last two decades the trend has been largely away from the use of the keyboard, or at least a minimization of the need to type or locate specific keys. When a test is designed properly, the response keys are easily identified and responses can be made without the need to look down at the keyboard. The goal is to remove any translation time from decision to response. The "heads up" approach offered by touchscreen and light pen devices is gaining considerable attention. Instead of selecting a key corresponding to "Same" or "Different," the subject presses a box on the screen labeled *Same* or *Different*. Mouse buttons are also frequently used as a response input device. Joysticks on the other hand, are far less popular and tend to only be used for specialized tracking tasks.

The type of video display used to present stimuli may also affect subjects' performance. Displays differ in size, flatness of the screen, resolution, contrast, and in the precision with which figures appear on the screen. For example, a figure that appears circular on one screen may present as an oval on another screen; test authors need to indicate the size of the video display used in the normatization process. Flat-screen monitors produce less peripheral field distortion than curved monitors, and are preferable when subjects' responses are influenced by stimuli in the periphery. Display clarity depends on the graphic standard used by the software. Software using earlier standards (i.e., Color Graphics Adapter, CGA) result in characters and figures with poor resolution. Stimuli needing finer detail or that attempt to portray dimensionality are best programmed using more advanced graphics standards (i.e., Enhanced Graphics Adapter, EGA; or Visual Graphics Array, VGA). As always, there are trade-offs. Lower resolution graphics can be drawn on the screen more quickly than can higher resolution graphics. However, today's faster computers and enhanced video display cards are able to display complex graphics in a fraction of the time needed just a few years ago.

Video monitors introduce a ± 14–20 millisecond error variance in reaction time measures unless the program has been written to disable the video, wait for retrace, enable the video, and then start or restart the clock. The display interval rate of monochrome liquid crystal displays produces even greater error. These rates are seldom documented and usually impossible to synchronize. The decay time of most inexpensive monochrome monitors and the on/off time of LCD elements introduce inaccuracies in RT measurements and prevent tachistoscopic presentations. Best results are achieved with color or fast phosphor monitors (Thorne, personal communication, June 8, 1992). SVGA monitors, which are now the standard for new computers, produce brilliant colors with a high degree of resolution and speed.

Normative data collected using one type of display may not apply if the type, quality, or size of the display is changed. This is especially true when changing from a cathode ray tube display used by "desktop" machines to liquid crystal displays used by most "laptop" machines.

Computers are especially proficient at recording, storing, and manipulating information. This is very beneficial in computerized testing and makes it possible for computers to automatically record all aspects of a subject's response: the response latency, response duration, and the characteristics of the actual response. The recorded responses can then be scored, entered into complex algorithms, and compared to normative data stored on the same computer. In addition, most commercial software programs now provide detailed automated reports of the subject's test performance. The computer provides more accurate, more complete, and more timely compilation and scoring of test data than is otherwise possible.

Neuropsychologists in many settings are finding it necessary to provide serial testing of patients. Periodic disability evaluations, drug trials, rehabilitation settings, and pre- and postoperative evaluations require repeated administration of neuropsychological tests. As previously stated, conventional tests rarely offer more than a single form. In contrast, computer-administered tests often can randomly generate items, thereby creating numerous forms of a test. This approach to creating alternate forms of a test is suitable for subtests in which the stimuli can be randomized, or for subtests in which the cognitive task remains fixed but for which the stimuli can be randomly substituted. For example, on an arithmetic test involving two-column addition, different numbers can be entered into the problems to create alternate forms. Nevertheless, the burden is on the test developer to demonstrate the equivalence of forms using appropriate statistical methodology.

Computerized testing applications also have facilitated testing of aspects of cognition that are otherwise difficult, if not impossible, to assess with conventional methods. The computer allows the examiner to administer tests of dual or multitasking capabilities. Although patients have long complained of difficulty performing simultaneous mental operations, it has been difficult to assess this important area of functioning. Computerized tests have now been developed that combine tasks from a single modality or across two or more modalities. The new multimedia computers with high fidelity audio and full motion video capability will permit simulations of everyday tasks and lead to an improvement in the ecological validity of neuropsychological testing.

Computerization greatly facilitates the entry of test data into a database for subsequent research, comparison, or both. The improved standardization and use of shared databases allows for collaboration across multiple laboratories and test sites.

Advanced graphics-oriented programming languages have made it possible for non-programmers to create new tests. Programs such as the Toolbook program that Cool Spring Software makes available for computers using the Windows operating system, Hypercard (a similar program for Apple Macintosh computers), and Borland's Delphi program create visual programming environments which are designed to be extremely user-friendly and which enable individuals with limited programming skills to create new tests.

The ease with which new computerized tests can be created is a double-edged sword. There are likely to be many "home-brewed" tests that lack adequate development for clinical application; unfortunately, some of these tests may reach the clinical market. These tests tend to lack adequate normative data, have unknown reliability and validity, and do not have test manuals that meet professional guidelines. Collection of normative data is an expensive activity which few individuals or test publishers are willing to capitalize—this inhibits independent development of new computerized measures.

EXAMPLES OF COMPUTERIZED TESTING APPLICATIONS

Computerization of Conventional Neuropsychological Tests

An informal survey of neuropsychologists conducted by a test publisher indicated a wide acceptance of the computer editions of the Halstead Category Test (Curtiss & Tuttle, 1993a) and the Wisconsin Card Sorting Test (Curtiss & Tuttle, 1993b). The advantages of computerization include standardization of test administration, error-free presentation of test stimuli, and collection of peripheral performance characteristics (such as response latency), which are not recorded in the traditional test format. However, when a conventional test is transfered to computer presentation a number of performance variables may be affected, and conventional norms should not be assumed to apply. Changes in test performance may result from the lack of flexibility in the order and rate of item presentation, the subject's inability to review prior test items or responses, the lack of human feedback and encouragement, the absence of a human test administrator, or any combination thereof. These effects may alter the absolute level of performance on a test, although there still might exist a very high correlation between the conventional and computerized versions (Mead & Drasgow, 1993). In the case where the two versions are producing different absolute levels of performance there is a need for separate norms. If there is a clear relationship between the scores, it may be possible to develop a set of scales for transforming computer-derived scores into conventional test scores, thereby allowing for the use of conventional norms.

Computer versions of the Halstead Category Test basically replace the slide presentation of items with computer graphics. Except for the replacement of the bell and buzzer sounds by other computer-generated tones, the two forms of this test are basically identical. Nevertheless, the extent to which computerized and conventional modes of administration of the HCT are equivalent is still under investigation. Results reported by Choca and Morris (1992) demonstrated no statistically significant difference between computerized and conventional test administrations for a group of cognitively impaired male inpatients. Subjects were tested on two separate days, and the order of test administration was counterbalanced. Their results demonstrated a high correlation between the two test versions (.90), with similar total error scores of 85.22 and 90.22 for the conventional and computerized versions, respectively. They also reported that the rank order of scores for the subjects was basically the same for the two versions. These findings suggest that one may be able to interpret scores from the computerized version in much the same way as one would interpret scores from the conventional slide version. On the other hand, some potential limitations to generalization of the Choca and Morris results would include the high number of errors and level of impairment of the subjects used in their study.

Results are still equivocal with respect to demonstrating the equivalence of the computerized and conventional (card) version of the Wisconsin Card Sorting Test. There are few published reports demonstrating the equivalence of the two forms of this test. Preliminary results have suggested that for some patient groups, and not others, the two forms may be equivalent (Hellman, Green, Kern, & Christenson, 1992). Note that the computerized edition of the WCST is still published as a "Research Edition" (Curtiss & Tuttle, 1993b). Use of research edition tests should be avoided in cases where the data may be used in a forensic setting. In those cases, the validity of test results obtained from so-called "research editions" may be considered legally questionable or even inadmissable in court, and a psychologist who administers these tests in a medicolegal context is likely to be severely chastised for performing "research" without consent.

It should be noted that for both the computerized and conventional test versions, all test instructions are administered by a trained examiner. Therefore the presentation of instructions is unchanged. However, the computerized WCST and HCT provide more accurate response scoring and greater control over certain aspects of stimulus presentation (e.g., the examinee cannot look back through the deck on the WCST) than the non-computerized forms.

There are a number of programs that provide "computer-assisted" administration of conventional tests. For example, a computerized version of the Paced Auditory Serial Addition Test offered by ForeThought (1993), presents the test items and allows the examiner to digitally record the examinee's responses for later scoring. The system provides a number of scoring dimensions otherwise unavailable using conventional methods. However, the utility of these added scoring dimensions has yet to be shown. The California Verbal Learning Test software (Delis, Kramer, Kaplan, & Ober, 1987) also has a computer-assisted administration mode. The administrator can enter the subject's responses with a keyboard or light pen. However, neither of these input modes appears to be popular with users of the CVLT software.

Computerized Tests Developed for the Computer

Although continuous performance tests predate the personal computer by close to 20 years, the hardware once required for this type of procedure has now been almost entirely replaced by software. Some of these tests, such as Conners' Continuous Performance Test (Conners, 1995) have extensive normative data. These programs administer, score, and interpret the test results. Generally, these tests involve the presentation of letters, one at a time, with one or more letters identified as the "target." When the target appears, the subject presses a specified key on the keyboard or a mouse button. Sometimes the subject presses the specified key only when the target letter is preceded by another specified letter. These tests measure sustained attention in terms of response latency, errors of omission and commission, and certain signal detection parameters. The primary application for these tests at present is in the assessment of attention deficit disorder (ADD) in children. However, research has also demonstrated the sensitivity of continuous peformance tests in evaluating solvent and lead neurotoxicity (Baker et al., 1985).

One of the most popular computerized continuous performance tests is the Test of Variables of Attention (TOVA; McCarney & Greenberg, 1990). TOVA was developed to assess attention deficit–hyperactive disorder (ADHD) and the effects of medication in treating this disorder. The test stimulus is a large colored square containing a small inner square. The inner square is either adjacent to the top or bottom edge of the larger square. The target condition occurs when the inner square is adjacent to the top of the larger square. Subjects are instructed to press a microswitch whenever a target appears. The TOVA is a fixed-interval test with a stimulus duration of 100 msec and an interstimulus interval of 2 seconds. The frequency with which targets appear varies throughout the test. A unique feature of the TOVA is that it requires the subject to monitor the screen for 23 minutes. The length of the test is considered important because boredom appears to be a potent variable in assessing attention failures in individuals with ADHD. At present, norms are available for 800 children ages 6 to 15 and for young adults.

The TOVA produces a series of scores for the entire test and for performance during each quarter of the test. These scores include: (a) omission errors, (b) commission errors, (c) mean response time for correct responses to targets, (d) standard deviation of mean correct response times, (e) incidents of multiple responses, and (f) frequency of anticipatory responses.

Computerized attention testing can also be found in a recently developed test designed to detect neuropsychological malingering. Tests for malingering are designed to detect conscious efforts at performing poorly on tests or a general lack of motivation to cooperate with neuropsychological testing.

The Symbol Attention and Memory Test (SAM; Kay, Starbuck, & Spector, 1993) is a computer-administered, forced-choice visual discrimination test. The test was designed to be sufficiently complex and demanding to assess a range of response tendencies associated with invalid neuropsychological test performance. The SAM test detects several different patterns of performance associated with malingering, including below-chance performance on measures of accuracy, slower than normal response speed (especially for incorrect responses), increased frequency of errors in response to positive feedback, lack of a normal relationship between complexity and performance, and the presence of rare responses.

The test consists of three modules. The format, which is common to all three modules, involves presentation of a series of shapes on the computer, screen. For example, a screen may consist of a square, a cross, a triangle, and a star. The stimuli are presented for 4 seconds. This presentation is followed by a blank screen that appears for a varying duration. The interstimulus interval is followed by another screen showing a series of shapes. The subject responds by indicating whether the series of shapes is identical to the one presented earlier. The patient's responses are examined using multiple performance criteria, each with empirical cutoffs, designed to discriminate malingering from nonmalingering subjects. The SAM test was designed to combine simplicity of presentation with complex and adaptive performance analyses to provide a sensitive measure of response integrity.

COMPUTERIZED TEST BATTERIES

CogScreen

CogScreen (Kay, 1995) is a computer-administered and -scored cognitive screening instrument that was initially designed to meet the Federal Aviation Administration's (FAA) need for an instrument which could detect subtle changes in cognitive functioning. Specifically, CogScreen has been found to assess attention, memory, visual perceptual processing, logical problem solving, and reaction time. CogScreen consists of a series of automated cognitive tests, each self-contained and presented with instructions and a brief practice segment. The battery was designed to take advantage of many of the benefits offered by computerization, including improved standardization of administration and scoring, superior timing resolution, and the presentation of dynamic and multiple test stimuli. The program automatically generates 12 alternate test forms needed for repeated test administration to the same individual. It also automatically records each test item, the respondent's response and the speed of the respondent's response. Software timing provides millisecond-level timing resolution.

The program allows the test user to select from among a variety of test report formats: a summary report of raw test scores; graphs and tables showing an individual's percentiles relative to a specified pilot normative data set; a data output file that can be used for exporting CogScreen results to a statistical package, database, or spreadsheet; and a detailed data output report listing the actual test items, responses, and response times. The battery runs on a standard IBM PC–AT compatible personal computer, with an EGA or VGA graphics card, color monitor, and a light pen. The light pen was chosen to be the primary response input device in order to reduce the advantage of prior computer experience and keyboard use. Furthermore, the light pen allows the examinee to maintain focus on the screen at all times.

The battery consists of 13 subtests (see Table 6.1). Each test begins with instructions that include examples of test items. This is followed by presentation of practice items. If the subject fails to meet a pre-established level of performance on the practice items, the instructions are repeated. If the practice criteria are met, the subject has the option of reviewing the instructions or proceeding with the test. Tests run for a set length of time or for a set number of items. The instructions are generally self-explanatory, and the test administrator rarely needs to provide further directions.

The normative database for the Aeromedical Edition of CogScreen (CogScreen–AE) consists of data collected from over 700 commercial aviators. Normative data collection for the general clinical edition is currently underway. Validity studies have demonstrated expected relationships with analog paper-and-pencil tests; factor analytic studies have demonstrated expected (and meaningful) cognitive constructs; and criterion-related studies have demonstrated high levels of sensitivity and specificity in comparison to traditional neuropsychological instruments.

CogScreen represents the culmination of a 7-year international effort aimed at developing a sensitive and specific instrument for the detection of cognitive changes resulting from mild

TABLE 6.1
CogScreen Subtests

Backward Digit Span
Math Test
Visual Sequence Comparison
Symbol Digit Coding (with Immediate and Delayed Paired Associate Recall)
Matching to Sample
Manikin (a test of visuospatial processing)
Divided Attention Test (combined Visual Monitoring and Sequence Comparison Test)
Auditory Sequence Comparison
Pathfinder (a Trail Making Test analog)
Shifting Attention Test (a test of executive functions)
Dual Task Test (a measure of tracking and working memory)

brain dysfunction. The first step in this process was an exploratory study which demonstrated that computer-based performance tests were as sensitive as traditional neuropsychological screening instruments in detecting the presence of brain dysfunction (Horst & Kay, 1988). This led to the earliest version of CogScreen, a computerized battery consisting of 11 subtests. The battery was evaluated by testing 40 pilots approximately balanced across four age groups, 40 age- and IQ-matched nonpilot normals, and 40 age- and IQ-matched patients with mild brain dysfunction secondary to head injury, tumor or stroke, substance abuse, or mild dementia. Respondents were administered a partial Wechsler Adult Intelligence Scale–Revised (Wechsler, 1981), the Paced Auditory Serial Addition Test (Gronwall, 1977), the Trail Making Test (Reitan & Wolfson, 1985), the Symbol Digit Modalities Test, and the 11 subtests of CogScreen. The conventional neuropsychological tests were selected for inclusion in the study based on their reported ability to detect brain dysfunction.

Pilots and nonpilot normals performed significantly better than patients on 38 of the 50 dependent measures derived from CogScreen. Using a five-variable cutoff rule, CogScreen was able to correctly classify 32 out of 40 patients with brain dysfunction and misclassified only three pilots. By comparison, the traditional neuropsychological tests correctly classified only 20 of the 40 patients and misclassified two pilots. Pilots outperformed nonpilot normals on many of the response time measures; however, these differences failed to reach statistical significance.

Construct validity was evaluated by comparing CogScreen performance with performance on paper-and-pencil analog tests. For example, the CogScreen Symbol Digit Coding test and the traditional Symbol Digit Modalities test correlated at .80, $p < .001$. The Number Pathfinder test correlated at .44 ($p < .001$) with Part A of the Trail Making Test, and Combined Pathfinder correlated at .73 ($p < .001$) with Part B of the Trail Making Test (Horst & Kay, 1991).

Two tests were added to the final version of CogScreen: one of concept formation and abstract reasoning, and one of divided attention employing tracking and memory components. Testing was conducted with over 460 commercial airline pilots at three major airports. In addition to CogScreen, all pilots were administered the WAIS–R and completed extensive demographic and medical history questionnaires. Approximately 200 of the pilots returned for 6-month and 12-month follow-up testing with CogScreen. An additional 100 pilots who were not tested at 6 months returned for follow-up testing only at the 12-month follow-up session. Data were analyzed to determine the battery's test–retest reliability.

Comparisons of CogScreen performance with scores from the WAIS–R, Symbol Digit Modalities Test, and Trail Making Test were used to determine the construct validity of the test. In addition, a modified Halstead–Reitan test battery was administered to 120 of the commercial pilot subjects who completed the first round of CogScreen testing. The results from this normative data collection process were used in further construct validation studies of CogScreen.

CogScreen has been used in a number of biomedical research applications. A version of CogScreen was designed for studying the effects of antihypertensive drugs on the orthostatic reflex with and without hypoxia (Kay, Eberle, Kaufman, & Hordinsky, 1996). The FAA's Civil Aeromedical Institute has used CogScreen to examine the effects of low dosages of alcohol on cognitive performance and to evaluate the influence of age on cognition and pilot flight performance. In the latter study, CogScreen was found to be significantly correlated with approach and landing performance in a Boeing-727 flight simulator. The test was also reported to be predictive of the number of performance errors per 100 hours of flying as measured by analysis of flight data recorder data (Yakimovich, Strongin, Govorushenko, Shroeder, & Kay, 1994). Versions of the battery have been used in studies of sleep apnea (Kay et al., 1990), diabetes, antihistamines, and in a study of eosinophilia myalgia syndrome. A keyboard version of the test has been used to track changes in cognitive functioning during balloon trial occlusion of the internal carotid artery (Spector, Kay, Geyer, Deveikas, & Sullivan, 1991) and to study the effects of HIV seropositivity on cognitive functioning (Mapou et al., 1995).

Neurobehavioral Evaluation System 2

The Neurobehavioral Evaluation System 2 (NES2; Letz, 1989) was developed to assess cognitive deficits associated with exposure to environmental toxins. Test selection was based on a literature review of the effects of neurotoxins on cognition and on the test authors' experience in assessing patients who were exposed to neurotoxins. The authors of the NES2 contributed to World Health Organization recommendations for a core set of neurobehavioral measures with which to study occupational hazards. Tests chosen for the NES2 assess a broad range of CNS functions, including psychomotor skill, memory, visuospatial ability, verbal ability, and mood (see Table 6.2). The battery was constructed to permit flexible selection of tests, depending on the needs of clinicians and investigators.

TABLE 6.2
NES2 Subtests

Finger Tapping
Visual Motor Tracking
Simple Reaction Time
Continuous Performance Test
Symbol–Digit/Code Substitution
Digit Recall
Switch/Shift Attention
Pattern Comparison
Serial Digit Learning
Associate Learning
Pattern Matching
Arithmetic Computation
Grammatical/Logical Reasoning
Vocabulary

The NES2 was developed for epidemiological research rather than for clinical practice, and the test manual does not contain normative tables. However, the NES2 has been given to a large number of control subjects who took part in various epidemiological studies (Letz, 1989). Consequently, data are available to construct normative tables.

Initial pilot studies were undertaken to field test equipment and methodology, and to collect normative data on industrial workers with no history of toxic exposure. Baker et al. (1985) studied the comparability of selected NES2 measures with manually administered tests of similar functions. Correlations ranged from .42 to .76. The lowest correlations were between visual and auditory digit span (forward) and between the NES2 Hand–Eye Coordination test and a manual aiming test. The highest correlation was between the standard and computerized versions of the WAIS–R Digit Symbol subtest ($r = .76$).

Rose et al. (1995) used the NES2 to examine performance factors in patients with Parkinson's disease (PD) and multiple sclerosis (MS). These patient groups were selected because many neurotoxins selectively target white matter and subcortical structures similar to those damaged in PD and MS. The investigators examined performance differences in 67 patients with PD and 61 patients with MS on 14 of the 17 NES2 subtests. Subtests were selected to reduce the overall test time while evaluating a broad range of cognitive functions. Test presentation and instructions were adapted on the basis of patient need, while holding all intratest parameters (e.g., ISI) constant. The study demonstrated that NES2 measures of motor speed were most sensitive to the global deficits in both patient groups. However, specific NES2 subtests appeared to be selectively sensitive to performance differences between groups. Specifically, measures of motor coordination, attention, and visual memory were more sensitive to white matter brain lesions characteristic of MS, whereas PD patients demonstrated performance differences on measures of motor speed and digit learning. These findings suggest that these NES2 subtests appear to be sensitive to deficits found in white matter disease and thus may be useful for the examination of cognitive deficits resulting from neurotoxic exposure.

The NES2 software appears to be reliable, and its subtests appear to be suitable for repeated administration. Overall, the NES2 contains a number of interesting tasks and has potential as a general clinical tool once norms become available.

MicroCog: Assessment of Cognitive Functioning

MicroCog (Powell et al., 1993) is intended as a screening device and a diagnostic tool for use as part of a general neuropsychological examination or any other clinical examination requiring the assessment of cognitive functioning efficiency. Initial development of MicroCog was funded by the Risk Management Foundation of the Harvard Medical Institutions. It was originally designed to assess cognitive status changes in physicians and other professionals that might interefere with occupational performance. The battery also was designed to be appropriate for testing of adults who are older than age 65. The test reportedly measures attention, memory, reasoning/calculation, spatial processing, information-processing speed and accuracy, reaction time, and general cognitive functioning. There are two versions: a Standard Form consisting of 18 subtests that require about 1 hour to complete, and a Short Form consisting of 12 subtests that can be completed in approximately 30 minutes. The publisher does not provide alternate forms for repeated testing; however, the Standard Form is reported to show relatively small practice effects with retest intervals of greater than 7 months.

Timing for the original version of the test, which was used to collect more than 60% of the normative data sample, was accomplished by program calls to the system clock. This generally provides only 100 msec timing resolution. The program was later modified to use

TABLE 6.3
MicroCog Subtests and Associated Assessed Cognitive Abilities

Subtest	*Assessed cognitive ability*
Numbers Forward/Reversed	Visual digit span
Alphabet	Letter sequencing
Wordlist 1 and 2	Verbal memory
Address	Verbal memory (immediate and delayed recognition)
Story 1 and 2	Verbal memory, immediate recall
Tic Tac 1 and 2	Visual working memory and visuoconstruction
Clocks	Telling time, visuospatial processing
Analogies	Verbal reasoning
Object Match A and B	Visuospatial problem solving
Math Calculations	Basic math skills
Timer 1 and 2	Simple reaction time

software timing routines. However, timing resolution is still diminished by the use of the keyboard as the response input device.

Different keys are used for different tasks. However, examinee interaction is simplified by restricting responses to the 0–9 keys on the numeric key pad, the <Enter> key, and the <BackSpace> key. The <P> key is used if the examinee wishes to take a break (pause) during testing. The software requires an MS–DOS compatible computer equipped with a 286 or more advanced processor. The system should have at least 640K of RAM, an EGA or better color graphics monitor, and a hard disk.

The nationally representative normative sample of 405 males and 405 females between the ages of 18 and 90 were stratified into three education levels: less than high school, high school, and greater than high school. Analysis of the 35–44 year age group in the normative sample shows that there were only 11 individuals with less than high school education in this sample, 33 with high school education, and 46 with greater than high school education. These relative sample sizes are roughly equivalent to those found in the demographic breakdown reported in the 1988 census. Nevertheless, the cell sizes appear to be too small for the purpose of comparison. The MicroCog subtests are indicated in Table 6.3.

The MicroCog subtests were designed to measure simple and choice reaction time, continuous performance, digit recall, pattern comparison, list recall and recogntion, memory for text, ability to read clock faces, spatial visualization, arithmetic computation, verbal analogies, and visual object matching. The battery begins with a brief introduction to the keyboard and a review of the keys necessary for completion of the test. Each subtest is preceded by an instruction screen, which in some cases includes task examples. Instructions are brief and are clearly written. The test does not provide practice trials prior to test administration; however, sequential errors made by the subject may result in a task being discontinued. The test authors noted that the test is generally self-administered following a brief introduction by the examiner.

Raw test scores are converted into scale scores and standard scores, domain index scores, and summary index scores. The output includes accuracy, response speed, and calculated scores known as "proficiency scores" that reflect the rate of accurate responding. Domain scores are reported for attention/mental control, memory, reasoning/calculation, spatial processing, and reaction time. There are also scores for general information-processing speed, general information-processing accuracy, proficiency, and general cognitive functioning.

The data output lists scores on an item-by-item basis, on a subtest-by-subtest basis, and according to each domain and summary index score.

The comprehensive test manual indicates a range of reliability coefficients for the different subtests for various age levels. Correlations between subtest scores are generally moderate and in the expected direction. MicroCog's Information Processing Accuracy Index and General Cognitive Proficiency Index both correlate .54 with the WAIS–R Full Scale IQ score. The MicroCog manual describes a number of studies that have demonstrated, with varying levels of success, MicroCog's ability to correctly classify patients into diagnostic categories.

Automated Neuropsychological Assessment Metrics

The Automated Neuropsychological Assessment Metrics (ANAM; Reeves, Kane, Winter, & Goldstone, 1995), unlike the normative-based CogScreen and MicroCog batteries, is a performance assessment battery for which the examinee typically serves as his or her own control. The battery was specifically designed for repeated administration of tests to the same person. ANAM represents a special adaptation of a test battery originally developed for NATO's Advisory Group for Aerospace Research and Development. The ANAM battery generally uses mouse buttons as the response input device. This test battery offers near-millisecond timing resolution.

Unlike the fixed battery format of CogScreen–AE and MicroCog, ANAM allows the examiner the option of running a set battery or selecting individual tests for a specific research purpose. Test instructions are in an ASCII text file that can be easily modified with a text editor or word-processing program. The examiner also has the option of modifying various test parameters, such as the inclusion or exclusion of test instructions. The ANAM software presently consists of 16 subtests. These are listed in Table 6.4.

A report of test results is generated automatically. The data report includes measures of response accuracy, test stimulus characteristics, response latencies for correct and incorrect

TABLE 6.4
ANAM Subtests

Stanford Sleepiness Scale
Mood Scale 2
Simple and Two-Choice Reaction Time
Sternberg Memory Search Tasks
Running Memory Continuous Performance Task
Mathematical Processing Task
Digit Set Comparison Task
Logical Reasoning (symbolic)
Tower of Hanoi (tower puzzle)
Stroop Color/Word Interference
Code Substitution (letter/symbol comparison)
Code Substitution (immediate and delayed recall)
Spatial Processing Task
Matching to Sample
Tapping (left and right index finger)
Modified Orientation and Amnesia Test

responses, an index of the number of correct responses per minute (i.e., throughput), and failures to respond within time limits.

The software includes standard and special purpose batteries that consist of different subsets and versions of ANAM subtests. The NCOG battery was designed for administration to normal and mildly impaired patients. In contrast, the MOD battery was designed for moderately impaired and geriatric patients. There is also an NTOX battery for use in neurotoxicology applications. These test batteries can be run in either a screening mode or in a repeated measures mode.

The current test manual (Reeves et al., 1995) provides clear software operation instructions and a description of each of the tests. In addition, the authors provide interpretive guidelines. These guidelines state that the emphasis of ANAM development was to create measures which stabilize with repeated administrations and which could thus be used to provide reliable (and stable) baselines. Collection of clinical normative data was viewed as appropriate for later phase development, and are just beginning. Nevertheless, the authors, based on clinical experience with the battery at several medical facilities, offer some guidance with respect to expected ranges of scores on a number of the ANAM tests.

The current version of the ANAM manual does not document the number of trials required for stabilization of test performance, the test–retest reliability of the subtests, the distribution of scores, or any evidence related to the sensitivity and specificity of the battery or its component subtests. With the addition of this information, the ANAM will become a far more useful instrument for clinical and experimental applications in neuropsychology.

Colorado Neuropsychology Tests

The Colorado Neuropsychology Tests is another battery of PC-compatible neuropsychological tests. The battery includes tests designed to assess explicit and implicit memory and are based on well-established cognitive tests (e.g., The Tower of Hanoi, Mirror Reading). The battery is designed to be flexible regarding the ability to set the order of presentation, number of items, trials, and delay intervals. The specific tests included in the battery are listed in Table 6.5.

The test authors provide normative data for individuals from age 20–80. However, the flexibility of the test battery, which allows the examiner to create test stimuli, change the order of presentation, and modify the duration of interstimulus intervals, would appear to undermine the applicability of the norms.

TABLE 6.5
The Colorado Neuropsychology Tests and Associated Assessed Cognitive Abilities

Test	*Assessed cognitive ability*
Memory Cards	Short term memory or working memory
Tower of Hanoi	Implicit memory and skill learning as well as executive functions
Repeat	Learning a sequential visual pattern
Mirror Reading	Implicit memory
Priming with Recall and Recognition	Implicit memory
Paired Association	Explicit memory (short- and long-term)
Temporal Order	Implicit memory for temporal order
Digit and Visual Span	Short term explicit memory

SUMMARY

This chapter has provided an overview of current computerized testing applications in neuropsychological assessment. These applications include computer analog versions of conventional paper-and-pencil tests as well as tests specifically designed for use with the computer. In this summary we question the value of computerization, review the advantages and drawbacks to computerized testing, offer some predictions regarding future technological advances in this area, and discuss the factors influencing the general acceptance (and nonacceptance) of computerized testing by neuropsychologists.

Have computerized test applications contributed anything significant to neuropsychological assessment? Or, are they simply novel ways of presenting conventional neuropsychological and cognitive tests? Computerized adaptations of paper-and-pencil tests probably represent only a minor advancement in neuropsychological assessment. For the most part, these tests are no more than automated test forms. However, to the extent that the measures reliably assess reaction time and yield valid reaction time measures, they are potentially offering an advancement over traditional test measures. These instruments have the capability of providing measures of response latency (i.e., the time taken before initiating a response) and measures of the time required to complete a response. This type of information can provide valuable insights into an examinee's test taking approach. Furthermore, because the actual timing is not as readily apparent to the examinee as it is when the examinee is being timed with a stopwatch, examinees are less likely to be distracted, concerned, or made anxious by being timed.

In comparison to conventional paper-and-pencil-type testing, computerization offers superior timing resolution, better stimulus control, greater suitability for repeated measures testing, and recording of multiple response parameters. In addition, it can present simultaneous tasks, has improved scoring accuracy, and provides automated reporting of results. These advantages result in improved standardization and allow laboratories to more accurately compare data obtained from different sites and by different examiners. There is also improved assessment of reaction time, attentional processes, and multitasking abilities. Finally, these measures enable neuropsychologists to better measure changes in performance resulting from disease, recovery of function, treatment effects, or responses to various stressors.

Computerized testing also has its drawbacks. Unscrupulous individuals may choose to exploit this methodology to provide unnecessary or incomplete neuropsychological evaluations. Clinicians who fail to take the time to carefully evaluate the reliability and validity of the computerized tests that they employ are especially likely to misuse this technology. Therefore, computerized testing, like other neuropsychological measures, are vulnerable to unethical misuse.

It should also be clear that computerized testing is not going to replace the human test administrator in the foreseeable future. The principal limitations of the computer environment are the lack of human-to-human interface and dependence on computer keyboard skills. The computer is not yet well suited for voice recognition and has limited utility in the assessment of language-related functions. The presentation of written instructions is also problematic. Some examinees are reluctant to read instructions, have difficulty following written directions, or both. In clinical practice it is generally necessary to have the test administrator observe the patient–computer interaction to monitor the examinee for problems comprehending instructions or responding to computerized feedback.

Another drawback is that many of the computerized tests have yet to be fully validated or are still considered experimental (e.g., research editions). For example, there are few equivalence studies comparing the computer versions of conventional tests with the original instruments. Also, many of the newly developed computerized tests lack adequate normative samples and clinical validation.

Many of these problems will no doubt be resolved over time. Test developers are beginning to use more intuitive input devices (such as light pens and touch screens), employ high-quality audio and state-of-the-art video graphics, and are exploring the use of multimedia in their applications. Furthermore, with improvements in computer hardware and programming tools there are a number of developments in computerized testing that are soon to be realized.

In the near future we are likely to see an increased use of adaptive testing methods (Weiss & Veil, 1987). Adaptive testing will allow for very efficient testing by automatically adapting to the examinee's capabilities. The computer can readily change test parameters such as stimulus presentation length, interstimulus interval, stimulus size, location of the stimulus on the screen, and the volume of auditory feedback, depending on an examinee's responses. In other words, a test can be automatically tailored to meet the examinee's specific needs. Adaptive testing can be used to perform item selection and to determine basal and ceiling levels of performance.

In addition, in the near future it is expected that computerized testing applications will fully exploit the computer's capabilities for multitasking, multimedia audio, and video presentation, and for vastly improved analysis and reporting of test findings. At present, very few of the available computerized test batteries truly incorporate the multitasking potential of computerized testing. When computerized tests begin to take advantage of multimedia systems, they will be able to better simulate real-world environments. The dramatic advances in sound card technology have made it possible to present and record highly intelligible and natural sounding speech. This will allow programs to provide audio instructions and not depend on the examinee to read test instructions. Furthermore, true-motion video will make it possible to present realistic problem-solving situations and high-quality demonstrations to examinees.

In spite of these advances, computerized testing appears to have had only minimal impact on the field of clinical neuropsychology. An informal survey of recently published articles showed very few neuropsychological studies to have utilized computerized testing. In contrast, a review of the experimental cognitive psychology literature, and especially the psychopharmacology literature, indicates that computerization has led to significant advances. The acceptance of this methodology in experimental cognitive psychology is probably attributable to the superiority of stimulus control and data recording that are afforded by computerized tests. For example, many of the studies investigating aspects of information processing have utilized computer-based chronometric methods (Posner, 1986).

Over time, computerized testing is likely to become more popular among clinical neuropsychological researchers as well. This is expected to be the case for neuropsychologists involved in treatment studies, for those involved in the investigation of processes underlying recovery of brain functioning, and for those involved in studies designed to detect subtle effects of various toxins or health conditions.

The major obstacles to the increased utilization of computerized tests by clinical neuropsychologists appear to be cost, "technophobia," and a general resistance to novel methods. Some psychologists will readily admit to a preference to use the low-cost or no-cost methods that they are presently using in their offices. Others express an interest in computerized testing but are uncomfortable with the use of computers beyond word processing. Other than by reducing the cost of programs and hardware, there probably is not a remedy for the expense obstacle. Fortunately, computer costs have dropped considerably over recent years. On the other hand, test publishers cannot be expected to give away their programs after investing in software development, normative data collection, and publication of APA-quality manuals. However, the test-use fees charged by some publishers are highly aversive to practitioners who are accustomed to one-time charges for test materials.

The technophobia obstacle will probably be remedied by increasingly more user-friendly programs and the replacement of the intimidating blinking DOS prompt with the popular Microsoft Windows operating system. The resistance to novel methods and computerphobia are obstacles that probably reflect personality characteristics and may not be very amenable to change. However, as graduate students receive training in the use of these instruments and become familiar with these tests during the early phases of their career, they likely will become more accepting of this methodology.

During this growth period of computerized testing, both test developers and test users will need to strictly apply professional testing standards (e.g., American Psychological Association, 1986) to these methods. Users need to determine if instruments meet professional guidelines. For example, computerized tests should only be used if the author or publisher provides a manual that meets APA test standards. Normative data should be made available and equivalence studies should be conducted for computer analogs of conventional tests. However, to a large extent, the acceptance and popularity of computerized neuropsychological testing will be a function of the creativity and effort of test authors to generate testing applications that are clearly superior to their conventional ancestors.

REFERENCES

American Psychological Association. (1986). *Guidelines for computer-based tests and interpretations*. Washington, DC: Author.

Baker, E. L., Letz, R. E., Fidler, A. T., Shalat, S., Plantamura, D., & Lyndon, M. (1985). A computer-based neurobehavioral evaluation system for occupational and environmental epidemiology: Methodology and validation studies. *Neurobehavioral Toxicology and Teratology, 7*, 369–377.

Banderet, L. E., Shukitt, B. L., Walthers, M. A., Kennedy, R. S., Bittner, A. L., & Kay, G. G. (1988, December). *Psychometric properties of three addition tasks with different response requirements*. Paper presented at the annual meeting of the Military Testing Association, Arlington, VA.

Choca, J., & Morris, J. (1992). Administering the Category Test by computers: Equivalence of results. *Clinical Neuropsychology, 6*, 9–15.

Conners, K. (1995). *Conners' continuous performance computer program 3.0: User's manual*. Canada: MHS.

Curtiss, G., & Tuttle, K. (1993a). *Category Test: Computer version. Research edition*. Odessa, FL: Psychological Assessment Resources.

Curtiss, G., & Tuttle, K. (1993b). *Wisconsin Card Sorting Test: Computer version—2*. Odessa, FL: Psychological Assessment Resources.

Delis, D. C., Kramer, J. H., Kaplan, E., & Ober, B. A. (1987). *California Verbal Learning Test*. New York: Psychological Corporation.

ForeThought (1993). *PASAT*. Nashua, NH: Author.

Graves, R. E., & Bradley, R. (1991). Millisecond timing on the IBM PC/XT/AT and PS/2: A review of the options and corrections for the Graves and Bradley algorithm. *Behavior Research Methods, Instruments, and Computers, 23*, 377–379.

Gronwall, D.M.A. (1977) Paced auditory serial addition task: A measure of recovery from concussion. *Perceptual and Motor Skills, 44*, 367–373.

Hellman, S. G., Green, M. F., Kern, R. S., & Christenson, C. D. (1992). Comparison of card and computer versions of the Wisconsin Card Sorting Test for psychotic patients. *International Journal of Methods in Psychiatric Research, 2*, 151–155.

Horst, R. L., & Kay, G. G. (1988). *Report of comparative studies on cognitive tests: Cognitive function evaluation in medical certification of airmen* (FAA/730–426). Federal Aviation Administration, Oklahoma City, OK.

Horst, R. L., & Kay, G. G. (1991). *Phase B final report: Cognitive function evaluation in medical certification of airmen: Development and validation of a prototype test battery*. Technical report submitted to the Federal Aviation Administration, Civil Aeromedical Institute (Contract No. FAA/933–014–90), Oklahoma City, OK.

Kaplan, E., Fein, D., Morris, R., & Delis, D. (1991). *WAIS–R as a neuropsychological instrument: Manual*. San Antonio: Psychological Corporation.

Kay, G. G. (1995). *CogScreen–Aeromedical edition: Professional manual*. Odessa, FL: Psychological Assessment Resources.

Kay, G. G., Starbuck, V. N., Heritage, L., Anderson, D., Yeh, R., & Potolicchio, S. J., Jr. (1990). *The role of sleep apnea induced hypoxia on cognitive performance* (Technical Report submitted to the United States Army Natick Research, Development and Engineering Center). Natick, MA: Author.

Kay, G. G., Starbuck, V. N., & Spector, J. (1995). *Symbol attention and memory test*. Unpublished manuscript.

Kay, G. G., Eberle, C. A., Kaufman, E., & Hordinsky, J. (1996, February). *Effects of antihypertensive medication, hypoxia and orthostatic stress on cognition*. Paper presented at the 24th annual meeting of the International Neuropsychological Society, Chicago, IL.

Letz, R. (1989). Quantitative neurobehavioral testing in humans for assessing potential effects of occupational exposure. *Journal of the American College of Toxicology, 8*, 303–309.

Mapou, R. L., Law, W., Kay, G. G., Clasby, S. G., Roller, T. L., & Temoshok, L. (1995, February). *Performance on conventional and computerized reaction time measures in HIV-1-infected individuals*. Papers presented at the 23rd annual meeting of the International Neuropsychological Society, Seattle, WA.

McCarney, D., & Greenberg, L. M. (1990). *Test Variables of Attention computer program, Version 5.01 for IBM PC or IBM compatibles: TOVA manual*. Minneapolis: University of Minnesota Press.

Mead, A. O., & Drasgow, F. (1993). Equivalence of computerized and paper-and-pencil cognitive ability tests: A meta-analysis. *Psychological Bulletin, 114*, 449–458.

Posner, M. I. (1986). *Chronometric explorations of mind*. New York: Oxford University Press.

Powell, D. H., Kaplan, E. F., Whitla, D., Weintraub, S., Catlin, R., Funkenstein, H. H. (1993). *MicroCog: Assessment of cognitive functioning*. San Antonio, TX: Psychological Corporation.

Reeves, D., Kane, R., Winter, K., & Goldstone, A. (1995). *Automated neuropsychological assessment metrics (ANAM)*. San Diego, CA: National Cognitive Recovery Foundation.

Reitan, R. M., & Wolfson, D. (1985). *The Halstead–Reitan Neuropsychological Test Battery*. Tucson, AZ: Neuropsychology Press.

Rose, F. E., White, R. F., Diamond, R., Eisen, E., Wegman, D., Krengel, M., Cyrus, P. A., Feldman, R. & Letz, R. (1995, February). *Validation of a computerized neuropsychological test battery in patients with subcortical lesions*. Poster presented at the annual meeting of the International Neuropsychological Society, Seattle, WA.

Spector, J., Kay, G. G., Geyer, C. A., Deveikas, J. P., & Sullivan, R. A. (1991). Neuropsychological screenning during trial balloon occlusion of the internal carotid artery [Abstract]. *Archives of Clinical Neuropsychology, 6*, 229.

Thorne, D., Grenser, S., Sing, H., & Hegge, F. (1985). The Walter Reed Performance Assessment Battery. *Neurobehavioral Toxicology and Teratology, 7*, 415–418.

Wechsler, D. (1981). *WAIS–R* manual. New York: Psychological Corporation.

Weiss, D., & Veil, D. (1987). Computerized adaptive testing for measuring abilities and other psychological variables. In J. Butcher (Ed.), *Computerized psychological assessment: A practitioner's guide*. New York: Basic Books.

Westall, R., Perkey, M. N., & Chute, D. L. (1986). Accurate millisecond timing on Apple's Macintosh using Drexel's millitimer. *Behavior research methods, instruments, and computers, 18*, 307–311.

Westall, R., Perkey, M. N., & Chute, D. L. (1989). Millisecond timing on the Apple Macintosh: Updating Drexel's research methods. *Behavior Research Methods, Instruments, and Computers, 21*, 540–547.

Yakimovich, N. V., Strongin, G. L., Govorushenko, V. V., Shroeder, D., & Kay, G. G. (1994, May). *CogScreen as a predictor of flight performance in Russian pilots*. Paper presented at the 65th annual meeting of the Aerospace Medical Association, San Antonio, TX.

7

Neuroimaging: Interface with Clinical Neuropsychology

Erin D. Bigler
Scott S. Porter
Christopher M. Lowry
Brigham Young University

Contemporary neuropsychology, in many respects, is very different than what it was prior to the advent of neuroimaging. The "early" days of clinical neuropsychology—circa 1930s through 1970s—were accomplished without the aid of any in vivo brain imaging technique. Although introduced in the early 1970s, computerized tomography (CT) did not become widely used clinically until the middle or end of that decade. Furthermore, the quality of CT imaging did not reach today's standards until the computer advances of the early to mid-1980s. At that time, nuclear magnetic resonance (NMR) or magnetic resonance (MR) imaging was introduced. Today we have two exceptional in vivo brain imaging techniques—CT and MR—that permit exquisite and detailed viewing of the living human brain. In addition to these contemporary standards of brain imaging, a variety of other imaging methods are available. These include metabolic (positron emission tomography—PET—single photon emission computed tomography—SPECT) electrophysiological (computerized electroencephalographic—EEG—mapping), energy metabolism (NMR spectroscopy), and MR functional activation (see Raichle, 1994a, 1994b). Each of these techniques has led to further understanding of brain–behavior relationships and is discussed in this chapter.

Because the pathologic brain could not be viewed, short of neurosurgical intervention, prior to the development of the aforementioned in vivo imaging techniques, clinical neuropsychology had to rely exclusively on inference in its formative years. There were a few studies that attempted to integrate neuropsychological studies completed years prior to death with autopsy findings, or to relate some neuropsychological finding with neurosurgical findings. Likewise, in part, a few studies attempted to relate neuropsychological results to findings on such diagnostic procedures as pneumoencephalography, radionuclide brain scan, or standard clinical EEG, but none of these measures actually represents an in vivo image of brain parenchyma. During these early years, the research and clinical work that probably came closest to some form of in vivo analysis was the work of Brenda Milner (1964, 1968). In her pioneering analyses, she studied the effects of various neurosurgical extirpations on neuropsychological outcomes. In much of her work, patient's pre- or post-surgical neuropsychological test performance (or both) was correlated with the location and amount of tissue removed. Despite the major contribution that this line of analysis provided and its key role in the evolution of very significant neuropsychological tenets, its major drawback was that it provided only a static look at the brain at the time of neurosurgical intervention. The amount of tissue removed at surgery is only one facet of the complex, interactive nature of brain lesions on behavior. For example, when an area of the brain is removed, there is usually scarring around the surgical lesion boundary and, of course, there is extensive anterograde as well as retrograde degeneration for all axons entering and exiting that region. Therefore, even by knowing the locus or extent of structural damage in one given region, the complete role of that region cannot be accounted for because of the disruption of interconnections between that part of the brain and other regions. Accordingly, *all* neuropsychological research conducted prior to CT/MR imaging had similar problems. Methods were not available in the past to control the actual extent and location of brain damage/dysfunction on neuropsychological outcome. The result of this lack of control made neuropsychological outcome findings difficult to interpret because the site, size, location, and diaschitic effects of the lesion could not be controlled.

In the early years (prior to the mid-1970s), neuropsychology was focused on another very different aspect of assessment than what is currently the case. Because the standard physical neurological exam was focused primarily on analysis of cranial nerves and reflex levels, it performed poorly in detecting a variety of cerebral disorders. Therefore, neuropsychological techniques were developed to test for "brain damage," "organic brain syndrome," or probable "neurological dysfunction," and so on. Much of this analysis was based on a unitary concept of "organicity" which posited that one could use "cut-off" scores to detect "brain damage" (see review by Lezak, 1976). Therefore, a given test instrument was administered and the patient's score would either fall into the "normal" or "brain-damaged" range. Accordingly, neurologic dysfunction was not viewed as quantifiable on some continuum, but rather as a dichotomous, qualitative variable. Entire rating schemes were developed and designed to not only "detect" this organic dichotomy (i.e., brain damage as either present or absent) but also to specify the presumed location of focal cerebral damage/dysfunction (see Russell, Neuringer, & Goldstein, 1970).

Although we continue to use many of the neuropsychologic instruments and measures that were developed during the aforementioned era, in contemporary clinical neuroscience imaging techniques that permit magnificent in vivo viewing of the living brain are now available (see Fox, 1993). The issue of cerebral lesion location based solely on neuropsychological assessment techniques has largely been supplanted by neuroimaging methods. For the first time, in vivo research or clinically applied imaging of the brain can be performed contemporaneously with the study of behavior (neuropsychological outcome). The neuropsychological assessment issues of the past (i.e., detection of "organicity") are no longer contemporary issues. However, neuropsychological assessment techniques remain the best descriptors of behavior and are essential to the mission of improved understanding of brain–behavior relationships. The task now at hand is to integrate the behavioral neuropsychological assessment with the various forms of neuroimaging analysis to provide a more refined understanding of human brain–behavior relationships.

Entire textbooks have been devoted to this one topic (see Bigler & Clement, in press). For the purposes of this chapter, an overview of the structure–function interface between neuroimaging and neuropsychological function is given. This chapter does not review imaging techniques in detail. The reader interested in a much more detailed review of the technical aspects of the imaging methods discussed in this chapter is referred to Hayman and Hinck (1992); Kucharczyk, Mosely, and Barkovich (1994); Osborn (1994); Stark and Bradley (1992); and Wolpert and Barnes (1992).

This chapter is divided into various sections that discuss the major brain imaging methods and ways in which that imaging information can be used to interface with neuropsychological analysis. The chapter concludes with a review of the major studies of the past 5 years that deal with neuroimaging findings as they relate to neuropsychological or behavioral outcome.

COMPUTERIZED TOMOGRAPHIC IMAGING

To depict the contemporary use and interrelationships of brain imaging, a case study is provided wherein a patient with traumatic brain injury is presented who has had CT, MR, and SPECT imaging performed. The CT findings are presented in this section and the MR and SPECT results are presented in subsequent sections.

In CT scanning, a computerized image of the brain is generated from brain/skull tissue density findings determined by attenuation of an X-ray beam passing through the brain (see Eisenberg, 1992; Oldendorf, 1980, for review of the development and technique of CT imaging). The four main constituents of the cranium and its contents are composed of bone, cerebrospinal fluid (CSF), white matter, and gray matter. Each of these has a different density and X-ray beam attenuation. Accordingly, on a gray scale, with CT imaging the convention is to represent bone as white, CSF as dark, with white matter dark gray and gray matter as gray (see Figs. 7.1 and 7.2).

This gray scale scheme provides a method to depict major structural and pathological states with CT imaging. For example, Fig. 7.1 readily depicts a skull fracture, underlying contused brain, presence of hemorrhage, and cerebral edema. CT imaging provides excellent identification of many of the acute variables in traumatic brain injury as well as other neurologic diseases/disorders (i.e., stroke). This methodology also permits the study of changes over time. When an acute lesion occurs (e.g., stroke, traumatic brain injury, acute infection), the pathology at lesion onset can be used to compare and contrast with the more permanent structural changes that may occur. For example, Figs. 7.1, 7.2, and 7.4 show the evolution of trauma-induced degenerative changes. Note the differences between the patient's day of injury CT in Fig. 7.1 and the CT in Fig. 7.2, which was taken several months following the injury. Fig. 7.2 shows pronounced enlargement of the ventricles as well as prominent sulci. (Fig. 7.4 is an MR of the same patient more than 1 year post-injury. The MR images, in comparison with the CT images, provide clear visualization of ventricular expansion as well as prominent sulci.) Additionally, in disorders like Alzheimer's disease, the degree of structural change (e.g., degree of degeneration) can be well documented by comparing scans over various time periods (Coffey et al., 1992; Wahlund et al., 1993).

The ability to graphically depict changes in brain morphology two-dimensionally (2-D) has been available since the onset of CT imaging. The larger challenge, from the neuropsychological standpoint, has been how to quantify these changes. Initially, CT findings were used to document presence or absence of pathology or the lateralization of a lesion. Most of CT imaging research performed prior to the 1990s was based on this premise (see Heaton &

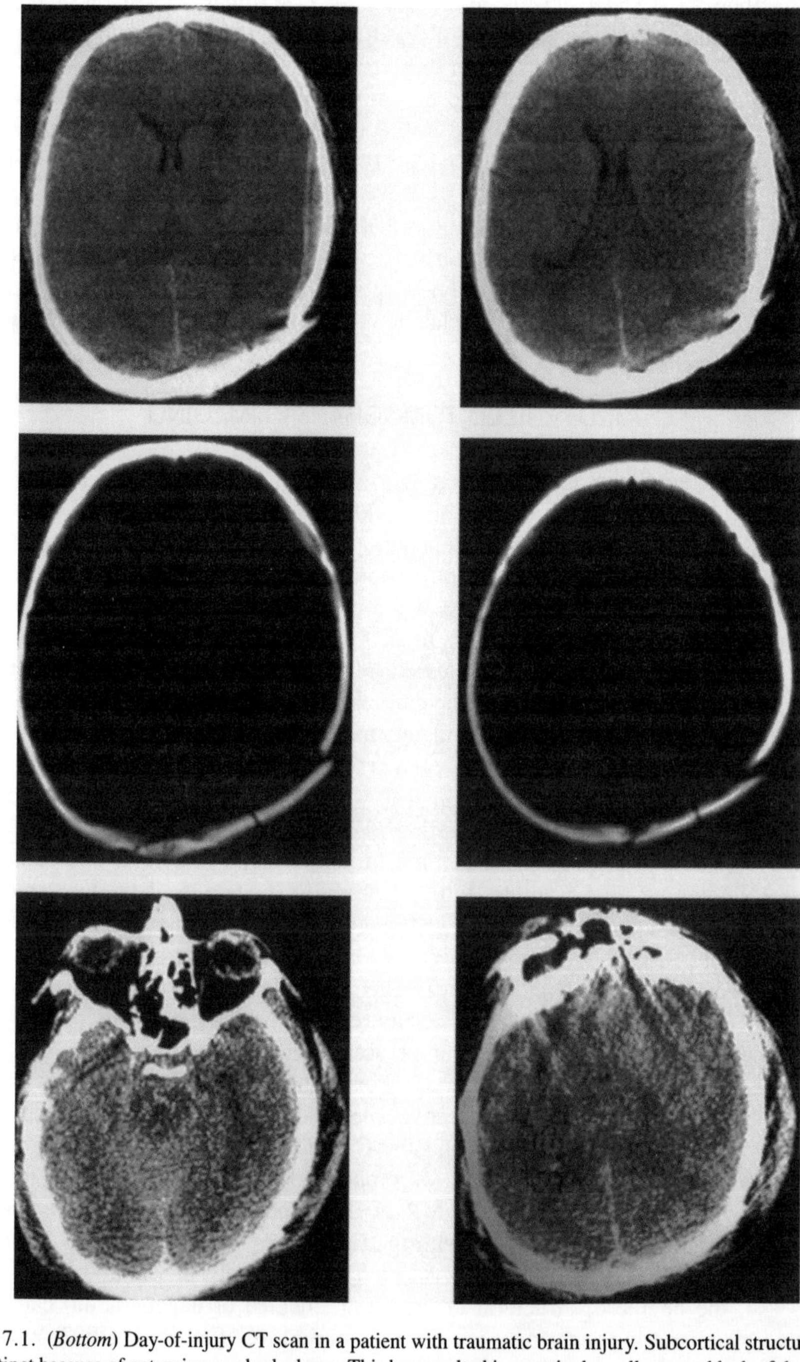

FIG. 7.1. (*Bottom*) Day-of-injury CT scan in a patient with traumatic brain injury. Subcortical structures are indistinct because of extensive cerebral edema. This has resulted in ventricular collapse and lack of demarcation of gray and white matter areas. (*Middle*) CT bone outline of the skull in axial (horizontal) plane depicting skull fracture. (*Top*) CT scan two days following injury and after intensive treatment for the cerebral edema showing a significant midline displacement (note the bend in the interhemispheric fissure and that it is off midline) and position of a hematoma (over the right frontal parietal region).

Bigler, 1993). The problem with this type of orientation was that it did not advance the interface of clinical neuropsychology with neuroimaging much because most of the anatomic changes were not quantified in any rigorous fashion. However, during that era (circa 1980s and earlier) there was not much of a choice other than use of these qualitative methods because there were no rapid, automatic analytic systems available, and essentially all analyses had to be performed by hand tracing and planimetric linear measurements. For example, one of the first quantitative measurements of the brain in Alzheimer's disease was performed by Turkheimer and colleagues in 1984. This required hand tracing of the cortical rim of each CT slice, interpolation between each slice, and manual calculation of brain volume and CSF space. Now, such tracings, calculations, and computations are performed automatically or in a semiautomated fashion (see Blatter et al., 1995). Likewise, the Alzheimer patient's imaging studies (see Fig. 7.3) can now be compared to normative data that are generated through semiautomated morphometric techniques (Blatter et al., 1995; Coffey et al., 1992; Wahlund et al., 1993).

With this history in mind, it is obvious that we are now only on the threshold of integration of quantitative image analysis with neuropsychological outcome. Returning to Figs. 7.1 and 7.2, the next step in image analysis of TBI (as well as a host of other neurologic disorders) is the quantification of pathologic change. For example, in the case presented in these two figures there are a multitude of pathologic changes that can now be quantitatively as well as qualitatively analyzed. For example, the degree of midline shift and sulcal effacement are indicators of the degree of cerebral edema. The hemorrhagic lesions can be counted, their volume calculated, and their locations specified. The relationship between the

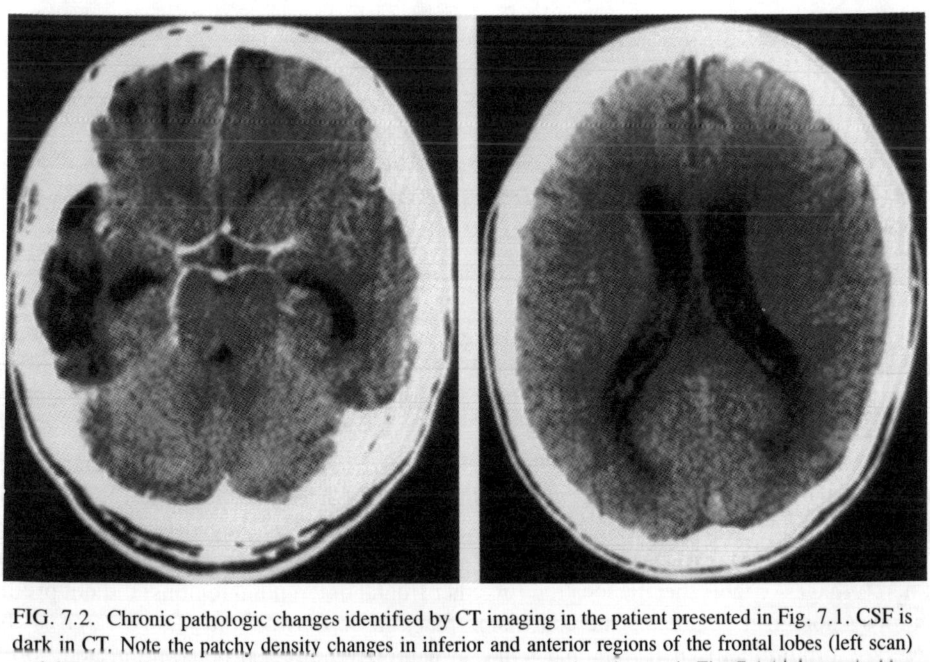

FIG. 7.2. Chronic pathologic changes identified by CT imaging in the patient presented in Fig. 7.1. CSF is dark in CT. Note the patchy density changes in inferior and anterior regions of the frontal lobes (left scan) and the generalized ventricular enlargement compared to the acute imaging see in Fig. 7.1 (right scan). Also note that the fissures have become more prominent. These images should be compared to those in Fig. 7.1, as the Fig. 7.1 images represent an estimate of the brain's preinjury status. The extensive ventricular enlargement is considered a sign of generalized cerebral atrophy (see Bigler et al., 1992).

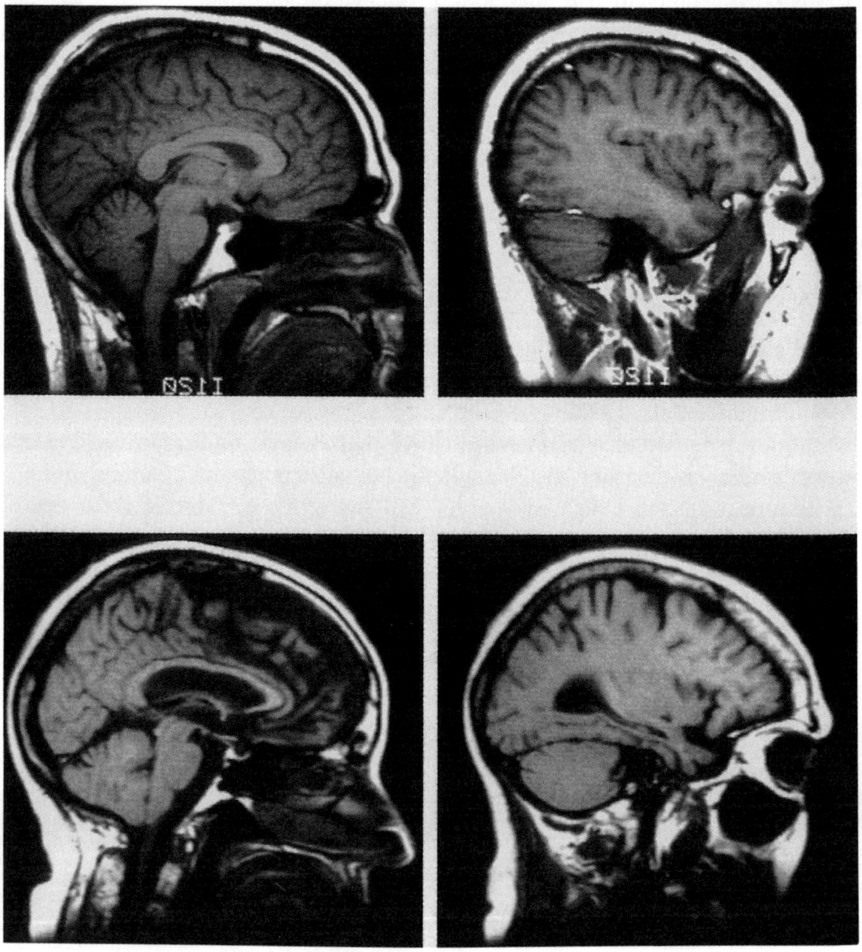

FIG. 7.3. Normal sagittal MR views (*top*) compared to an individual with Alzheimer's disease (*bottom*). Note the extensive atrophy of the cerebral cortex and especially the temporal lobe.

hemorrhagic lesions and cerebral edema also can be analyzed. Qualitatively, the presence or absence of skull fracture can be documented and related to the quantitative measurements mentioned previously. These are but a few of the quantitative methods that now can be explored empirically.

Preliminary research in this new domain is underway. Kurth, Blatter, and Bigler (1994) examined the relationship between acute (day-of-injury—DOI) intracerebral hemorrhages and neuropsychological outcome. This research demonstrated that the most common sites of trauma-induced hemorrhage were in the frontal and temporal regions; however, the number of hemorrhages or their specific location (in either frontal or temporal regions) did not predict neuropsychological outcome. One conclusion that can be drawn from this research is that there are a multiplicity of factors that relate to neuropsychological outcome in addition to location and number of lesion sites. For example, white versus gray matter changes as well as metabolic and neurotransmitter dysregulation effects remain to be explored. As is discussed later, we can now quantify the degree of white and gray matter changes using MR techniques. Such methods combined with the CT DOI information may be more predictive of outcome than current clinical evaluation methodologies.

With the advent of MR imaging, because of its superior anatomical detail some practitioners speculated that MR imaging would totally replace CT. However, that has not been the case. In many respects CT is superior to MR in imaging bone and abnormalities of bone, especially fractures. Many medical and life-support devices cannot be utilized in the MR environment (because strong magnetic fields disrupt some equipment and magnetizable objects cannot be in the same field), but these devices can readily be used with CT. CT remains less expensive than MR, CT is faster (although that is quickly changing), and CT is just as accurate as MR in screening for many of the major pathologic conditions of the brain. For example, as a rapid screening device to rule out major space occupying lesions in a patient presenting with dementia, CT scanning is comparable to MR imaging. Accordingly, CT imaging will likely remain the initial imaging modality for many neurologic disorders and, thereby, should continue to be the most common initial imaging technique available for quantification and structural–functional interface analyses with neuropsychological outcome and cognitive measures.

MAGNETIC RESONANCE IMAGING

MR imaging provides exquisite visualization of brain tissue (see Fig. 7.4, bottom views). This level of detail permits the visualization of all major cortical and subcortical nuclei and structures. As discussed earlier in the section on CT, Figs. 7.1 and 7.2 presented the data on the CT-based acute pathology in a TBI victim. Figure 7.4 presents his follow-up MR scan, which depicts significant degenerative changes that have occurred over time (compare Figs. 7.1, 7.2, and 7.4).

The MR, as well as the CT data, can also be analyzed in terms of three-dimensional (3-D) image presentation (discussed later and presented in Figs. 7.8–7.10). With MR imaging, there are typically three different types of image presentations: T1, T2, and Proton or Spin Density weighting (Newhouse & Wiener, 1991). T1-weighted images, on the standard gray scale, depict fat (i.e., white matter) or subacute hemorrhage as bright or white, whereas black represents fluid such as CSF. On T2-weighted images, fat appears gray, iron appears black, and fluid appears white. Substances that are always without signal because they have negligible magnetization include the cranium, air, blood, and CSF spaces. These three types of images are depicted in Fig. 7.5. A variety of methods now exist to quantify MR identified structures either in terms of surface areas or volumes. Figures 7.6 and 7.7 demonstrate some of the methods used to calculate surface areas and volumes. Through proper segmentation techniques, gray and white matter, as well as CSF spaces, can be shown. The upper right image in Fig. 7.6 shows the gray matter removed. Figure 7.7 illustrates full segmentation into white, gray, and CSF, any of which can have a surface area calculated. Stacking the surface areas for the individual slices allows the interpolation of volume. There are also various three-dimensional methods for image quantification (see Figs. 7.8–7.10).

MR, or as originally termed nuclear magnetic resonance (NMR), imaging is based on the magnetic properties of molecules, especially hydrogen nuclei, which in tissue basically act as randomly oriented bar magnets. When tissue is exposed to an external magnetic field, these nuclei tend to orient their magnetizations parallel to the magnetic field. The degree of orientation parallel to the main magnetic field is dependent on the strength of the external

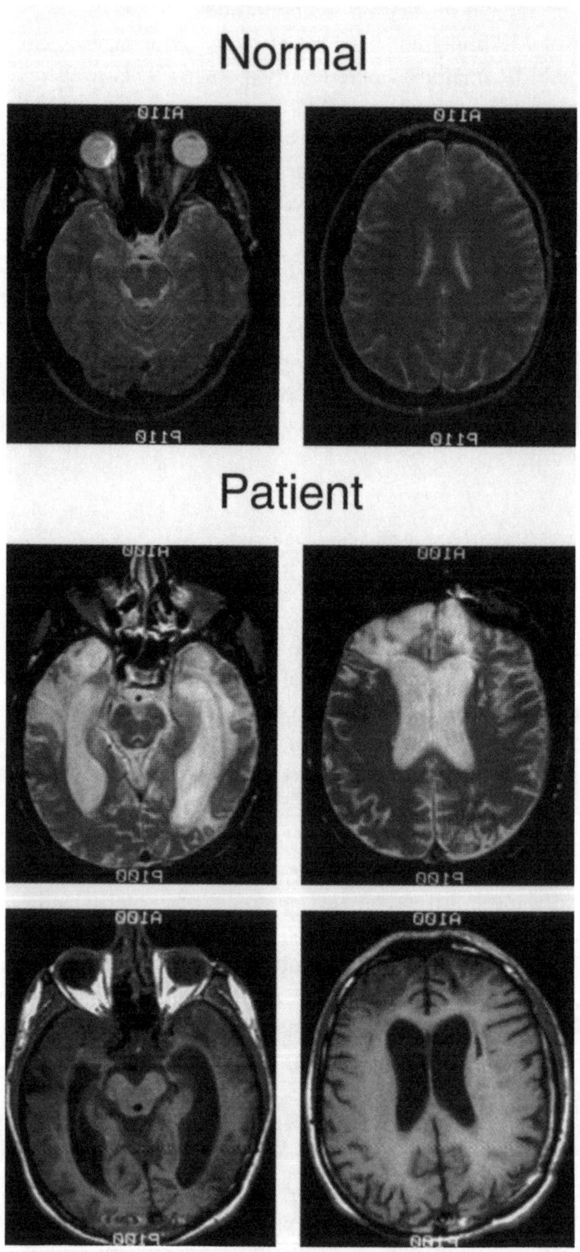

FIG. 7.4a. MR scans (axial views) over one year post-injury from the patient presented in Figs. 7.1 and 7.2. The pathologic images are presented below the normal comparison. Note the extensive enlargement of the ventricular system, tissue loss in both frontal lobes and extensive wasting of both temporal lobes, along with thinning of the corpus callosum and cerebellar atrophy. By comparing the scan to those presented in Figs. 7.1 and 7.2, the evolution of degenerative change in the traumatically injured brain can be readily visualized.

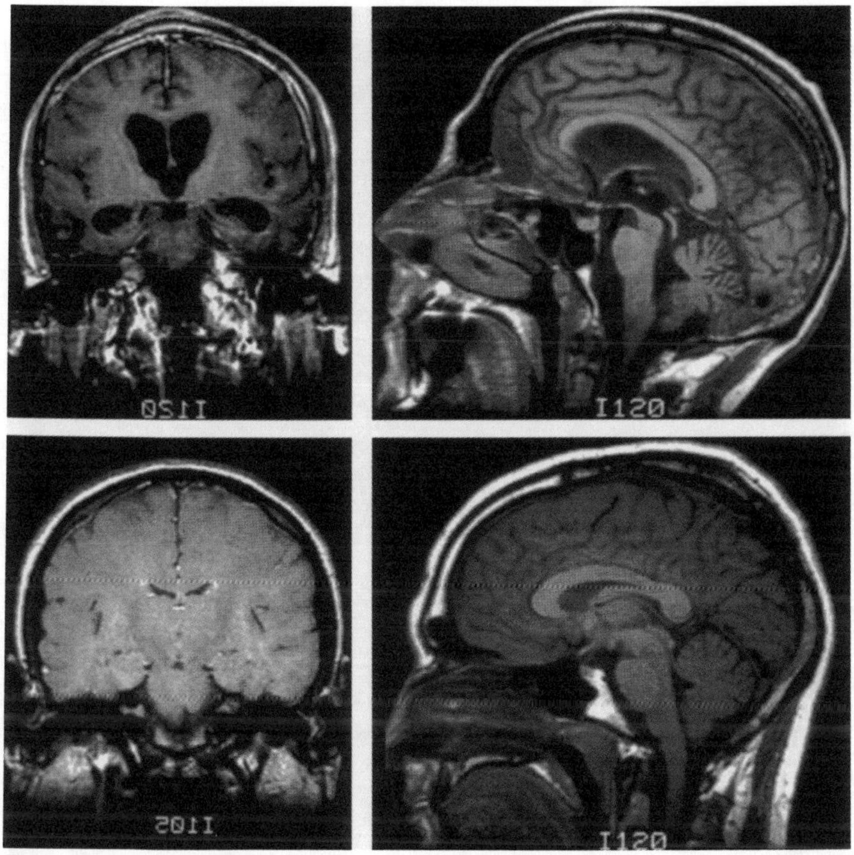

FIG. 7.4b. Normal comparisons are presented below each figure for the coronal and sagittal views of the same patient presented in Figs. 7.1, 7.2, and 7.4a. Note the extensive dilation of the lateral ventricles and temporal horns in comparison to the normal scan presented below. Also note the prominence of the gyri in the patient.

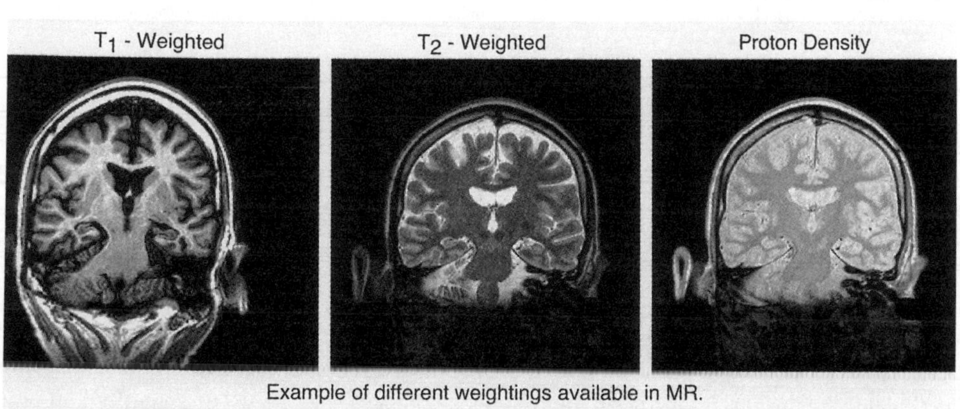

FIG. 7.5. Different weighting values in MR images demonstrating how the different weightings depict certain structures. For example, with T1 weighting, CSF is dark, whereas with T2 weighting, it is white. With a mixed weighted or proton density weighting, CSF is an intermediate gray.

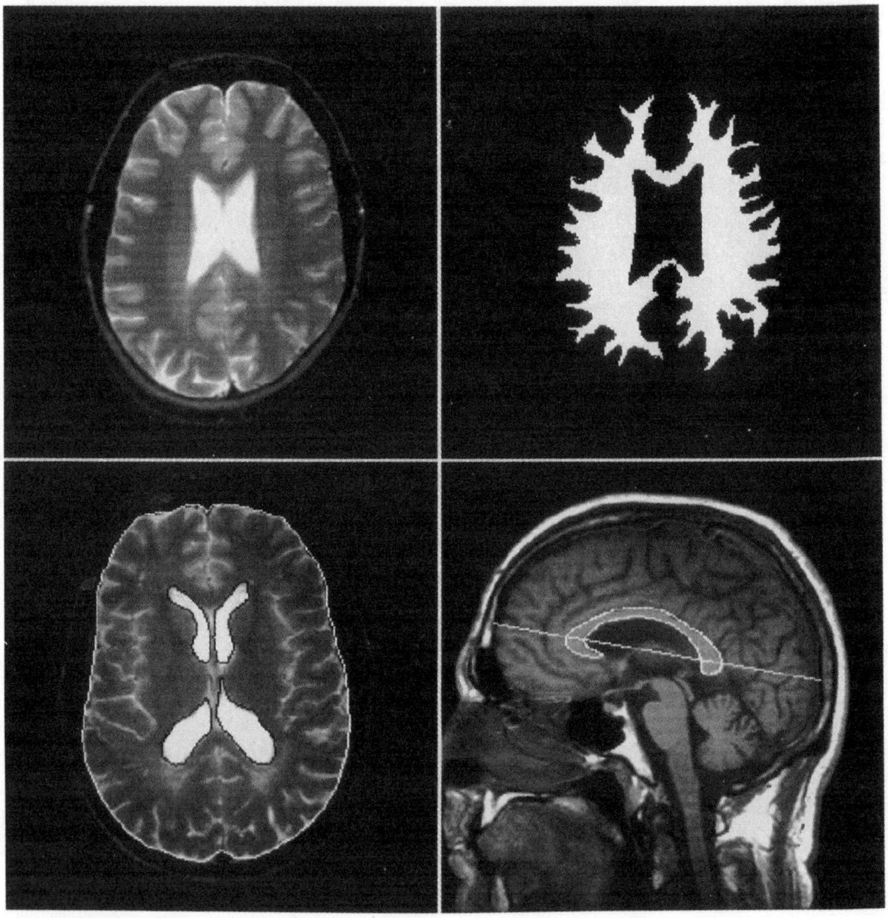

FIG. 7.6. Various methods using the threshold technique for image analysis. In the upper left, a T2 weighted image is presented, untouched. A threshold technique (upper right) is utilized to separate gray and CSF from white. Using this threshold principle, the surface area white matter at this slice level can be calculated (bottom left). The outer rim of cortical surface area is outlined (traced in white) and the ventricles are outlined (traced in black). (Lower right) Midsagittal view depicting a linear anterior-to-posterior measurement, typically used for head size correction, and a surface area tracing of the corpus callosum.

field and the magnetic properties of the tissue. Radio frequency energy, which can be detected and converted into an image, occurs in response to magnetization. Because hydrogen nuclei are particularly crucial to proton NMR imaging and the brain is largely composed of water (also, note that hydrogen atoms are contained in lipids), MR imaging provides a marvelous mechanism for imaging the brain (Newhouse & Weiner, 1991). Pathologic states give rise to MR signal differences due to changes in the distribution of water molecules, allowing a variety of neuropathological conditions to be diagnosed by MR imaging. As discussed earlier, we now have automated and semiautomated techniques to quantify most aspects of any MR image. As such, any of the pathological conditions that produce anatomically identified lesions or cerebral morphologic changes can now be quantified. These developments have led to the first in vivo studies that have examined quantitative relationships between certain pathological states, brain imaging, and neuropsychological outcome (see Blatter et al., 1995; Gale, Johnson, Bigler, & Blatter, 1995). All of these findings are discussed later in the chapter and in the tables that follow, but the following example illustrates the point.

Multiple sclerosis (MS) results in degeneration of the myelin coating of the axon. When these degenerative processes or lesions occur as an aggregate collection (plaques) in one region of the brain, an MR signal intensity change clearly occurs at the level of white matter (see Fig. 7.11). Although this has been recognized since the advent of MR imaging, because of technical problems in quantifying these lesions essentially all neuropsychological–MR imaging research in the past has been qualitative (presence/absence of white matter hyperintensities or some type of severity rating scale). However, with today's technology, lesions can be quantified in terms of location, size, and total amount of white matter change, and these

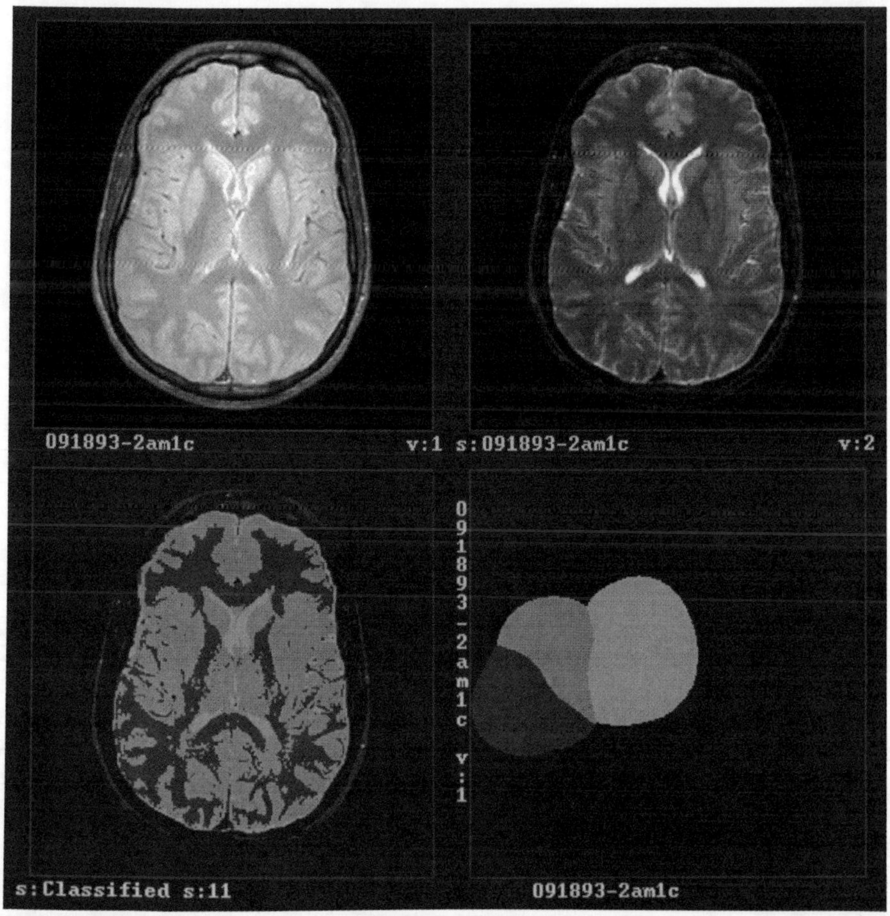

FIG. 7.7. Multispectral segmentation of MR images (*upper left*) intermediate and (*upper right*) T2 weighted spin-echo images at the level of the body of the lateral ventricles. (*Lower right*) A plot of two-dimensional feature space where each pixel is plotted with the signal intensity on the T2-weighted image as the x-axis and the signal intensity on the intermediate weighted image as the y-axis. The location and feature space on the pixels obtained in the user identified region are shown in their respective shades of gray. (*Lower left*) Application of the segmentation to the original image. By using this technique, the whole brain white, gray, and CSF values can be obtained. This segmentation is based on the ANALYZE program, which is a registered product of the Mayo Foundation/Clinic (200 First Street S. W., Rochester, MN 55905).

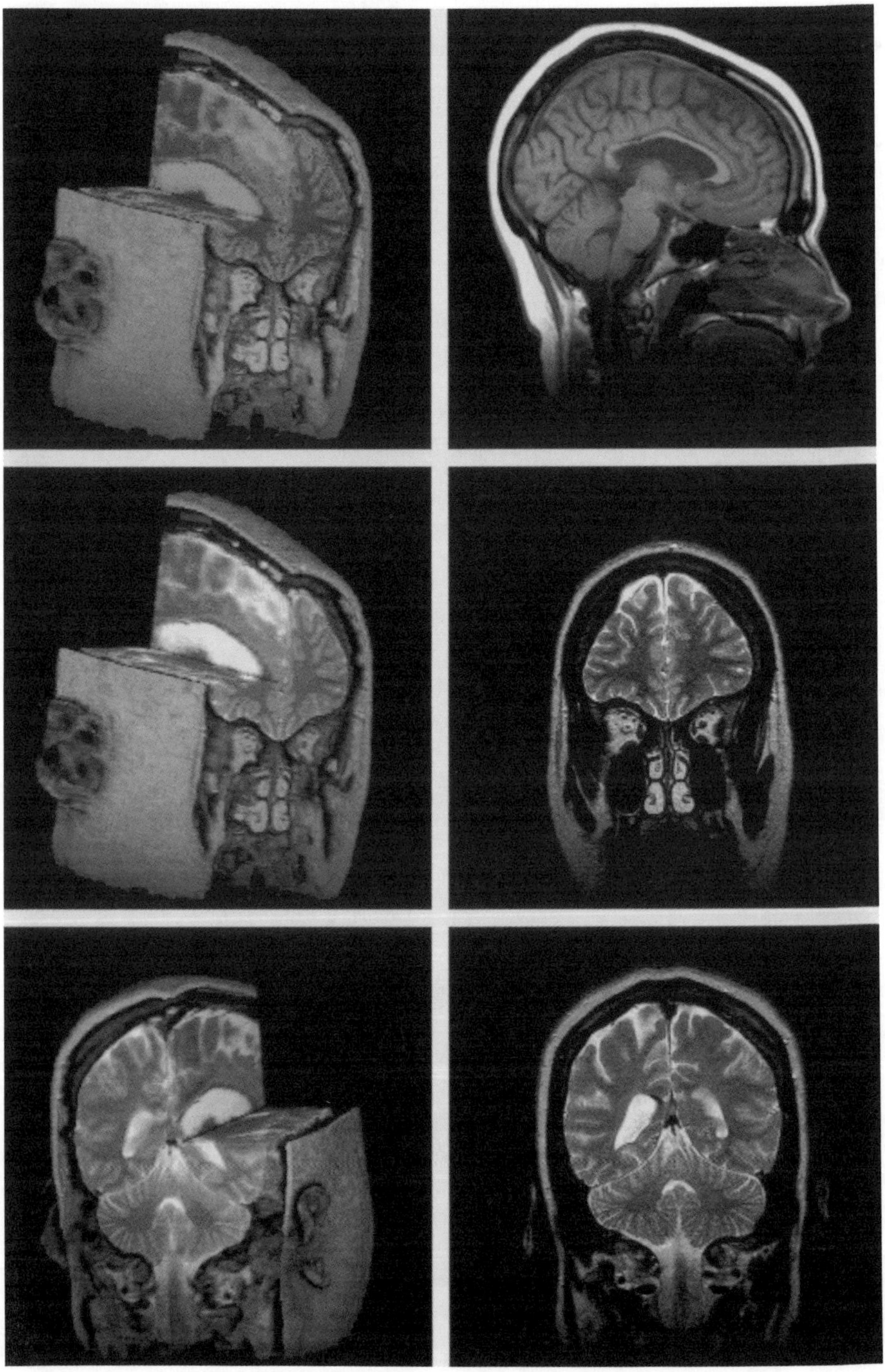

FIG. 7.8. Three-dimensional sections showing simultaneously the three different planes of the brain (coronal, axial, and sagittal) based on MR imaging. Using these techniques, simultaneous rendering of any 3-D section from a different plane of the brain based on MR imaging can be accomplished.

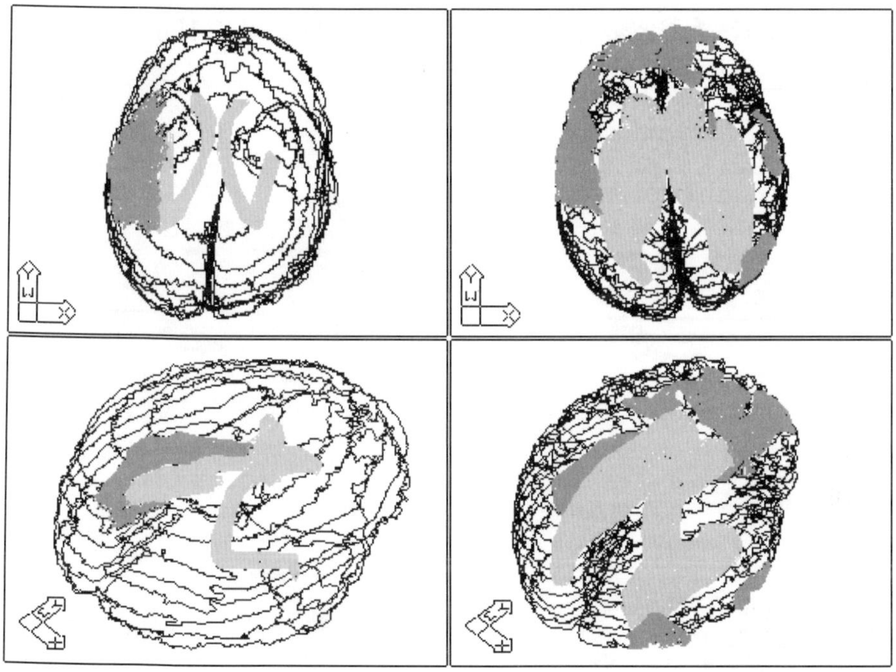

FIG. 7.9. Three-dimensional wire-framed depiction of ventricular dilation in the TBI patient presented in Figs. 7.1, 7.2, and 7.4. The two images on the left represent the wire-framed depiction based on the CT scan of injury and the one on the right depicts the similar views but indicating marked ventricular dilation in this patient.

parameters can be followed over time (Armspach et al., 1993; Barbosa, Blumhardt, Roberts, Lock, & Edwards, 1994). As this research progresses, the neuropsychologist and neuroradiologist should be able to make better predictions about functional status and therapeutic outcome in a variety of neurological disorders. For example, Lisk, Pasteur, Rhoades, Putnam, and Grotta (1994) have developed an outcome prediction formula for evaluation of the cognitive effects of intracerebral hemorrhage based on quantitative and semiquantitative measurements of brain imaging. It is predicted that as better quantification of pathologic neurologic states evolves with neuroimaging and this information is integrated with neuropsychological outcome, prediction models likely will be developed for most neurologic disorders based on initial and follow-up imaging data.

Another approach that has resulted from MR imaging is the development of normative databases. Because the dimensions of all major cerebral structures can now be quantified, a number of laboratories have been working toward normative standardization of the brain based on MR imaging (Blatter et al., 1995; Gur, Saykin, & Gur, 1991; Hayakawa et al., 1989; Jernigan, Archibald, et al., 1991; Pfefferbaum et al., 1994). For example, Blatter et al. (1995) have provided the most comprehensive normative analysis to date. The original intent of their study was to provide a normative data base for comparison of degenerative changes in patients with history of traumatic brain injury (TBI). This is illustrated in Figs. 7.12 and 7.13. By using the normative comparison, an estimate of change in brain size and its component structures can be made. Research is underway that may lead to a better understanding of neuropathologic changes that accompany craniocerebral trauma and other neurological diseases and disorders. The goal of such research is to elucidate the relationship between structural changes or functional outcome and the normative database. Hopefully,

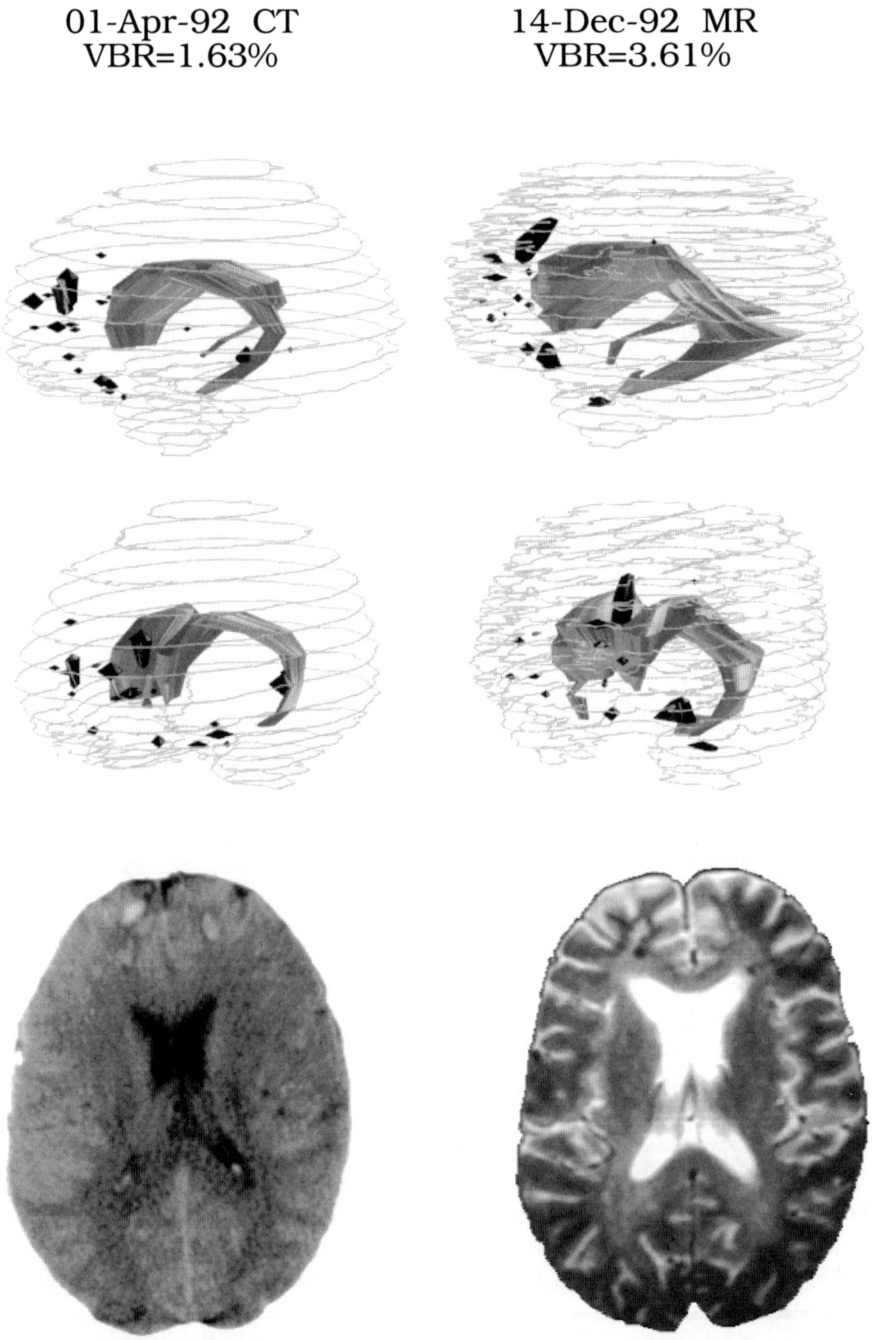

FIG. 7.10. Traumatic brain injury induced ventricular expansion and 3-D depiction of lesion location. (*Lower left*) Day-of-injury CT scan demonstrating numerous hemorrhagic lesions spread throughout the frontal lobes. 3-D depictions of these lesions are presented in wire frame format above (see Bigler, 1992b, for details of methodology). (*Lower right*) Follow-up MR demonstrating marked ventricular expansion (compared to day-of-injury scan on the left) with the chronic lesions identified in 3-D depiction as in Figs. 7.8–7.10.

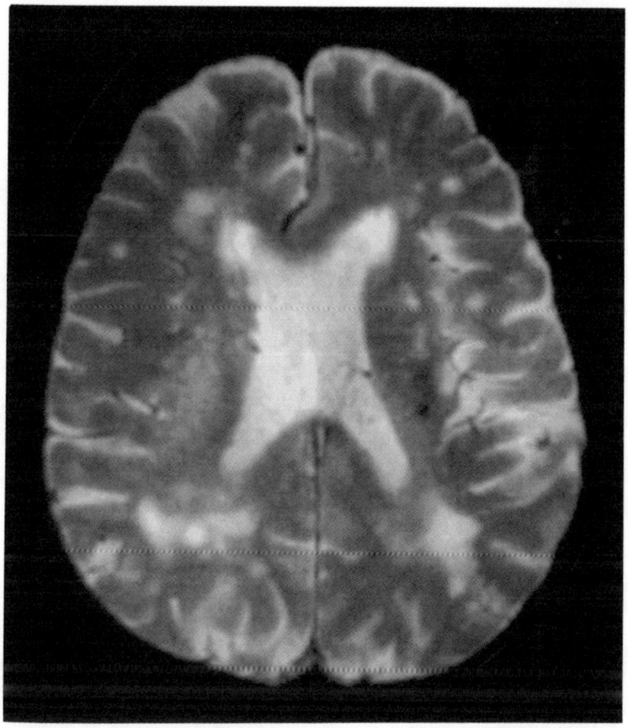

FIG. 7.11. MR imaging findings in multiple sclerosis. New methods provide for more refined analysis of white matter change (for details, see discussion in the text).

this line of research, which is already being utilized, will lead to increased understanding of neuropathologic changes that accompany various neurological diseases/disorders and craniocerebral trauma (see Fig. captions to Figs. 7.12 and 7.13 for further explanation).

As discussed in the last paragraph, Gale, Burr, Bigler, and Blatter (1993) and Gale, Johnson, Bigler, and Blatter (1995) have examined a variety of pathological changes that accompany TBI that might relate to functional outcome (see also Bigler, Kurth, Blatter, & Abildskov, 1992; Kurth et al., 1994). In this context, they found that lateral ventricular system temporal horn volume may be one of the key structures to monitor. Although the temporal horn is a CSF space and thereby only an indirect measure of parenchymal structures, it is strategically located. Part of the mesial wall of the temporal horn is comprised of the hippocampus with the amygdala situated just anterior to the tip of the horn. Additionally, temporal horn volume is somewhat of an indirect measure of temporal lobe integrity. Structural changes in the hippocampus, temporal lobe, or both that result in atrophy will also result in expansion of the temporal horn. Because the temporal lobe, and also the limbic structures in particular, play a critical role in cognitive and behavioral functioning, it comes as no surprise that temporal horn expansion in TBI patients is associated with poor neuropsychological outcome (see Gale, Johnson, Bigler, & Blatter, 1994).

The research examining the relationship between pathological brain changes and neuropsychological outcome has demonstrated many nonlinear relationships. Although the aforementioned research by Gale et al. demonstrated poor neuropsychological outcome in TBI patients with large temporal horn volume, the correlations were only modest (0.2 to 0.4 range) and often nonsignificant. Other research in our laboratories has shown no systematic

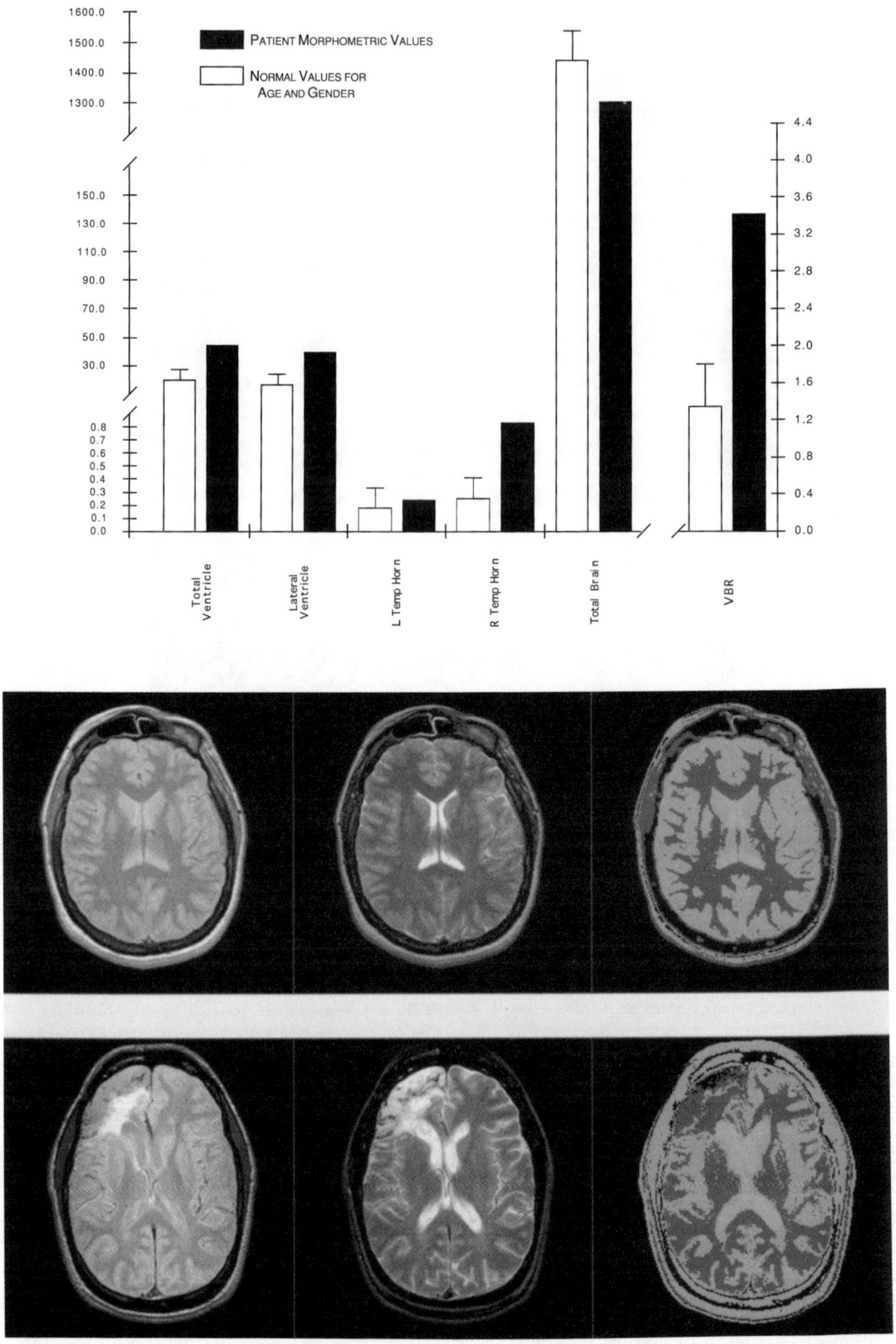

FIG. 7.12. Bar graph depicting aspects of the patient's quantitative neuroimaging findings of the ventricular system based on volumetric estimates from segmented images. The top row of MR images depict a medical control subject with proton density weighted MR scan on the left, T_2 weighted scan in the middle and the "segmented" image differentiating white, gray, and CSF space. The bottom row of images is from the TBI patient with similar level MR images and a large right frontal lesion (left is on the reader's right). The patient's neuropsychological data is presented in Fig. 7.13. These quantitative analyses indicate significant ventricular dilation, which in TBI, is a sign of white matter loss (see Bigler et al., 1994).

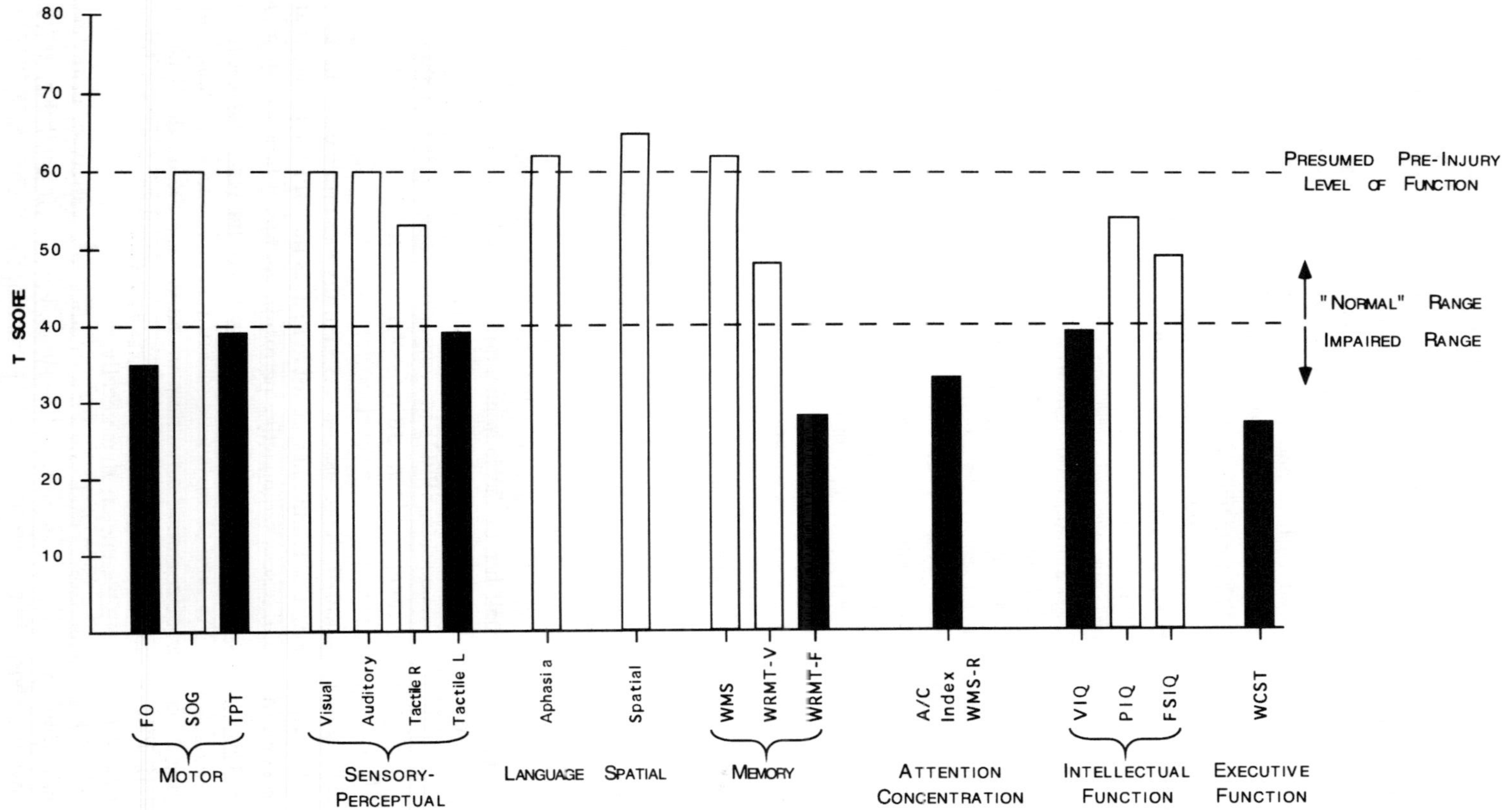

FIG. 7.13. Bar graphs of the patient's neuropsychological data (see Fig. 7.12 for the scans). Test results in the impaired range are indicated by black bars. The abbreviations are as follows: FO—Finger Oscillation, SOG—Strength of Grip, TPT—Tactual Peformance Test, WMS—Wechsler Memory Scale, WRMT–V—Warrington Recognition Memory Test–Verbal, WRMT–F—Warrington Recognition Memory Test–Faces, A/C—Attention Concentration Index, WMS–R—Wechsler Memory Scale–Revised, VIQ—Verbal Intelligence Quotient, PIQ—Performance Intelligence Quotient, WCST—Wisconsin Card Sorting Test.

relationship between certain structures that consistently demonstrate degenerative change in TBI and neuropsychological outcome. For example, Johnson, Bigler, Burr, and Blatter (1994) demonstrated that significant degenerative changes in the corpus callosum in TBI patients were related to the severity of injury, but the degree of degenerative change did not relate to intellectual outcome. Part of the explanation for this finding is that there is likely both anterograde as well as retrograde degeneration across the corpus callosum in TBI resulting from multiple injury sources in a multiplicity of cerebral regions. Until some additional methods can be developed for partialling out these multiple factors, there will likely be major neuropathological changes that can be quantified, but not necessarily related systematically to neurobehavioral and cognitive outcome states.

We also have sought to integrate brain imaging data with neuropsychological outcome in a two-dimensional probability map that outlines an importance function which is the relative value of a lesion in a given area to neuropsychological outcome (see Turkheimer, 1989; Yeo, Turkheimer, & Bigler, 1990). For example, a lesion in primary sensory cortex has a greater likelihood of producing sensory deficits than a lesion in association parietal cortex. Therefore, the importance function, relative to sensory deficits, gives more weight in the anatomic regions surrounding primary somatosensory cortex than adjacent areas. This work is very promising, but it has not progressed in the last several years because of the rapid changes in quantification image analysis. Now that we are entering an era of generally accepted and refined quantitative image analysis techniques for neuroimaging data, this approach holds great promise for the possibility of integrating neuropsychological outcome data with brain imaging parameters in two- or three-dimensional spatial models.

SPECT AND PET

Positron emission tomography (PET) has been primarily a research tool. Single photon emission computed tomography (SPECT), although serving as a research tool, has also been applied and utilized clinically in a much broader spectrum than PET (Holman & Devous, 1992; Volkow, Brodie, & Bendriem, 1991). The major problem with clinical applications using PET methodology is that a cyclotron is required to produce the necessary radionuclides. Because of the short half-life of the radionuclides, the cyclotron has to be very close to the imaging laboratory. As a consequence, only a few large research medical centers have PET scanning capabilities. In contrast, SPECT imaging is based on cerebral blood flow via tomographic scintigraphic techniques. Standard radiopharmaceuticals that are used in SPECT imaging do not require on-site cyclotron development. Accordingly, SPECT imaging has become widely used in neuroradiologic assessment of a diverse array of neurologic disorders. The problem with SPECT scanning, in contrast to PET, is that SPECT provides an image at a single point in time to assess radionuclide perfusion via blood flow in all brain regions simultaneously. PET scanning, however, permits the study of the temporal sequence of metabolic activity, typically the cerebral metabolic rate of regional glucose metabolism, over time or during some type of cognitive activation procedure (see Démonet, Wise, & Frackowiak, 1993). PET scanning also can examine oxygen metabolism, cerebral blood flow, and neurotransmitter density parameters dynamically.

Table 7.1 (see p. 190) summarizes SPECT and PET findings in a variety of disorders. Because PET is primarily a research tool at this time (see Heiss, Pawlik, Holthoff, Kessler, & Szelies, 1992; Pawlik & Heiss, 1989), the focus of this portion of the discussion will be on SPECT. It is likely that by the end of this decade a variety of SPECT–neuropsychological outcome relationships will be well established.

Figure 7.14 depicts a normal SPECT in a 45-year-old female. Note the even distribution

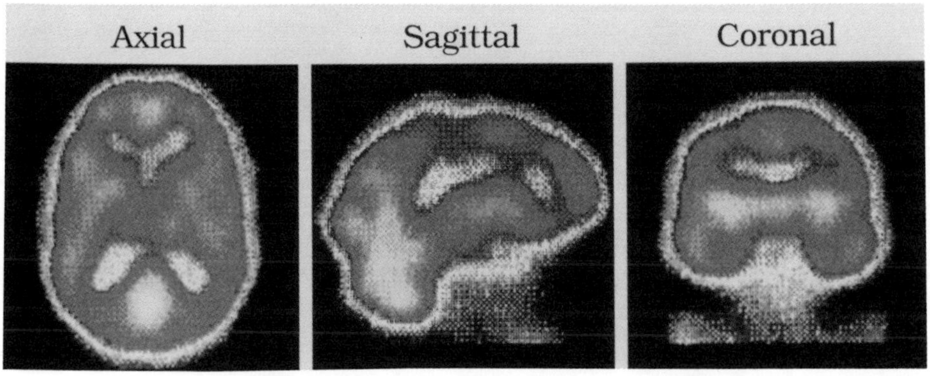

FIG. 7.14. Axial, sagittal, and coronal views of the SPECT imaging. The color scheme (in this illustration, gray scale) is utilized to depict various areas of metabolic functioning. Note the general uniformity and symmetry of these SPECT images which have been interpreted to be within normal limits.

of radiopharmaceutical perfusion. The symmetry and intensity of perfusion defines the normal distribution. In contrast, asymmetric changes or regions of diminished perfusion mark potential areas of metabolic/functional abnormality. To illustrate this principle, Fig. 7.15 presents the SPECT data from a patient with Alzheimer's disease. (The interested reader is referred to Holman, Johnson, Gorada, Carvalho, & Satlin, 1992, for a general discussion of SPECT imaging in Alzheimer's disease.) Note the marked areas of hypoperfusion in the parietal areas bilaterally and to some degree, in the frontal regions as well. Figure 7.16 presents SPECT imaging data from the patient who sustained a severe traumatic brain injury

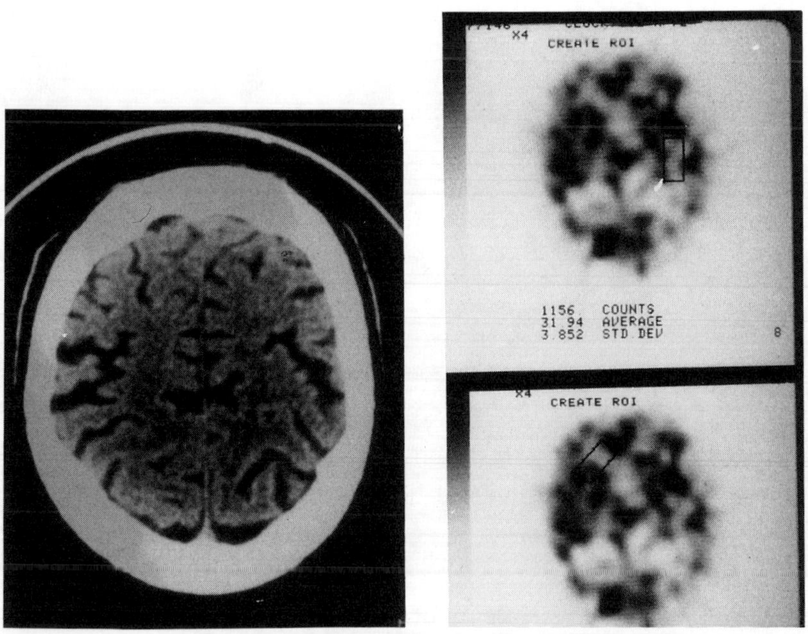

FIG. 7.15. Clinical SPECT scanning. Alzheimer's SPECT depicting bilateral parietal hypometabolism (*right*) in comparison to CT scan, which depicts generalized atrophy (*left*).

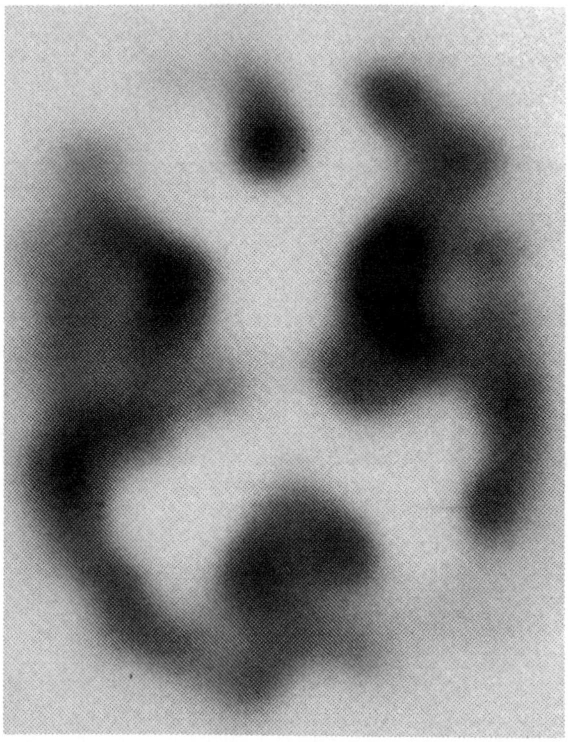

FIG. 7.16. SPECT imaging in the patient in Figs. 7.1 and 7.2 done at approximately the same time as the MR imaging in Fig. 7.4 (see Fig. 7.9 also). Note the absence of homogeneous metabolic absorption in the anterior frontal and posterior parietal occipital areas.

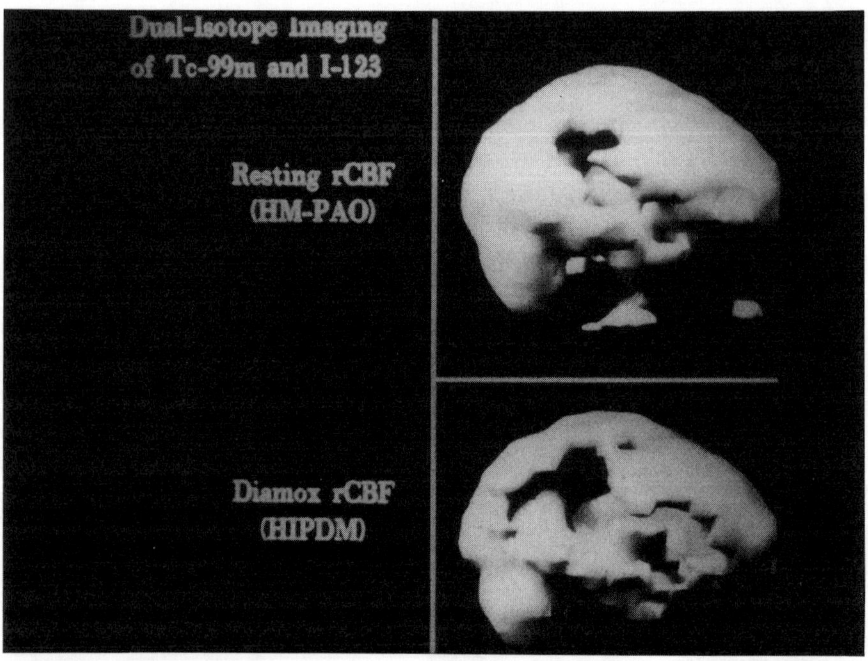

FIG. 7.17. Application of three-dimensional imaging to SPECT scanning in a patient with stroke. These three-dimensional surface rendered images show a right frontal parietal resting regional cerebral blood flow (RCBF) deficit with expansion following vasodilation with Diamox in a stroke patient (bottom scan). The difference in affected areas in the resting and vasodilated studies represents the area of failed vasodilatory reserve. From Holman and Devous (1992). © 1992 by the Society of Nuclear Medicine. Reprinted with permission.

from a fall and whose CT and MR images previously have been viewed in Figs. 7.1, 7.2, 7.4, and 7.9. Note that the findings depicted in Fig. 7.16 coincide with the deficits seen anatomically, but also suggest a much larger area of physiologic abnormality than would be predicted specific to the areas of anatomic damage. SPECT imaging can be performed in any cerebral plane (axial, coronal, and sagittal). The images can be reconstructed to form a 3-D image of the damaged brain (see Fig. 7.17), they can be registered in a fashion to superimpose the CT or MR on the SPECT scan image so that specific lesion foci can be compared to areas of metabolic abnormality, or both. Simultaneous registration of anatomic structures with metabolic function provides a method of verifying the anatomic structures that are affected metabolically (compare Fig. 7.16 with Fig. 7.4).

As of this writing, large sample size studies that illustrate the relationship between SPECT and neuropsychological outcome are lacking. It is anticipated that as SPECT scanning achieves greater clinical acceptance, studies of this type will be conducted. The work to date is summarized in the tables that follow.

ACTIVATION OR FUNCTIONAL MR IMAGING (fMRI)

Belliveau et al. (1991) demonstrated an MR-based method to examine blood volume changes over time that correspond to focal cerebral activation. For example, in response to light flash an activation of visual cortex can be demonstrated by using the techniques reported by Belliveau et al. Their study, along with several others (Ogawa, Lee, Nayak, & Glynn, 1990; Rosen, Belliveau, Vevea, & Brady, 1990), utilized a contrast media—Gadolinium-DTPA (diethylenetriaminepentaacetic acid)—to enhance the detection of time-related changes in the magnetic susceptibility of tissue. The contrast agents produce magnetic field gradients around blood vessels. The concomitant changes in NMR signal intensity are measurable and proportional to the tissue's concentration of contrast agent. The concentration of contrast agent passing through the tissue is related to blood flow; therefore, contrast agents can be used indirectly in assessing blood flow (for a more in-depth discussion see Turner & Jezzard, 1994). More recently, others (see Schad, Trost, Knopp, Müller, & Lorenz, 1993; Schad et al., 1994) have used an even less invasive approach to functional MR imaging (fMRI) as well as using standard MR imaging systems (Connelly et al., 1993; Constable, McCarthy, Allison, Anderson, & Gore, 1993). This approach capitalizes on the paramagnetic effects of hemoglobin wherein deoxygenated hemoglobin, being paramagnetic, slightly distorts the magnetic field around it, whereas oxygenated hemoglobin is not paramagnetic. A paramagnetic substance is magnetizable but has only a small positive susceptibility that varies little with the intensity of the magnetizing force. As can be seen in Fig. 7.18, this technique permits the imaging of activation patterns using the standard MR apparatus. Such imaging possibilities hold great promise for the in vivo study of brain–behavior relationships because they provide a method of simultaneous visualization of anatomic structures along with an indirect visualization of physiologic changes. In this context, it may soon be the case that neuropsychological studies can be administered to a patient wherein part of the examination is given under fMRI activation procedures.

The MR procedure has achieved, within the decade since its introduction, exceptional imaging resolution of brain tissue. Anatomic structure, however, is only one part of the puzzle. Without knowing the concomitant "function" or physiologic integrity of a structure, even the immense precision of anatomic MR imaging is incomplete. The interface of anatomy, physiological function, and behavior represents one of the major challenges of this, the "decade of the brain." One avenue to accomplish the goal of a more comprehensive interface between understanding brain and behavior may be provided by fMRI procedures. For exam-

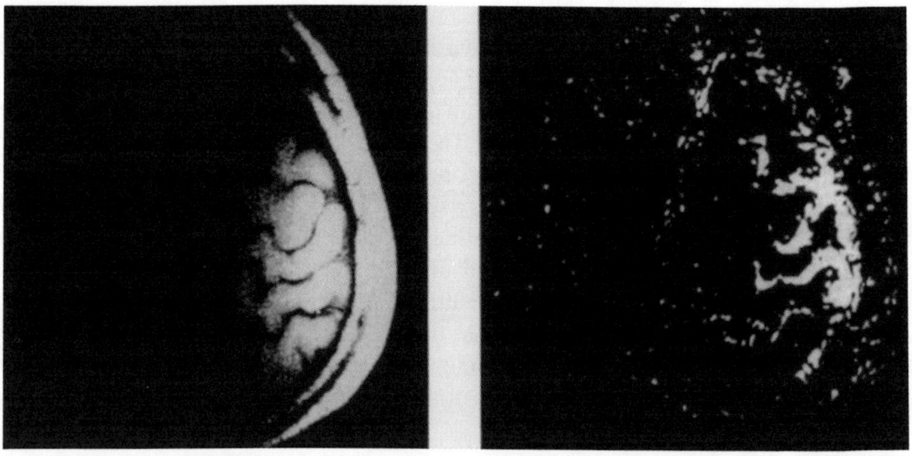

FIG. 7.18. Activation MR. 2D stimulation experiment. (*Left*) Oblique (axial to coronal: 10°) SE image (TR/TE 600/15) of a normal volunteer with high spatial resolution (FOV = 150 mm, TH = 2 mm, matrix = 256 × 256) using the surface coil. (*Right*) Difference image (FOV = 150 mm, TH = 2 mm, matrix = 128 × 128) between averages of all stimulation (30 images) and nonstimulation (30 images) images showing signal increase produced by the stimulation (touching each finger to thumb) occurred in areas predominantly occupied by the grey matter of primary left motor and sensory cortex. Reprinted from Schad et al., 1993, with kind permission from Elsevier Science, Ltd, The Boulevard, Langford Lane, Kidlington OX5 1GB, UK.

ple, Kosslyn et al. (1993) recently demonstrated significant PET abnormalities in brain regions outside the boundary of focal tissue damage. Accordingly, if we focused solely on the structural boundaries of damage, Kosslyn et al.'s research demonstrates that part of the functional significance of the damage is missed. Hopefully, fMRI will provide a means of investigating these indirect effects of a focal lesion, while retaining the exquisite detail of MR visualization.

Because fMRI is such a new technique, there are no major neuropsychological outcome studies available that correlate structural and functional deficits with clinical syndromes. However, some very exciting research has been published (see Casey et al., in press; Rao et al., 1993) that demonstrates very interesting relationships between speech and fMRI findings. For example, the areas of the brain actually involved in language can now be studied with the anatomic precision of MRI coupled with simultaneous monitoring of physiologic changes in the brain as they relate to various aspects of language function.

MR SPECTROSCOPY

NMR spectroscopy (see Fig. 7.19) provides a means to study energy metabolism in vivo (Cohen, 1987; DeCertaines, Bovee, & Podo, 1992; Frahm et al., 1989; Longo, Giorgini, Magnaldi, Pascazio, & Ricci, 1993). NMR spectroscopy holds great promise for the in vivo study of various aspects of brain metabolism, energy dynamics, and basic chemical constituency of the normal and pathological brain. Whereas fMRI only allows an indirect measure, NMR spectroscopy allows a direct measure. Currently, NMR spectroscopy or magnetic resonance spectroscopy (MRS) provides techniques for assessing concentrations of phosphorous metabolites, lactate, both amino as well as fatty acids, and a variety of the metabolically relevant compounds including some neurotransmitters. Unfortunately, as for application in

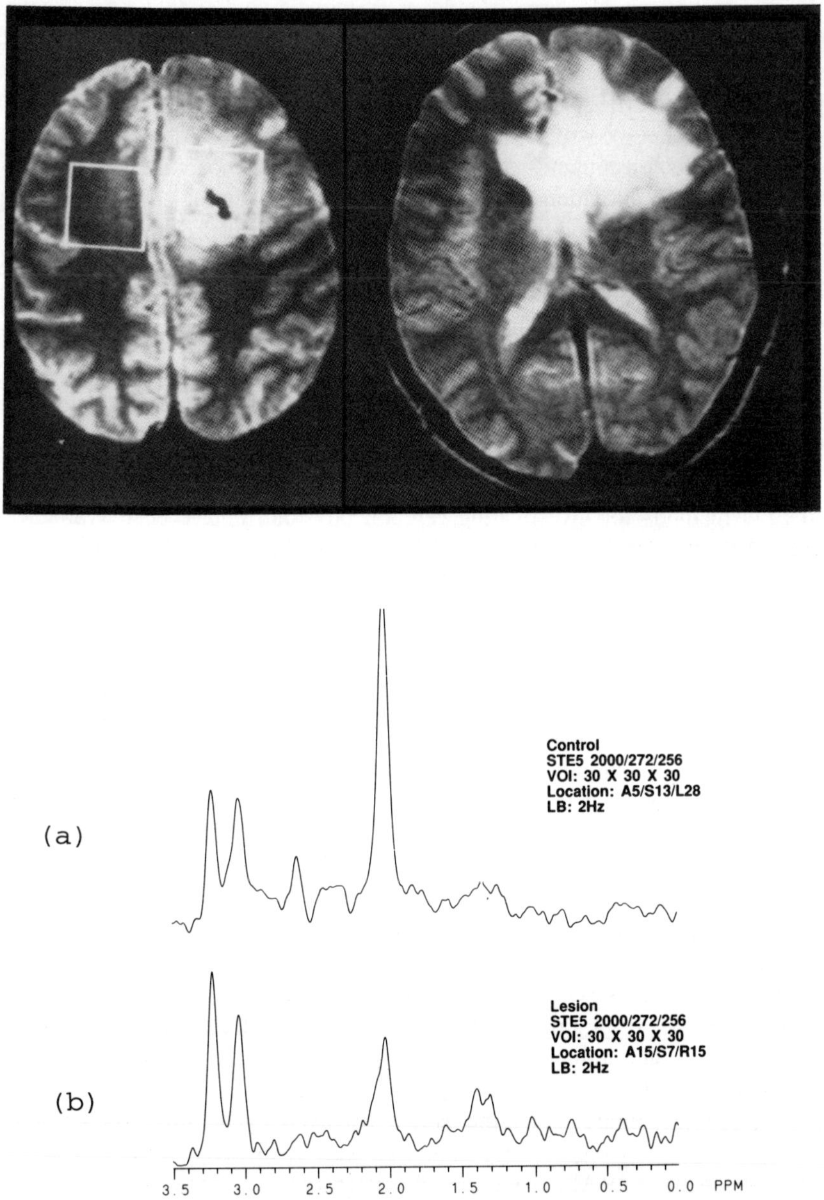

FIG. 7.19. MR images and spectra from an untreated low-grade astrocytoma. Axial T2-weighted images showing a tumor in the right frontal lobe, extending across the midline. Short flip angle image shows MR spectroscopic volumes of interest (squares) of the tumor (*right*) and the mainly normal contralateral brain (*left*). (Note that the brain image is presented with right hemisphere on the reader's right.) *Bottom*: Hydrogen MR spectra from control tissue (*a*) and the lesion (*b*). There is elevation of the choline (3.25 ppm) and creatine (3.05 ppm) levels and a marked decrease in the NAA peak (2.02 ppm) in the lesion spectra compared with the control. From Alger et al., 1990. © 1990 by the Radiological Society of North America. Reprinted with permission.

neuropsychology, the same disclaimer previously mentioned needs to be reiterated here. This is a very new technique. No large sample or systematic studies that have examined the relationship between NMR spectroscopy findings and neuropsychological outcome across a broad spectrum of neurologic disorders have been published. Techniques are currently being developed to integrate NMR spectroscopy with 3-D MR image rendering of the brain (Cao et al., 1993). Such a technique will permit an integrated 3-D depiction of brain surface anatomy and biochemistry. Such techniques should have a significant impact on neuropsychological studies in the future by providing a method of examining pathological changes in specific brain regions and by examining the relation of those pathological changes to neuropsychological outcome. For example, disorders such as Alzheimer's Disease could be studied by examining the hippocampus anatomically, functionally, and metabolically in relation to neuropsychological performance. The brain will no longer be the "black box," and neuropsychologists will no longer look at "behavior" alone.

QUANTITATIVE ELECTROENCEPHALOGRAPHY (EEG) AND BRAIN MAPPING

Standard EEG methods for investigating cerebral physiology have been available for approximately half a century. In the past, the typical EEG was read by an electroencephalographer who visually scanned the EEG patterns emanating from multiple electrode sites. It has always been recognized by electroencephalographers (see Finitzo, Pool, & Chapman, 1991) that quantitatively there were a tremendous amount of data embedded in the EEG tracings, but these data were inaccessible, for the most part, via traditional visual and clinical inspection. With the advent of averaging techniques (including evoked response averaging), various filtering methods and the onset of computerized assisted EEG analysis, this analytic ambiguity began to change in the early 1970s (see Gevins & Illes, 1991). This research has led to a variety of techniques to map electrophysiologically or "image" physiological activity of the brain (see Zappulla, LeFever, Jaeger, & Bilder, 1991). Such procedures provide a distinct advantage in analyzing the extensive data embedded in the EEG tracing data that may provide important insights into normal and aberrant physiological functioning in a variety of neurologic disorders (see Thatcher, Cantor, McAlaster, Geisler, & Krause, 1991).

Figure 7.20 illustrates several important points concerning EEG topographic mapping. This map was obtained from a patient with a history of significant cerebral trauma (loss of consciousness, coma, and initially left-side hemiplegia) as a consequence of a motorcycle–motor vehicle accident (he was the motorcyclist). Neuropsychologically, when first tested 6 weeks post-closed head injury (CHI), the patient displayed a generalized reduction in cognitive functions (VIQ = 91, PIQ = 80, FSIQ = 85 and WMS MQ = 86) but with particular deficits in visual memory (WMS visual reproduction score = 3 [2 after 15-minute delay] and 11 errors on the Benton Visual Retention Test, BVRT). At nearly a year postinjury his hemiplegia had resolved but he continued to display significant neuropsychological deficits in nonverbal visual–spatial functions that are presumed to be related to residual right hemisphere injury (WMS visual reproduction score = 7 [3 after 15-minute delay] and 7 errors on the BVRT). MR studies (see Fig. 7.20) demonstrated no major structural abnormalities. However, quantitative electroencephalography did demonstrate abnormalities over the right posterior hemisphere.

These types of quantitative EEG map findings may even provide important electrophysiological information in more subtle forms of brain dysfunction than those that are presented in the aforementioned TBI case. For example, it has long been assumed that the left hemisphere mediates language function and that left hemisphere irregularities are the basis for learning disabilities (Bigler, 1992a; Galaburda & Kemper, 1979). Duffy and colleagues (see Duffy & McAnulty, 1990) have spent over a decade studying with EEG topography methods various irregularities that may accompany reading disorders. Figure 7.21 presents a composite quantitative EEG map based on a sample of individuals with dyslexia. Duffy and McAnulty's dyslexia-pure appears to be associated with an electrophysiologic "difference" in all regions normally involved in language function, including the medial

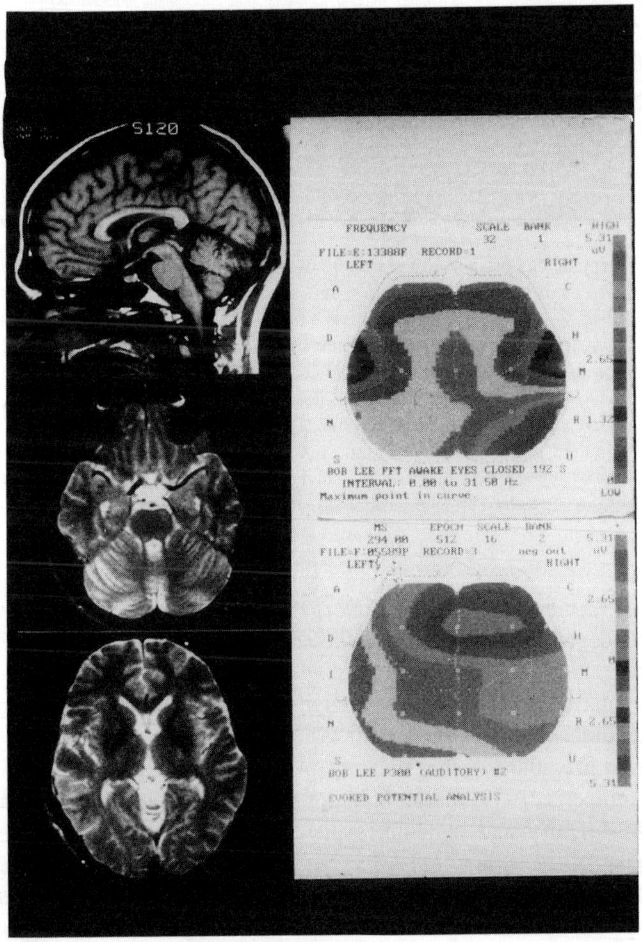

FIG. 7.20. EEG mapping. (*Left*) MRI views in sagittal (*top*) and horizontal planes (*middle and bottom*) taken from a 42-year-old high school educated motorcycle police officer who sustained a closed head injury as a result of a car–motorcycle collision. Initially he was rendered comatose and left hemiparetic. Note that the MRI findings do not depict any gross structural damage. (*Right*) Electrophysiological topography mapping studies indicating the presence of a lateralized deficit in the right posterior quadrant. The neuropsychological test results are suggestive of residual right temporal lobe dysfunction even though MRI studies were negative. However, note that there is a slight asymmetry of the temporal horns with the right temporal horn being slightly larger than the left, which may be a sign of tissue loss. Taken together, the combination of EEG and neuropsychological abnormalities clearly implicate right hemisphere dysfunction in this CHI victim. From Bigler, 1991. © 1991 by Pergamon Press Ltd. Reprinted with permission.

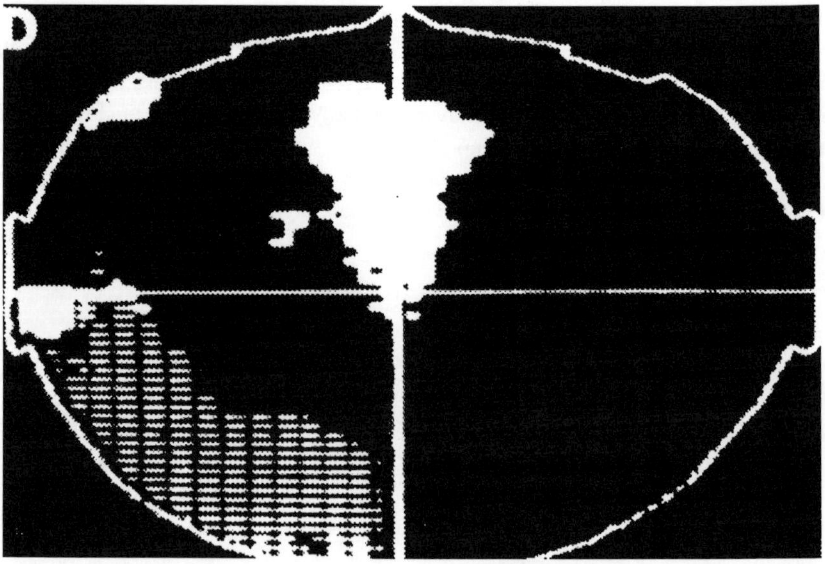

FIG. 7.21. EEG mapping of a brain from a child with dyslexia. This image shows a schematic outline of the head–nose above, left ear to the left, right ear to right, vertex (crown of the head) in the center, and occiput (back of the head) below—taken from Duffy and McAnulty, 1990, displaying all regions of between group differences that differentiated boys with dyslexia-pure from normal readers in white. Note that those areas represent a distortion from the normal background in control subjects. Regions shown reached or exceeded the $p < 0.02$ two-tailed probability level across all EEG and/or EP state. Note that the regions delineated include the classic left midtemporal and left anterior temporal regions typically associated with language function. Note, also, the prominent bilateral medial frontal involvement. The very same regions were delineated elsewhere by blood flow studies during language functions in nondisabled subjects. From Duffy and McAnulty 1990. © 1990 by Pergamon Press Ltd. Reprinted with permission.

frontal region (see further discussion in Bigler, 1992a). The implications of such findings are that there is some degree of dysfunction in the dominant left hemisphere regions of the brain as well as frontal region. The clinical interpretation of such findings has been that the left hemispheric irregularities are likely to be related to the central language processing elements of the reading disorder and that the frontal lesion findings may be related to attentional or response execution irregularities that may accompany a developmental reading disorder. As Galaburda and Kemper's (1979) research demonstrated neuropathologic evidence for dyslexia, the research of Duffy and colleagues provides parallel physiologic evidence for the neurobiologic basis of dyslexia.

As described previously, when examining the biological basis of a given behavior there are two major parts—one anatomic, the other physiologic. An anatomic irregularity or abnormality can occur without a concomitant physiologic abnormality and vice versa. The case presented in Fig. 7.15 is an excellent example of this principle. In this case of a patient with confirmed Alzheimer's Disease, his CT scan demonstrates only generalized atrophy, whereas his SPECT scan demonstrates focal changes in parietal and frontal areas. It is likely that research that achieves the greatest application in integrating neuroimaging findings and neuropsychological outcome will come from studies where both structure and physiology are examined simultaneously with some facet of neuropsychological function. The research by Gevins and colleagues (see Gevins & Illes, 1991) exemplifies this approach. By using a 128-

electrode array integrated by MR registration, this type of research paradigm permits the interface of brain imaging with electrophysiological mapping of the physiologic findings on 2-D and 3-D brain images. Gevins' work has, as of this writing, focused on a functional network approach with a variety of cognitive tasks and an attempt to isolate the earliest electrophysiological components of cognition. This approach has not been applied to clinical populations or in conjunction with traditional neuropsychological assessment methods. This will be accomplished in future research.

MAGNETOENCEPHALOGRAPHY

Electric currents in the human brain generate magnetic fields. These magnetic fields are extremely small in the magnitude of 50 to 500 femtotesla (fT = 10^{-15} Tesla), but can be detected by sensors from a special device with the eponym of SQUID (Superconducting Quantum Interference Device). This emerging technology and study of human magnetic field changes has been labeled "magnetoencephalography" (MEG). The technique appears to be well suited for source localization of magnetic field changes (i.e., 3-D identification of generation sites). Accordingly, MEG investigations looking at sensory processing differences (Sams & Hari, 1991), various aspects of cognitive processing (Papanicolaou, Rogers, & Baumann, 1991), and seizure focus have been reported. Papanicolaou and Tarkka's (1995) research holds great promise in terms of a variety of MEG findings in cognition that may have particular relevance to neuropsychological outcome. These investigations are underway (see also Mäkelä et al., 1993).

CURRENT STATUS OF BRAIN IMAGING STUDIES IN THE LAST FIVE YEARS

Table 7.1 summarizes the imaging and functional outcome research of the past 5 years. Imaging research has become so technology-driven that studies prior to the late 1980s should be viewed very critically and many of the conclusions may have to be dismissed. Therefore, it was decided not to include any research prior to 1989. The table is organized by disorder states rather than by neuroimaging method. With each entry the type of imaging method is clearly listed. In some cases, multiple imaging modalities were utilized and each is listed. This table is certainly not exhaustive of the field, but is representative of the current status of brain imaging in neuropsychological functioning or outcome in a variety of neuropsychological diseases.

SUMMARY

Development of neuroimaging technology has greatly changed and enhanced clinical neuropsychology as well as neuroscience research in general. The combination of neuropsychological assessment techniques and neuroimaging allows neuropsychologists to begin to elucidate the complex relationships between brain structure/physiology and behavior. Current imaging methodologies as well as future imaging techniques will become the tools used by neuropsychologists to provide a more refined understanding of human brain–behavior relationships. This will lead to improved diagnostic criteria and intervention techniques for neurologic disorders.

TABLE 7.1
A Summary of Recent Studies of Brain Imaging Research

Author	*Year*	*Imaging Method*	*Disorder*	*Anatomic focus*	*Subjects/ Participants*	*Conclusions that relate to neuropsychology*
				Clinical syndromes		
Byring et al.	1991	qEEG	spelling disorders	parietooccipital	23 patients 21 controls	Patients had an excess of abnormal electrical activity.
Cappa et al.	1991	CT	unilateral neglect	temporoparietal	24 patients	Temporoparietal lesions were the most common. The severity of neglect correlated with size of lesion.
Laloux et al.	1992	SPECT	transient global amnesia	general vasculature	5 patients	Transient global amnesia occurred due to vascular mechanisms. SPECT was used to examine blood flow changes.
Marciani et al.	1991	EEG, MR	prosopagnosia	right temporo-occipital	1 patient	Computerized EEG showed impairment of brain posterior regions. Partial recovery of neuropsychological deficit coupled with improved EEG readings were observed at 2 months.
Plante et al.	1991	MR	language impairment	perisylvian asymmetries	boys with language impairment	Atypical perisylvian asymmetries were identified on MR. Prenatal alteration of brain development underlying specific language impairment is discussed.
Wang et al.	1992	MR	Down's and Williams syndromes	cerebrum,neo-cerebellar tonsils	DS patients, WS patients as matched controls	Cerebellar tonsils were larger in proportion to cerebrum in Williams' syndrome patients than in Down's patients and controls. Language function also was relatively preserved in Williams' syndrome.
				Degenerative disorders		
Angelini et al.	1992	MR	Hallervorden Spatz disease	general brain abnormalities	11 patients	All patients had behavioral changes followed by dementia. MR identified hyperintensities and proposed iron deposits.

Barth et al.	1989	CT, MR	Schilder's diffuse myelinoclastic sclerosis	white matter anomalies	1 patient, 6-year-old female	CT and MR revealed stable amyelinic lesions. An arrest in neuropsychological performance contrasted with EEG findings and motor control.
Blansjaar et al.	1992	MR	Korsakoff's syndrome	brain lesions and atrophy	10 patients (5 Korsakoff, 5 alcoholics)	Both groups exhibited lesions, atrophy and lesions thought to be more related to Korsakoff's syndrome.
Chang et al.	1993	MR, SPECT	myotonic dystrophy (MD)		22 MD (11 paternal MD & 8 maternal MD), 10 controls	The maternal MD group had earlier onset and lower IQ's than the paternal MD group. Cerebral perfusion in the maternal MD group was consistent with a diffuse brain injury while more minor cerebral perfusion differences were noted in the paternal MD.
Comi et al.	1993	MR	multiple sclerosis	corpus callosum, ventricles	100 patients	Ventricular dilation and corpus callosum atrophy were observed in patients with lower performance on neuropsychological measures.
Dietrich et al.	1990	MR	myelin disorder	white matter	25 children and young adults	This study was conducted to assess the correlation between MR findings and severity of disease.
Eberling et al.	1993	SPECT	Alzheimer's disease	frontal and parietal regions	12 AD mild & 38 AD moderate patients, 8 controls	The results of this study support *a priori* grouping of neuropsychological tests into frontal and visuoconstructive clusters and suggest that those two clusters are good measures of frontal and parietal lobe function respectively.
Feinstein et al.	1992	MR	multiple sclerosis	CNS lesions, ventricular system	10 w/psychosis, 10 patients w/o psychosis	Patients with higher incidence of psychotic symptoms had larger lesion scores, especially around the periventricular regions.
Goldenberg et al.	1989	SPECT	Parkinson's disease	frontal and parietal regions	28 non-demented W/PD, 21 matched controls	Middle frontal and parietal region flow rates correlated significantly with several test scores.

(*continued*)

TABLE 7.1 (*Continued*)

Author	*Year*	*Imaging Method*	*Disorder*	*Anatomic focus*	*Subjects/ Participants*	*Conclusions that relate to neuropsychology*
Huber et al.	1989	MR	Parkinson's disease	atrophy	68 patients, 28 controls	Neuropsychological performance was lower in patients but was not associated with any specific pattern of MR abnormalities.
Hunt et al.	1989	MR	aging	white matter	46 normals	Normal aging adults were found to have white matter lesions, 9% severe lesions, and moderate lesions in 22%. White matter lesions in the elderly may not always be significant.
Izquierdo et al.	1991	MR	multiple sclerosis	CNS lesions	35 patients	MR detection of lesions was related to neuropsychological outcome.
Jagust et al.	1992	SPECT	Parkinson's disease & Alzheimer's disease	frontal and temporal lobe regions	20 non-demented W/PD, 21 mildly demented W/ AD, 24 controls	PD patients performed more poorly than controls in all cognitive domains and were intermediate to AD patients on memory and overall cognitive functioning. PD poor performers showed lowest (rCBF) ratios in left and right temporal lobes.
Jambaque et al.	1991	MR	tuberous sclerosis	CNS lesions	23 patients	Lesions and neuropsychological data were interrelated.
Jernigan et al.	1991	MR	Korsakoff's syndrome	ventricular system, atrophy	8 patients, alcoholics, controls	Tissue volume loss in the diencephalic areas in Korsakoff's patient's was more severe than non-amnesic alcoholics.
Kessler et al.	1991	PET	Alzheimer's disease	general	7 patients, 7 controls	Metabolic rate at rest reflected the extent of morphologic damage. Metabolism in Alzheimer's disease patients was more impaired during activation than at rest.
Leli et al.	1992	SPECT	Alzheimer's disease	general	15 patients	Decreased perfusion on SPECT scans was correlated with the severity of Alzheimer's disease, and neuropsychologic test scores correlated with lateralized perfusion deficits on SPECT scans.

McDonald et al.	1991	MR	Alzheimer's disease	white matter abnormalities	22 patients, 16 matched controls	MR revealed abnormalities related to normal aging more so than disease. Abnormalities in both groups are discussed.
Moore et al.	1989	MR	hepatic encephalopathy	cerebrum	19 patients, 19 matched controls	Neuropsychological performance correlated poorly with measures although pathology was present.
Murphy et al.	1993	proton NMR, PET	Alzheimer's disease	general abnormalities	9 patients, 8 matched controls	AD patients demonstrated hypometabolism. There was no correlation between phosphorus metabolite concentration and dementia or glucose metabolism.
Peppard et al.	1992	PET	Parkinson's disease	temporoparietal	14 patients, 20 controls	Widespread cortical glucose hypometabolism was evident in non-demented patients. Demented patients had a global decrease in glucose metabolism; the most severe abnormalities were in the temporoparietal regions.
Pozilli et al.	1991	MR	multiple sclerosis	corpus callosum	18 patients, 18 age & sex matched controls	Anterior corpus callosum area was strongly related to performance on verbal fluency tasks. The anterior corpus callosum is implicated in the transferring of information relative to verbal fluency.
Primavera et al.	1990	qEEG	Alzheimer's disease	general abnormalities	AD patients, normal elderly controls	A significant correlation was observed between the Mini Mental State score and some qEEG parameters. QEEG may reduce the amount of false positives resulting from neuropsychological exams in identifying Alzheimer's disease.
Pugnetti et al.	1993	MR	multiple sclerosis	white matter abnormalities	64 patients	MS patients with parenchymal changes had a less favorable outcome than those who had lesions without parenchymal changes.
Ron et al.	1991	MR	multiple sclerosis	general abnormalities	58 MS patients, 46 disabled, 40 controls	MR abnormalities related to overall performance on psychometric tests.
Scheltens et al.	1992	MR	Alzheimer's disease	temporal lobe, hippocampus	21 patients 21 matched controls	Medial temporal lobe atrophy identified by MR correlated with scores on the mini-mental state examination and memory tests.

(continued)

TABLE 7.1 (*Continued*)

Author	*Year*	*Imaging Method*	*Disorder*	*Anatomic focus*	*Subjects/ Participants*	*Conclusions that relate to neuropsychology*
Schmidt	1992	MR	Alzheimer's disease, vascular dementia	Parenchyma	27 AD patients, 31 VD patients, 18 controls	Alzheimer's patients had frequent signal abnormalities in the uncal-hippocampal, and insular regions. Cortical and ventricular atrophy were discriminators between groups.
Schmitt et al.	1992	rCBF	Alzheimer's disease	general abnormalities	7 patients, 7 controls	Decreased perfusion was related to the severity of AD on SPECT. Neuropsychological data correlated with lateralized perfusion deficits. SPECT perfusion deficits were also related to global changes in intellectual functioning.
Swirsky-Sacchetti et al.	1992	MR	multiple sclerosis	CNS lesions, corpus callosum	MS patients	Frontal lobe abnormalities best predicted word fluency, memory and abstract problem solving tasks. Lesions of the left parieto-occipital region best predicted poorer performance on verbal learning and complex visual-integrative tasks.
				Developmental disorders		
Berthier et al.	1990	MR	autism	cortex	2 patients	Asperger's syndrome (a form of autism) in two patients; One patient had left frontal macrogyria and the other had polymicrogyria. A close relative with bipolar disorder also showed a cortical migration anomaly.
Courchesne et al.	1993	MR	autism	brain atrophy	21 patients, 52 controls in 3 groups	In a part of the autistic population volume loss in the parietal region was observed.

Flowers et al.	1991	rCBF	reading disability	left hemisphere	69 normals 83 ability known	This study shows that left hemisphere cerebral activation is anomalous in adults who were dyslexic as children.
Hagman et al.	1992	PET	dyslexia	medial temporal lobe	10 dyslexic 10 matched controls	A significant difference in medial temporal lobe in dyslexic patients having higher absolute and relative brain metabolism along an anterior-posterior gradient was observed.
Piven et al.	1992	MR	autism	ventricles, pons, cerebellum	15 autistic, 15 matched controls, 15 male matched controls	Autistic patients had smaller cerebellar lobules than controls. The pons and fourth ventricle were not significantly different between groups. Autistic children had larger mid-sagittal brain area than did the controls.
Rumsey et al.	1992	PET	dyslexia	left temporoparietal region	14 male dyslexic, 14 matched controls	In this study, dyslexic men failed to activate left temporo-parietal regions that were activated in controls during rhyme detection.
Zametkin et al.	1993	PET	attention & hyperactivity	frontal lobe	10 ADHD patients, 10 controls	Six of 60 specific areas of the brain demonstrated significant reduction in normalized glucose metabolism. Lower metabolism in the left frontal lobe inversely correlated with the severity of symptoms.
				Epilepsy		
Bromfield et al.	1992	PET	epilepsy	frontal lobe	23 patients	A significant non-lateralized mood by region interaction was observed. The only significant difference in normalized regional metabolic rates between depressed and non-depressed patients was in the frontal cortex.
Henry et al.	1993	PET	epilepsy	temporal lobe and thalamus	27 temporal lobe epileptics, 10 controls	Thalamic hypometabolism in patients suggested a pathophysiologic role for the thalamus in initiation or propagation of temporal lobe seizures or in the interictal cognitive dysfunction.

(continued)

TABLE 7.1 (*Continued*)

Author	*Year*	*Imaging Method*	*Disorder*	*Anatomic focus*	*Subjects/ Participants*	*Conclusions that relate to neuropsychology*
Kirkpatrick et al.	1993	SPECT	epilepsy	temporal lobe	6 patients	There was a significant increase in the activation index in various cortical regions. The medial temporal cortices were positively correlated with a word memory score.
Lencz et al.	1992	MR	epilepsy	temporal lobe	25 epileptics, 14 controls	MR measures and some neuropsychological memory results were significantly correlated.
Marciani et al.	1992	EEG, MR	epilepsy	CNS lesions	22 patients	EEG with other parameters such as MR lesion localization were found to be useful in comparison with neuropsychological tests of lateralization of function.
Njemanzc et al.	1992	CBF	epilepsy		1 patient	This study suggests that mean blood flow velocity may be a useful parameter for monitoring functional brain activity in epilepsy.
				Miscellaneous		
Adams et al.	1993	MR	alcoholism	general	31 patients	Impaired function of cerebral tissue in the medial frontal region was found to relate to chronic alcohol intake.
Battistini et al.	1991	EEG, MR	phenylketonuria (PKU)	white matter abnormalities	1 patient	A diet low in phenylalanine lowered psychiatric disturbances and revoked neurophysiological and MRI changes.
Baum et al.	1993	MR	lupus	CNS lesions	21 patients	MR was useful in detecting lesions in CNS lupus. Some patients exhibited poor neuropsychological performance.
Berardi et al.	1991	PET	normative study (memory and age)	parietal lobe region	11 elderly normals	Parietal and hemispheric metabolic asymmetries were related to long-term memory discrepancies, such that subjects with better visual than verbal memory had higher right than left brain glucose metabolism. The opposite pattern was exhibited in others.

Bernsen et al.	1992	CT, MR	toxic poisoning	brain atrophy, ventricles	1 34-year-old male patient	MR and CT scanning of the brain revealed enlarged ventricles and generalized atrophy. Neuropsychological and behavioral assessments were indicative of an organic brain syndrome.
Bornstein et al.	1992a	MR	HIV	white matter	243 HIV+ and HIV− males	AIDS patients had a slightly higher incidence of hyperintensities.
Callender et al.	1993	CT, MR, PET, SPECT	toxic encephalopathy	lobes, subcortical	33 patients	CT, MR, and EEG were found to be less sensitive to this type of patient in this study. Metabolic imaging studies are recommended.
Cantor-Graal	1993	rCBF	normative study	frontal lobes	22 normals	Significant flow augmentations in the left dorsolateral cortex were exhibited during performance of the word fluency test.
Carbotte et al.	1992	CT, MR, PET	lupus	general abnormalities	3 patients	Reassessment changes on PET related with changes in cognitive function. Localized abnormalities were not observed on CT.
Caselli et al.	1991	SPECT	thalamic infarctions	thalamus	7 patients	Thalamic deafferentation of cerebral cortex may result in focal reduction of rCBF and cognitive dysfunction; however, clinical recovery can occur despite persistence of cortical diaschisis.
Charlot et al.	1992	SPECT	normative study	left hemisphere	69 normals	Imagery tasks produced an rCBF increase in the left visual association and left frontal cortices in both groups. The authors discuss differences between high and low imagers.
Dal·Pan et al.	1992	MR	HIV	brain atrophy	116 HIV+, 23 HIV−	Cerebral atrophy and caudate atrophy were observed in patients experiencing dementia.
Dejgaard et al.	1991	MR	diabetes	subcortical regions, CNS lesions	39 patients, 40 matched controls	This study observed evoked potential abnormalities and subcortical white matter lesions in relation to neuropsychological outcome in diabetic patients. Long term patients were compared with short term patients and controls.

(*continued*)

TABLE 7.1 (*Continued*)

Author	*Year*	*Imaging Method*	*Disorder*	*Anatomic focus*	*Subjects/ Participants*	*Conclusions that relate to neuropsychology*
Démonet et al.	1992	SPECT	normative study	general	6 male normals 6 female normals	No significant CBF changes were observed across conditions. Word monitoring in sentences was investigated.
Duffy et al.	1993	qEEG	normative study	brain mapping	202 normals	This study correlated qEEG data with psychological factors. Visual assessment was done on multidimensional image graphics.
Frith et al.	1991	PET	normative study	prefrontal and temporal cortices	4 normals	Intrinsic generation of a word was associated with an increase in left dorsolateral prefrontal cortical activity and a bilateral decrease in activity in auditory and superior temporal cortices. There was an increase in superior temporal activity associated with lexical decisions about words that were presented auditorily.
Gallen et al.	1993	fMRI, MEG, MR	normative study	postcentral, superior temporal	7 normals	Magnetic source imaging, a technique that combines magnetoencephalography and magnetic resonance imaging, was used to localize the auditory and somatosensory cortices in normals.
Garrido et al.	1993	MR	altitude sickness	general brain abnormalities	26 climbers, 21 controls	Neuropsychological deficits were experienced by all climbers during the ascent with residual problems following the return to sea level. MR showed abnormalities on 46% of the climbers, five of which had characteristic atrophy.
Gazzaniga et al.	1989	MR	commissurotomy	corpus callosum	2 patients, normal controls	A commisurectomy patient's performance on rhyming word tasks was compared to normals.
Goldenberg et al.	1991	SPECT	normative study	left occipital region and thalamus	18 male normals 10 female normals	Acoustic rather than visual imagery conditions were associated with larger flow increases in both hippocampal regions and the right inferior and superior temporal regions.

Gottschalk et al.	1991	PET	anxiety and hostility during dreaming and waking	all lobes	30 normals	Significant correlations for anxiety scales were found for different cerebral areas. Significant correlations were more frequent in waking and REM than NREM conditions and were more common in the frontal, parietal, and temporal lobes than in the occipital lobe.
Grasby et al.	1993	PET	normative study	general	18 normals	The study identified a number of neuroanatomical components of a distributed system for signal processing and storage relevant to auditory-verbal memory functions.
Hockerstedt et al.	1992	MR	liver disease	lesions	8 patients	MR revealed cerebral lesions in two patients. The majority of neurological impairment disappeared after liver transplantation.
Hodges et al.	1991	CT, MR	cyst	fornix	2 patients	Verbal memory has remained impaired and nonverbal anterograde memory improved over time. These two patients' specific deficits implicate the role of the fornix in memory function.
Jacobson et al.	1993	qEEG	encephalopathy	brain mapping	34 elderly patients	This study was performed to examine the usefulness of qEEG in the diagnosis of encephalopathy in elderly patients with delirium and/or dementia.
Kingma et al.	1993	MR	leukemia	general brain abnormalities	35 juvenile patients	Children with acute lymphoblastic leukemia treated with cranial irradiation and intrathecal and intravenous methotrexate showed both cognitive deficits and MR abnormalities.
Kirk et al.	1991	CT, MR	lupus	white matter abnormalities	1 58-year-old patient	MR revealed hyperintensities in cerebral and cerebellar white matter regions. CT revealed no abnormalities.
Kohn et al.	1989	CT, MR	cysts		8 patients	This study illustrates the relationship between intracranial cysts with atypical neuropsychiatric disorders.
Kosslyn et al.	1993	PET	normative study	brain mapping	exp 1: 14 exp 2: 13 exp 3: 16	This study suggests that imagery activates topographically mapped cortex. It explores several types of imagery and their effects on activation patterns.

(*continued*)

TABLE 7.1 (*Continued*)

Author	*Year*	*Imaging Method*	*Disorder*	*Anatomic focus*	*Subjects/ Participants*	*Conclusions that relate to neuropsychology*
Leira et al.	1992	MR,CT	encephalopathy	CNS lesions	9 patients	MR was used as the modality of choice in the clinical makeup of solvent induced encephalopaths.
Levin, Goldstein et al.	1989	MR	decompression sickness	CNS lesions	2 patients	Both divers had subcortical white matter lesions revealed by MR. Disturbances in memory, divergent thinking and visuospatial and motor deficits were observed.
Levin et al.	1990	MR	HIV	brain atrophy	25 patients, 7 controls	The slowing of information processing speed and cerebral atrophy were related to the stage of HIV infection, as identified on MR.
Lu et al.	1993	MEG	normative study	auditory cortex	normals	Auditory memory is explored in this study using MEG.
Martin et al.	1991	PET	mental disorders with alcoholism	cortex	10 alcoholics, 7 matched controls	Normalized CMRglu (glucose) levels were increased in the left cerebellar and parietal cortical regions and decreased in the right posterior white matter and anterior temporal regions of alcoholics.
McEvoy et al.	1993	MEG	normative study	right temporal cortex	normals	This study used MEG to enhance the understanding of auditory cortex.
Pardo et al.	1993	PET	normative study	cortex	7 normals	This study investigated the importance of inferior and orbitofrontal cortices in normal emotional cognitive processes.
Pool et al.	1991	SPECT	stuttering	cingulate and middle temporal gyri	20 stutterers	Stutters showed global absolute flow and reduction relative flow asymmetries (left $<$ right) in anterior cingulate and superior and middle temporal gyri. Milder changes were noted in left frontal gyrus.
Primavera et al.	1993	qEEG	amnesic syndrome	temporo-parietal	13 patients, 13 controls	Transient global amnesic patients had an implicated disturbance of the temporo-parietal regions.
Rezai et al.	1993	SPECT	normative study	frontal regions	60 normals	Significant increases in frontal regions were noted during the continuous performance test, Wisconsin Card Sort test (WCST), and Tower of London. Specific regions are discussed.

Rogers	1993	MEG	visual perception	superior temporal sulcus	normals	MEG was used to study visual processing in the inferior regions of the temporal lobe.
Schad et al.	1994	fMRI	normative study	motor cortex	normals	During motor cortex stimulation, there was a 10–20% increase in signal order in the motor and sensory cortices.
Sergent et al.	1992	PET	normative study (face recognition tasks)	see conclusion	7 normals	rCBF changes were demonstrated in the striate and extrastriate cortex on visual orientation tasks. Specific cortical regions are implicated in the various tasks.
Tonkonogy	1991	CT, MRI	temporal lobe lesion	temporal lobes	23 organic mental syndrome, (14 violent 9 non-violent)	There were 5 cases of local lesions in the anterior-inferior temporal lobe in the violent group. This study suggested that release of programs for violent behavior may result from unilateral destruction of the amygdaloid nuclei or adjacent structures.
van Gorp et al.	1992	PET	AIDS	basal ganglia, thalamus and temporal lobe	17 patients, 14 controls	The AIDS group had relative regional hypometabolism in the basal ganglia and thalamus. There was a significant relationship for AIDS group between temporal lobe metabolism and severity of dementia.
van Sweiten et al.	1991	MR	cerebral lesions	white matter	42 patients, 42 matched controls	Strokes and chronic end-organ damage of the brain in the form of demyelination of the white matter identifiable on MR, with cognitive decline may result from long term hypertension.
Wang et al.	1993	MR, PET	alcoholism	atrophy, ventricles	10 patients 10 controls	PET detected early functional changes related to alcohol use and/or age before structural changes could be detected on MR.
Warkentin et al.	1991	rCBF	normative study	see conclusion	39 normals	Significant flow augmentation was found in the left dorsolateral prefrontal cortex during speech production.
Wilson et al.	1991	MR	leukemia	white matter abnormalities	25 patients	Children under the age of 5 undergoing cancer treatment are at risk for neuropsychological decline and may exhibit white matter changes.

(continued)

TABLE 7.1 *(Continued)*

Author	*Year*	*Imaging Method*	*Disorder*	*Anatomic focus*	*Subjects/ Participants*	*Conclusions that relate to neuropsychology*
Yang et al.	1993	MEG, MRI	normative study	Somatosensory cortex	normals	High resolution mapping of somatosensory cortex during sensory tasks was conducted using MEG.
				Psychiatric disorders		
Andreasen et al.	1992	SPECT	schizophrenia	frontal region	13 neuroleptic naive, 23 non-naive, 15 controls	The left mesial frontal cortex was not activated in neuroleptic naive and non-naive subjects on Tower of London task. Decreased activation was found only in patients with high negative symptom scores. Therefore, hypofrontality may be related to negative symptoms.
Berman et al.	1992	rCBF	schizophrenia	frontal region	21 pairs	Significant differences were only found between affected and unaffected discordant monozygotic twins on a prefrontal task. Schizophrenic patients were hypofrontal.
Bornstein et al.	1992b	MR	schizophrenia	ventricles	72 patients, 31 controls	The third ventricle dilation and neuropsychological outcome correlated significantly.
Botteron et al.	1992	MR	affective disorder	white matter abnormalities	1 patient	A young adolescent manic patient had subcortical focal signal hyperintensities on brain MR. Etiology, pathophysiology and clinical relationships of these lesions is reviewed.
Brown et al.	1992	MR	psychiatric	white matter abnormalities	229 patients, 154 controls	The prevalence of hyperintensities on MR in bipolar patients was not significantly different than controls. Higher rates of deep white matter hyperintensites in relation to bipolar illness occurred.
Buchsbaum et al.	1992	PET	schizophrenia	basal ganglia, frontal region	18 neuroleptic naive, 20 matched controls	Hypofrontality was observed with significantly reduced ratios of inferior and medial frontal regions compared to occipital cortex; lower metabolism was noted in the basal ganglia.

Coffman et al.	1990	MR	bipolar disorder	midsagittal structures	30 patients, controls	Bipolar patients had significantly lower cognitive functioning than controls. A correlation was found between a reduction in mid-sagittal areas of the brain and impairment.
Filley et al.	1990	MR	toluene abuse	white matter abnormalities	14 patients	In such patients, a strong correlation (p less than .01) was found between white matter abnormality and neuropsychological performance. The relationship between dementia and toluene abuse is discussed.
Friston et al.	1992	PET	schizophrenia	see conclusion	30 patients	High correlations between the left medial temporal regions, mesencephalic, thalamic, and left striatal structures and psychopathology and neurophysiology were exhibited. The highest correlation was with the left parahippocampal region.
Holsenbeck et al.	1992	CT	schizophrenia	ventricle and brain volume	33 patients, 45 neurological controls	A significantly higher ventricle to brain ratio (VBR) was noted in patients with a neurological diagnosis of vertigo or syncope. Psychotic and the Schizophreniform patients had a higher VBR.
Klausner et al.	1992	CT	schizophrenia	ventricles	88 patients, 14 controls	Patients had a larger VBR of the anterior portion of the lateral ventricles. Larger frontal horns were associated with more severe negative symptoms and poorer premorbid childhood adjustment.
Laplane et al.	1989	CT, MR, PET	obsessive compulsive disorder	basal ganglia	8 patients	Obsessive compulsive patients shared the combination of basal ganglia lesions with frontal lobe-like syndrome. The frontal associative cortex and basal ganglia system are believed to be involved in this group's syndrome.
Mattson et al.	1992	EEG, MR	fetal alcohol syndrome	basal ganglia, corpus callosum, thalamus	2 children with FAS	These two boys had IQ measures in the mentally deficient range with other accompanied deficits. MR identified abnormalities of the corpus callosum, basal ganglia and thalamic structures were found.

(*continued*)

TABLE 7.1 (*Continued*)

Author	*Year*	*Imaging Method*	*Disorder*	*Anatomic focus*	*Subjects/ Participants*	*Conclusions that relate to neuropsychology*
Neppe et al.	1992	MR	psychiatric illness	cerebrum	45 psychiatric patients	Results from BROCAS SCAN, a bedside neuropsychiatric exam correlated well with MR changes in pathology.
Raine et al.	1992	MR	schizophrenia	prefrontal atrophy	17 schizophrenic, 18 psychiatric controls, 19 controls	Significantly smaller prefrontal areas were found in the Schizophrenic patients as compared to both the psychiatric controls and the normal controls. Schizophrenics also had poorer performance on neuropsychological exams.
Raz	1993	CT	schizophrenia	cortical and subcortical regions	56 schizophrenics, 16 psychiatric controls, 31 controls	Schizophrenics had generalized cortical and subcortical enlargement of the spaces filled with CSF, except in the occipitoparietal cortex. Significant differences in perisylvian atrophy were noted between Schizophrenics and patients with mood disorders.
Siegel et al.	1993	PET	schizophrenia	see conclusions	70 schizophrenia 30 matched controls	Low metabolic rates were confirmed in the medial frontal cortical regions as well as the basal ganglia of Schizophrenics. Correlations with negative symptoms and group differences were more prominent in medial than lateral frontal cortex.
Tamminga et al.	1992	PET	schizophrenia	cingulate cortex and hippocampus	12 patients, 12 matched controls	This study demonstrated a lower regional cerebral metabolic rate of glucose in the hippocampus and anterior cingulate cortex of Schizophrenics.
Vita et al.	1991	CT	schizophrenia	ventricles	18 patients	Cortical atrophy is associated with poor outcome in several areas of clinical and social functioning.
Weinberger et al.	1992	MR, CBF	schizophrenia	prefrontal region, hippocampus	9 pairs of monozygotic twins	This study implicates a dysfunction within the widely distributed neocortical-limbic neural network involved in Schizophrenia.

Wolkin et al.	1992	PET	schizophrenia	frontal region	22 patients	A relationship between negative symptoms and hypofrontality was noted in Schizophrenics. Hypometabolism especially in right dorsolateral convexity was found in patients.
				Traumatic injuries		
Anderson et al.	1994	MR	TBI	caudate and corpus callosum	17 male, 13 female patients	This study compared day of injury CT to post injury MR. Results suggest that atrophy is more so associated with white matter rather than grey matter structures following TBI. Ventricular dilation related to memory scores.
Bigler	1992b	CT, MR	TBI	ventricles	1 male	3-D reconstruction of CT findings are compared with postinjury MR. Neuropsychological decline coincided with parenchymal tissue loss.
Bigler et al.	1994	CT, MR	TBI	ventricle and brain volume	15 TBI, 21 controls	Day of injury CT was compared to post injury MR and controls. Both day of injury and control ventricle to brain ratios (VBR) were significantly different than postmorbid VBR.
Boldrini et al.	1992	MR	TBI	corpus callosum	1 patient	A callosal lesion of the middle and posterior third of the truncus was found in a patient with an interhemispheric mediation for praxis, right-left transfer of spatial information, and a left-sided apraxia.
Ettlin et al.	1992	EEG, MR	whiplash	cerebrum	21 patients	Neuropsychological findings are discussed as being compatible with possible damage to basal frontal and upper brain stem structures after whiplash injury of the neck.
Gale et al.	1993	MR	TBI	fornix	27 patients, 18 controls	TBI patients had a significantly reduced fornix to brain ratio compared with controls. Fornix damage in TBI and possible neuropsychological relationships are discussed.

(continued)

TABLE 7.1 (*Continued*)

Author	*Year*	*Imaging Method*	*Disorder*	*Anatomic focus*	*Subjects/ Participants*	*Conclusions that relate to neuropsychology*
Godersky et al.	1990	MR	TBI	CNS lesions	31 patients	A positive correlation was found between neurobehavioral assessment and findings on MRI. Specific lesions were also found to correspond with neurobehavioral impairments.
Johnson et al.	1994	MR	TBI	corpus callosum, ventricles, brain volume	31 female, 33 male TBI patients	Males exhibited more damage than females. A relationship between VBR, performance IQ and the Digit Symbol subtest of the Wechsler Adult Intelligence Scale Revised (WAIS-R) was observed.
Kawahata et al.	1989	CT, MR	TBI	CNS lesions	1 61-year-old male right-handed patient	CT revealed subcortical hematomas in the temporo-occipital regions and MR revealed lesions in the lingual, fusiform and posterior inferior temporal gyri of both hemispheres. Neuropsychological evaluations revealed impairment in verbal memory, alexia, agraphia, object agnosia, color naming difficulty, prosopagnosia, and visuospatial construction.
Koeda and Takeshita	1992	MR	preterm birth with spastic diplegia	CNS lesions	18 patients (children)	The researchers propose that visuoperceptual impairment is caused by cerebral lesions and that the measurement of peritrigonal white matter by MRI is useful for detecting potential visuoperceptual impairment at an early age.
Levin, Amparo, et al.	1989	MR	closed head injury	CNS lesions	21 patients (children)	MR revealed high intensity in the parenchyma in 8 of the 11 severely injured patients. MR findings were normal in the 10 patients with mild-moderate head injuries. Lesions were strongly associated with neuropsychological outcome in the severe group.
Shores et al.	1990	CBF, EEG, MR	blunt head injury	frontal lobes	1 patient	A 43 year old man had frontal lobe damage with a Korsakoff-like syndrome.

Vilkki et al.	1992	CT	closed head injury	parenchymal lesions	53 patients	Parenchymal lesions were associated with poor test results. Spatial and verbal deficits were related to parenchymal lesions in the right and left hemispheres respectively. Cognitive inefficiency, in late CT, was related to ventricular enlargement.
Wilson et al.	1992	MR	closed head injury	CNS lesions	43 patients	Certain lesions and general damage correlated with specific subtests of the WAIS. Hemispheric sites significantly related to neuropsychological measures and showed significant intercorrelations.
Zihl et al.	1991	MR	traumatic injury	bilateral lesions	1 patient	The occipital gyri, cortical fiber pathways are implicated in this patient's visual motion deficit following injury.
				Vascular disorders		
Baumgartner and Regard	1993	MR	infarct	CNS lesions	5 patients	5 patients exhibited dysfunction implicating the frontotemporal hemispheric structures unilateral to the thalamic lesion. Neuropsychological deficits point to non MR detected lesions as well.
Eberling et al.	1992	SPECT	multiple infarct dementia (MID) & Alzheimer's	frontal, parietal, and temporal	11 MID patients, 22 AD patients, 12 controls	Blood flow pattern in MID and Alzheimer's disease was similar showing hypoperfusion in the temporal area. Alzheimer's disease is characterized by hypoperfusion in the temporal and parietal areas.
Evrard et al.	1992	MR, CT	infarct	right-left hemisphere comparisons	24 patients	Resultants of infarct are aphasia, quadrantanopsia, spatial dyscalculia, Gertsmann syndrome, and frontal syndrome. Right-left hemisphere relationships are correlated with neuropsychological and neurobehavioral measures.

(*continued*)

TABLE 7.1 (*Continued*)

Author	*Year*	*Imaging Method*	*Disorder*	*Anatomic focus*	*Subjects/ Participants*	*Conclusions that relate to neuropsychology*
Heide et al.	1990	CT, MR	infarct	thalamus	2 patients	Patients had a vertical gaze palsy and apraxia of head movements, attention disorder, memory and affective deficits. Bilateral post-ischemic lesions in the dorsomedial thalamus and the mesodiencephalic junction, dorsomedial to the red nucleus were identified.
Kugler et al.	1993	MR	infarcts (sickle cell)	infarct region, general	8 w/infarcts, 8 w/o infarcts	The presence of cognitive abnormalities in the absence of MR-identified pathology was seen in patients. MR abnormalities were also seen on patients with asymptomatic clinical observations.
Lisovoski et al.	1993	MR	infarct	tubero-thalamic region	1 patient	A reduced voice volume and verbal memory trouble, aspontaneity, loss of self-activation and affective drive were observed. The neurobehavioral disturbances disappeared within 15 days after the onset of the troubles as the mass lesion decreased.
Malamut et al.	1992	MR	stroke	thalamus	1 patient	The memory deficit in this case results from a disconnection of the diencephalon from the medial temporal region.
Mielke et al.	1992	PET	Alzheimer's dementia, vascular dementia (VD)	see conclusion	28 VD, 20 matched AD patients, 24 normal controls	Vascular and Alzheimer's patients demonstrated metabolic impairment in the temporoparietal and frontal association cortex. Metabolism was also reduced in patients with vascular dementia only. Differences between both pathology groups is discussed.
Paquier et al.	1992	CT, MR	hemorrhage	right hemisphere	1 52-year-old female patient	Right subarachnoid hemorrhage identified on CT and MR was compared with prominence of auditory hallucinations. A discussion on verbal versus musical hallucinations is presented.

Perani et al.	1993	PET	stroke & ischemic lesion	right–left hemisphere comparisons	2 patients	Functional metabolic recovery in both the undamaged left hemisphere and the unaffected regions of the right hemisphere may lead to remission of unilateral neglect.
Fujol et al.	1991	MR	vascular disease	white matter	22 patients	4 vascular patients with periventricular white matter changes showed left ear extinction on dichotic listening tests.
Romner et al.	1989	MR	aneurism surgery	tissue damage	20 patients	MR pathological findings following aneurism rupture and cognitive malfunctioning was observed in patients.
Sakurai et al.	1992	MR	infarct	upper middle cerebral artery territory	1 patient	An infarction in the right middle cerebral artery, including areas homologous to Broca's and Wernicke's areas was observed on MR. Cerebral blood flow in the same areas remained reduced even after language activation. A dissociated aphasia is implicated.
Selnes et al.	1991	MR, CT	stroke	left cerebral artery territory	1 male right-handed patient	This patient had a massive left middle cerebral stroke. Extensive damage of both anterior and posterior areas typically associated with language was identified on CT and MR. Limb apraxia, dyscalculia, dense right visual neglect, and anosognosia were observed.
Verslegers et al.	1991	CT, MR	infarct	basilar region	3 patients	Three cases of bilateral posterior cerebral artery infarction showed slow progressive neuropsychological deterioration.

Note. AD = Alzheimer's disease, CBF = cerebral blood flow, CT = computed axial tomography, HIV = Human Immuno-Deficiency Virus, HD = Huntington's disease, MEG = magnetoencephalography, MR = magnetic resonance imaging, NMR = nuclear magnetic resonance, qEEG = quantitative electroencephalography, PD = Parkinson's disease, PET = positron emission tomography, SPECT = Single photon emission computed tomography, TBI = traumatic brain injury

REFERENCES

Adams, K. M., Gilman, S., Koeppe, R. A., Kluin, K. J., Brunberg, J. A., Dede, D., Berent, S., & Kroll, P. D. (1993). Neuropsychological deficits are correlated with frontal hypometabolism in positron emission tomography studies of older alcoholic patients. *Alcoholism, Clinical and Experimental Research*, *17*, 205–210.

Alger, J. R., Frank, J. A., Bizzi, A., Fulham, M. J., Desouza, B. X., Duhuney, M. D., Iscue, S. W., Black, J. L., van Zijl, P. C., Monnen, C. T., & Giovanni, D. C. (1990). Metabolism of human gli-omas: Assessment with H-1 spectroscopy and F-18 fluorodeoxyglucose PET. *Radiology, 177*,633–641.

Anderson, C. V., & Bigler, E. D. (1994). The role of the caudate nucleus and corpus callosum in trauma enduced anterior horn dilation. *Brain Injury*, *8*, 565–569.

Andreasen, N. C., Rezai, K., Alliger, R., Swayze, V. W., II, Flaum, M., Kirchner, P., Cohen, G., & O'Leary, D. S. (1992). Hypofrontality in neuroleptic-naive patients and in patients with chronic schizophrenia. Assessment with Xenon 133 single-photon emission computed tomography and the Tower of London. *Archives of General Psychiatry*, *49*, 943–958.

Angelini, L., Nardocci, N., Rumi, V., Zorzi, C., Strada, L., & Savoiardo, M. (1992). Hallervorden–Spatz disease: Clinical and MRI study of 11 cases diagnosed in life. *Journal of Neurology*, *239*, 417–425.

Armspach, J. P., Gounot, D., Namer, I. J., Ohlenbusch, H. H., Rumbach, L., & Chambron, J. (1993). Quantitative cerebral magnetic resonance imaging during ACTH treatment of multiple sclerosis. *Magnetic Resonance Imaging*, *11*, 1147–1153.

Barbosa, S., Blumhardt, L. D., Roberts, N., Lock, T., & Edwards, R. H. T. (1994). Magnetic resonance relaxation time mapping and multiple sclerosis: Normal appearing white matter and the "invisible" lesion load. *Magnetic Resonance Imaging*, *12*, 33–42.

Barth, P. G., Derix, M. M., de Krom, M. C., Valk, J., & Theunissen, P. M. (1989). Schilder's diffuse sclerosis: Case study with three years' follow-up and neuro-imaging. *Neuropediatrics*, *20*, 230–233.

Battistini, S., De Stefano, N., Parlanti, S., & Federico, A. (1991). Unexpected white matter changes in an early treated PKU case and improvement after dietary treatment. *Functional Neurology*, *6*, 177–180.

Baum, K. A., Hopf, U., Nehrig, C., Stover, M., Schorner, W., (1993). Systemic lupus erythematosus: Neuropsychiatric signs and symptoms related to cerebral MRI findings. *Clinical Neurology and Neurosurgery*, *95*, 29–34.

Baumgartner, R. W., & Regard, M. (1993). Bilateral neuropsychological deficits in unilateral paramedian thalamic infarction. *European Neurology*, *33*, 195–198.

Belliveau, J. W., Kennedy, D. N., Jr., McKinstry, R. C., Buchbinder, B. R., Weisskoff, R. M., Cohen, M. S., Vevea, J. M., Brady, T. J., & Rosen, B. R. (1991). Functional mapping of the human visual cortex by magnetic resonance imaging. *Science*, *254*, 716–719.

Berardi, A., Haxby, J. V., Grady, C. L., & Rapoport, S. I. (1991). Asymmetries of brain glucose metabolism and memory in healthy elderly. *Developmental Neuropsychology*, *7*, 87–97.

Berman, K. F., Torrey, E. F., Daniel, D. G., & Weinberger, D. R. (1992). Regional cerebral blood flow in monozygotic twins discordant and concordant for schizophrenia. *Archives of General Psychiatry*, *49*, 927–934.

Bernsen, H. J., Verhagen, W. I., de Bijl, M. A., & Heerschap, A. (1992). Magnetic resonance studies on brain dysfunction induced by organic solvents. *Acta Neurologica Belgica*, *92*, 207–214.

Berthier, M. L., Starkstein, S. E., & Leiguarda, R. (1990). Developmental cortical anomalies in Asperger's syndrome: Neuroradiological findings in two patients. *Journal of Neuropsychiatry and Clinical Neuroscience*, *2*, 197–201.

Bigler, E. D. (1991). Neuropsychological assessment, neuroimaging, and clinical neuropsychology: A synthesis. *Archives of Clinical Neuropsychology*, *6*, 113–132.

Bigler, E. D. (1992a). The neurobiology and neuropsychology of adult learning disorders. *Journal of Learning Disabilities*, *25*, 488–506.

Bigler, E. D. (1992b). Three-dimensional image analysis of trauma induced degenerative changes: An aid to neuropsychological assessment. *Archives of Clinical Neuropsychology*, *7*, 449–456.

Bigler, E. D. (1994). Neuroimaging in neuropsychology. In R. E. Kelley (Ed.), *Functional neuroimaging*. Armonk, NY: Futura Publishing.

Bigler, E. D., Burr, R., Gale, S., Norman, M., Kurth, S., Blatter, D., & Abildscov, T. (1994). Day-of-injury CT scan as an index to preinjury brain morphology. *Brain Injury*. *8*, 231–238.

Bigler, E. D., & Clement, P. (in press). *Diagnostic clinical neuropsychology.* Austin: University of Texas Press.

Bigler, E. D., Kurth, S. M., Blatter, D. D., & Abildskov, T. J. (1992). Degenerative changes in traumatic brain injury: Post-injury magnetic resonance identified ventricular expansion compared to pre-injury level. *Brain Research Bulletin*, *28*, 651–653.

Blansjaar, B. A., Vielvoye, G. J., van Dijk, J. G., & Rijnders, R. J. (1992). Similar brain lesions in alcoholics and Korsakoff patients: MRI, psychometric and clinical findings. *Clinical Neurology and Neurosurgery*, *94*, 197–203.

Blatter, D. D., Bigler, E. D., Gale, S. D., Johnson, S., Anderson, C., Burnett, B., Parker, N., Kurth, S. & Horn, S. (1995). Quantitative neuroimaging: Normative MR database spanning 5 decades. *American Journal of Neuroradiology, 16*, 241–251.

Boldrini, P., Zanella, R., Cantagallo, A., & Basaglia, N. (1992). Partial hemispheric disconnection syndrome of traumatic origin. *Cortex, 28*, 135–143.

Bornstein, R. A., Chakeres, D., Brogan, M., Nasrallah, H. A., Fass, R. J., Para, M., & Whitacre, C. (1992a). Magnetic resonance imaging of white matter lesions in HIV infection. *Journal of Neuropsychiatry and Clinical Neuroscience, 4*, 174–178.

Bornstein, R. A., Schwarzkopf, S. B., Olson, S. C., & Nasrallah, H. A., (1992b). Third-ventricle enlargement and neuropsychological deficit in schizophrenia. *Biological Psychiatry, 31*, 954–961.

Botteron, K. N., Figiel, G. S., Wetzel, M. W., Hudziak, J., & VanEerdewegh, M. (1992). MRI abnormalities in adolescent bipolar affective disorder. *Journal of the American Academy of Child and Adolescent Psychiatry, 31*, 258–261.

Bromfield, E. B., Altshuler, L., Leiderman, D. B., Balish, M., Ketter, T. A., Devinsky, O., Post, R. M., & Theodore, W. H. (1992). Cerebral metabolism and depression in patients with complex seizures. *Archives of Neurology, 49*, 617–623.

Brown, F. W., Lewine, R. J., Hudgins, P. A., & Risch, S. C. (1992). White matter hyperintensity signals in psychiatric and nonpsychiatric subjects. *American Journal of Psychiatry, 149*, 620–625.

Buchsbaum, M. S., Haier, R. J., Potkin, S. G., Neuchterlein, K., Bracha, H. S. Katz, M., Lohr, J., Wu, J., Lottenberg, S., Jerabek, P. A., Trenary, M., Tafalla, R., Reynolds, C., & Bunney, W. E., Jr. (1992). Frontostriatal disorder of cerebral metabolism in never-medicated schizophrenics. *Archives of General Psychiatry, 49*, 935–942.

Byring, R. F., Salmi, T. K., Sainio, K. O., & Orn, H. P. (1991). EEG in children with spelling disabilities. *Electroencephalography and Clinical Neurophysiology, 79*, 247–255.

Callender, T. J., Morrow, L., Subramanian, K., Duhon, D., & Ristovv, M. (1993). Three-dimensional brain metabolic imaging in patients with toxic encephalopathy. *Environmental Research, 60*, 295–319.

Cantor-Graae, E., Warkentin, S., Franzén, G., & Risberg, J. (1993). Frontal Lobe challenge: A comparison of activation procedures during rCBF measurements in normal subjects. *Neuropsychiatry, Neuropsychology and Behavioral Neurology, 6*, 83–92.

Cao, Y., Levin, D. N., Gregory, C. D., Raidy, T., So, G. J., & Pelizzari, C. A. (1993). Integrated 3D display of brain surface anatomy and MR spectral data. *Magnetic Resonance Imaging, 11*, 1043–1049.

Cappa, S. F., Guariglia, C., Messa, C., Pizzamiglio, L., & Zoccolotti, P. (1991). Computed tomography correlates of chronic unilateral neglect. *Neuropsychology, 5*, 195–204.

Carbotte, R. M., Denburg, S. D., Denburg, J. A., Nahmias, C., & Garnett, E. S., (1992). Fluctuating cognitive abnormalities and cerebral glucose metabolism in neuropsychiatric systemic lupus erythematosus. *Journal of Neurology, Neurosurgery and Psychiatry, 55*, 1054–1059.

Caselli, R. J., Graff-Radford, N. R., & Rezai, K. (1991). Thalamocortical diaschisis: Single-photon emission tomographic study of cortical blood flow changes after focal thalamic infarction. *Neuropsychiatry, Neuropsychology and Behavioral Neurology, 4*, 193–214.

Casey, B. J., Cohen, J. D., Noll, D. C., Schneider, W., Giedd, J., & Rapoport, J. L. (in press). Functional magnetic resonance imaging. In E. D. Bigler (Ed.), *Handbook of human brain function: Neuroimaging*. New York: Plenum Press.

Chang, L., Anderson, T., Migneco, O. A., Boone, K., Mehringer, C. M., Villanueva-Meyer, J., Berman, N., & Mena, I. (1993). Cerebral abnormalities in myotonic dystrophy: Cerebral blood flow, magnetic resonance imaging, and neuropsychological tests. *Archives of Neurology, 50*, 917–923.

Charlot, V., Tzourio, N., Zilbovicius, M., Mazoyer, B., & Denis, M. (1992). Different mental imagery abilities result in different regional cerebral blood flow activation patterns during cognitive tasks. *Neuropsychologia, 30*, 565–580.

Coffey, C. E., Wilkinson, W. E., Parashos, I. A., Soady, S. A., Sullivan, R. J., Patterson, L. J., Figiel, G. S., Webb, M. C., Spritzer, C. E., & Djang, W. T. (1992). Quantitative cerebral anatomy of the aging human brain: A cross-sectional study using magnetic resonance imaging. *Neurology, 42*, 527–536.

Coffman, J. A., Bornstein, R. A., Olson, S. C., Schwarzkopf, S. B., & Nasrallah, H. A. (1990). Cognitive impairment and cerebral structure by MRI in bipolar disorder. *Biological Psychiatry, 27*, 1188–1196.

Cohen, S. M. (1987). Physiological in MR spectroscopy: From isolated cells to man. *Annals of the New York Academy of Sciences, 508*, 1–537.

Comi, G., Filippi, M., Martinelli, V., Sirabian, G., Visciani, A., Campi, A., Mammi, S., Rovaris, M., & Canal, N. (1993). Brain magnetic resonance imaging correlates of cognitive impairment in multiple sclerosis. *Journal of Neurological Science, 115* (Suppl.), 66–73.

Connelly, A., Jackson, G. D., Frackowiak, R. S., Belliveau, J. W., Vargha-Khadem, F., & Gadian, D. G. (1993).

Functional mapping of activated human primary cortex with a clinical MR imaging system. *Radiology*, *188*, 125–130.

Constable, R. T., McCarthy, G., Allison, T., Anderson, A. W., & Gore, J. C. (1993). Functional brain imaging at 1.5 T using conventional gradient ECHO MR imaging techniques. *Magnetic Resonance Imaging*, *11*, 451–459.

Courchesne, E., Press, G. A., & Yeung-Courchesne, R. (1993). Parietal lobe abnormalities detected with MR in patients with infantile autism. *American Journal of Roentgenology*, *160*, 387–393.

Dal Pan, G. J., McArthur, J. H., Aylward, E., Selnes, O. A., Nance-Sproson, T. E., Kumar, A. J., Mellits, E. D., & McArthur, J. C. (1992). Patterns of cerebral atrophy in HIV-1-infected individuals: Results of a quantitative MRI analysis. *Neurology*, *42*, 2125–2130.

DeCertaines, J. D., Bovee, W. M. M. J., & Podo, F. (1992). *Magnetic resonance spectroscopy in biology and medicine: Functional and pathological tissue characterization*. New York: Pergamon.

Dejgaard, A., Gade, A., Larsson, H., Balle, V., Parving, A., & Parving, H. H. (1991). Evidence for diabetic encephalopathy. *Diabetic Medicine*, *8*, 162–167.

Démonet, J. F., Celsis, P., Nespoulous, J. L, Viallar, G., Marc-Vergnes, J. P., & Rascol, A. (1992). Cerebral blood flow correlates of word monitoring in sentences: Influence of semantic incoherence. A SPECT study in normals. *Neuropsychologia*, *30*, 1–11.

Démonet, J. F., Wise, R., & Frackowiak, R. S. J. (1993). Language functions explored in normal subjects by positron emission tomography: A critical review. *Human Brain Mapping*, *1*, 39–47.

Dietrich, R. B., Vining, E. P., Taira, R. K., Hall, T. R., & Phillipart, M. (1990). Myelin disorders of childhood: Correlation of MR findings and severity of neurological impairment. *Journal of Computer Assisted Tomography*, *14*, 693–698.

Duffy, F. H., & McAnulty, G. (1990). Neuropsychological heterogeneity and the definition of dyslexia: Preliminary evidence for plasticity. *Neuropsychologia*, *28*, 555–571.

Duffy, F. H., McAnulty, G. B., Jones, K., Als, H., & Albert, M. (1993). Brain electrical correlates of psychological measures: Strategies and problems. *Brain Topography*, *5*, 399–412.

Eberling, J. L., Jagust, W. J., Reed, B. R., Kwo-on-Yuen, P. F., & Martin, E. M. (1992). Single-photon emission computed tomography studies of regional cerebral blood flow in multiple infarct dementia. *The Journal of Neuroimaging*, *2*, 79–85.

Eberling, J. L., Reed, B. R., Baker, M. G., & Jagust, W. J. (1993). Cognitive correlates of regional cerebral blood flow in Alzheimer's disease. *Archives of Neurology*, *50*, 761–766.

Eisenberg, R. L. (1992) *Radiology: An illustrated history*. St. Louis: Mosby.

Ettlin, T. M., Kischka, U., Reichmann, S., Radii, E. W., Heim, S., Wengen, D., & Benson, D. F. (1992). Cerebral symptoms after whiplash injury of the neck: A prospective clinical and neuropsychological study of whiplash injury. *Journal of Neurology, Neurosurgery and Psychiatry*, *55*, 943–948.

Evrard, S., Woimant, F., Le Coz, P., Polivka, M., Cousin, C., & Haguenau, M. (1992). Watershed cerebral infarcts: Retrospective study of 24 cases. *Neurological Research*, *14*, 97–99.

Feinstein, A., du Boulay, G., & Ron, M. A. (1992). Psychotic illness in multiple sclerosis. A clinical and magnetic resonance imaging study. *British Journal of Psychiatry*, *161*, 680–685.

Filley, C. M., Heaton, R. K., & Rosenberg, N. L. (1990). White matter dementia in chronic toluene abuse. *Neurology*, *40*, 532–534.

Finitzo, T., Pool, K. D., & Chapman, S. B. (1991). Quantitative electroencephalography and anatomoclinical principles of aphasia. A validation study. *Annals of the New York Academy of Sciences*, *620*, 57–72.

Flowers, D. L., Wood, F. B., & Naylor, C. E. (1991). Regional cerebral blood flow correlates of language processes in reading disability. *Archives of Neurology*, *48*, 637–643.

Fox, P. T. (1993). Human brain mapping: A convergence of disciplines. *Human Brain Mapping*, *1*, 1–2.

Frahm, J., Bruhn, H., Gyngell, M. L., Merboldt, K. D., Hannicke, W., & Sauter, R. (1989). Localized proton NMR spectroscopy in different regions of the human brain in vivo: Relaxation times in concentrations of cerebral metabolites. *Magnetic Resonance Medicine*, *11*, 47–63.

Friston, K. J., Liddle, P. F., Frith, C. D., Hirsch, S. R., & Frackowiak, R. S. J. (1992). The left medial temporal region and schizophrenia. A PET study. *Brain*, *115*, 367–382.

Frith, C. D., Friston, K. J., Liddle, P. F., & Frackowiak, R. S. J. (1991). A PET study of word finding. *Neuropsychologia*, *29*, 1137–1148.

Galaburda, A. M., & Kemper, T. L. (1979). Cyto-architectonic abnormalities in developmental dyslexia: A case study. *Annals of Neurology*, *6*, 94–102.

Gale, S. D., Burr, R. B., Bigler, E. D., & Blatter, D. D. (1993). Fornix degeneration and memory in traumatic brain injury. *Brain Research Bulletin*, *32*, 345–349.

Gale, S. D., Johnson, S. C., Bigler, E. D., & Blatter, D. D. (1994). Traumatic brain injury and temporal horn enlargement: Correlates with tests of intelligence and memory. *Neuropsychiatry, Neuropsychology & Behavioral Neurology*, *7*(3), 160–165.

Gale, S. D., Johnson, S. C., Bigler, E. D., & Blatter, D. D. (1995). Nonspecific white matter degeneration following traumatic brain injury. *Journal of the International Neuropsychological Society, 1*, 17–28.

Gallen, C. C., Sobel, D. F., Lewine, J. D., Sanders, J. A., Hart, B. L., Davis, L. E., & Orrison, W. W., Jr. (1993). Neuromagnetic mapping of brain function. *Radiology, 187*, 863–867.

Garrido, E., Castello, A., Ventura, J. L., Capdevila, A., & Rodriguez, F. A. (1993). Cortical atrophy and other brain magnetic resonance imaging (MRI) changes after extremely high-altitude climbs without oxygen. *International Journal of Sports Medicine, 14*, 232–234.

Gazzaniga, M. S., Kutas, M., Van Petten, C., & Fendrich, R. (1989). Human callosal function: MRI-verified neuropsychological functions. *Neurology, 39*, 942–946.

Gevins, A. S., & Illes, J. (1991). Neurocognitive networks of the human brain. *Annals of the New York Academy of Sciences, 620*, 22–44.

Godersky, J. C., Gentry, L. R., Tranel, D., Dyste, G. N., & Danks, K. R. (1990). Magnetic resonance imaging and neurobehavioural outcome in traumatic brain injury. *Acta Neurochirurgica Supplementum' (Wien), 51*, 311–314.

Goldenberg, G., Podreka, I., Müller, C., & Deecke, L. (1989). The relationship between cognitive deficits and frontal lobe function in patients with Parkinson's disease: An emission computerized tomography study. *Behavioral Neurology, 2*, 79–87.

Goldenberg, G., Podreka, I., Steiner, M., Franzen, P., & Deecke, L. (1991). Contributions of occipital and temporal brain regions to visual and acoustic imagery—a SPECT study. *Neuropsychologia, 29*, 695–702.

Gottschalk, L. A., Buchsbaum, M. S., Gillin, J. C., Wu, J., Reynolds, C. A., Herrera, D. B. (1991). Positron-emission tomographic studies of the relationship of cerebral glucose metabolism and the magnitude of anxiety and hostility experienced during dreaming and waking. *The Journal of Neuropsychiatry and Clinical Neurosciences, 3*, 131–142.

Grasby, P. M., Frith, C. D., Firston, K. J., Bench, C., Frackowiak, R. S., & Dolan, R. J. (1993). Functional mapping of brain areas implicated in auditory–verbal memory function. *Brain, 116*, 1–20.

Gur, R. C., Saykin, A. J., & Gur, R. E. (1991). Neuropsychological study of schizophrenia. *Schizophrenia Research, 1*, 153–162.

Hagman, J. O., Wood, F., Buchsbaum, M. S., Tallal, P., Flowers, L., & Katz, W. (1992). Cerebral brain metabolism in adult dyslexic subjects assessed with positron emission tomography during performance of an auditory task. *Archives of Neurology, 49*, 734–739.

Hayakawa, K., Konishi, Y., Matsuda, T., Kuriyama, M., Konishi, K., Yamashita, K., Okumura, R., & Hamanaka, D. (1989). Development and aging of brain midline structures: Assessment with MR imaging. *Radiology, 172*, 171–177.

Hayman, L. A., & Hinck, V. C. (1992). *Clinical brain imaging*. St. Louis: Mosby.

Heaton, T. B., & Bigler, E. D. (1993). Neuroimaging techniques in neuropsychological research. *Bulletin of the National Academy of Neuropsychology, 9*, 14–17.

Heide, W., Fahle, M., Koenig, E., Dichgans, J., & Schroth, G. (1990). Impairment of vertical motion detection and downgaze palsy due to rostral midbrain infarction. *Journal of Neurology, 237*, 432–440.

Heiss, W. D., Pawlik, G., Holthoff, V., Kessler, J., & Szelies, B. (1992). PET correlates of normal and impaired memory functions. *Cerebral Vascular and Brain Metabolism Reviews, 4*, 1–27.

Henry, T. R., Mazziotta, J. C., & Engel, J., Jr. (1993). Interictal metabolic anatomy of mesial temporal lobe epilepsy. *Archives of Neurology, 50*, 582–589.

Hockerstedt, K., Kajaste, S., Muuronen, A., Raininko, R., Seppalainen, A. M., & Hillbom, M. (1992). Encephalopathy and neuropathy in end-stage liver disease before and after liver transplantation. *Journal of Hepatology, 16*, 31–37.

Hodges, J. R., & Carpenter, K. (1991). Anterograde amnesia with fornix damage following removal of IIIrd ventricle colloid cyst. *Journal of Neurology, Neurosurgery and Psychiatry, 54*, 633–638.

Holman, B. L., & Devous, M. D. (1992). Functional brain SPECT: The emergence of a powerful clinical method. *Journal of Nuclear Medicine, 33*, 1888–1904.

Holman, B. L., Johnson, K. A., Gorada, B., Carvalho, P. A., & Satlin, A. (1992). The scintigraphic appearance of Alzheimer's disease: A prospective study using technetium-99m HMPAO SPECT. *Journal of Nuclear Medicine, 33*, 181–185.

Holsenbeck, L. S., III, Davidson, L. M., Hostetter, R. E., Casanova, M. F., Taylor, D. O., Kelley, C. T., Perrotta, C., Jr., Borison, R. L., & Diamond, B. (1992). Ventricle-to-brain ratio and symptoms at the onset of first-break schizophrenia. *Schizophrenia Bulletin, 18*, 427–435.

Huber, S. J., Shuttleworth, E. C., Christy, J. A., Chakeres, D. W., Curtin, A., & Paulson, G. W. (1989). Magnetic resonance imaging in dementia of Parkinson's disease. *Journal of Neurology, Neurosurgery and Psychiatry, 52*, 1221–1227.

Hunt, A. L., Orrison, W. W., Yeo, R. A., Haaland, K. Y., Rhyne, R. L., Garry, P. J., & Rosenberg, G. A. (1989). Clinical significance of MRI white matter lesions in the elderly. *Neurology, 39*, 1470–1474.

Izquierdo, G., Campoy, F., Jr., Mir, J., Gonzalez, M., & Martinez Parra, C. (1991). Memory and learning disturbances in multiple sclerosis. MRI lesions and neuropsychological correlation. *European Journal of Radiology, 13*, 220–224.

Jacobson, S. A., Leuchter, A. F., & Walter, D. O. (1993). Conventional and quantitative EEG in the diagnosis of delirium among the elderly. *Journal of Neurology, Neurosurgery and Psychiatry, 56*, 153–158.

Jagust, W. J., Reed, B. R., Martin, E. M., Eberling, J. L., & Nelson-Abbott, R. A. (1992). Cognitive function and regional cerebral blood flow in Parkinson's disease. *Brain, 115*, 521–537.

Jambaque, I., Cusmai, R., Curatolo, P., Cortesi, F., Perrot, C., & Dulac, O. (1991). Neuropsychological aspects of tuberous sclerosis in relation to epilepsy and MRI findings. *Developmental Medicine and Child Neurology, 33*, 698–705.

Jernigan, T. L., Archibald, S. L., Berhow, M. T., Sowell, E. R., Foster, D. S., & Hesselink, J. R. (1991). Cerebral structure on MRI, Part I: Localization of age-related changes. *Biological Psychiatry, 29*, 55–67.

Jernigan, T. L., Schafer, K., Butters, N., & Cermak, L. S. (1991). Magnetic resonance imaging of alcoholic Korsakoff patients. *Neuropsychopharmacology, 4*, 175–186.

Jernigan, T. L., Zisook, S., Heaton, R. K., Moranville, J. T., Hesselink, J. R., & Braff, D. L. (1991). Magnetic resonance imaging abnormalities in lenticular nuclei and cerebral cortex in schizophrenia. *Archives of General Psychiatry, 48*, 881–890.

Johnson, S. C., Bigler, E. D., Burr, R. B., & Blatter, D. D. (1994). White matter atrophy, ventricular dilation and intellectual function following traumatic brain injury. *Neuropsychology, 8*, 307–315.

Kawahata, N., & Nagata, K. (1989). A case of associative visual agnosia, neuropsychological findings and theoretical considerations. *Journal of Clinical and Experimental Neuropsychology, 11*, 645–664.

Kessler, J., Herholz, K., Grond, M., & Heiss, W. D. (1991). Impaired metabolic activation in Alzheimer's disease: A PET study during continuous visual recognition. *Neuropsychologia, 29*, 229–243.

Kingma, A., Mooyaart, E. L., Kamps, W. A., Nieuwenhuizen, P., & Wilmink, J. T. (1993). Magnetic resonance imaging of the brain and neuropsychological evaluation in children treated for acute lymphoblastic leukemia at a young age. *American Journal of Pediatric Hematology/Oncology, 15*, 231–238.

Kirk, A., Kertesz, A., & Polk, M. J. (1991). Dementia with leukoencephalopathy in systemic lupus erythematosus. *Canadian Journal of Neurological Sciences, 18*, 344–348.

Kirkpatrick, P. J., Morris, R., Syed, G. M., & Polkey, C. E. (1993). Cortical activation during cognitive challenge in patients with chronic temporal lobe epilepsy—a dynamic SPECT study. *Behavioral Neurology, 6*, 187–192.

Klausner, J. D., Sweeney, J. A., Deck, M. D., Haas, G. L., & Kelly, A. B. (1992). Clinical correlates of cerebral ventricular enlargement in schizophrenia. Further evidence for frontal lobe disease. *The Journal of Nervous and Mental Disease, 180*, 407–412.

Koeda, T., & Takeshita, K. (1992). Visuo–perceptual impairment and cerebral lesions in spastic diplegia with preterm birth. *Brain and Development, 14*, 239–244.

Kohn, R., Lilly, R. B., Sokol, M. S., & Malloy, P. F. (1989). Psychiatric presentations of intracranial cysts. *Journal of Neuropsychiatry and Clinical Neuroscience, 1*, 60–66.

Kosslyn, S. M., Alpert, N. M., Thompson, W. L., Maljkovic, V., Weise, S. B., Chabris, C. F., Hamilton, S. E., Rauch, S. L., & Buonanno, F. S. (1993). Visual mental imagery activates topographically organized visual cortex: PET investigations. *Journal of Cognitive Neuroscience, 5*, 263–287.

Kosslyn, S. M., Daly, P. F., McPeek, R. M., Alpert, N. M., Kennedy, D. N., & Caviness, V. S. (1993). Using locations to store shape: An indirect effect of a lesion. *Cerebral Cortex, 3*, 567–582.

Kucharczyk, J., Mosley, M., & Barkovich, A. J. (1994). *Magnetic resonance neuroimaging*. Boca Raton, FL: CRC.

Kugler, S., Anderson, B., Cross, D., Sharif, Z., Sano, M., Haggerty, R., Prohovnik, I., Hurlet-Jensen, A., Hilal, S., Mohr, J. P., & De Vivo, D. C. (1993). Abnormal cranial magnetic resonance imaging scans in sickle-cell disease. Neurological correlates and clinical implications. *Archives of Neurology, 50*, 629–635.

Kurth, S. M., Blatter, D. D., & Bigler, E. D. (1994). Neuropsychological outcome and quantitative image analysis of acute hemorrhage in traumatic brain injury: Preliminary findings. *Brain Injury, 8*(6), 489–500.

Laloux, P., Brichant, C., Cauwe, F., & Decoster, P. (1992). Technetium-99m HM-PAO single photon emission computed tomography imaging in transient global amnesia. *Archives of Neurology, 49*, 543–546.

Laplane, D., Levasseur, M., Pillon, B., Dubois, B., Baulac, M., Mazoyer, B., Tran-Dinh, S., Sette, G., Danze, F., & Baron, J. C. (1989). Obsessive–compulsive and other behavioral changes with bilateral basal ganglia lesions. A neuropsychological, magnetic resonance imaging and positron tomography study. *Brain, 112*, 699–725.

Leira, H. L., Myhr, G., Nilsen, G., Dale, L. G. (1992). Cerebral magnetic resonance imaging and cerebral computerized tomography for patients with solvent-induced encephalopathy. *Scandinavian Journal of Work, Environment and Health, 18*, 68–70.

Leli, D. A., Falgout, J. C., Hannay, H. J., Katholi, C. R., Halsey, J. H., Harrell, L. E., Wills, E. L., & White, A. (1992). Focal cognitively mediated blood-flow activation in Alzheimer's disease patients. *Neuropsychology, 6*, 137–148.

Lencz, T., McCarthy, G., Bronen, R. A., Scott, T. M., Inserni, J. A., Sass, K. J., Novelly, R. A., Kim, J. H., & Spencer, D. D. (1992). Quantitative magnetic resonance imaging in temporal lobe epilepsy: Relationship to neuropathology and neuropsychological function. *Annals of Neurology*, *31*, 629–637.

Levin, H. S., Amparo, E. G., Eisenberg, H. M., Miner, M. E., High, W. M., Jr., Ewing-Cobbs, L., Fletcher, J. M., & Guinto, F. C., Jr. (1989). Magnetic resonance imaging after closed head injury in children. *Neurosurgery*, *24*, 223–227.

Levin, H. S., Goldstein, F. C., Norcross, K., Amparo, E. G., Guinto, F. C., Jr., & Mader, J. T. (1989). Neurobehavioral and magnetic resonance imaging findings in two cases of decompression sickness. *Aviation Space and Environmental Medicine*, *60*, 1204–1210.

Levin, H. S., Williams, D. H., Borucki, M. J., Hillman, G. R., Williams, J. B., Guinto, F. C., Jr., Amparo, E. G., Crow, W. N., Pollard, R. B. (1990). Magnetic resonance imaging and neuropsychological findings in human immunodeficiency virus infection. *Journal of Acquired Immune Deficiency Syndrome*, *3*, 757–762.

Lezak, M. D. (1976). *Neuropsychological assessment*. New York: Oxford University Press.

Lisk, D. R., Pasteur, W., Rhoades, H., Putnam, R. D., & Grotta, J. C. (1994). Early presentation of hemispheric intracerebral hemorrhage: Prediction of outcome and guidelines for treatment allocation. *Neurology*, *44*, 133–139.

Lisovoski, F., Koskas, P., Dubard, T., Dessarts, I., Dehen, H., & Cambier, J. (1993). Left tuberothalamic artery territory infarction, neuropsychological and MRI features. *European Neurology*, *33*, 181–184.

Longo, R., Giorgini, A., Magnaldi, S., Pascazio, L., & Ricci, C. (1993). Alzheimer's disease histologically proven studied by MRI and MRS: Two cases. *Magnetic Resonance Imaging*, *11*, 1209–1215.

Lu, Z. L., Williamson, S. J., & Kaufman, L. (1992). Behavioral lifetime of human auditory sensory memory predicted by physiological measures. *Science*, *258*, 1668–1670.

Mäkelä, J. P., Ahonen, A., Hämäläinen, M., Hari, R., Ilmoniemi, R., Kajola, M., Knuutila, J., Lounasmaa, O. V., McEvoy, L., Salmelin, R., Salonen, O., Sams, M., Simola, J., Tesche, C., & Vasama, J.-P. (1993). Functional differences between auditory cortices of the two hemispheres revealed by whole-head neuromagnetic recordings. *Human Brain Mapping*, *1*, 48–56.

Malamut, B. L., Graff-Radford, N., Chawluk, J., Grossman, R. I., & Gur, R. C. (1992). Memory in a case of bilateral thalamic infarction. *Neurology*, *42*, 163–169.

Marciani, M. G., Carlesimo, G. A., Maschio, M. C., Sabbadini, M., Stefani, N., & Caltagirone, C. (1991). Comparison of neuropsychological, MRI and computerized EEG findings in a case of prosopoagnosia. *International Journal of Neuroscience*, *60*, 27–32.

Marciani, M. G., Stefanini, F., Stefani, N., Maschio, M. C., Gigli, G. L., Roncacci, S., Caltagirone, C., & Bernardi, G. (1992). Lateralization of the epileptogenic focus by computerized EEG study and neuropsychological evaluation. *International Journal of Neuroscience*, *66*, 53–60.

Martin, P. R., Rio, D., Adinoff, B., Johnson, J. L., Bisserbe, J. C., Rawlings, R. R., Rohrbaugh, J. W., Stapleton, J. M., & Eckhardt, M. J. (1991). Regional cerebral glucose utilization in chronic organic mental disorders associated with alcoholism. *Journal of neuropsychiatry and clinical neuroscience*, *4*, 159–167.

Mattson, S. N., Riley, E. P., Jernigan, T. L., Ehlers, C. L., Delis, D. C., Jones, K. L., Stern, C., Johnson, K. A., Hesselink, J. R., & Bellugi, U. (1992). Fetal alcohol syndrome: A case report of neuropsychological, MRI and EEG assessment of two children. *Alcoholism, Clinical and Experimental Research*, *16*, 1001–1003.

McDonald, W. M., Krishnan, K. R., Doraiswamy, P. M., Figiel, G. S., Husain, M. M., Boyko, O. B., & Heyman, A. (1991). Magnetic resonance findings in patients with early-onset Alzheimer's disease. *Biological Psychiatry*, *29*, 799–810.

McEvoy, L., Hari, R., Imada, T., & Sams, M. (1993). Human auditory cortical mechanisms of sound lateralization: II. Interaural time differences at sound onset. *Hearing Research*, *67*, 98–109.

Mielke, R., Herholz, K., Grond, M., Kessler, J., & Heiss, W. D. (1992). Severity of vascular dementia is related to volume of metabolically impaired tissue. *Archives of Neurology*, *49*, 909–913.

Milner, B. (1964). Some effects of frontal lobectomy in man. In J. M. Warren & K. Akert (Eds.), *The frontal granular cortex and behavior* (pp. 313–334). New York: McGraw-Hill.

Milner, B. (1968). Visual recognition and recall after right-temporal lobe excision in man. *Neuropsychologia*, *6*, 191–209.

Moore, J. W., Dunk, A. A., Crawford, J. R., Deans, H., Besson, J. A., De Lacey, G., Sinclair, T. S., Mowat, N. A., & Brunt, P. W. (1989). Neuropsychological deficits and morphological MRI brain scan abnormalities in apparently healthy non-encephalopathic patients with cirrhosis. A controlled study. *Journal of Hepatology*, *9*, 319–325.

Murphy, D. G., Bottomley, P. A., Salerno, J. A., Decarli, C., Mentis, M. J., Grady, C. L., Teichberg, D., Giacometti, K. R., Rosenberg, J. M., Hardy, C. J., Schapiro, M. B., Rapoport, S. I, Alger, J. R., & Horwitz, B. (1993). An in vivo study of phosphorus and glucose metabolism in Alzheimer's disease using magnetic resonance spectroscopy and PET. *Archives of General Psychiatry*, *50*, 341–349.

Neppe, V., Chen, A., Davis, J. T., Sawchuk, K., & Geist, M. (1992). The application of the Screening Cerebral Assessment of Neppe (BROCAS SCAN) to a neuropsychiatric population. *Journal of Neuropsychiatry and Clinical Neuroscience*, *4*, 85–94.

Newhouse, J. H., & Wiener, J. I. (1991). *Understanding MRI*. Boston: Little, Brown.

Njemanzc, P. C., Mirza, W. U., Rosenfeld, W. E., & Njemanz, V. U. (1992). Cerebral blood flow velocity and electroencephalography amplitude in generalized seizures: A case study. *The Journal of Neuroimaging*, *2*, 151–155.

Ogawa, S., Lee, T.-M., Nayak, A. S., & Glynn, P. (1990). Oxygenation-sensitive contrast in magnetic resonance image of rodent brain at high magnetic fields. *Magnetic Resonance in Medicine*, *14*, 68–78.

Oldendorf, W. H. (1980). *The quest for an image of brain*. New York: Raven.

Osborn, A. G. (1994). *Diagnostic neuroradiology*. St. Louis: Mosby.

Papanicolaou, A. C., & Tarkka, I. M. (1995). Magnetoencephalography. In E. D. Bigler (Ed.), *Handbook of human brain function*. New York: Plenum.

Papanicolaou, A. C., Rogers, R. L., & Baumann, S. B. (1991). Applications of magnetoencephalography to the study of cognition. *Annals of the New York Academy of Sciences*, *620*, 118–127.

Paquier, P., van Vugt, P., Bal, P., Cras, P., Parizel, P. M., van Haesendonck, J., Creten, W., & Martin, J. J. (1992). Transient musical hallucinosis of central origin: A review and clinical study. *Journal of Neurology, Neurosurgery and Psychiatry*, *55*, 1069–1073.

Pardo, J. V., Pardo, P. J., & Raichle, M. E. (1993). Neural correlates of self-induced dysphoria. *American Journal of Psychiatry*, *150*, 713–719.

Pawlik, G., & Heiss, W. D. (1989). Positron emission tomography and neuropsychologic function. In E. D. Bigler, R. A. Yeo, & E. Turkheimer (Eds.), *Neuropsychological function and brain imaging* (pp. 65–138). New York: Plenum.

Pfefferbaum, A., Mathalon, D. H., Sullivan, E. V., Rawles, J. M., Zipursky, R. B., & Lim, K. O. (1994). A quantitative MRI study of changes in brain morphology from infancy to late adulthood. *Archives of Neurology*, *51*, 874–887.

Peppard, R. F., Martin, W. R., Carr, G. D., Grochowski, E., Schulzer, M., Guttman, M., McGeer, P. L., Phillips, A. G., Tsui, J. K., & Calne, D. B. (1992). Cerebral glucose metabolism in Parkinson's disease with and without dementia. *Archives of Neurology*, *49*, 1262–1268.

Perani, D., Vallar, G., Paulesu, E., Alberoni, M., & Fazio, F. (1993). Left and right hemisphere contributions to recovery from neglect after right hemisphere damage—An [$_{18}$F]FDG PET study of two cases. *Neuropsychologia*, *31*, 115–125.

Piven, J., Nehme, E., Simon, J., Barta, P., Pearlson, G., & Folstein, S. E. (1992). Magnetic resonance imaging in autism: Measurement of the cerebellum, pons, and fourth ventricle. *Biological Psychiatry*, *31*, 491–504.

Plante, E., Swisher, L., Vance, R., & Rapcsak, S. (1991). MRI findings in boys with specific language impairment. *Brain and Language*, *41*, 52–66.

Pool, K. D., Devous, M. D., Sr., Freeman, F. J., Watson, B. C., & Finitzo, T. (1991). Regional cerebral blood flow in developmental stutterers. *Archives of Neurology*, *48*, 509–512.

Pozzilli, C., Bastianello, S., Padovani, A., Passafiume, D., Millefiorini, E., Bozzao, L., & Fieschi, C. (1991). Anterior corpus callosum atrophy and verbal fluency in multiple sclerosis. *Cortex*, *27*, 441–445.

Primavera, A., Novello, P., Finocchi, C., Canevari, E., & Corsello, L., (1990). Correlation between mini-mental state examination and quantitative electroencephalography in senile dementia of Alzheimer type. *Neuropsychobiology*, *23*, 74–78.

Primavera, A., Novello, P., & Stara, S. (1993). Transient global amnesia: A quantified electroencephalographic study. *Acta Neurologica Scandinavia*, *87*, 115–117.

Pugnetti, L., Mendozzi, L., Motta, A., Cattaneo, A., Biserni, P., Caputo, D., Cazzullo, C. L., & Valsecchi, F. (1993). MRI and cognitive patterns in relapsing-remitting multiple sclerosis. *Journal of Neurological Science*, *115* Suppl., 59–65.

Pujol, J., Junque, C., Vendrell, P., Garcia, P., Capdevila, A., & Marti Vilalta, J. L. (1991). Left-ear extinction in patients with MRI periventricular lesions. *Neuropsychologia*, *29*, 177–184.

Raichle, M. E. (1994a). Images of the mind: Studies with modern imaging techniques. *Annual Review of Psychology*, *45*, 333–356.

Raichle, M. E. (1994b). Visualizing the mind. *Scientific American*, *270*, 58–64.

Raine, A., Lencz, T., Reynolds, G. P., Harrison, G., Sheard, C., Medley, I., Reynolds, L. M., & Cooper, J. E. (1992). An evaluation of structural and functional prefrontal deficits in schizophrenia: MRI and neuropsychological measures. *Psychiatry Research*, *45*, 123–137.

Rao, S. M., Binder, J. R., Bandettini, P. A., Hammeke, T. A., Yetkin, F. Z., Jesmamowicz, A., Lisk, L. M., Morris, G. L., Mueller, W. M., Estkowski, L. D., Wong, E. C., Haughton, V. M., & Hyde, J. S. (1993). Functional magnetic resonance imaging of complex human movements. *Neurology*, *43*, 2311–2318.

Raz, S. (1993). Structural cerebral pathology in schizophrenics: Regional or diffuse? *Journal of Abnormal Psychology, 102*, 445–452.

Rezai, K., Andreason, N. C., Alliger, R., Cohen, G., Swayze, V., II, & O'Leary, D. S. (1993). The neuropsychology of the prefrontal cortex. *Archives of Neurology, 50*, 636–642.

Rogers, R. L., Basile, L. F., Papanicolaou, A. C., Bourbon, T. W., & Eisenberg, H. M. (1993). Visual evoked magnetic fields reveal activity in the superior temporal sulcus. *Electroencephalography and Clinical Neurophysiology, 86*, 344–347.

Romner, B., Sonesson, B., Ljunggren, B., Brandt, L., Saveland, H., & Holtas, S. (1989). Late magnetic resonance imaging related to neurobehavioral functioning after aneurysmal subarachnoid hemorrhage. *Neurosurgery, 25*, 390–397.

Ron, M. A., Callanan, M. M., & Warrington, E. K. (1991). Cognitive abnormalities in multiple sclerosis: A psychometric and MRI study. *Psychological Medicine, 21*, 59–68.

Rosen, B. R., Belliveau, J. W., Vevea, J. M., & Brady, T. J. (1990). Perfusion imaging with NMR contrast agents. *Magnetic Resonance in Medicine, 14*, 249–265.

Rumsey, J. M., Andreason, P., Zametkin, A. J., Aquino, T., King, C., Hamburger, S. D., Pikus, A., Rapoport, J. L., & Cohen, R. M. (1992). Failure to activate the left temporoparietal cortex in dyslexia: An oxygen 15 positron emission tomographic study. *Archives of Neurology, 49*, 527–534.

Russell, E. W., Neuringer, C., & Goldstein, G. (1970). *Assessment of brain damage. A neuropsychological key approach.* New York: Wiley–Interscience.

Sakurai, Y., Kurisaki, H., Takeda, K., Iwata, M., Bandoh, M., Watanabe, T., & Momose, T. (1992). Japanese crossed Wernicke's aphasia *Neurology, 42*, 144–148.

Sams, M., & Hari, R. (1991). Magnetoencephalography in the study of human auditory information process. *Annals of New York Academy of Sciences, 620*, 102–117.

Schad, L. R., Trost, U., Knopp, M. V., Müller, E., & Lorenz, W. J. (1993). Motor cortex stimulation measured by magnetic resonance imaging on a standard 1.5 T clinical scanner. *Magnetic Resonance Imaging, 11*, 461–464.

Schad, L. R., Wenz, F., Knopp, M. V., Baudendistel, K., Muller, E., & Lorenz, W. J. (1994). Functional 2-D and 3-D magnetic resonance imaging of motor cortex stimulation at high spatial resolution using standard 1.5 T imager. *Magnetic Resonance Imaging, 12*, 9–15.

Scheltens, P., Leys, D., Barkhof, F., Huglo, D., Weinstein, H. C., Vermersch, P., Kuiper, M., Steinling, M., Wolters, E. C., & Valk, J. (1992). Atrophy of medial temporal lobes on MRI in "probable" Alzheimer's disease and normal aging, diagnostic value and neuropsychological correlates. *Journal of Neurology, Neurosurgery and Psychiatry, 55*, 967–72.

Schmidt, R. (1992). Comparison of magnetic resonance imaging in Alzheimer's disease, vascular dementia and normal aging. *European Neurology, 32*, 164–169.

Schmitt, F. A., Shih, W. J., & DeKosky, S. T. (1992). Neuropsychological correlates of single-photon emission computed tomography (SPECT) in Alzheimer's disease. *Neuropsychology, 6*, 159–171.

Selnes, O. A., Pestronk, A., Hart, J., & Gordon, B. (1991). Limb apraxia without aphasia from a left sided lesion in a right handed patient. *Journal of Neurology, Neurosurgery and Psychiatry, 54*, 734–737.

Sergent, J., Ohta, S., & MacDonald, B. (1992). Functional neuroanatomy of a face and object processing. A positron emission tomography study. *Brain, 115*(1), 15–36.

Shores, A., Kraiuhin, C., Zurynski, Y., Singer, A., Gordon, E., Marosszeky, J., & Fearnside, M. R. (1990). Neuropsychological assessment and brain imaging technologies in evaluation of the sequelae of blunt head injury. *Australian and New Zealand Journal of Psychiatry, 24*, 133–138.

Siegel, B. V., Jr., Buchsbaum, M. S., Bunney, W. E., Jr., Gottschalk, L. A., Haier, R. J., Lohr, J. B., Lottenberg, S., Najafi, A., Nuechterlein, K. H., Potkin, S. G., & Wu, J. C. (1993). Cortical–striatal–thalamic circuits and brain glucose metabolic activity in 70 unmedicated male schizophrenic patients. *American Journal of Psychiatry, 150*, 1325–1336.

Stark, D. D., & Bradley, W. G. (1992). *Magnetic resonance imaging*. St. Louis: Mosby.

Swirsky-Sacchetti, T., Mitchell, D. R., Seward, J., Gonzales, C., Lublin, F., Knobler, R., & Field, H. L., (1992). Neuropsychological and structural brain lesions in multiple sclerosis: A regional analysis. *Neurology, 42*(7), 1291–1295.

Tamminga, C. A., Thaker, G. K., Buchanan, R., Kirkpatrick, B, Alphs, L. D., Chase, T. N., & Carpenter, W. T. (1992). Limbic system abnormalities identified in schizophrenia using positron emission tomography with fluorodeoxyglucose and neocortical alterations with deficit syndrome. *Archives of General Psychiatry, 49*, 522–530.

Thatcher, R. W., Cantor, D. S., McAlaster, R., Geisler, F., & Krause, P. (1991). Comprehensive predictions of outcome in closed head injured patients: The development of prognostic equations. *Annals of the New York Academy of Sciences, 620*, 82–101.

Tonkonogy, J. M. (1991). Violence and temporal lobe lesion: Head CT and MRI data. *The Journal of Neuropsychiatry and Clinical Neurosciences, 3*, 189–196.

Turner, R., & Jezzard, P. (1994). Magnetic resonance studies of brain functional activation using echo-planar imaging. In R. W. Thatcher, M. Hallet, T. Zeffiro, E. R. John, & M. Huerta (Eds.), *Functional neuroimaging: Technical foundations* (pp. 69–78). San Diego: Academic Press.

Turkheimer, E. (1989). Techniques of quantitative measurement of morphological structures of the central nervous system. In E. D. Bigler, R. A. Yeo, & E. Turkeheimer (Eds.), *Neuropsychological Function and Brain Imaging* (pp. 47–64). New York: Plenum.

Turkheimer, E., Cullu, C. M., Hubler, D. W., Paver, S. W., Yeo, R. A., & Bigler, E. D. (1984). Quantifying cortical atrophy. *Journal of neurology, neurosurgery, and psychiatry*, *47*, 1314–1318.

van Gorp, W. G., Mandelkern, M. A., Gee, M., Hinkin, C. H., Stern, C. E., Paz, D. K., Dixon, W., Evans, G., Flynn, F., Frederick, C. J., Ropchan, J. R., & Blahd, W. H. (1992). Cerebral metabolic dysfunction in AIDS: Findings in a sample with and without dementia. *The Journal of Neuropsychiatry and Clinical Neurosciences*, *4*, 280–287.

van Swieten, J. C., Geyskes, G. G., Derix, M. M., Peeck, B. M., Ramos, L. M., van Latum, J. C., & van Gijn, J. (1991). Hypertension in the elderly is associated with white matter lesions and cognitive decline. *Annals of Neurology*, *30*, 825–830.

Verslegers, W., De Deyn, P. P., Saerens, J., Marien, P., Appel, B., Pickut, B. A., & Lowenthal, A. (1991). Slow progressive bilateral posterior artery infarction presenting as agitated delirium, complicated with Anton's syndrome. *European Neurology*, *31*, 216–219.

Vilkki, J. Holst, P., Öhman, J., Servo, A., & Heiskanen, O. (1992). Cognitive test performances related to early and late computed tomography findings after closed-head injury. *Journal of Clinical and Experimental Neuropsychology*, *14*, 518–532.

Vita, A., Dieci, M., Giobbio, G. M., Azzone, P., Garbarini, M., Sacchetti, E., Cesana, B. M., & Cazzullo, C. L. (1991). CT scan abnormalities and outcome of chronic schizophrenia. *American Journal of Psychiatry*, *148*, 1577–1579.

Volkow, N. D., Brodie, J., & Bendriem, B. (1991). Positron emission tomography: Basic principles and applied applications in psychiatric research. *Annals of the New York Academy of Sciences*, *620*, 128–144.

Wahlund, L. O., Andersson-Lundman, G., Basun, H., Almkvist, O., Björkstén, K. S., Sääf, J., & Wetterberg, L. (1993). Cognitive functions in brain functions: A quantitative study of CSF volumes on Alzheimer patients and healthy control subjects. *Magnetic Resonance Imaging*, *11*, 169–174.

Wang, G. J., Volkow, N. D., Roque, C. T., Cestaro, V. L., Hitzemann, R. J., Cantos, E. L., Levy, A. V., & Dhawan, A. P. (1993). Functional importance of ventricular enlargement and cortical atrophy in healthy subjects and alcoholics as assessed with PET, MR imaging, and neuropsychologic testing. *Radiology*. *186*, 59–65.

Wang, P. P., Hesselink, J. R., Jernigan, T. L., Doherty, S., & Bellugi, U. (1992). Specific neurobehavioral profile of Williams' syndrome is associated with neocerebellar hemispheric preservation. *Neurology*, *42*, 1999–2002.

Warkentin, S., Risberg, J., Nilsson, A., Karlson, S., & Graae, E. (1991). Cortical activity during speech production: a study of regional cerebral blood flow in normal subjects performing a word fluency task. *Neuropsychiatry, Neuropsychology and Behavioral Neurology*, *4*, 305–316.

Weinberger, D. R., Berman, K. F., Suddath, R., & Torrey, E. F. (1992). Evidence of dysfunction of a prefrontal–limbic network in schizophrenia: A magnetic resonance imaging and regional cerebral blood flow study of discordant monozygotic twins. *American Journal of Psychiatry*, *149*, 890–897.

Wilson, D. A., Nitschke, R., Bowman, M. E., Chaffin, M. J., Sexauer, C. L., & Prince, J. R. (1991). Transient white matter changes on MR images in children undergoing chemotherapy for acute lymphocytic leukemia: Correlation with neuropsychologic deficiencies. *Radiology*, *180*, 205–209.

Wilson, J. T., Hadley, D. M., Wiedmann, K. D., & Teasdale, G. M. (1992). Intercorrelation of lesions detected by magnetic resonance imaging after closed head injury. *Brain Injury*, *6*, 391–399.

Wolkin, A., Sanfilipo, M., Wolf, A. P., Angrist, B., Brodie, J. D., & Rotrosen, J. (1992). Negative symptoms and hypofrontality in chronic schizophrenia. *Archives of General Psychiatry*, *49*, 959–965.

Wolpert, S. M., & Barnes, P. D. (1992). *MRI in pediatric neuroradiology*. St. Louis: Mosby.

Yang, T. T., Gallen, C. C., Schwartz, B. J., Bloom, F. E. (1993). Noninvasive somatosensory homunculus mapping in humans by using a large-array biomagnetometer. *Proceeding of the National Academy of sciences of the United States of America*, *90*, 3098–3102.

Yeo, R. A., Turkheimer, E., & Bigler, E. D. (1990). Neuropsychological methods of localizing brain dysfunction: Clinical versus empirical approaches. *Neuropsychiatry, Neuropsychology, and Behavioral Neurology*, *3*, 290–303.

Zametkin, A. J., Liebenauer, L. L., Fitzgerald, G. A., King, A. C., Minkunas, D. V., Herscovitch, P., Yamada, E. M., & Cohen, R. M. (1993). Brain metabolism in teenagers with attention-deficit hyperactivity disorder. *Archives of General Psychiatry*, *50*, 333–340.

Zappulla, R. A., LeFever, F. F., Jaeger, J., & Bilder, R. (1991). Windows on the brain: Neuropsychology's technological frontiers. *Annals of the New York Academy of Sciences*, *620*.

Zihl, J., von Cramon, D., Mai, N., & Schmid, C. (1991). Disturbance of movement vision after bilateral posterior brain damage. Further evidence and follow up observations. *Brain*, *114*, 2235–2252.

8

Cognitive Retraining in a Milieu-Oriented Outpatient Rehabilitation Program

Pamela S. Klonoff
David G. Lamb
Dennis A. Chiapello
Susan K. Kime
Janet Shepherd
Marie Cunningham
Adult Day Hospital for Neurological Rehabilitation
Barrow Neurological Institute,
St. Joseph's Hospital and Medical Center,
Phoenix, AZ

Cognitive remediation has been defined traditionally as activities that improve brain-injured patients' higher cerebral functioning, including disorders of perception, memory, and language (Butler & Namerow, 1988; Gianutsos & Gianutsos, 1979). Others have assigned a more global definition, which incorporates: (a) the enhancement of problem-solving abilities; (b) development and utilization of appropriate compensatory strategies; and (c) improvement of the patients' awareness of brain-injury-related difficulties (Ben-Yishay & Diller, 1993; Ben-Yishay & Prigatano, 1990; Klonoff, O'Brien, Prigatano, Chiapello, & Cunningham, 1989).

Cognitive retraining has been viewed from two different conceptual orientations (see Ben-Yishay & Diller, 1993 for review). The first is the *restorative* model, originally proposed by Zangwill (1947, cited in Ben-Yishay & Diller, 1993). This approach proposes to remediate specific cognitive functions with systematic retraining. With repeated practice, it is hoped the targeted cognitive function will be relearned or reacquired (see Butler & Namerow, 1988, for a review). Similarly, Luria, Naydin, Tsvetkova, and Vinarsky (1969) proposed that the cognitive deficit should be analyzed into modular components. With practice and overlearning, functional reorganization of neural pathways occurs, a process that is hypothesized to be related to brain "plasticity."

The second model emphasizes teaching patients strategies to solve functional problems of daily life (Ben-Yishay & Diller, 1993). It has been referred to as the *substitutive* or *compensatory* approach (Ben-Yishay & Diller, 1993) and *skill acquisition training* (Butler & Namerow, 1988). This improves the functional adaptation of the patient in the face of his or her deficits by relying on preserved cognitive processes. This approach focuses on *metacognition*, by which patient functioning is improved through the use of control processes, that is, executive functions that help the patient better plan, prioritize, organize, and self-monitor his or her problem-solving behavior (Ben-Yishay & Diller, 1993).

No matter how inclusive the definition, cognitive remediation presupposes a number of assumptions. First, there must be a model of the cognitive processes to be treated. In addition, it is necessary to generate specific hypotheses regarding the impact of brain damage on these cognitive processes. Finally, there should be hypotheses specifying how interventions modify the patient's functional status (Carmazza & Hillis, 1993; Wilson & Patterson, 1990). The first two considerations have been addressed extensively through cognitive neuropsychology and are not addressed specifically as part of this chapter (see Carmazza & Hillis, 1993, for a review).

This chapter focuses on the third element; namely, how to elicit change in the patient's functional status using cognitive retraining tasks. To this end, some important considerations are presented, including: (a) further clarification of the goal and intent of cognitive remediation exercises in the context of our outpatient milieu-oriented day-treatment program; (b) the role of the neuropsychological assessment in determining appropriate candidates for milieu-oriented therapy; (c) description of general patient characteristics that promote "successful" cognitive remediation; (d) description of treatment plans, with emphasis on improving the patients' awareness and use of compensations; (e) description of cognitive retraining techniques to address specific neuropsychological disorders; (f) interface of the multidisciplinary treatment team with cognitive retraining; and (g) techniques to assess the outcome and efficacy of cognitive retraining exercises, using case study examples and preliminary empirical research.

TREATMENT CONSIDERATIONS IN COGNITIVE RETRAINING

The Milieu-Oriented Approach to Cognitive Remediation

A unique aspect of our outpatient day-treatment program at the Adult Day Hospital for Neurological Rehabilitation (ADHNR), Barrow Neurological Institute, Phoenix, AZ, is the emphasis on the milieu approach (Prigatano, 1989; Prigatano with Fordyce et al., 1986). This has aptly been described as an active therapeutic environment that promotes and facilitates positive change (Gunderson, 1978). Within this context, the cognitive retraining session becomes an invaluable source of data regarding the patients' capacity to function appropriately as part of a treatment community. It closely simulates what would be expected in the work or school environment, where the patient is also part of a small community. In such settings, he or she will be expected to be cooperative and responsible, that is, arrive on time, bring the necessary tools, and interact appropriately with peers and authority figures. Evaluation of the patients' performance and behavior in a therapeutic milieu therefore affords powerful and clinically reliable information of what would be observed in other community settings. As such, it is similar to the "multimodal" approach of Ben-Yishay (Ben-Yishay & Diller, 1993), who found patients receiving cognitive retraining and who participated in interpersonal skills models showed the optimal outcome.

In our clinical experience, the problems identified in the milieu of cognitive retraining also exist outside the treatment setting, and typically are found in a more severe form. This is because there is less structure, understanding, and tolerance of brain-injury-related problems in the "real world." Therefore, the manner in which the patients function in the treatment milieu provides an opportunity for the patients (and staff) to become better educated and equipped to deal with the complex sequelae of the injury, beyond what can be expected in the more isolated traditional treatment environment. More specific examples of the quantitative and qualitative data obtained from cognitive retraining sessions are provided later.

The Role of the Neuropsychological Assessment in Identifying Appropriate Candidates for Milieu-Oriented Therapy

Techniques and issues related to the neuropsychological assessment of traumatic brain injured patients have been described elsewhere (Prigatano, Pepping, & Klonoff, 1986). As part of the evaluation of patients' appropriateness for the ADHNR program, all prospective patients undergo a detailed neuropsychological examination. Table 8.1 summarizes the tests and procedures most commonly employed to evaluate the patients' neuropsychological status. Areas addressed include speed of information processing, general intellectual functioning, memory, attention and concentration, and "executive functions" (including planning, problem solving, and organization). Note the inclusion of various personality measures. Personality tests have proven to be an invaluable source of information regarding the behavioral and psychosocial sequelae of the injury.

We recognize the formal neuropsychological examination is useful, yet limited (Prigatano et al., 1986). The exam yields information about selected cognitive skills based on standardized tests in a well-controlled setting. Confounding variables include lack of access to other "untapped" areas of intellectual functioning and the artificial nature of the testing environment that can mask significant behavioral and psychosocial influences. The evaluation also depends on the examiner's capacity to quickly develop a good working alliance and perceive clinically relevant observational data.

Given the aforementioned limitations of formal testing, an extended clinical interview is critical. This requires detailed information gathering from *both* patient and family members. Topics discussed include the patient's description of the injury and his or her perceived injury-related changes. Inquiry is made into changes in cognition, personality, leisure activ-

TABLE 8.1
Neuropsychological Tests Used in Core Battery

Wechsler Adult Intelligence Scale–Revised (Wechsler, 1981)
Wechsler Memory Scale–Revised (Wechsler, 1987)
California Verbal Learning Test (Delis, Kramer, Kaplan, & Ober, 1987)
Rey–Osterrieth Complex Figure (Osterrieth, 1944)
Halstead Reitan Battery (Reitan & Davison, 1974)
1. Finger Tapping
2. Category Test
3. Trails A and B
4. Tactual Performance Test
Symbol Digit Modalities Test, Oral Administration (Smith, 1982)
FAS Word Fluency (Spreen & Benton, 1969)
Porteus Maze Test (Porteus, 1950)
Wisconsin Card Sorting Test (Heaton, 1981)
Wide Range Achievement Test–Revised (Jastak & Wilkinson, 1984)
Patient Competency Rating Scale (Prigatano with Fordyce et al., 1986)
Relative's Competency Rating Scale (Prigatano with Fordyce et al., 1986)
Relative's Katz Adjustment Scale (Katz & Lyerly, 1963)
Minnesota Multiphasic Personality Inventory–2 (Butcher, Dahlstrom, Graham, Tellegen, & Kaemmer, 1989)

ities, and work/school status. All questions are addressed first to the patient and then to the family member. This allows the examiner to see to what extent there is concurrency in responses as well as how the patient reacts to differences of opinion. A detailed preinjury history is also obtained, including work/school history, other medical illnesses, drug and alcohol use, trouble with the law, psychiatric history, family history, and presence or absence of injury-related litigation. Last, the patient's and family's perceived goals and expectations of the rehabilitation process are discussed.

An important piece of data from the interview is the patient's level of awareness and distress about the injury-related problems. This often influences the degree to which the patient engages the rehabilitation process. For example, patients who are unaware of or disavow problems will often be more resistant during cognitive retraining sessions and less likely to consistently utilize compensatory strategies. They are also more prone to setting unrealistic expectations of the therapy process. Conversely, patients who are overwhelmed or distressed about their deficits may experience "catastrophic reactions" (Goldstein, 1952; Klonoff, Lage, & Chiapello, 1993) during neuropsychological testing, cognitive retraining exercises, or both. This type of behavioral data becomes important when examining patients and evaluating their appropriateness for cognitive retraining exercises. Therefore, we have found both the extensive initial interview with the patient and his or her family and the formal neuropsychological assessment to be important tools for formulating an initial understanding of the patient's needs and goals for the rehabilitation process.

General Patient Characteristics That Promote "Successful" Cognitive Remediation

As stated previously, patients are screened for their appropriateness for the ADHNR program. One important consideration is whether he or she will engage the broad intent of the program, namely: (a) improved independent functioning in the home and community, (b) return to productive work or school activities, or both. The latter includes active willingness to participate in work trials or school coursework as part of the rehabilitation process. Patients who are not motivated toward these goals typically do not make measurable progress in the rehabilitation setting. In addition, any gains they may have attained are rarely maintained postdischarge.

Patients must be medically stable and have considerable stamina if they are to realistically engage in the daily therapy demands. The etiological basis of the brain injury is varied, with approximately 66% having sustained traumatic brain injuries and the others suffering from various types of cerebrovascular insults (e.g., strokes, ruptured aneurysms, arteriovenous malformations), tumors, and infections. The typical patient displays moderate to moderately severe deficits on neuropsychological testing, often most directly affecting speed of information processing, higher level reasoning skills, and memory. The severity of injury must not preclude the patient from using compensations. Therefore, patients with significant confusion or disorientation (e.g., in posttraumatic amnesia) are not considered appropriate candidates.

Overall, patients need to have sufficient cognitive and personality skills to participate and benefit from small-group interaction within 4 to 6 weeks of entering into the program. They must have the capacity and willingness to increase their awareness and acceptance of their problem areas and to develop realistic goals with respect to independent functioning and productive work/school. Major psychiatric disturbance (e.g., antisocial personality, paranoia, psychotic behavior) usually significantly interferes with such progress in the milieu treatment environment. This is because patients are expected to cooperate with fellow patients and staff and act as responsible community members.

Family participation and involvement is mandatory in the program. Our clinical experience has been that the capacity of the patient to adjust and cope with his or her injury is directly linked to the family's level of support and adaptation (Klonoff & Lage, 1991; Prigatano with Fordyce et al. 1986). Families are expected to attend weekly family meetings and/or "Relatives' Groups." In addition, family members are invited to observe treatment days on a monthly basis to better acquaint themselves with the specific therapies and goals relevant to the patient in their family.

Development of a Cognitive Remediation Plan

As we have discussed elsewhere (Klonoff et al., 1989; Prigatano with Fordyce et al. 1986), our approach to cognitive retraining focuses on developing the patient's awareness of deficits. This requires a sophisticated understanding of the patient's needs and capacity to flexibly shift and adapt treatment procedures. There are three aspects of the cognitive retraining session which provide opportunities for this: (a) interpretation of patient performance; (b) the introduction, practice, and generalization of compensatory strategies; and (c) requirements of the session that are extraneous to performance on the cognitive exercises but relevant in settings outside the therapy milieu, particularly the work environment.

Interpretation of Patient Performance. A primary emphasis of cognitive retraining is helping patients better appreciate their areas of cognitive strength and difficulty (Klonoff et al., 1989). Discussion of how performance levels reflect the effects of the injury and their application to home, community, and work activities is often done on a daily basis. Having patients work together also facilitates the awareness process, because patients can compare their level of performance to others. Patients will often ask therapists to perform tasks, which provides another source of comparison. "Expected" scores also are provided for patients so they may judge their level of performance relative to non-brain-injured persons.

With the generalization of therapists' observations regarding task performance, patients gradually develop more realistic goals regarding work and school. They may be asked to anticipate their level of performance previous to doing the task. They often substantially underestimate their deficit areas.

The Home Independence and Work Re-Entry Programs each have a separate assortment of cognitive retraining tasks, distinguished primarily by level of difficulty. Within each program, however, the patient begins by confronting a standard set of exercises, designed to cover a range of cognitive requirements. The first exercises to be presented are rather basic in terms of content. As these are completed, more complex ones are introduced.

The cognitive retraining session is deliberately set as the first session of the morning, so that the treatment day can begin promptly and precisely. Before performing any exercise, the patient is first asked to name, either from memory or by referring to notes, the specific purposes of the exercise. For instance, a basic letter-cancellation task is said to work on attention and concentration, visual scanning, and striking a balance between speed and accuracy. As a matter of principle this step is never omitted, although the extended repetition of these somewhat abstract terms tends to blunt its effectiveness over time. Therefore, it is often helpful to introduce "real-life" applications of these skills. For example, the cancellation task can be viewed as being similar to using an index or dictionary.

When patients are encouraged to generate their own ideas, the tasks are likely to become even more meaningful to them. For example, a patient of ours who worked as an auto mechanic found the letter-cancellation task similar to looking up information in a parts manual. Another patient, planning to return to her job as a check-out clerk at a supermarket, was confronted with the prospect of memorizing about 100 numeric codes for produce items.

She saw a close similarity between this task and a cognitive retraining exercise based on the Symbol Digit test of the WAIS–R.

As patients work their way through the dozen or so cognitive retraining exercises that occupy their first 4–5 months in the program, they may find them all to be somewhat difficult. More commonly they will discover some exercises (or certain aspects of them) are especially difficult, whereas others are relatively easy.

It should be noted that tasks, procedures, and expectations often need to be modified to accommodate individual patients. For example, the speech and language pathologists typically work with aphasic patients in cognitive retraining, as their expertise may be required to modify activities appropriately. Patients with significant right hemisphere injury or hemiplegia may require task modification or simplification. At times, certain cognitive retraining activities may be omitted, particularly if they may heighten the patient's level of frustration and cause a "catastrophic reaction" (Goldstein, 1952).

Another consideration is the degree to which a given patient is able to confront their deficits. With patients who are less able emotionally to handle feedback, less direct emphasis is placed on the implications of the cognitive retraining scores until they begin to show signs of increased tolerance for feedback.

Occasionally, we may decide a patient must work one-on-one with his or her therapist rather than in the usual configuration of two patients to a therapist. This may be due to the patient's distractibility, jealousy over a therapist's divided attention, or simply to the amount of attention required by the level of impairment. In such cases, if possible, we help the patient advance to working with another patient. In our experience, the "success" of cognitive retraining is based more on the expertise and clinical sensitivity of the therapist than the specific tasks and procedures.

Often, patients report this group as the most enjoyable aspect of therapy. This is because it is easy for them to appraise their performance level and evaluate first hand their cognitive strengths and difficulties.

Compensatory Strategies. Whether or not patients see the broader purpose of the exercises in cognitive retraining, they usually perceive deficiencies in task performance. This is where we ideally begin to introduce compensatory strategies. However, it is important to present compensations in a way the patient will appreciate; that is, in a way that will make the patient more likely to: (a) adopt the strategy in cognitive retraining, and (b) carry the strategy over to practical activities outside the session.

When a patient is doing a task for the first time, we generally do not make reference to any compensatory methods, preferring instead to obtain something close to a baseline measure. Our next step will be to ask the patient what method he or she thinks might improve performance. If the patient cannot think of one, we will, of course, suggest an appropriate strategy and encourage the patient to use it.

Ideally, improvement in scores will begin when the patient adopts the compensatory strategy, making its effectiveness quite clear. From a practical standpoint, we are unable to apply all the rigors of a controlled study during treatment and therefore effectiveness is not always so clearly shown. However, this approach is usually a sufficient demonstration to the patient. As the patient adopts strategies in cognitive retraining, therapists may begin encouraging them to carry these strategies over to other activities in the program. For example, a patient using a ruler to help in a visual scanning task may be asked to use the same method to help keep their place while following a recipe in a home management task.

We have found that even when the positive effect is very clear, some patients remain reluctant to use the compensation. This issue itself may become an important focus of subsequent sessions. Helping the patient recognize the need for compensations and develop a willingness to use them is a vital goal of cognitive retraining. It is not just the use of strategies in cognitive retraining that is at stake, but the patient's willingness to later apply it to other important functional activities.

We may begin by proposing a comparison of scores with and without the strategy, so that the patient has the opportunity to judge the effectiveness of the strategy without necessarily being pressured into adopting it. Other approaches draw on aspects of the milieu setting: Patients naturally have many opportunities to observe fellow patients employing compensations effectively, and therapists likewise have many opportunities to encourage the use of compensations in other program sessions.

We have often heard patients voice the concern that using a compensatory strategy (especially for memory problems) will become a "crutch" and actually cause their skills to deteriorate. At this point we emphasize the functional importance of these tools and remind them that cognitive deficits are often longstanding. Aside from a patient's reluctance to use them, other problems may arise with compensatory strategies. Some patients may be willing to use the methods but are sometimes unable to initiate the behavior or remember to use them independently. In this situation, the therapist helps devise notes or checklists to guide the patient through the procedures of cognitive retraining tasks. For example, we worked with a young woman who was very cooperative but severely amnestic. She relied on written notes to guide her through the steps and compensations for each task. Gradually, more and more steps were incorporated into her procedural memory until she consistently used the compensation.

What this patient could not do, however, was generalize any of her cognitive retraining strategies to other activities. Difficulty generalizing compensatory strategies is a problem many patients may face for reasons other than memory deficits. Patients with rigid thinking or impaired problem-solving ability may show poor generalization of skills developed in cognitive retraining. In such a case, we know the patient will require a greater degree of assistance outside the program, with a slim probability of gainful employment.

It must be acknowledged that there are practical limitations to all compensatory strategies. Even with compensations, a patient's scores might improve to a certain point but remain below the normal range. In addition, our clinical impression is that most compensations are more successful at improving accuracy of performance than increasing speed.

Application of Cognitive Retraining to Work and School Settings. Patients in cognitive retraining often complain that the tasks at hand are so far removed from the demands of their job or school work that there is little value in working on them. Some patients even reject exercises which are highly similar to their work duties simply because of their conviction that, once back at the job, they will not make the same errors that have been plaguing them in cognitive retraining. Such an outlook reflects the patient's difficulty seeing the "big picture" of cognitive retraining; that is, whatever difficulties the patient experiences in this session are likely to resurface at work or school.

The therapist's challenge is to avoid too narrow a focus on the somewhat routine and repetitive cognitive retraining exercises. By broadening his or her observations to all relevant aspects of the patient's behavior in this session, the patient is helped to see the larger context. With patients who are early in their recovery, these observations mainly serve as an assessment of the patient's recovery. However, for patients who are further on, especially those planning to return to work, we present our observations to the patient as matters of concern and help target them for active intervention.

We have already discussed the importance of compensatory strategies within the cognitive retraining session and how a patient's resistance to using them may become a proper focus of therapy. Such resistance may be manifest in a number of behaviors based on clinical observa-

TABLE 8.2
Cognitive Retraining Behaviors Relevant to Problematic Work/School Re-Entry

Failure to arrive on time for the session.
Difficulty learning/remembering procedures for specific tasks.
Frequent errors in calculating scores.
Frequent errors in recording data.
Difficulty working in the presence of mild distractions.
Inability to modify speed of performance when cued.
Difficulty initiating, requiring cues from therapist to proceed through exercises.
Disorganized working methods.
Reluctance to use compensatory methods.
Inability to generalize compensatory methods from one task to another.
Difficulty perceiving relevance of cognitive retraining tasks to job-related skills.
Jealous reaction when therapist's attention is divided between two patients.
Negative emotional reactions to poor task scores.
Defensive responses to feedback about task performance.
Difficulty handling changes in routine (e.g., working with a substitute for an absent therapist).
Expression of irritation or anger under mildly stressful conditions.

tions in cognitive retraining (see Table 8.2) and should caution the therapist about the patient's readiness for work or school.

Cognitive Retraining: Remediation of Specific Neuropsychological Disorders

Although the primary value of cognitive retraining is the clinically relevant data derived from behavioral observation, a variety of cognitive skills are more formally addressed as part of the cognitive retraining sessions. These areas are discussed in this section.

Attention and Concentration. The patient's capacity to attend to tasks is addressed in several ways. First, as described earlier, patients work in a group environment, with each therapist assigned to two patients. Patients must "screen out" the visual and auditory distractors of another patient working close by on a different task, as well as the ambient noise created by the larger group's presence. This simulates the environmental stimulation typically observed in most work and school environments. Furthermore, successful completion of all cognitive retraining tasks requires the patient to sustain his or her attention for a significant allotted time period.

Memory and Learning. An important aspect of cognitive retraining is the emphasis on learning and recall. As stated earlier, the purpose of each task is reviewed on a daily basis. This allows an opportunity to see to what extent each patient recalls the purpose without the assistance of notes. Similarly, each task has a scoring procedure consisting of several steps and a protocol for graphing scores on a weekly basis. Procedural memory can be assessed by seeing to what extent the patient recalls these protocols independently.

As each activity is performed over several trials, information regarding the learning slope is obtained. In addition to general procedural recall, several cognitive retraining tasks directly incorporate memory as a training skill (e.g., a variant of the Digit Symbol subtest of the Wechsler Adult Intelligence Scale–Revised (WAIS–R) and a task requiring the patient to write down the first letter of each word in a sentence read aloud by the therapist).

Language. Although all cognitive retraining tasks incorporate language skills to some extent, some tasks focus specifically on language abilities. For example, verbal fluency is addressed through oral and written variations of word generation tasks. Reading skills are addressed using activities requiring visual scanning for words. All tasks, whether primarily verbal or visuospatial in nature, require scores to be recorded on scoresheets and a master ledger. The patient's reading skills are employed in order to review the purpose of all tasks.

Visuospatial Abilities. Some cognitive retraining activities focus specifically on visuospatial abilities. Visual scanning is addressed using letter, number, and symbol cancellation tasks. Other exercises require construction skills (constructing designs using multicolored blocks) and rapid pattern recognition and position recall (shape matching).

Visual neglect is addressed as part of all scanning activities. Cognitive retraining allows ample opportunity to assess this deficit as well as to practice appropriate compensatory strategies. These include using colored borders and rulers to help guide vision.

Impulsivity. This general skill area emerges across all cognitive retraining tasks. Its impact on eventual productive work and school can easily be assessed given the milieu environment of cognitive retraining. For example, because patients work together, the effect of impulsivity on interpersonal communication can be observed by staff. Patients are expected to work cooperatively with one another. At times, this means one patient will need to wait for the therapist to finish with another patient. This teaches patients the importance of self-monitoring and turn taking.

Impulsivity often affects task performance. A frequently stated goal of cognitive retraining tasks is the balance between speed and accuracy. Often the impulsive patient will sacrifice accuracy for speed, particularly on timed tasks such as Block Design and various cancellation activities. Alternatively, he or she will perform or score a task without taking adequate time to think through the necessary steps.

Planning and Organization. These skills permeate many aspects of cognitive retraining. They are important to consider when evaluating the patient's capacity to function independently and productively in the community. Is the patient on time to sessions? Does he or she know the tasks to be performed? Is there anticipation of the tools needed as compensatory devices? The capacity to perform scoring procedures sequentially and to maintain cognitive retraining books in an organized fashion are also important indicators of adequate daily functioning. Intact organizational skills are often helpful in ameliorating memory deficits. For example, performance on Block Design typically improves if the different colored blocks are consistently arranged in the same sequence and placed in the same area of the table. Typically the more organized and independent the patient functions in the cognitive retraining sessions, the higher the level of independence and productive work or school obtained.

Abstract Thinking and Mental Flexibility. The role of abstract thinking is critical in helping patients to appreciate how observations derived from cognitive retraining apply to their daily functioning outside of the therapy environment. Often patients will view the cognitive retraining activities concretely, complaining they will not be expected to "scan letters" or "build designs" at work or school. This is often a hallmark sign of frontal lobe damage where the patient is unable to see "the big picture" benefits of cognitive retraining. We continually emphasize the value of general skill building, increasing patient's awareness and realistic appraisal of deficits, and developing compensatory strategies as therapeutic goals of cognitive retraining.

Mental flexibility is addressed directly through several tasks. For example, word search, word fluency, and Stroop activities all require shifting of mental set. The milieu of cognitive retraining also requires cognitive/conceptual flexibility; patients must interact appropriately with other patients. At times, their particular requests or needs must be postponed to accommodate other patients. Problems with pragmatics (e.g., turn taking) and self-centeredness can be directly discussed in cognitive retraining, as well as individual and group speech/language therapies.

Interface of Different Treatment Disciplines With Cognitive Retraining

Occupational Therapy. Behavior in cognitive retraining usually affects home functioning. If the patient displays poor memory for tasks/procedures in cognitive retraining, we often note difficulty with bill paying, compliance with the medication regime, and making and following through with appointments. For example, during a home visit of a severely impaired patient, the occupational therapist found approximately 100 bills that were unopened. This resulted in several collection agencies becoming involved.

When a disorganized approach to the cognitive retraining tasks is observed, inefficient management of daily activities is often seen. For example, there may be difficulty following directions or recipes, filling out forms, or financial chaos with checkbook and personal financial management. Poor visual scanning during tasks often is correlated with difficulty using a phone book, dictionary, or encyclopedia, using schedules/calendars, and finding items when grocery shopping. Distractibility affects safety during activities such as cooking, driving, and child care. If a patient displays inflexibility with cognitive retraining tasks, they may encounter problems when adapting to changes in routines at home or when traveling.

The overall goal of occupational therapy is to help establish a systematic, structured approach to daily tasks to maximize the patient's independence. Often, use of compensations such as daily calendars, watches that chime hourly, and checklists are practiced in cognitive retraining and then applied directly to the home environment.

Speech and Language Therapy. As stated earlier in this chapter, all cognitive retraining tasks incorporate communication skills to a degree, and some activities are specifically designed for that purpose. Therefore, a speech/language therapist working with a patient during the cognitive retraining hour can derive valuable information that correlates with formal language test results. Such supplementary information can provide valuable input for discussions and activities conducted during individual and group speech therapy sessions. Particular areas of interest for the speech/language therapist may include attention and concentration, short-term memory, organization of thought, verbal fluency, reading skills, and the ability to understand task purposes and procedures. Specific problems in one or more of these areas during cognitive retraining may be approached during individual speech/language therapy using workbook and computer tasks, graded reading exercises, or Attention Process Training (Sohlberg & Mateer, 1987).

Speech and language therapists can apply observations from cognitive retraining to decisions regarding vocational placement. For example, a 45-year-old woman who suffered a cerebrovascular accident resulting in significant receptive and expressive aphasia required modification of some of the cognitive retraining tasks due to her aphasia. At the same time, she also showed difficulties attending to activities in the presence of noise or distractions that are typically present during the cognitive retraining hour. These factors made it impossible for her to return to her former position of nurse and department head at a large metropolitan hospital. Over time, however, with therapeutic assistance and counseling, she was able to assume two volunteer positions, one in a medical library and the other doing basic clinical work. These positions relied less on her communication skills and could be modified and enhanced by strategies to help her to cope with distractibility and organizational difficulties.

A growing role of speech and language therapy is the reintegration of patients into high school and college coursework. Observations from cognitive retraining often help to determine the number and setting of classes (special education vs. mainstream) that a patient should choose for enrollment.

A patient's ability to interact socially and use language effectively during cognitive retraining is carefully noted by therapists and affords the speech therapist an additional area of focus or interface. *Pragmatics* refers to a system of rules that clarify the use of language in situational and social contexts (Sohlberg & Mateer, 1989). Disturbances of communication pragmatics may include hyperverbality, tangentiality, peculiar phraseology, interrupting, turn-taking difficulties, inappropriate comments and use of humor, and an inability to interpret social cues. Prigatano (with Fordyce et al., 1986) stated that these problems compromise an individual's ability to interact and communicate appropriately or effectively in social and work settings, and may eventually lead to social alienation, isolation, and unemployment. For example, a 24-year-old woman who had a brain injury in a motor vehicle accident was frequently verbally blunt and argumentative during cognitive retraining and other therapy sessions. On an international flight (7 months postadmission to ADHNR) she was involved in an altercation with another passenger over her desire to occupy two seats in order to sleep. Reportedly, the situation escalated to such a point that the pilot and other crew members were involved before the patient gave up the extra seat.

With the cognitive retraining hour serving as a "microcosm" of the actual world, these issues can be addressed by the speech/language therapist either on an individual basis (i.e., through discussion) or during group therapy (i.e., role playing, videotaping, or both).

Recreation Therapy. Behavior during cognitive retraining tasks provides valuable insight into potential problem areas in the community. The recreation therapist applies these observations to such activities as community outings and selection of appropriate leisure activities. Important problems addressed through recreation therapy include impulsivity, visual inattention, and reduced sensitivity to social cues.

In cognitive retraining tasks, the impulsive patient may begin without waiting for instructions or a cue to begin. In one case, a patient was observed starting the stopwatch and timing himself on a task because a therapist was attending to another patient. In the community setting, the problem of impulsivity could have serious safety implications. Patients may step off the curb too soon and expect a vehicle to stop, or bump into other shoppers in a mall while walking too quickly. Patients have also been observed recklessly steering and zig-zagging a shopping cart through a crowded grocery store.

Visual inattention (Heilman & Valenstein, 1985) is often exhibited in cancellation tasks or in record-keeping activities. Visual inattention in the community precludes a patient from safely operating a motor vehicle, getting around obstacles, navigating through doorways, or safely crossing the street.

Reduced sensitivity to social cues is often observed during cognitive retraining and over time can lead to social isolation (Prigatano, 1992; Prigatano with Fordyce et al. 1986). For example, during cognitive retraining a patient often interrupted another patient at a nearby table by talking loudly or making jokes when the other patient was actively concentrating on an exercise. The same patient was later seen on a zoo outing feeding the birds and tapping on animals' cages, although signs clearly prohibited these behaviors. Other examples include patients spitting off of a balcony during a community outing, eating from another patient's plate and a trash container, and wandering out of a theater during a movie (with a therapist in tow). Initially, friends and family may tolerate or even be amused by such behavior. However, over time these inappropriate behaviors often have a wearing effect.

Helping the patient to appreciate how his or her cognitive problems impact community functioning is particularly important given the patient's desire to return to a variety of complex and sometimes dangerous activities (e.g., driving, crossing intersections).

ASSESSMENT OF OUTCOME AND EFFICACY OF COGNITIVE RETRAINING

We are committed to evaluating the efficacy of cognitive retraining in improving brain-injured patients' eventual level of productivity. The following case study observations and pilot study data illustrate how cognitive retraining behavioral and quantitative data facilitate return to work and school.

Case Studies

AB: Predictive Value of Cognitive Retraining. This case study illustrates the importance of behavioral observations derived through the "milieu" of cognitive retraining in determining interpersonal functioning at the work place.

AB was a 42-year-old man who was employed in marketing for a hazardous waste management company. He had been with the company 2–3 years when an industrial container exploded into his face. In addition to extensive facial trauma, AB suffered swelling of the brain as well as bleeding in the left parietal and temporal lobes. With the exception of double vision and reduced stamina, AB made a good physical recovery. Postinjury, AB showed mild to moderate deficits in the areas of memory for visual and verbal information, visuospatial skills, and speed of information processing.

AB achieved generally good scores on cognitive retraining tasks, with the exception of some slowed speed of performance. However, he clearly demonstrated behavioral difficulties that negatively impacted his participation in cognitive retraining sessions. He was highly distractible, cognitively rigid (with categorically narrow, "black-and-white" thinking), explosive, hyperverbal, and frustration intolerant. One morning, the staff was discussing a change in the schedule related to a therapist's absence. AB became sarcastic and then enraged, and went on to accuse the staff of being disorganized and unprofessional. This rage reaction continued throughout the morning and attempts to calm AB were to no avail. In other cognitive retraining sessions, AB would initiate a good-natured, but inappropriate and distracting banter with a patient at the next table. When this was brought to his attention, he became angry and expressed resolve to discontinue the cognitive retraining exercises, questioning the validity of the therapy.

Approximately 12 weeks after program admission, similar patterns were observed at work. As with cognitive retraining, AB showed good use of compensatory strategies for memory and was highly organized. Nonetheless, there was evidence of reduced productivity that was primarily related to reduced efficiency and slowed problem solving. Of greater diagnostic saliency was the supervisor's report of impulsivity and low frustration tolerance. Impatience and cognitive inflexibility were particularly marked and problematic. On several occasions AB had become explosively angry at work, verbally attacking co-workers and his supervisor.

In this case, cognitive retraining was helpful in identifying cognitive changes (e.g., slower speed of information processing) that affected work productivity. More importantly, the "milieu approach" afforded observation of behavioral changes that were critical in foreshadowing adjustment problems at work. Due to the incompatibility of AB's symptom pattern and job requirements, AB terminated his job and returned to the ADHNR program. He is now successfully involved in another job domain.

CD: Correlation to Positive Outcome. This case study illustrates how a patient's positive performance and adaptation to his injury through cognitive retraining related to a smooth transition back to school.

CD was a 15-year-old high school student injured during a motor vehicle accident when, as a restrained backseat passenger, his head hit a metal bar. He experienced loss of consciousness and had to be extricated from the car. CT scans and X-rays revealed a left parietal depressed skull fracture. CD had cerebral contusions around the wound area and a left temporal subarachnoid hemorrhage. His initial Glasgow Coma Scale score was 9. CD required tube feedings initially because of dysphagia; he also required ventilation. At the time of injury, CD was enrolled in a 9th-grade gifted student's program. Academic testing with the Iowa Test of Basic Skills ranged from the 91st to 98th percentiles. CD was also a member of the swim team.

Initial neuropsychological testing results were consistent with his traumatic brain injury and revealed mild to moderate difficulties in the areas of fine motor control, abstract reasoning, problem solving, rate of learning, memory, bilateral tactile perception, and awareness of deficits.

CD was admitted to ADHNR 1 month postinjury. He participated in daily cognitive retraining sessions for 9 weeks, which was the length of his stay in our program. Generally, CD showed a fairly rapid recovery and a positive learning curve with practice. He was a very hard worker, achievement-oriented, and sensitive to feedback. Areas of strength included visual scanning, rate of learning with practice, and visuospatial problem solving. Relative areas of difficulty included flexible problem solving (on a word fluency task) and overall speed of information processing. These few difficulties were also reflected in speech and language therapy sessions, where CD showed deficits on measures of perceptual speed and verbal ability relative to his overall above average scores on cognitive abilities. Early on, CD showed an ability to understand the purpose of each task, and to complete scoring and record keeping relatively independently. He also discussed compensatory strategies and the potential impact of his injury on returning to school.

CD had a very supportive family, and regular contact took place between his mother and stepfather and the staff through a relative's counseling group and individual meetings. A consistent rating of "excellent" was derived for our "Working Alliance" over time.

CD made a rapid recovery from a physical and cognitive standpoint, and his overall progress seemed positively related to his performance during the cognitive retraining hour. Within 2 weeks of starting the program (6 weeks postinjury), CD was able to pursue two academic courses, algebra and science, on a homebound basis. By 2 months postinjury he had returned to his former high school to begin two additional classes. Shortly thereafter, CD was discharged from the program for transition back to school full time. For several months he continued to receive select therapies, including occupational therapy, speech therapy, and psychotherapy.

As of 1 year postinjury, CD has returned to the program on several occasions for brief reevaluation and consultation subsequent to formal discharge. By his report, he completed the 9th-grade gifted program with a 4.0 average. He is continuing to take honors classes, is the layout editor for the school newspaper, and participates on the swim team. During testing, CD did display some residual deficits in speed of information processing, as well as verbal learning and recall, which mirrored the difficulties observed with his performance in cognitive retraining while in the program. Also reflective of previous performance during the cognitive retraining hour was his excellent performance on tests of nonverbal logical reasoning, visual problem solving, and overall verbal intellectual functioning.

CD remains a sensitive young man with some understandable emotional feelings of sadness relative to his residual difficulties. At the same time, he has made a relatively rapid and good cognitive recovery, which was predicted in large measure by the quantitative and behavioral data gathered during formal cognitive retraining sessions.

Preliminary Research Findings

Empirical research is paramount for determining the efficacy of cognitive retraining efforts with brain injured patients. The following represents some preliminary data, based on a pilot study conducted at ADHNR. The goal was to identify aspects of cognitive retraining that, in the context of milieu therapy, best predict successful productive outcome at the time of program discharge.

Subjects. A total of 16 patients were examined in the study. Of those, 13 sustained traumatic brain injuries and 3 suffered cerebrovascular accidents. A rating of severity of injury was obtained using input from various treatment disciplines regarding the extent of the neurological, motor, cognitive, behavioral, and language deficits. A 10-point scale was devised based on the staff's experience with our rehabilitation population, with 1 equaling the least functional patient seen at the ADHNR and 10 being the mildest level of functional impairment seen among our program patients. Each patient was assigned a rating of functional severity using this scale. The mean age of the subjects was 28 (range 14–48). The mean education was 13 years (range 8–20). The mean time period from injury until program admission was 3.33 months (range .75–19.95 months). The average length of program participation was 5.92 months (range 1.03–10.95 months).

Methods. All patients participated in cognitive retraining exercises as part of their program therapies. Selected cognitive retraining tasks were identified a priori as potential predictors of vocational outcome. Specific scores computed for these tasks were the mean of the first 3 trials, the mean of the last 3 trials, and a difference (delta) score reflecting the degree of change between these 2 mean scores. In addition, some cognitive retraining tasks are stratified into progressively more difficult levels (e.g., Stroop and Digit Symbol—I, II, & III). On these tasks, scores were derived for the first and last levels only, in order to maximize the difference scores. In addition, all patients underwent admission neuropsychological testing, and selected test scores from these evaluations also were identified for inclusion a priori. Only nine patients had discharge neuropsychological testing, because of either abrupt discontinuation or short length of stay. Scores were also computed for these patients that reflected change from admission to discharge administrations. Table 8.3 lists the cognitive retraining tasks and relevant neuropsychological test scores used in the analyses.

Variables that were considered to be important based on the milieu treatment approach were incorporated in two ways. First, working alliance data were obtained for each patient and his or her family. These numerical values are based on a 100-point scale and are gathered on a monthly basis. Ratings are divided into quadrants (1–25 = needs work; 26–50 = fair; 51–75 = good; 76–100 = excellent) and represent the staff's global view of the quality of the working relationship with the patients and their families. A more detailed description of the definition and components of the working alliance is contained in an outcome study by Prigatano et al. (1994). However, generally these scores represent the extent to which the patient (and family) work in consonance with the staff. Attendance, follow through with assignments, willingness to embrace compensations, and perceptions of the injury-related strengths and difficulties are considered in assigning scores. For purposes of this study, a mean of all ratings and the final month's rating were used for analysis.

The second measure that was employed to assess the contribution of the interpersonal or milieu therapeutic interventions was a Cognitive Retraining Behavioral Checklist. This

TABLE 8.3
Dependent Measures Used in ADHNR Outcome Study

Neuropsychological Tests
WAIS-R:
Verbal IQ
Performance IQ
Full scale IQ
Vocabulary —Raw Score
—Scale Score
Digit symbol—Raw Score
—Scale Score
California Verbal Learning Test:
Sum: Trials 1–5 (*T* score) × Trials
Delayed/free recall (*Z* score)
Cognitive Retraining Tasks
Word Fluency
Digit Symbol (I & III)
Stroop (I & III)
Matching Shapes

checklist contains eight behaviors that were defined a priori by the staff as relevant to patient outcome (see Table 8.4). For the purpose of this study, mean ratings of the staff were obtained for each patient, based on a 5-point scale.

Vocational and school outcome was recorded based on a 10-point scale, depending on whether the patients returned to paid work/school or volunteer activities on a full- or part-time schedule (see Table 8.5). Also, several patients ($n = 6$) discontinued the program without completing the goals and their outcome was recorded as such.

Results and Discussion. Given the small sample size, use of multiple regression was unsuitable, so a correlation matrix was obtained. Significant and clinically relevant correla-

Table 8.4
Cognitive Retraining Behavioral Checklist

	Characteristic	*Score*
1.	Timeliness	_____
2.	Organization	_____
3.	Independence in scoring & record keeping	_____
4.	Recall of task purposes	_____
5.	Initiates & uses compensations	_____
6.	Pragmatics	_____
7.	Distractibility	_____
8.	Sees "BIG" picture	_____

Score	*Description*
1	Unable to carry out independently
2	Completes with 75% cuing
3	Completes with 50% cuing
4	Completes with 25% cuing
5	Independent in functioning

TABLE 8.5
Scoring and Criteria for Outcome Measures

Category	*Score*	*Description of outcome*
Good	10	Returns to previous level of work/school
	9	Full-time paid work/school (job modifications or new placement)
	8	Part-time paid work/school and part-time volunteer work
	7	Part-time paid work/school
Fair	6	Full-time volunteer work
	5	Part-time volunteer work
	4	Some paid/volunteer work with problems in adjusting
Poor	3	Some paid/volunteer work resulting in termination
	2	Discharge from program with work trial
	1	Discharge from program without work trial

tion coefficients are provided in Table 8.6. Note the significant contribution of age ($r = -.64$, $p = .008$) and level of education ($r = -.77$, $p = .001$), with younger and less educated patients showing a better outcome that may reflect superior ability to physically recover from injury. This suggests that the school reentry patients are showing a more positive global cognitive outcome.

Of the neuropsychological tests included, only the WAIS–R PIQ difference score (discharge vs. admission) ($r = .71$, $p = .03$) and the WAIS–R Digit Symbol raw score at discharge ($r = .69$, $p = .04$) correlated significantly with outcome. Similarly, initial performance on the third level of the Digit Symbol cognitive retraining exercise correlated significantly ($r = .83$, $p = .05$) with productive outcome. This result suggests that overall speed of information processing (and motor speed) are important determinants of return to work and school. The Stroop III test, a facsimile of Part C of the Stroop Test (Stroop, 1935) that relies

TABLE 8.6
Correlation of Outcome With Selected Descriptive, Cognitive Retraining, Neuropsychological, and Behavioral Data

	Outcome[a]	
	r	*p*
Descriptive data:		
Education	−.77	.001
Age	−.64	.008
Neuropsychological data:		
WAIS–R—Digit symbol—Discharge[b]	.69	.04
WAIS-R: PIQ—Difference score[c]	.71	.03
Cognitive Retraining:		
Stroop I—Difference score	.59	.02
Digit symbol III[d]	.83	.003
Behavioral Data:		
Final Working Alliance		
rating of patient	.52	.04
Behavioral Checklist		
Item 5—"initiates and uses compensations"	.44	.09
Item 8—"sees the 'big picture'"	.57	.02

Note. [a]$n = 16$. [b]Raw Score. [c]Discharge minus admission. [d]Average of the first 3 trials.

on response inhibition, also correlated with outcome (r = .59, p = .02), perhaps reflecting the negative impact of disinhibition on outcome.

Other variables that represented the milieu-oriented intervention showed significant correlations. The last recorded working alliance with the patient was one indicator (r = .52, p = .04). This result suggests that by the end of the rehabilitation process, if the working alliance is positive, a more successful outcome is likely. Two of the items on the Behavior Checklist also correlated with outcome: (a) initiates and uses compensations (r = .44, p = .09) and (b) sees the "big picture" purpose of the cognitive retraining exercises (r = .57, p = .02). Although the first result is not statistically significant, it offers some support for our clinical impression that successful outcome is related to the capacity of the patient to actively embrace compensatory cognitive strategies. Being able to "see the big picture" is directly related to a patient's ability to improve his or her awareness of the effects of the injury on work or school functioning and thus experience a better outcome at discharge.

Although this research project is ongoing, these initial results appear to be promising in implicating an important role for the milieu-oriented approach (above and beyond simple test scores) in successful vocational outcome.

SUMMARY

Cognitive retraining is an integral component of the rehabilitation process at ADHNR. Even though research as yet has not convincingly demonstrated that it enhances physiological recovery, we feel cognitive retraining can provide valuable rehabilitative assistance within a milieu setting. Beyond the potential ameliorative effects of the tasks per se, the experienced and clinically astute therapist can learn a great deal from how the patient copes with the demands of cognitive retraining sessions. Such behavioral observations act as a rehabilitative behavioral barometer, which is immediately sensitive to the patient's overall mood, attitude toward rehabilitation, and ability to tolerate feedback. It also provides a clinically reliable forecast of the patient's ability to successfully reintegrate socially into work or school. These are valuable benefits of milieu-based cognitive retraining with practical applications to rehabilitation, which generalize to the work or home environments. As data accumulates, we will continue to explore the relationship between specific behaviors seen in cognitive retraining (within a milieu-oriented program) and eventual patient outcome.

REFERENCES

Ben-Yishay, Y., & Diller, L. (1993). Cognitive remediation in traumatic brain injury: Update and issues. *Archives of Physical Medicine Rehabilitation, 74*, 204–213.

Ben-Yishay, Y., & Prigatano, G. P. (1990). Cognitive remediation. In M. R. Rosenthal & J. D. Miller (Eds.), *Rehabilitation of the adult and child with traumatic brain injury* (2nd ed., pp. 393–409). Philadelphia: F. A. Davis.

Butcher, J. N., Dahlstrom, W. G., Graham, J. R., Tellegen, A., & Kaemmer, B. (1989). *Manual for the Restandardized Minnesota Multiphasic Personality Inventory—MMPI–2: An administrative and interpretive guide*. Minneapolis: University of Minnesota Press.

Butler, R. W., & Namerow, N. S. (1988). Cognitive retraining in brain injury rehabilitation: A critical review. *Journal of Neurological Rehabilitation, 2*, 97–101.

Carmazza, A., & Hillis, A. (1993). For a theory of remediation of cognitive deficits. *Neuropsychological Rehabilitation, 3*, 217–234.

Delis, D. C., Kramer, J. H., Kaplan, E., & Ober, B. A. (1987). *California Verbal Learning Test manual*. San Antonio: Psychological Corporation.

Gianutsos, R., & Gianutsos, J. (1979). Rehabilitating the verbal recall of brain injured patients by mnemonic training: An experimental demonstration using single case methodology. *Journal of Clinical Neuropsychology, 1*, 117–122.

Goldstein, K. (1952). The effect of brain damage on the personality. *Psychiatry, 15*, 245–260.
Gunderson, J. G. (1978). Defining the therapeutic process in psychiatric milieus. *Psychiatry, 41*, 327–335.
Heaton, R. K. (1981). *A manual for the Wisconsin Card Sorting Test*. Odessa, FL: Psychological Assessment Resources.
Heilman, K. M., & Valenstein, E. (1985). *Clinical neuropsychology* (2nd ed.). New York: Oxford University Press.
Jastak, S., & Wilkinson, G. (1984). *The Wide Range Achievement Test—Revised: Administration manual*. Wilmington, DE: Jastak Associates.
Katz, M. M., & Lyerly, S. B. (1963). Methods for measuring adjustment and social behavior in the community. I. Rationale, description, discriminative validity and scale development. *Psychology Reports, 13*, 503–535.
Klonoff, P. S., & Lage, G. A. (1991). Narcissistic injury in patients with traumatic brain injury. *Journal of Head Trauma Rehabilitation, 6*, 11–21.
Klonoff, P. S., Lage, G. A., & Chiapello, D. A. (1993).Varieties of the catastrophic reaction to brain injury: A self-psychology perspective. *Bulletin of the Menninger Clinic, 57*, 227–241.
Klonoff, P. S., O'Brien, K. P., Prigatano, G.P., Chiapello, D. A., & Cunningham, M. (1989). Cognitive retraining after traumatic brain injury and its role in facilitating awareness. *Journal of Head Trauma Rehabilitation, 4*, 37–45.
Luria, A. R., Naydin, F. L., Tsvetkova, L. S., & Vinarsky, E. N. (1969). Restoration of higher cortical function following local brain injury. In P. J. Vinken & G. W. Bruyn (Eds.), *Handbook of clinical neurology* (Vol. 3, pp. 368–433). Amsterdam: North-Holland.
Osterrieth, P. A. (1944). Le test de copie d'une figure complexe: *Archives de Psychologie, 30*, 206–356; [J. Corwin & F. W. Bylsma, Trans., 1993] *The Clinical Neuropsychologist, 7*, 9–15.
Porteus, S. D. (1950). *The Porteus Maze Test and intelligence*. Palo Alto, CA: Pacific.
Prigatano, G. P. (1989). Bring it up in milieu: Toward effective traumatic brain injury rehabilitation interaction. *Rehabilitation Psychology, 34*, 135–144.
Prigatano, G. P. (1992). Personality disturbances associated with traumatic brain injury. *Journal of Consulting and Clinical Psychology, 60*, 360–368.
Prigatano, G. P., with Fordyce, D. J., Zeiner, H. K., Roueche, J. R., Pepping, M., & Wood, B. C. (1986). *Neuropsychological rehabilitation after brain injury*. Baltimore: Johns Hopkins University Press.
Prigatano, G. P., Klonoff, P. S., O'Brien, K. P., Altman, I. M., Amin, K., Chiapello, D. A., Shepherd, J., Cunningham, M., & Mora, M. (1994). Productivity after neuropsychologically oriented, milieu rehabilitation. *Journal of Head Trauma Rehabilitation, 9*(1), 91–102.
Prigatano, G. P., Pepping, M., & Klonoff, P. S. (1986). Cognitive, personality and psychosocial factors in the neuropsychological assessment of brain-injured patients. In B. P. Uzzell & Y. Gross (Eds.), *Clinical neuropsychology of intervention* (pp. 135–166). Boston: Martinus Nijhoff.
Reitan, R. M., & Davison, L. A. (1974). *Clinical neuropsychology: Current status and applications*. Washington, DC: Winston.
Smith, A. (1982). *Symbol Digit Modalities Test manual—revised*. Los Angeles: Western Psychological Services.
Sohlberg, M. M., & Mateer, C. A. (1987). Effectiveness of an attention training program. *Journal of Clinical and Experimental Neuropsychology, 9*, 117–130.
Sohlberg, M. M., & Mateer, C. A. (1989). *Introduction to cognitive rehabilitation: Theory and practice*. New York: Guilford.
Spreen, O., & Benton, A. L. (1969). *Neurosensory Centre Comprehensive Examination for Aphasia (NCCEA)*. Victoria, BC: University of Victoria Neuropsychological Laboratory.
Stroop, J. R. (1935). Studies of interference in serial verbal reaction. *Journal of Experiemental Psychology, 18*, 643–662.
Wechsler, D. (1981). *Manual for the WAIS–R*. New York: Psychological Corporation.
Wechsler, D. (1987). *Wechsler Memory Scale—Revised*. New York: The Psychological Corporation.
Wilson, B., & Patterson, K. (1990). Rehabilitation for cognitive impairment: Does cognitive psychology apply? *Applied Cognitive Psychology, 4*, 247–260.

9

The Role of Self-Regulation Therapy With the Brain-Injured Patient

Bruce K. Schefft
University of Cincinnati
James F. Malec
Mayo Clinic
Beverly K. Lehr
University of California, San Francisco
Frederick H. Kanfer
University of Illinois

The growing interest of neuropsychologists in methods of intervention has been accompanied by an increasing recognition of the potential utility of self-regulation procedures. Self-regulation refers to behavior sequences in which the individual actively participates in generating and maintaining newly learned responses. Self-regulation models and clinical strategies have enjoyed considerable popularity and success in application to neurologically normal patient groups, and in application to the brain-impaired patient has increased in recent years. The focus of this chapter is on the assessment, the theoretical foundations, and empirical support that surround the clinical application of self-regulation therapy with brain-injured (BI) patients.

We begin with a review of the many factors that influence the utilization of self-regulatory therapy with the patient. Subsequently, current types of psychological interventions used with BI patients that vary in their emphases on self-regulatory processes are critically reviewed. This is followed by a presentation of our self-regulation approach with a description of its clinical application and current status.

ASSESSMENT OF FACTORS AFFECTING SELF-REGULATION

Self-regulatory therapy is a nonlinear, iterative, and recursive process. In self-regulatory therapy, the initial assessment of the patient leads to systematic interventions that in turn reveal other patient characteristics or precipitate changes in the patient's behavior which require alterations of the therapeutic strategy. In this type of process, it is unrealistic to think that an initial evaluation will identify all factors that are critical for the success of therapeutic intervention. Nonetheless, initial therapeutic contacts and ongoing assessment will be enhanced by a thorough initial evaluation. The need for a thorough initial assessment is particularly critical for self-regulatory treatment with BI individuals, who typically present a complex of interrelated emotional, physical, cognitive, and behavioral impairments and disabilities.

Definitions

The International Classification of Impairments, Disabilities, and Handicaps (World Health Organization, 1980) recommends specific definitions to distinguish among *impairment, disability,* and *handicap.* ICIDH defines *impairment* as a limitation of a physical or mental function because of disease or injury. *Disability* is defined as the loss of the ability to participate in some activity because of an impairment. ICIDH further differentiates impairment and disability from *handicap,* which is a loss of a social role because of disability or impairment. According to the ICIDH schema, impairments do not necessarily lead to disabilities. The existence of handicap usually implies an environmental or social barrier. For instance, a paraplegic may overcome ambulatory impairment through the use of a wheelchair with the net result of virtually no disability in mobility. However, if the environment includes structures that are not wheelchair-accessible, the individual will be handicapped.

The distinction between impairment and disability is particularly relevant to a discussion of self-regulation, because some form of self-regulation is frequently the element that allows individuals to minimize disability despite significant impairments. For example, following BI, an individual may experience significant memory impairment. However, if that person is able to learn appropriate self-regulatory skills to systematically use a memory notebook to compensate for this memory impairment (Sohlberg & Mateer, 1989b), the impact of the memory impairment on her or his daily life may be minimal, resulting in little effective disability.

The concept of handicap is also relevant to the practice of self-regulatory therapy with individuals with BI. Cognitive impairment may be handicapping in therapy, creating barriers to a therapeutic process. However, a knowledgeable therapist can assist the patient in reducing this handicap by using special techniques to be described in this chapter. A working knowledge of the patient's cognitive strengths and weaknesses will assist the therapist to determine appropriate therapeutic tasks and goals for the patient. In some cases, specific interventions to improve or to assist the patient to compensate for cognitive impairments may be required before a therapeutic process directed at improving self-regulation will be effective.

POTENTIAL DISABILITIES AND HANDICAPS

Impairments following BI may: (a) precipitate distress, (b) lead to behavioral disability, (c) directly interfere with self-regulation, (d) interfere with attempts to improve self-regulatory capacities, (e) interfere with social support and adjustment, or any combination thereof. The potential for a kind of negative synergism among these five potential results of impairment is clear. Increased distress may further interfere with self-regulation through immobilizing depression, anger, or anxiety. Anxiety, depression, and anger may also exacerbate cognitive impairments and associated disabilities and contribute to social handicaps. Increased distress may increase behavioral disability, decrease social adjustment, and further decrease self-regulatory capacities. Conversely, increased disability, decreased social support and adjustment, and decreased self-regulatory capacity will increase distress.

This negative synergism is often described subjectively by patients as "a vicious circle" or "spinning out of control." Although such self-perpetuating destructive processes are familiar to most therapists working with non-BI individuals, such processes can be more complex for BI patients. To understand this complexity, additional clinical elements must be considered in evaluating BI patients for treatment. For instance, in assessing non-BI individuals, it is assumed that limited self-regulation is a consequence of inadequate prior learning experiences that may be exacerbated by current distress. In contrast, impaired self-regulation in BI individuals may be a direct consequence of the BI instead of, or in addition to, inadequate prior learning and current distress.

Kay's Model

Kay, Newman, Cavallo, Ezrachi, and Resnick (1992) and Kay (1993) have proposed a neuropsychological model for functional disability following mild traumatic BI (see Fig. 9.1). Kay's model illustrates the negatively synergistic relationships among neurological, physical, and psychological factors in creating disability following mild BI. In mild BI, neurologic and associated objective cognitive factors leading to disability often disappear during the first few months after injury. The potential for these elements to have minimal impact on psychological experience and functional disability after the first few months postinjury is illustrated by dashed lines in the model. However, as the model indicates, psychological factors, such as distress and a susceptible personality structure, may lead to a subjective sense of impaired cognition that in turn feeds back to exacerbate psychological factors that contribute to, or sustain, functional disability. Additionally, the existence of disability feeds back through the personal system, causing increased distress and confirming the subjective sense of impaired cognition.

With only minor modification, Kay's model may be applied to moderate and severe BI as well as to mild BI. In moderate and severe BI, neurological and objective cognitive factors may remain active in the model in the long term, contributing to the prolonged impact of psychological and subjective cognitive factors on functional disability. The potential for perceived disability to increase subjective distress and subjective cognitive impairment also remains. Kay (personal communication, Winter, 1994) suggests that in the individual case, regardless of severity of injury, the relative contribution of each component of the model to

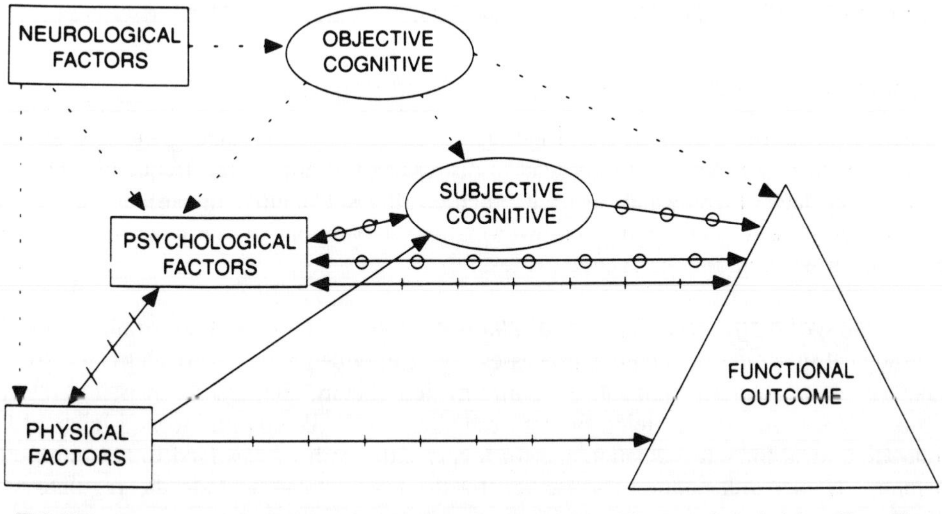

FIG. 9.1. A neuropsychological model of functional outcome after mild traumatic brain injury. From Kay (1993). ©1993 by Aspen Publishers, Inc. Reprinted with permission.

the functional outcome should be evaluated. This type of assessment will result in a profile for each patient in terms of components of the model that will assist in determining the most appropriate clinical intervention.

TARGET AREAS FOR BEHAVIORAL ASSESSMENT

The initial assessment of an individual with BI should examine for impairment, disability, and handicap in a number of areas in both the intrapersonal and the social domains. The following sections review the most commonly recommended areas for such assessment.

Physical Impairments and Disabilities

A variety of physical impairments caused by BI may result in distress and interfere with valued activities (i.e., lead to disability or handicap). With more severe injuries, severe impairments in ambulation and manual dexterity may be present. Even in mild and moderate injuries, bilateral coordinated movements may become difficult and disturbances of gait and fine motor skills may occur. Lip and tongue movements that are necessary for speech articulation are arguably some of the most complex movements the human body is required to make. Even mild BI may result in articulatory impairment that either interferes with communication or causes changes in the quality of the voice that are distressing to the patient because he or she "no longer sounds like me." In evaluating speech problems, it is important for the clinician to determine whether such motorically based articulatory problems are associated with language impairment or other higher level communication disabilities.

In traumatic BI, the frequency of frontal brain trauma is associated with frequent damage to the olfactory bulbs, causing reduced smell and taste. Visual impairments may occur either because of direct damage to visual centers in the brain or because of damage to peripheral nerves regulating eye coordination. In the latter case, disturbances such as diplopia may occur.

An additional physical impairment that merits particular note is posttraumatic pain. Posttraumatic pain, which most frequently occurs as posttraumatic headache, may at times become totally disabling so that it interferes with basic self-regulatory capacities in addition to causing distress and disability. Posttraumatic headache frequently frustrates both pharmacologic and behavioral attempts to provide symptomatic (or distress) amelioration.

Cognitive Impairments—Related Disabilities and Handicaps

Cognitive impairments after BI are of particular concern in self-regulatory therapy because these types of impairments not only lead to distress and disability, but frequently interfere with self-regulatory therapy and other rehabilitation efforts. Cognitive impairments should be thoroughly assessed to allow the therapist to tailor interventions to minimize the impact of these impairments on the therapeutic process.

Neuropsychology and Functional Neuroanatomy. Only a short summary of the neurological substrates of cognitive processes can be provided here. The reader is referred to other volumes for more comprehensive information (Levin, Benton, & Grossman, 1982; Lezak, 1983; Luria, 1973; Meier, Benton, & Diller, 1987). Briefly, the frontal lobes of the brain are critical for self-regulation and for higher order abilities involved in reasoning and planning. Higher order abilities subserved by the frontal lobes include the regulation of attention and the integration of new information for memory storage.

Although the frontal brain system plays an important role in both memory and attention, other brain structures are more basic to these processes. The reticular activating system, near the base of the brain, is the primary mechanism supporting arousal, alertness, and attention. The hippocampi, residing deep in the temporal lobes on both sides of the brain, and the diencephalon, including the thalamic structures, are critical to developing new memories. The parietal and occipital cortices are primary to sensation and perception. Simply put, information acquired through the sense organs is received and integrated in the posterior brain and then fed forward to be further integrated by the anterior brain into an action plan. At the same time, this information begins to be processed through the hippocampi for memory storage. For most people, the left hemisphere of the brain is the primary processor for verbal information, whereas the right hemisphere of the brain is primarily responsible for nonverbal information processing.

In cases of traumatic BI, especially those sustained in motor vehicle accidents, frontal and anterior temporal brain regions are most likely to be injured due to mechanical force factors that cause scraping of the brain against the rough inside surface of the skull (contusions). Stretching and shearing forces throughout the brain during traumatic BI often also may cause diffuse axonal injuries which partially disconnect the brain stem systems that are necessary for alertness and attention (reticular activating system) from the frontal lobe integrative and regulatory system.

Attentional Impairments. The capacity to attend and concentrate is frequently impaired after BI. Sohlberg and Mateer (1989a) identified a number of dimensions within this area of impairment. *Focused attention,* for instance, to a digit repetition or alphabet recitation task, may be impaired. More frequently after mild BI, attentional focusing is preserved, but impairments of more complex attentional processes that are required for *selective, alternating, divided,* and *sustained attentional skills* are present. Selective attention is the ability to focus on a stimulus while disregarding irrelevant and distracting stimuli in the environment. Alternating attention is the ability to rapidly shift attention between two stimulus sets. Divided attention is the process of simultaneously attending to two stimulus sets. Sustained attention identifies the process of maintaining appropriate focus to a changing set of stimuli over an extended period of time.

Ponsford and Kinsella (1992) have shown that, after severe BI, individuals do not make more attentional errors, but are slower in performance than demographically similar normals. These investigators conclude that the various types of deficits in complex attention noted clinically are all related to a fundamental impairment in speed of information processing. Thus "attentional deficits" that have been traditionally observed among individuals with BI may be more aptly described as "intentional deficits." That is, individuals with BI are able to adequately focus and sustain attention to perceptual information, but have difficulty organizing and effecting an appropriate response on a timely basis.

Attention: Disabilities and Handicaps. From the perspective of the patient, whether impairment is attentional or intentional in nature is primarily an academic question. Whether because of poorly regulated attention or slowness of response, individuals with BI find that they are unable to perform adequately at tasks that require speed, timely response, or frequent shifting of response. Such impairments lead to significant disabilities in activities such as communicating in noisy environments or in the context of multiple conversations; reliably performing rapid, repetitive tasks, such as supermarket checking; taking an order being made under the highly distracting environment of a fast-food restaurant; alternately responding to household chores and children's demands; or alternately responding to a counter customer at a convenience store and the adolescents who are beginning to create a disturbance at the magazine rack. Subtle attentional impairments may be less apparent in the distraction-free, highly structured, and highly cued context in which self-regulatory therapy occurs than in the patient's everyday life. Nonetheless a skilled therapist will need to be sensitive to the patient's capacity to attend in order to prevent attentional impairments from becoming a significant handicap in therapy.

Memorial Impairment. Memorial impairment is perhaps the most frequent complaint of BI patients and their families. Disorders of recent memory may be distinguished from those that include impairment of both *recent* and *remote memory.* Recent memory is the ability to learn and retain new information. Remote memory is the ability to access information that has been overlearned over many years. An important distinction can also be made between *procedural* and *declarative memory.* Declarative memory is the ability to recall circumscribed, often linguistic, information. Most memory tests, such as recall tests of stories, figural designs, or word lists, assess declarative memory. Procedural memory is the ability to learn a skill. More frequently assessed through functional than through psychometric evaluation, procedural memory may be evaluated, for instance, by noting the degree to which a patient's performance on a motor-skills task (e.g., a pegboard task or a videogame) improves from day to day. If the person can begin performing such a task at the level that she or he quit performing the task on the previous day, relatively intact procedural memory is inferred.

Memory: Disabilities and Handicaps. In many cases, remote memory is preserved after BI. Because for adults verbal intelligence is heavily influenced by prior learning, many BI individuals with significant cognitive impairments nonetheless demonstrate a fund of information, vocabulary knowledge, and other elements of measured verbal intelligence that are within the average range (N. Brooks, 1989; Malec, Machulda, & Smigielski, 1993). This intact store of information may offer an area of competency that is useful to the individual in compensating for other cognitive impairments.

Procedural memory may remain intact even in cases of severely compromised declarative memory. Glisky and Schachter (1986) have described cases in which patients who were totally amnestic, in terms of declarative memory, were able to learn the relatively complex procedure of computer data entry. This type of domain-specific learning has potential application in self-regulatory therapy. In our Brain Injury Outpatient Rehabilitation Program, we have seen a dramatic case of a young woman with BI who was able to learn the procedure of responding to her negative self-statements with an immediate retort of a more accurate and positive self-statement, even though here inability to describe this procedure to others confirmed an absence of declarative memory for the procedure.

In some cases, neuropsychological evaluation reveals that a memory disability is primarily due to impairment of attention. A memory disability may also be secondary to higher order cognitive impairments affecting the ability to integrate and consolidate new information for memory storage. Therefore, memory disorders that are *secondary* to attentional or organizational impairment may be distinguished from *primary* memory disorders in which fundamental memory storage and retrieval processes are impaired, presumably in association with damage to primary memory (i.e., mesial temporal or diencephalic structures). In secondary memory disorders, the individual may show improved learning and retention of new information if his or her attention and organizational activity during learning is facilitated through environmental or self-regulatory interventions.

Language Impairment: Communication Disabilities/Handicaps. Because of the typically frontal brain trauma occurring in traumatic BI, primary language impairment, or *aphasia,* is less common following traumatic BI than it is in more lateralized brain lesions resulting, for instance, from stroke. Even in the absence of aphasia after BI, secondary communication disabilities may be present in association with impaired word finding or impairments in formulating and organizing thoughts. Appropriate self-regulation of the communication process may also be compromised, resulting in social communication disabilities. At one extreme, the BI individual may be limited in the initiation of communication. At the other extreme, he or she may be garrulous, poorly organized, tangential, and rambling in his or her verbalizations. Social communication skills have been collectively described as the *pragmatics* of communication (Prutting & Kirchner, 1987). Pragmatic communication skills that may be compromised after BI additionally include sensitivity to both verbal and nonverbal interpersonal cues, nonverbal and gestural aspects of expressive communication, voice prosody, and turn taking.

Visuospatial Impairment and Disabilities. Visual-perceptual and constructional abilities are also less frequently impaired after traumatic BI than after lateralized brain damage. When these or peripheral visual disturbances occur, they can create barriers to valued activities, such as, constructional, assembly, and mechanical work; route finding; or driving. In the interpersonal domain, visual and visual-perceptual impairments may interfere with accurate perception of nonverbal emotional cues, resulting in significant social disabilities.

Impairment of Higher Order Abilities. As mentioned previously, the frontal lobes have been implicated as critical for abstract reasoning and other higher order executive cognitive functions involved in novel problem solving (Cicerone & Giacino, 1992; Stuss & Benson, 1986). Because of the frequency of frontal lobe damage in BI, impairment of abstract abilities, reasoning, and novel problem solving is common.

Guilford (1967) has made a useful distinction between *divergent thinking* and *convergent thinking*. Both underlie the reasoning and problem-solving process. Following BI, patients may show prominent impairment in one or both of these critical processes. *Divergent thinking* is the ability to develop a number of alternative solutions to a novel problem, as in brainstorming. *Convergent thinking* is the subsequent process of prioritizing the alternative solutions in order to select the single solution with the greatest probability of leading to a successful resolution of the problem.

Higher Order Abilities: Disabilities and Handicaps. The process of divergent–convergent reasoning may be automatic in many non-BI patients involved in self-regulatory therapy, and consequently taken for granted. However, these basic reasoning processes often need to be prompted and systematically guided in working with a BI patient. Impairment of higher order, abstract abilities may create another barrier to self-regulatory therapy. A BI patient may simply be unable to work at a conceptual level in self-regulatory therapy and consequently be unable to grasp the therapist's "models" for self-regulation or other therapeutic interventions at a conceptual level. Instead, the BI patient may require numerous concrete examples and behavioral exercises, as more constructively self-regulatory behaviors are built behaviorally from the "bottom up" rather than conceptually from the "top down."

Related to impairment in abstraction is a common limitation in the ability to generalize learning from one situation to another. Learning that is demonstrated during self-regulatory therapy may not be transferred to real life. This is not an uncommon problem even among self-regulatory therapy patients without BI. However, among BI patients, the solution to generalization problems is usually not adequately addressed by the standard exhortation to "plan for generalization." When one is working with BI patients, often no degree of "planning" will prevent a lack of generalization of learning. A failure to generalize behaviors from one situation to another often can be assumed. Following behavioral practice in the office or clinic setting, some retraining of the behavior in the problematic situation either by the therapist or by a therapeutic ally within the patient's family or social network must be a standard feature of self-regulatory therapy for BI patients with this type of cognitive impairment.

Emotional Impairments, Disabilities, and Handicaps. Individuals with BI may experience significant emotional distress that is characterized by feelings of anxiety, depression, or anger. In some cases, this distress may occur in reaction to perceived impairments. In other cases, impaired self-awareness (discussed later) interferes with accurate perception of BI-related impairments and mitigates emotional reactions. However, with the passage of time or with specific interventions, self-awareness and reactive emotional distress increase. Godfrey, Partridge, Knight, and Bishara (1993) documented this process and the reciprocal relationship between self-awareness and emotional distress. If memory of the aspects of the traumatic event associated with the injury is accessible, as is sometimes the case in mild traumatic BI, symptoms of a posttraumatic stress disorder may be present.

Although precise neural mechanisms are not completely understood, the organic impact of BI may also directly cause emotional disorders such as depression, episodes of anger or rage, and other experiences of limited emotional control. In such cases, pharmacologic treatment (O'Shanick, 1988; Zasler, 1992) may be a useful adjunct to self-regulatory therapy.

Behavioral Disabilities and Handicaps. As mentioned previously, cognitive and emotional dysfunction after BI may be associated with social communication disabilities. In some cases, social skill disabilities are severe. The patient's behavior may be frequently inappropriate and impulsive, at times self-centered and childish, and episodically moody, irritable, or aggressive. These types of behavioral changes are typically very distressing to the patient's spouse and family (D. Brooks, 1984; D. Brooks & Aughton, 1979; Brooks, Campsie, Symington, Beattie, & McKinlay, 1986; Florian, Katz, & Lahav, 1989; Godfrey, Knight, & Bishara, 1991; Lezak, 1978, 1986, 1988; Livingston, 1987, 1990) and are the most frequent barriers to the patient's successful return to work (Weddell, Oddy, & Jenkins, 1980).

In contrast to those patients whose behavior is primarily impulsive and inappropriate, another group of patients show severely limited behavioral initiation. *Abulia,* a syndrome characterized by a lack of appropriate behavioral and emotional response, is easily mistaken for depression, although such patients almost by definition experience little emotional distress. Working with the abulic patient toward more behavioral initiation and participation in activities can be extremely frustrating for therapists as well as for family and other social partners. Although there is no reliable intervention to reduce abulia, abulic patients may show more initiation in very highly valued activities. For instance, an abulic woman with BI in her 50s who had worked all her life frequently indicated during rehabilitation therapies that she wanted most of all to return to work. This woman became much more responsive and initiated much more frequently in a supported work setting than in any other therapeutic activity.

In many cases, behavioral disturbances are due to a complex of cognitive, emotional, and social factors. In some cases, however, it may be possible to identify specific cognitive impairments that underlie behavioral disturbances (Malec, 1984), such as impaired perception of verbal or nonverbal communications, impaired reasoning, impaired organization of communication, impaired shifting of attention or cognitive set, or memory impairment. An example is provided by a young adult woman whose behavior had deteriorated dramatically when she moved from residential to foster placement. Her disturbed behavior appeared primarily in reaction to her severely impaired new learning ability. The new environment presented an extreme challenge to her memory abilities. Frequent memory failures in the new environment resulted in significant distress and aggressive behavior toward her foster mother. With more frequent memory prompts and reminders from the foster mother, the patient quickly became more comfortable in the new environment and her behavior became more appropriate.

Behavioral disorders after BI are also regularly associated with dramatically impaired self-awareness. Cerebral neural mechanisms underlying this type of global *anosognosia,* or unawareness of illness and impairment, are described by McGlynn and Schacter (1989). Patients with impaired self-awareness typically base their actions and plans on an understanding of themselves that predates their injuries. Because their self-assessments do not consider current cognitive, behavioral, or emotional restrictions resulting from their injuries, their actions often appear to be grossly inappropriate. Impaired self-awareness may be the single most significant barrier to social and work adjustment following BI. Impaired self-awareness provides a significant obstacle to interventions directed at increasing self-regulatory behaviors and may preclude individual therapy directed at increasing self-regulation. Improvement in self-awareness and associated improvements in behavioral self-regulation often requires an intensive, multimodal rehabilitation approach based on group therapy. Such comprehensive-integrated outpatient BI rehabilitation utilizes peer and other types of direct feedback regarding personal behavior and its consequences (Ben-Yishay & Prigatano, 1990; Malec, Schafer, & Jacket, 1992; Malec, Smigielski, DePompolo, & Thompson, 1993; Prigatano, 1986; Smigielski, Malec, Thompson, & DePompolo, 1992).

More severe cognitive–behavioral abnormalities, such as hallucinations, paranoia, and delusions, may occur infrequently as a consequence of BI. These types of symptoms may respond to pharmacologic intervention.

Disabilities and Handicaps Involving Valued Activities. The disabilities and handicaps that are most distressing and discouraging to BI individuals are usually those that interfere with participation in valued routine self-care activities, such as dressing, hygiene, cooking, eating, and toileting. The inability to perform these tasks that have become automatic since early childhood undermine personal autonomy and independence and can be particularly distressing to patients and families. Other independent living skills, including driving and money management, may be restricted following BI. Lost valued activities also frequently include participation in work or school as well as independent leisure and recreational activities.

Some of the most valued activities that are disrupted after BI involve relationships with other people. Impairments, distress, and disability may interfere with relationships within the family as well as with friends and acquaintances. The distress that a disruption of a relationship causes within the context of that relationship can further contribute to the negative synergism of distress, impairment, and disability.

Patients may enter into a pattern of substance abuse or dependence in an attempt to reduce distress or to enhance social comfort and contact. Substance abuse will ultimately lead to increased disability, social maladjustment, and distress. Estimates are that between one-quarter to over one-half of persons involved in severe motor vehicle injuries are intoxicated at the time of injury (Lowenfels & Miller, 1984; Rimel, 1981). Therefore, the BI population likely also includes a substantial proportion of individuals with preinjury histories of substance abuse or dependency.

EVALUATION

In assessing areas of potential impairment, disability, and handicap, several other considerations are important. In addition to deficit areas, areas of strength should be noted. These areas often form the basis for further developing coping and compensation strategies. Additionally, an assessment that focuses solely on deficits can leave the patient, whose self-worth is already threatened by the effects of injury, feeling even more vulnerable and possibly worthless or hopeless.

With traumatic brain injuries, the initial assessment should consider the severity of the BI and the amount of time that has elapsed since injury. As rule of thumb, BI that results in coma of one-half hour or less with less than 24 hours of posttraumatic amnesia is classified as mild ("Definition," 1993; Kolb & Whishaw, 1990). BI with longer coma and posttraumatic amnesia is classified as moderate to severe.

As mentioned previously, objective cognitive impairments often resolve during the first few months after a mild BI. Objective cognitive impairments and self-awareness can be expected to significantly improve during the first 1 to 2 years after moderate to severe BI. Improvements in self-awareness and cognition may continue after the second year, although typically this resolution proceeds at a slower rate. This is not to imply that interventions should be delayed waiting for "spontaneous recovery" during the first 2 years. In general, patients who have had access to early rehabilitation have shown most successful outcomes in the long term (Cope, Cole, Hall, & Barkan, 1991; Malec, Smigielski et al., 1993). During the early period after injury, consistency of rehabilitative or psychotherapeutic interventions and prevention of psychosocial factors that exacerbate distress and disability may be more important than intense and focused psychological interventions. By comparison, impairments and disabilities that have resulted in a number of years of unsatisfactory adjustment following BI are likely to require intense, focused intervention for remediation. Finally, therapeutic planning will be facilitated by an assessment that differentiates between the relative extent to which the current distress and impairment are due primarily to the effects of injury rather than the preinjury effects attributable to personality or other personal, social, and environmental characteristics.

Patient Interview

An interview with the patient is a reasonable place to begin an assessment. However, impairments in cognition and self-awareness often interfere with the accuracy of a BI patient's self-report. In conducting an interview with a person with BI, the interviewer must be sensitive to impairments of attention, of memory, and of other cognitive abilities as described previously. The interviewer will need to quickly evaluate if the patient is paying attention before asking each question. Open-ended questions are very useful for interviewing but may be overly challenging for some patients who have difficulty conceptually or linguistically formulating thoughts. Such patients may require a series of questions about concrete situations to be able to communicate relevant aspects of their current situation. The interviewer will often need to allow BI patients extra time to formulate responses. An experienced examiner may find other creative ways to facilitate verbal or nonverbal communication in the interview with a BI patient.

Interviewers will always need to determine the reliability of information obtained from patients with memory problems. The behavior of some patients with severe memory or other cognitive problems is determined primarily by elements of his or her current environment rather than by memories or consistent concerns. Therefore, such patients may behave quite differently in the interview than in other contexts.

Psychological Tests

A patient's responses to self-report personality and cognitive measures may be helpful, particularly in milder injuries, to assess the degree of current psychological distress and maladaptive behavior. However, the results of these inventories may also either overestimate or underestimate current adjustment problems because of distortions resulting from impaired cognition and self-awareness. Although impaired self-awareness may be less problematic with projective measures, other cognitive and perceptual impairments may distort results toward signifying more disturbed adjustment than objectively exists. A neuropsychological evaluation (Malec, 1990), performed by a qualified neuropsychologist and including psychometric assessment of intellectual and cognitive abilities, will be necessary to clarify the intricate brain–cognitive–behavior relationships that must be understood before effective planning of self-regulatory therapy and rehabilitation with patients with BI can begin.

Interviews With Others

Direct behavioral observations of patients in medical or vocational rehabilitation settings or reports of the clinical observations of other professionals often are helpful in identifying problem areas of which the patient is unaware. Interviews with families or significant others can give a perspective of patients from individuals who observe them in intimate settings on a daily basis. The observations of families and significant others, however, should not be considered to be unbiased. Often, family members also are distressed by the patient's impairments and may respond to this distress either with exaggeration or minimization of the patient's cognitive deficits.

Mayo–Portland Adaptability Inventory

The Mayo–Portland Adaptability Inventory (MPAI; Malec & Thompson, 1994; see Appendix, this chapter) provides a useful checklist for the clinician to profile areas of BI-related impairment and disability. The MPAI is also a useful tool for collating the observations of a number of different professionals who have regular contact with the patient.

Patients and families sometimes feel that rehabilitation staff overemphasize the patient's cognitive impairments and are unaware of the patient's strengths in their assessments. Staff often feel patients and families tend to be unaware of or minimize cognitive impairments. We have recently developed versions of the MPAI that can be completed independently by the patient and by a family member or significant other. In reviewing results of the MPAI completed separately by staff, patients, and families on a small group of patients (n = 20) that have been evaluated to date, the somewhat different perspectives of staff, patients, and families on evaluation of the patient's situation are apparent (Malec & Machulda, 1994). Relative to staff, some patients exaggerate and some minimize their problems, just as some families exaggerate and some minimize the patient's impairments and disabilities. However, our MPAI data show no consistent trend for staff, patients, or families to differ in their overall ratings; that is, overall MPAI mean ratings for the group were not significantly different among these three types of raters.

TREATMENT MODELS OF PSYCHOTHERAPY WITH BI

Based on the review of factors affecting social adjustment and self-regulation after BI, a picture emerges not only of the many possible impairments related to BI but also of the many targets for intervention. Premorbid, psychosocial, and injury-related factors all contribute to the variability of disability after BI and to the amenability of specific cognitive impairments to treatment. Not surprisingly, psychotherapists have been reluctant to work with brain-injured adults due to the seemingly immutable nature of these individuals' problems. This attitude relates not only to the organic damage but perhaps also to a related sense of feeling overwhelmed by the range of problems. For example, the therapist might be confronted with an individual with a pre-existing personality disorder and associated family turmoil who now also has defects in such basic cognitive processes as perception and memory. Developing a therapeutic relationship and treatment goals with such an individual is often a challenging task even for the sophisticated clinician who is knowledgeable about brain injury and skilled in psychotherapy with BI patients.

Controversial Issues

The role of the patient in treatment is an issue that has recently assumed greater significance with the demand for more consumer-based rehabilitation programs. After the trauma, the patient often cannot participate in treatment due to coma or a confusional state and the medical team turns to the family for assistance. Consequently, family members become more involved in the patient's goal setting and treatment than the patient early in the rehabilitation program. As the patient improves and becomes better able to understand and communicate, he or she also becomes better able to participate in treatment planning. If there are conflicts about the direction that treatment should take between the patient and family or the patient and staff, there may need to be a determination of the patient's decisional capacity and ability to act on her own behalf in negotiating care. For example, the patient may insist on ambulating on the ward, even though the physical therapist has determined that the patient would be unsafe and needs to work on preambulation activities.

Another dilemma is created when the patient wishes to engage in sexual activity (perhaps with another patient) and there is a question about either patient's capacity to understand or engage in such behavior and to appreciate all the possible consequences. Because the patient is continuing to recover cognitively, the determination of decisional capacity is difficult and cannot be considered to be completed at one point in time; it must be ongoing. Consequently, it is a difficult therapeutic balancing act to help the patient to become more of an active treatment participant while guiding independent decisions. Therapists must guard against their own tendencies to be too protective or permissive so that the patient can resume duties and responsibilities as they are able. Some treatment teams utilize consultants (e.g., psychiatrists or psychologists) to evaluate a patient's decision-making capability. This can protect the team's therapeutic alliance with the patient, because the consultant is making the determination about the patient's cognitive status rather than the team. A significant limitation to this practice, however, is that the professional making the determination has had the least exposure to the patient and may not have the same information about the patient's background or recovery course as a team physician or psychologist.

Proactive models have been proposed for coordinating goal setting among the patient, family, and staff so that potential conflicts are identified at the beginning of treatment and ongoing dialogue is established between all parties (Becker, Abrams, & Onder, 1974; Malec, Smigielski, & DePompolo, 1991). Becker et al., for example, have described a process by which each party completes a goal sheet at the beginning of treatment so that the various expectations for recovery can be discussed openly, goals can be prioritized, and compromises between conflicting goals can be developed. Compromise is important so that all parties remain motivated and involved in the treatment process, although the patient and family may often feel that the rehabilitation staff are not being sufficiently optimistic about the patient's potential for recovery. The rehabilitation staff, in turn, may feel that the patient and family are not being realistic about the patient's likely residual cognitive deficits (McLaughlin & Carey, 1993). Malec et al. (1991) have developed a formal goal-setting process which improves the measurement of progress and the attainment of goals that can be utilized for ongoing treatment planning, communication about the patient's functioning to the patient and family, and for program evaluation.

Deciding to "empower" patients with mild cognitive impairment to be active members of their own treatment team is not a difficult choice. However, it becomes increasingly difficult to know how to empower patients when their cognitive impairments are much more severe or generalized. O'Hara and Harrell (1991), as one option, have addressed this in terms of providing severely impaired persons with structure and information so that they have some basic tools for better functioning and improved self-advocacy. For patients with lack of awareness of deficits and unrealistic expectations for long-term outcomes, the focus may need to shift to daily interactions and tasks over which they have more control and a greater possibility of acting successfully on their own behalf.

There is often the implicit assumption that the goal of treatment is to keep the family together and to send the patient home. This can also pose special problems for the treatment team. Because rehabilitation programs are structured for community discharge, there can often be intense pressure on family members to take the patient back into their home once the rehabilitation program is completed. Unfortunately for the family, this may not be the best outcome for them; however, they may have great difficulty expressing their concerns about placement options for their brain-injured family member to the treatment staff. For example, the family may not have functioned as a cohesive unit for many years. In addition, the BI patient is often perceived as a different person and the BI patient's priorities may have changed significantly since the injury. The family may be put in the position of trying to reincorporate someone who has become a stranger to them.

This dilemma is especially difficult for spouses who may feel trapped in the caregiving role (Lezak, 1978, 1988). There may be intense pressure on the spouse who may feel martyred and unappreciated. In terms of graded interventions for the family as a unit, there at least should be permission given to family members to discuss some of these possible areas of concern so they do not feel that options are being denied by the treatment team. While rehabilitation efforts are directed toward return of the patient to a noninstitutional setting, treatment staff should be sensitive to family concerns and ambivalence about living with a cognitively impaired family member.

Important factors for the rehabilitation staff to consider when planning for discharge include the type and amount of supervision that the patient will require, the medical needs of the patient, the behavioral management issues, daily or weekly activities of the patient (e.g., outpatient therapy, school, work), and the family's physical, emotional, and economic ability to provide for these needs (DePompei & Zarski, 1991). In addition, a premorbid history of problematic family relationships should be included. Therapy for the patient and the family can help to clarify the issues involved and help them come to a decision that they all can accept (Sachs, 1991).

The Psychotherapy Candidate: Selection Criteria

Special mention should be made of how psychotherapists determine who is appropriate for psychological therapy. Most agree that the BI patient needs adequate attentional and language skills in order to effectively participate in dialogue over the course of the session and to understand and stay focused on a given topic (Lewis & Rosenberg, 1990; Miller, 1993; O'Hara & Harrell, 1991; Prigatano, 1986). Beyond these points, variability emerges as to the cognitive and emotional skills that must be relatively intact in order for the clinician to consider therapy as a treatment option. Prigatano (1986), for example, described the following criteria that must be met in order for a patient to be considered appropriate for his neuropsychological rehabilitation program within which psychotherapy is a standard treatment component: (a) IQ not less than 75; (b) WAIS or WAIS–R Digit Symbol score not less than 5; (c) WMS Quotient not less than 75; (d) absence of psychotic disorder or severe characterological disturbance; (e) preserved ability to talk about painful issues and has intact motivation for treatment; and (f) has an ability to keep appointments and to engage in cognitive retraining and psychotherapeutic tasks. Lewis and Rosenberg (1990) outlined the following criteria for psychotherapy: (a) the patient is motivated to engage in psychotherapy; (b) has had one close, positive relationship in the past; (c) has had some attainment of success in their life through their own efforts; (d) does not have severe frontal lobe damage with associated behavioral changes of apathy, decreased awareness, perseveration, and impulsivity; (e) does not have extreme emotional distress that might require psychotropic medications and supportive therapy rather than psychotherapy; and (f) has preserved expressive and receptive linguistic abilities.

Although others have emphasized memory functioning as an important factor in assessing BI patients' appropriateness for therapy, Lewis and Rosenberg (1990) have found that even patients with severe memory or perceptual–motor deficits have substantially benefited from psychoanalytic psychotherapy. Others have defined even more stringent criteria for psychotherapy that include demonstration of adequate abstraction, generalization, and self-reflection abilities in order to benefit from the transference relationship (Miller, 1993). Clearly, criteria will vary depending on a clinician's treatment model and goals for therapy. However, there are indications that clinicians feel they are experiencing treatment success even with patients who show significant cognitive impairment. Therefore, a "trial" of therapy is probably recommended for BI patients whose suitability for psychotherapy cannot be clearly established during evaluation.

Therapy Approaches Prominent in BI Literature

Therapy approaches for treatment of BI patients are categorized broadly here in terms of the extend to which they require involvement of the patient's self-regulatory processes. For example, although traditional psychotherapy is not self-regulation therapy per se, it has features that are self-regulatory in nature. In contrast, pharmacotherapy does not have these features. Consequently, in this discussion, all psychological interventions are considered "therapy," although a distinction is made between those that emphasize self-regulatory processes and that directly involve the BI patient as a participant and those that do not place demands for self-regulation and direct involvement on the patient. Clearly, therapies that involve self-regulation may not be an appropriate treatment option for some BI patients at any point in their recovery, whereas other patients may progress through available psychological interventions as they improve.

Therapies That Are Not Self-Regulatory

Behavior Modification. The initial forays by psychologists into treatment of BI patients were not typically of a counseling nature but were more often developed from a behavior modification approach that altered the patient's environment to affect adaptive change. Regardless of the patient population, behavior modification follows a standardized process through which the patient and the environment are assessed and interventions are implemented (Wesolowski & Burke, 1988). Desired behaviors are identified as goals of treatment. The occurrences of the patient's targeted behaviors are measured to establish baseline frequencies. An analysis of environmental contingencies is conducted to clarify *antecedents* that are associated with certain patient responses (e.g., a noisy room is associated with a patient's outbursts) and *consequences* that reinforce and maintain them (e.g., a therapist attends to a patient primarily when inappropriate sexual remarks are made).

A behavioral intervention is developed that alters the environmental contingencies so that desirable behaviors are systematically reinforced and increase. The result of the intervention is evaluated by establishing the frequency of patient behaviors, desired and undesired, and by comparing this frequency to the baseline measurements. Generalization of the intervention is planned by carrying it out in the environment in which the patient will work or live or, if that is impossible, in the closest approximation to that environment to maximize learning generalization (Wesolowski & Burke, 1988).

When it is utilized in a preventive manner, behavior modification can increase the orderliness and predictability of a patient's responses to the environment as recovery takes place. It also enhances the emotional and cognitive functioning of that patient so that other treatments can be effectively delivered. For example, controlling such antecedents as the noise level in the patient's room and the tone of voice of staff can increase the probability that a patient will act calmly during morning nursing care. Ensuring that social attention is provided for appropriate behaviors can increase the likelihood that they will occur more frequently and consistently. Such contingent learning also establishes the predictability of the environment for the patient. This approach also helps to prevent a vicious cycle from developing in which staff primarily attend to a patient's disruptive behavior and then inadvertently ignore the patient's appropriate behavior.

Behavior modification also may be used to treat undesired patient behaviors that have become established during recovery or that have persisted prior to onset of the injury. Behavioral excesses, such as aggression, and behavioral deficits, such as lack of initiation, can be targeted for intervention. Problems that reflect behavioral excess are more likely to be treated because of the immediate difficulties that they pose for those persons who are living or working with the BI patient. Behavioral deficits, although better tolerated, can be equally problematic for the patient in terms of setting and accomplishing goals. The success of behavior modification can be seen in case reports and single case studies which have shown that BI patients respond appropriately to this type of behavioral intervention in increasing appropriate behavior and decreasing inappropriate behavior (e.g., Jacobs, 1993; Murphy, 1976).

Although clinicians are now beginning to utilize psychotherapeutic approaches (e.g., Miller, 1993), behavior modification remains an important psychological intervention methodology for the rehabilitation of BI patients (Eames, Haffey, & Cope, 1989; Hollon, 1973; Miller, 1993). Patients who are too disoriented or agitated to benefit from techniques involving verbal interchange (such as those patients who are emerging from coma) and patients who cannot assume full responsibility for their behavior (such as disinhibited and aggressive patients) can still be helped by this approach.

Pharmacotherapy. Although it is not a psychological intervention, pharmacotherapy is addressed here briefly because it is often an important treatment component in the management of BI patients' behavior disturbances and emotional lability. In BI patients, behavioral and emotional disturbances can be produced by a variety of factors including central nervous system (CNS) damage, metabolic and endocrine changes, withdrawal syndromes from substances of abuse, and side effects of treatments used acutely to stabilize them medically (O'Shanick, 1987). Pharmacotherapy attempts to restore normal functioning or homeostasis to the BI patient's neurophysiological milieu, and thus it can affect behavior change.

A close collaboration between the physician and the psychologist who are jointly responsible for the patient's treatment is essential for the successful management of difficult or potentially dangerous behavioral disturbances in the BI patient. This interactive collaboration can be especially effective in alleviating symptomatology in the BI patient (Eames, Haffey, & Cope, 1989). A review of possible drug interventions is beyond the scope of this chapter and the reader is referred to comprehensive reviews of this literature (Gualtieri, 1988; O'Shanick, 1988; Zasler, 1992).

Therapies That Improve Self-Regulation in Others Who Affect the Identified Patient

Family Therapy. Treatment directed at the patient's family members is another intervention approach that targets persons or situations that are external to the patient. Family interventions, including education, supportive counseling, and family therapy, have been components of the rehabilitation of the BI patient as family members also are in acute distress and in need of information and support (Muir, Rosenthal, & Diehl, 1990). The family is often confronted with a life-and-death situation in the emergency room and then maintains a vigil until their relative emerges from coma. The relief when this happens can be replaced by grief, anxiety, and anger as the profound trauma-related changes in their relative are appreciated (Grahame, 1991).

A number of models for family intervention have been proposed (e.g., Muir et al., 1990; Sachs, 1991; Williams & Kay, 1991). These models are based in family systems theory, which sees the family, not the individual, as the unit for assessment and intervention. It is assumed that family members are psychologically interdependent and that the effects of a change in one member will be felt by all. Even in the most stable families, a brain injury to one family member can have profound effects because of changes in role functioning, economic status, and social relationships.

Factors that influence the family therapist's choice of interventions and treatment strategies can include the premorbid psychological functioning of the family, their cultural and ethnic identity, the severity of the patient's brain injury, socioeconomic status, educational level of the family members, the stage of the family life cycle (e.g., young parents with an injured infant, middle-aged parents with a previously college-bound BI teenager), and the reaction of the family to the trauma (DePompei & Zarski, 1991). Themes to family intervention can include mourning the many losses related to the BI (e.g., permanent changes in the BI patient's personality, loss of the patient's role in the family), developing effective coping strategies for managing the initial crisis and the many long-term changes in the family, and reorganizing the family system to incorporate the new, brain-injured member (Muir et al., 1990; Sachs, 1991).

The type of intervention chosen will depend on the desired goals for a given family and their ability to participate in a particular type of treatment. Typically, most families will want or need education about BI so that they can reinforce the treatment team's efforts and make informed decisions.

When the severity of the patient's injury-related deficits is great, the direct behavior modification and supportive family therapy paradigms are the only approaches that can be utilized. Due to profound cognitive changes early in the course of recovery, many patients cannot be meaningfully engaged in their own change process. Providing a consistent, structured environment and supportive counseling and education to distressed family members is beneficial to the patient immediately, as he or she is provided with the best situation in which to recover, and in the future, as expectations have been set appropriately and family members have begun to develop skills in behavior management.

Although the family often receives some sort of counseling during the recovery process, the patient has been less routinely involved in these sessions. There have been various reasons for this, including the patient's cognitive impairments, which may impede interactions between the staff and family and may cause frequent interruptions to sessions. In addition, due to the patient's lack of awareness of deficits, staff and family may be reticent to discuss problematic areas in front of the patient because of the potential for eliciting an angry outburst from the patient (O'Hara & Harrell, 1991). However, there has been a movement to include the patient in family therapy sessions because the family system does include the patient and must accommodate to the changes in this person if this system is to retain him or her as a member. The decision to include the patient with the family in therapy sessions rests on the therapeutic judgment that the family, including the patient, can benefit from such an arrangement (Zarski & DePompei, 1991). As others have suggested (e.g., Miller, 1993), treatment of the entire family system can also be usefully directed at helping the system to accommodate to changes in an impaired member and may help to prevent problems such as other family members (e.g., children, siblings, or spouses) ignoring, inappropriately controlling, or unnecessarily protecting the BI patient.

Therapies That Reduce Factors That Interfere with Self-Regulation

Support and Information. Standard components of most psychotherapy approaches include education and emotional support, but these also are essential components on their own for providing BI patients with the necessary basis for interacting effectively with their environments (Miller, 1993; O'Hara & Harrell, 1991; Prigatano, 1986). It cannot be assumed that the patient has been exposed to important information about his mental and physical condition or that he will recall such information from previous interactions with staff. Patients' lack of current knowledge about their life situations and their mental and physical conditions can contribute significantly to inappropriate responding. Support and information can correct otherwise problematic misperceptions. Frequent and repeated demonstrations and explanations in terms that the patient can understand can be effective methods to help the patient to understand what has happened to her, where she is, and what treatment is being provided. In addition, emotional support should be provided to communicate reassurance and acceptance of the BI patient who may be feeling confused and frightened (O'Hara & Harrell, 1991). When combined with environmental stability and predictability, support and information provide the conditions that are necessary to permit the BI patient to make more effective use of self-regulatory strategies.

Substance Abuse Treatment. New theoretical models have been introduced recently that are having a significant impact on BI rehabilitation. Substance abuse is a common problem with BI patients and it is often a contributing factor to the accident that resulted in the brain injury (Reitan & Wolfson, 1986). However, a National Head Injury Foundation survey in 1988 did not find a single treatment facility that was systematically addressing this issue. Fortunately, this situation is beginning to change (Miller, 1993). Some facilities are beginning to incorporate substance abuse treatment as a standard component of rehabilitation. The psychological intervention is typically modeled after a form of CB therapy called *relapse prevention training* (Marlatt & Gordon, 1985). This approach helps the patient to identify high-risk situations, to develop coping behaviors to replace drinking in these situations, and to learn to manage relapses should they occur. The goal for substance abuse can be abstinence or legal substance use in moderation. The inclusion of substance abuse treatment components for BI patients may play both therapeutic and preventive roles.

Therapies That Improve the Identified Patient's Capacity for Self-Regulation

These approaches share the common element that the patient is involved, at least in part, in regulating his or her own behavior change process. Consequently, self-regulatory processes are involved. Typically, patients are seen in session with a therapist and the expectation is that they will carry some of the responsibility for their own behavioral learning by means of their in-session work and by carrying out whatever strategies or programs for change on which they have agreed. Although the targets for behavioral intervention may vary widely depending on the theoretical orientation of the therapist, there is an assumption that the patient has some capacity for negotiating these goals and the course of treatment. Therapy can occur individually, in a peer-group setting (e.g., other BI patients), or with family members.

Cognitive-Behavioral Therapy. Cognitive-behavioral (CB) therapy utilizes behavioral techniques within an ongoing therapeutic relationship. CB therapy is based in learning theory which proposes that a person's behavior is developed and maintained according to principles of operant and classical conditioning. The primary difference between behavior modification, discussed earlier, and CB therapy is the role that is assigned to the patient's cognitions and emotions. In behavior modification, environmental factors are considered to be responsible for changes in the person's behavior, whereas in CB therapy, the person's cognitions and emotions are considered to be of equal if not greater importance than these environmental factors in understanding the patient's behavior (Calhoun & Turner, 1981). The patient's cognitions and emotions are assumed to reflect self-regulatory processes by which he plans, executes, and evaluates his own behavior. These self-regulatory processes are then targeted for intervention in order to help the patient to gain greater control over his or her environment and to realize improved cognitive, emotional, and social functioning.

Although the brain-injury may have created obstacles to the change process (e.g., impaired memory, making skill learning more difficult), the underlying principles of behavior change are still considered to be valid. Patients are trained in the use of techniques such as accurate self-monitoring and realistic goal setting in order to build self-regulatory skills and to improve or correct deficits in cognitive, emotional, or social functioning. In addition, they are likely to undergo some form of coping skills training which helps them to prepare for and effectively deal with the numerous stressful situations that they are likely to encounter. This principle is illustrated by the description of a stress-inoculation procedure that was employed with a brain-injured man who had significant anger control problems (Lira, Carne, & Masri, 1983). His treatment was staged in three phases. The cognitive preparation phase provided him with an explanation for the function of anger and provided a rationale for treatment. He then was taught the stress-inoculation procedure, which involved making positive self-statements in order to counter and replace the negative self-statements and feelings that he was experiencing when he became angry. Finally, he was given opportunities in role play and in situations out of session to practice his new skills.

With respect to group intervention, Ben-Yishay and Lakin (1989) have described a format for CB therapy that involves the patient receiving feedback and advice from staff and peers. A staff person, working closely with the patient in the group session, helps titrate communications made to the patient and helps modulate the patient's emotional reactivity. Through this group process, the patient improves in her realistic awareness of her situation and in her ability to engage in appropriate social skills.

Dynamic Therapy. Psychodynamic psychotherapy has also been extended to intervention with BI patients (e.g., Leichtman, 1992; Lewis & Rosenberg, 1990; Stern, 1985). It is assumed that although the brain-injury may have caused cognitive and emotional deficits in the patient, it did not erase that patient's unconscious (Lewis & Rosenberg, 1990). It is also assumed that the previous level of psychological development and nature of intrapsychic conflicts will determine, along with the nature of the neurological insult, the patient's postinjury clinical presentation. From a psychodynamic point of view, patients who have a higher level of ego organization, with an accompanying improved sense of self and stronger ego functions (such as an improved ability to experience and cope with conflict), will present differently than those who have not achieved this level of psychological development. Clinicians from other theoretical frameworks are likely to agree with the general notion that patients with greater psychological resources prior to injury have an increased probability of a positive outcome postinjury, with all other factors such as the type of neurological insult being equal.

Although the nature of the patient's cognitive and emotional deficits is likely to dictate some modification of treatment delivery, the psychodynamic techniques of transference, interpretation, and catharsis are still employed by psychodynamic therapists and are felt to benefit BI patients in ways that are similar to their use with neurologically intact patients (Leichtman, 1992). The transference relationship in which the patient inappropriately projects feelings, attributes, and ideas from past relationships (especially parental) onto the therapist is felt to be an important vehicle for exploring the core psychological conflicts of the patient and for examining delays or failures of development in self-identity and relationships with others. BI patients also are believed by this group of theoreticians to be capable of benefiting from therapeutic interpretations that promote insight into these putative conflicts which can be amplified or redintegrated by the trauma of the brain injury (Klonoff & Lage, 1991). Finally, emotional catharsis techniques are used to help patients to release emotional conflicts and, in doing so, to experience relief and possibly better emotional control.

According to Lewis (1991a, 1991b), two issues dominate psychodynamic psychotherapy: anxiety and affect management, and self-esteem and identity. It has been noted that BI patients' sensitivity to distress can increase over time and that anxiety may appear postacutely when it had not been present immediately postinjury (Prigatano, 1992). Rather than being directly caused by the brain injury, these events may reflect the patient's reaction to the situation and problems in long-term adaptation. In terms of psychodynamic psychotherapy, the patient is assisted to make use of the anxiety as a signal that repressed psychological conflicts are emerging and one is encouraged to explore the meaning behind the experience of anxiety. It is felt that once the conflict is identified and worked through, the anxiety will dissipate.

Affect management refers to the broader goal of helping the patient to develop an improved ability to experience and modulate emotion. Instead of distracting patients when they are distressed and redirecting them to another topic, Lewis and Rosenberg (1990) recommended helping patients to reflect on and adaptively use their painful emotions as they experience them. Distraction and redirection are used only for catastrophic reactions that require de-escalation.

By focusing on self-esteem and identity issues, the psychodynamic psychotherapist hopes to help the patient to develop a realistic self-concept. This goal is accomplished in part by having the patient recognize the commonalities between his preinjury and postinjury "selves" while mourning the loss of those preinjury characteristics that will likely never return (Stern, 1985). By developing a positive relationship with the therapist, the patient can idealize this individual and attribute many positive qualities to him or her. The patient's self-esteem is raised when he begins to identify with the idealized therapist, starts to see the two of them as alike, and incorporates into his self-identity the positive qualities once attributed only to the therapist.

Self-Awareness/Existential. Prigatano (1986, 1991a) has developed a rehabilitative approach to BI patients within which psychotherapy occurs. Although Prigatano's psychotherapy approach has been conceptualized as supportive counseling within a dynamic framework (Christensen & Rosenberg, 1991), he described a more eclectic approach that also utilizes behavioral management techniques. The therapeutic goals are consistent with an existential approach. According to Prigatano (1986), successful therapy would result in the patient objectively viewing and accepting her impaired cognitive status, finding a meaning and commitment to life, and developing a realistic hope for the future. Although treatment can target a variety of impairments for improvement, the patient needs to regain a feeling of being worthwhile as an individual. Toward this end, Prigatano (1991a) has suggested that work, love, and play become important symbols in the patient's treatment because these are avenues for increasing a sense of meaningfulness.

Prigatano (1986) recommended both individual and group psychotherapy for addressing these issues. Private contact with the therapist provided in individual psychotherapy is viewed as necessary because BI patients are so unique in their particular constellations of premorbid personality, psychosocial situation, and injury-related characteristics. Group therapy is recommended to address interpersonal behavior and the commonalities of BI experiences, and to discuss and learn to cope with catastrophic reactions as they occur in a group. Awareness of BI deficits is addressed throughout group treatment as patients examine their in-group behavior and discuss their own and their families' reactions to their cognitive deficits after brain injury.

The use of symbolism figures importantly into Prigatano's (1986) approaches for individual and group psychotherapy. Because of diminished capacity for abstract reasoning, Prigatano feels that therapists may underutilize symbolic methods, such as art and music, with BI patients. He has illustrated through case reports that BI patients can communicate through songs, poetry, and paintings the psychological issues that they might otherwise have difficulty discussing in a therapy session.

Empowerment Approach. Also newly emerging is the empowerment rehabilitation model proposed by O'Hara and Harrell (1991). BI support groups, such as the National Head Injury Foundation, were originally conceived as self-help groups for family members. In the rehabilitation literature there has been a growing awareness that the consumer, in this case the BI patient, must play a central role in the treatment rather than being only a passive recipient of interventions.

O'Hara and Harrell (1991) have presented an advocacy model for treatment that focuses on helping the BI patient overcome his victim status (as a victim of BI), regain internal control, and redefine himself as a survivor. Called *empowerment rehabilitation,* they have identified its components as structure, information, acceptance, skills, and motivation. Although it can be used in a variety of ways in a rehabilitation program, its emphasis in psychotherapy is to facilitate emotional recovery. *Structure* is provided at the beginning of therapy in the form of a written contract (if the patient is able to understand this) to identify the boundaries of therapy, expectations for participation, the responsibilities of the patient and the therapist, and treatment goals. *Information* is given to the patient not only about their condition but about the choices and control they have. The therapist may train involved staff and family members about how to negotiate with the patient by providing choices and lessening dependency.

In this model, *acceptance* refers to the patient's acceptance of a new postinjury identity. Even severely impaired BI patients are believed to be able to go through the process of perceiving their losses as well as development of a new sense of self. The *skills* component focuses on enhancing self-awareness and developing coping skills for improved long-term adjustment. Finally, *motivation* addresses the patient's desire and ability to adaptively change their behavior. O'Hara and Harell feel that the therapist provides external reinforcement for change and eventually identifies the BI patient's hopes and goals that will provide internal motivation. Although many of these components overlap with other therapy approaches, unique features of this approach appear to be its emphasis on self-advocacy and its ability to be adapted to treatment of even severely injured patients.

Therapy Modifications for BI Patients

All treatment models that emphasize self-regulatory processes have had to adapt interventions because of the BI patient's unique behavioral, cognitive, physical, and emotional limitations. Although different therapeutic approaches may have different goals and different means for achieving them, common modifications have been proposed by each group of therapists and theorists to adapt the traditional form of therapy to the needs of the BI patient. In traditional therapy, if patients fail to do assigned homework, forget important information from one session to the next, or miss sessions, issues of motivation, denial, or repression are raised as possible explanations. With the BI patient, it is often difficult to separate the behavioral deficits from their neurological bases. Consequently, some modifications of common therapy structures may be needed to minimize the negative impact of BI deficits on treatment progress.

In the discussion that follows, specific psychotherapy approaches are only mentioned if they would recommend a departure from what is generally proposed. It should be noted that a number of the recommended modifications for treatment could apply to a wide variety of disciplines that work with BI patients (e.g., occupational therapy, physical therapy), but as they are presented here, they are intended for the delivery of psychological therapy for BI patients.

Identification of "Client"/Treatment Format. The question, "Who should participate in treatment?" is a special consideration given the variability among BI patients in their capacity to communicate, understand, remember, and make decisions. When the BI patient is unable to participate because of the inability to comprehend and communicate with others, significant others should be involved in treatment for their own personal needs (e.g., grieving the loss of a partner or dealing with the often-associated lifestyle changes after BI) as well as for the patient's needs (e.g., learning behavior-modification techniques to enhance the patient's adaptive functioning at home). Even when the patient can participate in treatment, it may still be beneficial to include a significant other. This person can serve many functions, including that of reliable observer and historian (although certainly the therapist needs to be mindful of the potential for biased reporting). The significant other can also function as the patient's source of "working memory" for what was discussed in the session, and can assist in the use and generalization of change strategies between sessions. The significant other can benefit by observing an effective interactional style that is modeled by the therapist with the BI patient and can be sensitized to the patient's unique constellation of neuropsychological strengths, weaknesses, and conflicts.

Significant others can also be included with the patient if treatment focuses on the patient's important social relationships, which is consistent with a family systems approach. For example, a husband and wife may be treated in couples therapy to confront the changes in their lives after brain injury. How this injury impacts their relationship, whether their marriage can withstand these changes, and their future plans are among the issues to be explored. The clinician may also wish to consider friends of the patient for inclusion in treatment. If the patient permits this, such involvement can serve both educational and treatment goals. At the very least, information about the patient's condition may enhance understanding and acceptance of the patient postinjury and may help to maintain relationships. Inclusion of the patient's friends can be important in some instances. For example, if friends encouraged or condoned substance abuse in the patient preinjury and are likely to remain a significant influence in the patient's life postinjury, their involvement in treatment may be very important so that this destabilizing influence can be effectively confronted and corrected.

Whether a patient should be treated individually or in a group of peers is another issue for the therapist to consider. Group therapy can be very useful, because there are some treatment issues that may be more effectively dealt with in a peer group, such as denial and lack of awareness of deficits. The BI patient may be more receptive to feedback from others that they perceive to be in similar circumstances. If the patient can engage in conversational turn taking, can attend adequately for the length of the group meeting, and can derive some personal benefit from this format, then his inclusion should be considered. Prigatano (1986) has provided suggestions both for the structure of the group therapy session and for the progression of topics that could be covered in these sessions. He has recommended that the hour begin by stating the purpose of the group and by reviewing the difficulties in doing psychotherapy with BI patients (e.g., impaired memory that affects carryover between sessions) so that these problems are openly and regularly discussed in the group. The group work then begins and can focus on a scheduled topic such as denial of illness, sexual dysfunction, or social isolation, or on an issue that has been presented by the members.

Yalom's (1983) recommendations for group sessions with lower functioning psychiatric inpatients (e.g., psychotic patients) may also have relevance for group work with BI patients whose communication skills and interpersonal behaviors are poor and prevent social interactions except in highly structured situations. Yalom's outline for a session includes an orientation to the group's structure and purpose, a warm-up exercise (e.g., a brief relaxation procedure) as an "ice breaker" for group members, structured exercises designed to facilitate self-disclosure and empathy, and then a review of the session. Offering two levels of group therapy to BI patients can be a useful approach. At the lower level, initially a structured group could use this format not only to work on areas of personal concern, but also to improve social interactional skills. Eventually, these patients might then be shifted from the structured to a more freely interactional group to enhance therapeutic progress.

Session Structure/Therapist Behavior. Graded interventions are typically recommended. This involves an assessment of the type of psychological intervention that is most appropriate for the patient and the form that a therapeutic strategy should take in treatment. Important factors include the patient's willingness to engage in treatment as well as the ability to participate in cognitively and emotionally demanding treatment interventions. For example, Muir et al. (1990) adapted the PLISSIT model for sexuality treatment to BI patients. This approach grades psychological interventions on a continuum from those involving the least amount of commitment and effort on the part of the patient to those involving the most effort. PLISSIT stands for Permission, Limited Information, Specific Suggestions, and Intensive Therapy. Patients can be provided the opportunity to talk about matters of concern, they can be provided information about their condition, they can be given specific suggestions on ways to manage focal problems (e.g., shown deep-breathing techniques in order to interrupt or decrease episodes of emotional lability), or they can be engaged in psychotherapy. This continuum of interventions helps the therapist to accommodate to the patient's readiness for treatment. An easily distracted and agitated patient may simply be encouraged to express his distress in order to help that patient to feel understood by the therapist, even though he may not be able to tolerate a more active verbal interaction. Conversely, a patient may be at a point in recovery where she can discuss problems, tolerate potentially negative feedback, learn new strategies, and try them out between sessions. This person might then be offered psychotherapy.

Therapeutic strategies that are utilized within a given treatment approach may also need to be graded in order to enhance their successful utilization with BI patients. The strategy may need to be presented to the patient in small, sequential steps in order for the patient to understand it and master it most effectively. For example, in social skills training, a neurologically intact individual may be able to work on several areas simultaneously, such as body language, verbal assertiveness, and active listening skills. However, the BI patient may need to work on these areas sequentially, and each area may need to be broken down further to make the tasks more discrete, specific, and manageable. Body language may be addressed in terms of physical hygiene, grooming, appearance of clothing, posture, facial expression, and physical movement.

Providing negative feedback to the patient is often a treatment strategy that has to be graded when it is used with BI patients. For example, a patient may not be able to tolerate hearing a negative statement from the therapist but could entertain a question that required reflection on potentially negative aspects of the current situation. Another patient might be able to listen to a therapist's negative statement as long as it was "balanced" by a positive statement. A patient with greater emotional control and cognitive abilities might be able to discuss at length and in detail some aspect of their condition or situation that was highly aversive (e.g., the poor prognosis for recovery of a particular deficit or the inability to return to a previous occupation).

Therapists also need to change their own in-session behavior to accommodate the patient's deficits and maximize the effectiveness of treatment interventions. More concrete feedback and fewer abstract concepts need to be introduced to the patient to foster clear communication and minimize confusion. Unstructured time (e.g., therapeutic silence) and open-ended questions are less likely to be utilized effectively by the patient because initiation of novel responses and tolerance of ambiguity may be reduced. For BI patients the session should be structured with a clear beginning, middle, and end, and the goals of treatment may need to be repeated because patients may be easily distracted and lose the focus of treatment. Consequently, the therapist has to be more directive in providing structure, prompts, and redirection to the patient. Therapy must also be more supportive than explorative in the early stages as the patient becomes acclimated to the demands of therapy.

Common Issues/Treatment Expectations. The therapist may need to alter expectations of the patient. Carry-over between sessions cannot be assumed and the therapist must be involved in helping the patient to utilize external memory aids that facilitate recall of important therapeutic issues and to facilitate execution of homework assignments. More time will have to be spent on treatment issues due to the need for repetition of information and the extended time that it may take to learn behavioral change strategies. There may be greater involvement of professional staff and family members to encourage progress on therapeutic goals and generalization of treatment gains, even if the patient is being seen individually.

One of the critical issues in treatment is to help the BI patient to develop emotional control. Rather than encouraging a BI patient to express emotions (when there may already be a problem with emotional lability), the therapist may need to select interventions to reduce emotional reactance and to teach the patient coping skills to control heightened affective arousal. Most approaches recommend graded feedback and gradual confrontation, rather than directly confronting the patient at a time of distress, to help foster emotional control. In a manner that is similar to neurologically intact patients who present emotional control problems, BI patients need to learn their signs of emotional arousal so that they can utilize therapeutic techniques for deescalation and for maintaining emotional stability when they are faced with a stressor. Techniques such as stress inoculation training, systematic desensitization, and relaxation training (Turner, Calhoun, & Adams, 1981) can help the patient to reduce their level of emotional distress and to learn more effective coping behaviors for managing life's difficulties.

SELF-REGULATION THERAPY: A MODEL AND CLINICAL STRATEGIES

The self-regulation approach we describe in this section grows from a body of empirical and conceptual work that has been developed with several different clinical populations, including psychiatric as well as some neurologic groups (cf. Kanfer, 1979, 1985; Schefft & Kanfer, 1986, 1987). This approach has been widely used in the treatment of neurotic disorders (Kanfer & Schefft, 1988). It has also been applied to the treatment of addictive behaviors (Kanfer, 1986), geriatric nursing home residents, cardiac rehabilitation patients (Lehr & Schefft, 1987), elderly rehabilitation patients (Schefft & Lehr, 1990, 1994) and Alzheimer's disease patients (Schefft & Zueck, 1987). The major emphasis of the approach is on helping the patient to share responsibility for the change process by participating actively in creating conditions that favor adaptive behavior change. A formulation of dysfunctional behavior together with a seven-stage treatment model are described. The model focuses heavily on motivation, response generalization, and maintenance as crucial processes in therapeutic behavior change.

In this section we describe the major features of this therapeutic model, including therapist style and strategies for facilitating clinical change with the BI patient. The major goal of this treatment approach is one of creating conditions that are favorable for the acquisition of new skills and behaviors which permit more effective cognitive, emotional, and behavioral control and independence for the patient in daily life situations. Utilization of self-regulatory techniques with commonly encountered clinical problems is presented and illustrated with reference to clinical case examples. Future directions for clinical practice and empirical research are then discussed in the context of a summary of the current status of self-regulation therapy for the brain-injured.

A Self-Regulation Model

Although the conceptual and empirical literature that documents the development and efficacy of psychotherapy is extensive (cf. Frank, 1985; Garfield & Bergin, 1994), little systematic attention has been paid to the application of psychotherapeutic strategies for BI patients (Cicerone, 1989; Horton & Barrett, 1988; Lewis, 1991a; Lewis & Rosenberg, 1990; Lovell & Starratt, 1992). Recent literature on psychotherapeutic intervention with brain-injured patients highlights the emerging interest of neuropsychologists in this area, which was forecast over a decade ago by Satz and Fletcher (1981) and Costa (1983). Putnam and DeLuca's (1990) review of professional practice in neuropsychology further confirms the growing interest of clinicians and researchers in psychotherapy for the neuropsychologically impaired.

Our application of the self-regulation model to the BI patient extends this emerging interest. The model is based on a blend of knowledge derived from both empirical work and practical clinical experience. It provides an organizing structure for selecting and sequencing strategies and methods that are needed to accomplish clinical change with the brain-injured patient. The model offers a systematic approach to therapeutic goals and tasks by which to attain these goals from the beginning to the end of treatment.

The potential utility of this approach for treating the brain-injured patient is underscored by three important elements that have been present in settings in which the approach has been previously used successfully. First, the patient comes to the attention of a health professional because of a dissatisfaction with his current behavioral coping state and the expectation that this behavioral dysfunction can be altered. The concept of change is therefore of critical importance to this approach, which emphasizes, as the central purpose of psychotherapy, a change form the current dysfunctional state toward a more desirable adaptive state. The second important element in self-regulation therapy is the continuous effort to stimulate patients toward self-direction and exercise of an active role in producing more desirable outcomes. The third element is the clinician's emphasis on flexibility and probabilistic thinking. Recognizing the multiple determinants of the diverse problems that patients present and the potential for multiple solutions, the self-regulation approach conceptualizes therapy as a dynamic, recursive, and iterative process that requires continual evaluation and adjustment of both goals and methods as the patient acquires new skills.

Sources of Behavioral Influence. Our perspective on the nature of dysfunctional behavior in brain injury is based on a recognition of the impact of three classes of variables: (a) environmental, (b) intrapersonal, and (c) biological. Dysfunctional behavior is considered to be the net result of the interactive effect of three classes of variables: (a) events that originate in the patient's social environment (environmental); (b) cognitive processes, which include perceptions, memories, expectations and other cognitions influenced by prior learning (intrapersonal); (c) contributions of the peripheral and central nervous systems and other biological systems that affect the relationship between brain and behavior (biological).

This probabilistic framework highlights the interaction of these three classes of variables and their constant change over time, recognizing that the relative contribution of each of these components will fluctuate in a patient across situations. The operation of these variables can be illustrated by the case of Mr. P., a patient who had a traumatic brain injury 18 years ago with a coma of 4 weeks and posttraumatic amnesia of over 3 months. On presentation for treatment, he showed a proclivity for becoming enraged at motorists who were not courteous to him both in his role as a pedestrian and as a driver. He reported numerous situations in which he chased motorists in a heated rage, eventually engaging in verbal and physical aggression, the unfortunate outcome of which, in hindsight, he invariably regretted.

In this case, we would view the environmental variables as the presence of a motorist who acts in ways perceived as discourteous and insensitive. The intrapersonal variables might include cognitions and self-reactions such as "How dare he cut me off like this!" or "How dare he tailgate me!" along with other cognitive responses that represent Mr. P.'s resources for coping with emotionally arousing and unpleasant situations. The biological variables would be represented by the behavioral loss of control he experiences as a result of severe closed head-injury and consequent lesions to the fronto-temporal regions bilaterally, decreasing the regulatory influence Mr. P. can exercise over limbic-generated emotional arousal. The environmental, intrapersonal, and biological variables interact to escalate the intensity of the response and nature of the dysfunctional behavior. For example, the presence of a discourteous motorist may trigger Mr. P.'s memories of unpleasant previous experiences in similar circumstances. The limbic activity that attends these cognitions may facilitate development of maladaptive self-generated cognitions which heighten limbic activity already poorly modulated by Mr. P.'s compromised frontal lobes (cf. Schefft, Moses, & Schmidt, 1985). Application of self-management techniques to treatment of the cognitive deficits and maladaptive behavior of this patient is presented in a subsequent section of this chapter.

Automatic Versus Controlled Processing. Despite the dynamic and interactive complexity of environmental, intrapersonal, and biological variables in determining the nature of the dysfunctional behavior in question, our model suggests that there will be a considerable degree of predictability and consistency of the patient's dysfunctional behavior across similar circumstances. Although this implies a regularity in the connection between stimulus conditions and response outcomes, it also represents what we conceptualize as automatic and well-rehearsed stereotypic responding that has become habitual and overlearned with time.

In daily routines, *automatic responses* make up a necessary and effective repertoire for dealing with many routine situations. The habitual nature of these responses reduces cognitive demands, decreases response latency, and facilitates execution of daily routines. However, when a patient's automatic responses are elicited under inappropriate conditions, they constitute dysfunctional behavior. Automatic, overlearned, rigid motor and verbal responses that are part of a well-conditioned behavioral repertoire are difficult to alter. This is especially true for the brain-injured patient because the anatomic substrate for new learning, impulse control, and novel problem solving has been altered.

In contrast to automatic processing, *controlled processing* refers to behaviors that require novelty, attention, and nonstereotypic responding. A central concept for self-regulation therapy is that it involves cognitive behavior which demands continuous attention and choice making among alternatives (cf. Kirschenbaum, 1987). This controlled processing mode is required for the patient to effectively interrupt the dysfunctional automatic response patterns that result in commonly observed behavioral sequelae such as rigidity, depression, anxiety, and withdrawal. We have noted elsewhere:

> If a universal rule for therapy can be stated at all, it is that during the change process the client must be aided to produce verbal and motor behaviors in interactions and self-reactions that are predominantly non-stereotyped, relatively new, and initially low in frequency of occurrence and that have the characteristics of controlled processing. (Kanfer & Schefft, 1988, p. 45)

The distinction we have drawn between controlled and automatic processing reflects a well-established body of knowledge in the cognitive psychology literature (e.g., LaBerge, 1981; Posner & Snyder, 1975; Schneider & Shiffrin, 1977). Cognitive psychologists have long observed that the human cognitive system can engage in these two fundamental types of activities. Indeed, the distinction between these concepts also parallels a neuroscientific–anatomic model advanced by Mishkin and his coworkers (Mishkin, Malamut, & Bachevalier, 1984; Mishkin & Petri, 1984). These investigators have noted that learning can involve the human cognitive system as habits stored in the cortico–striatal system or as memories stored in the cortico–limbic system. One can conceptualize that the former system represents the anatomic substrate for automatic processing, whereas the latter may constitute the neuroanatomic basis for controlled processing. Mishkin's theoretical formulation has been used to interpret and understand distinctions that have been drawn between procedural knowledge and declarative knowledge (Kolb & Whishaw, 1990; Mishkin, 1993). In turn, the participation of the cortico–striatal and cerebellar systems has been empirically linked to procedural memory in numerous animal and human studies that examine lesion effects. Declarative memory has been linked through similar research efforts to the cortico–limbic system (Cohen & Squire, 1980; Goldberg & Barr, 1992; Moscovitch, 1992; Petri & Mishkin, 1994). These specific domains of knowledge suggest the possibility that although automatic processing may have parallels to procedural learning with similar anatomic substrates, controlled processing may reflect operation of the declarative memory system and the cortico–limbic substrate.

Our model suggests that controlled processes are activated when individual response sequences are interrupted and the patient must learn new behaviors. Control of cognitive and verbal responses becomes increasingly rule-governed as effortful and novel responses with a low initial probability of occurrence are generated with increasing facility during the therapeutic change process. Ultimately, newly learned responses, initiated by controlled processing, must become automatic so that complex intervening decisional behaviors are not continuously required for the patient to behave adaptively. The clinician therefore guides the patient through a process of disrupting and abandoning old automatic dysfunctional behavior sequences in favor of generating new, more adaptive, response patterns that become well-learned and stable with practice.

A Conceptual Framework for the Therapy Process

Self-regulation therapy involves a framework which systematically structures treatment so that automatic dysfunctional behavior sequences can be eliminated while new, initially difficult, but more adaptive response patterns can be gradually integrated into the patient's daily routine. The change process for the brain-injured patient will typically involve a correction of automatic and problematic behavior patterns for impulse control, emotional modulation, self-esteem, and negative affect such as depression and anxiety. Therapy can also involve the development of new skills related to the patient's goals and life pursuits.

We have developed a treatment model (Kanfer & Grimm, 1980; Kanfer & Schefft, 1987, 1988) that sequentially orders a series of phases in the treatment process, each of which is defined by several subgoals. The first four phases are intended to prepare the patient for the change process. Establishing a strong and effective therapeutic relationship together with building a commitment to the change process are the essential features addressed in these phases. The last three phases are focused on administering that aspect of therapy which is typically considered to be the treatment program per se. Specific skills focused on particular target behaviors are administered with gradual attention to response maintenance and generalization with eventual termination of therapeutic support. The phases, together with their related subgoals, are summarized in Table 9.1.

Several features about the conceptual framework should be noted. First, the phases are interrelated, overlapping, and nondiscrete aspects of treatment by design. The phases of therapy represent a dynamic and recursive model in which the effects of change efforts are carefully monitored in relation to intended effects, and corrections are made to increase the effectiveness of subsequent interventions. In this sense, the larger conceptual framework parallels the process of human self-regulation in which response outcomes are compared against goals, and future responding becomes altered by self-corrective feedback to maxi-

TABLE 9.1
The Seven Phases of Therapy and Their Goals

Phase	*Goals*
1. Role structuring and creating a therapeutic alliance	1. Facilitate the person's entry into the role of patient 2. Define patient and therapist roles including modes of treatment interactions, rules of conduct, and the patient's responsibility for change 3. Establish motivation to continue therapy 4. Form a working relationship by reducing the patient's reluctance to assume responsibility and developing control (by verbal impact of therapist) first over the patient's in-session behavior and gradually over outside-of-session activities 5. Model covert thinking behaviors and break up the patient's automatic cognitive and motor responses and shift to hypothesis-forming-and-testing approach
2. Developing a commitment for change	1. Reduce demoralization and increase confidence that change is possible 2. Prompt the patient to consider positive consequences of change 3. Relate possible goal options to the patient's values and beliefs by goal and value clarification 4. Develop new incentives for change and explore available options and their limits
3. The behavioral analysis	1. Engage the patient in refinement and restatement of problem definition and initial analysis of current and desired states 2. Collect data needed to resolve remaining questions about objectives and applicable methods 3. Re-evaluate role of therapist and best resources for change 4. Identify relevant functional relationships and their significance in target selection and treatment choice
4. Negotiating treatment objectives and methods	1. Seek agreement on problem areas 2. Establish priorities for change, specify change methods, and design program sequence 3. Negotiate a contract for initiation of a change procedure
5. Implementing treatment and maintaining motivation	1. Conduct treatment program 2. Assess effects on nontarget behaviors or persons 3. Initially encourage adherence to "learning aids" and problem-solving approach, gradually dropping out supports as new behaviors become automatic 4. Assess and maintain motivation to comply with program and contracts
6. Monitoring and evaluating progres	1. Monitor changes in patient and environment 2. Assess coping-skill increases and related effect on self and others 3. Use data to review and strengthen progress and reassess objectives and methods 4. Attend to new "natural" reinforcers that can promote or defeat change effort
7. Maintenance, generalization, and termination of treatment	1. Foster self-management skills for new and future problem situations 2. Initiate relapse-prevention procedures 3. Prepare for therapy termination and arrange for other supports or transient supports, if needed 4. Avoid exceeding "minimum intervention" and reduce reinforcement for patient role 5. Encourage acceptance of new situation and termination of therapeutic change process

From Kanfer and Schefft (1988). © 1988 by F. H. Kanfer and B. K. Schefft. Adapted by permission.

mize goal attainment on subsequent solution attempts (Kanfer, 1971; Schefft & Lehr, 1985). Implementation of the approach is therefore done in a problem-solving fashion with continual assessment of the patient's response to treatment efforts and corresponding adjustment of therapeutic goals and techniques. Second, although the conceptual framework is structured to recognize the dynamic recursive nature of treatment, it does underscore the importance of enhancing the patient's capacity to participate actively in treatment prior to the introduction of specific techniques that are intended to alter skills and behavior patterns. The essence of this view is captured by Marks' (1978) statement: "Both motivating and executing factors are crucial. An effective treatment is of little use if patients cannot be motivated to carry it out" (p. 497).

A third feature to note is that the application of the model requires the presence of several basic cognitive capacities of the patient including: (a) the ability to understand and communicate with the clinician; (b) the ability to eventually form a relationship with the clinician or other health professionals who assume a therapeutic support role; and (c) the capacity to acquire the essential emotional, cognitive, and behavioral responses demanded by the environment in which the patient will be eventually expected to function following treatment.

Contributions of Self-Regulation Therapy

The self-regulation approach that we are describing emphasizes a core group of features that constitute its defining elements. Among these features are systematic attention to active patient participation and motivation, a therapeutic process and structure that focuses on the instigation of change, and a framework for implementation that targets response generalization and maintenance, not only as eventual outcomes of treatment but also as ongoing components of all behavior change efforts throughout the treatment process. Each of these features of our approach is described and illustrated here to convey both their conceptual underpinnings and the clinical strategies that derive from the model for therapeutic application with BI patients.

Patient participation has been clearly identified as an important variable that leads to patient change (cf. Gomes-Schwartz, 1978; Saltzman, Luetgert, Roth, Creaser, & Howard, 1976; Sloane, Staples, Cristol, Yorkston, & Whipple, 1975), and in controlled investigations of outcome and process effects of our self-regulation approach we have demonstrated the relationship between patient participation and positive behavior change outcomes. Specifically we have shown that behavioral ratings of active patient involvement in treatment are associated with magnitude of behavioral gains and positive patient self-reactions, and between-session indices of therapeutic involvement such as assignment completion have also been related to therapeutic gains and maintenance (Schefft & Kanfer, 1986, 1987). These findings underscore the potential importance of creating and maintaining patient involvement with therapeutic tasks and goals.

Furthermore, a growing empirical literature with implications for clinical effectiveness demonstrates beneficial learning and emotional effects of procedures that require active attention, effort, and involvement with material to be learned (Kanfer & Schefft, 1988). For example, we have conducted several studies which suggest the clinical utility of procedures that require the subject to generate the information to be remembered rather than only to listen. In the first experiment with college students, when subjects self-generated a response, both recall and recognition memory for the material was superior to a condition in which the response was provided by the experimenter. In addition, the self-generation condition led to decreases in negative affect relative to the didactic condition, over the course of the experiment (Schefft & Biederman, 1990). In a follow-up study with elderly rehabilitation patients, we found a similar and significant advantage for self-generation procedures both with regard to learning and affective state (Schefft & Lehr, 1994). The findings that highlight the learning advantage of self-generation have been replicated (Basso, Schefft, & Hoffmann, 1994), and follow-up studies have also shown that this learning advantage of self-generation is accompanied by enhanced somatic and autonomic arousal patterns during the learning process (Schefft & Basso, 1994). Recently, Schefft, Backscheider, and O'Dell (1996) have demonstrated the potential clinical utility of self-generation procedures by showing a significant incremental learning effect on recognition memory in a study with 20 BI patients. Consequently, the available knowledge base underscores the usefulness of procedures that maximize strategic cognitive involvement with the change process.

Specific Clinical Strategies

The description and brief illustration of several clinical strategies that may be used to achieve subgoals associated especially with the first several phases of our conceptual model may help to clarify the critical importance and purpose of these early phases. Strategies for motivating the patient to continue with treatment are followed by a discussion of our six "Think Rules." Goals and value clarification techniques are then described. Strategies from each of these areas may be used to achieve some of the overlapping goals associated with the various phases of therapy described in the model.

Motivating the Patient to Participate in Therapy. In the outpatient context, it is of course impossible to do therapy with a patient who does not return for treatment. In the inpatient context, uncooperative, resistive, and otherwise "unmotivated" efforts on the part of significantly compromised brain-injured patients can sabotage the efforts of even the most skilled clinicians. For these and other reasons, it is critical to maximize the patient's interest in participating in therapeutic change efforts. For many brain-impaired individuals, demoralization and hopelessness are part of a larger clinical picture characterized by fear and depression that is related to loss of cognitive skills and life opportunities. As we have suggested earlier, the severity and nature of the injury will partly moderate the intensity of emotional responses and the capacity for cognitive control (Sullivan, Schefft, Warm, & Dember, 1994; Sullivan et al., 1995). Although patients will vary greatly according to combinations of premorbid resources, severity of brain injury, neurobehavioral skills affected, and other factors discussed in the first section of this chapter, it is important to work on increasing the patient's sense of hope and positive expectations for therapeutic change.

Reducing demoralization and enhancing expectations for change are in fact components that have been identified as critical ingredients that are shared by all effective psychotherapies (cf. Frank, 1985). Small interventions on the part of the clinician which give the patient the message that change is possible are therefore important aspects of this phase of treatment. For example, in the case of Mr. P., in the 10 years prior to the start of our treatment with him, he had various experiences with analytic and insight-oriented psychotherapists. He reported that these experiences had helped him to understand more about his personality but that they did not assist him to change his behavior adaptively. Consequently, he was quite skeptical about the possibility of changing any of his behaviors, including the tendency to become enraged and chase motorists. To assist Mr. P. to change this behavior very early in treatment would therefore represent evidence that adaptive behavior change is possible. It also would help to increase his sense of hope and positive expectations for future sessions.

In effecting this alteration in his rage and car-chasing behavior, a series of small and sequential strategies were tried in our first session. First, a subjective units of disturbance (S.U.D.S.) monitoring technique was described (cf. Wolpe, 1982), modeled, and then practiced by the patient to teach him how to assign a numeric value (ranging from a low of 1 to a high of 100) to his general arousal level. Several stress-inducing exercises were then used to help Mr. P. to practice the application of this self-monitoring technique in the session. In this process, we attempted to link increased arousal responses with an evaluative rating using the S.U.D.S. technique. The major between-session assignment was to use this technique systematically, practicing it during two agreed-on times each day.

At the beginning of our second session, Mr. P. reported that this was the first time since he could remember that he had not chased "rude" motorists. He reported that a driver nearly cut him off as he was about to step from the curb to cross a street. In this instance, however, he found himself becoming aware that his arousal level had significantly increased. This self-awareness distracted him sufficiently to pause and then realize that the negative consequences of chasing the driver outweighed the highly probable urge to act on his angry impulses. In effect, the introduction of this S.U.D.S. monitoring technique assisted Mr. P. in interrupting the well-learned, automatic response pattern that included rage and then pursuit, which was a behavior pattern that he had identified as chronic, problematic, and very upsetting to him.

The fact that Mr. P. was able to alter this maladaptive behavior during the first week of our treatment provided him with several pieces of evidence. First, he concluded that change was possible for him, even though years of prior treatment had not led to significantly different behavior. Second, he was more optimistic about the possibility that further positive change could occur, and his hope for general improvement increased. There was a collateral decrease in his overall sense of demoralization. These co-occurring events interacted to alter his perceptions about the potential efficacy of treatment. They also served to increase the energy and effort he was willing to invest into the therapeutic process, including the very important but difficult task of completing between-session assignments.

In reviewing the success that Mr. P. had had with this technique, it was important to assist him to feel positive about the accomplishment. In this regard, it was interesting to note that although he felt quite happy that he had done something differently this week, he was appropriately skeptical about his ability to sustain this improvement. His skepticism was associated with a number of spontaneous, ostensibly automatic, and severely self-punitive comments that negatively characterized his overall competence and effectiveness as a person.

The first target identified on the basis of Mr. P.'s presentation involved increasing the probability that he would utilize the S.U.D.S. technique in future similar circumstances over the coming week. Toward this end, we anticipated and rehearsed several scenarios through role play and other experiential exercises to strengthen the newly learned response and its effectiveness in altering his earlier well-learned and automatic pattern of dysfunctional behavior. A second important target identified on the basis of Mr. P.'s remarks was yet another pattern of automatic and clearly dysfunctional behavior: his propensity for self-punitive and self-degenerating comments. In a manner which was similar in process to that described for altering the rage response and chasing of motorists, his self-deprecatory comments became another target for intervention. At first this dysfunctional response pattern was interrupted only in small ways by the clinician during the therapy session. This demonstration provided the opportunity to introduce cognitive controlling responses that Mr. P. could rehearse and utilize on his own between sessions to change his self-statements. This method also consequently served to reinforce the belief that adaptive behavior change was indeed possible for him.

The Six Think Rules. The six Think Rules are guides for behavior change that derive from our self-regulation model (Kanfer & Schefft, 1988). They assist in early phases and throughout the therapeutic course as a means of initiating and maintaining change efforts in the patient. For the BI patient, the utilization of these rules helps to minimize the disabling effects of cognitive impairment so that, for example, modest behavioral routines are able to be enacted and carried out with more consistent success. Our Think Rules also function as techniques to provide a focus for accomplishing tasks and goals during treatment. This focus allows the patient to actively participate in the therapeutic process.

The six Think Rules are: (a) Think behavior; (b) Think solution; (c) Think positive; (d) Think small steps; (e) Think flexible; and (f) Think future. These rules are typically introduced very early in the therapeutic process and they are explained, modeled, and then illustrated by helping the patient to rehearse their application during the treatment session and then apply them to appropriate life situations. Between-session assignments are made that enable the patient to incorporate the rules into his daily life. Especially in the treatment of BI patients, the rules are written into the patient's memory notebook that he carries at all times.

The Think Rules serve several specific functions in the treatment of BI patients with self-regulation therapy. First, the rules are techniques for bolstering the patient's reduced capacity for processing information efficiently and quickly. The application of the rules assists the patient to organize, select, and effect appropriate responses. As such, the rules help the clinician to assist the patient to reduce the negative impact of impaired attention on in-session and between-session behavior. Second, the rules help the patient to organize ideas so that material is more easily learned and more readily accessible for later use. Third, the rules are guides to help the BI patient deal with defects in higher reasoning and problem solving. For example, "Think flexible" helps the patient cope with problems in divergent thinking by training him to avoid becoming stuck on one single idea. "Think solution" assists in overcoming obstacles associated with reduced capacity for convergent thinking, so that the patient is helped to evaluate and select actions that are supported by his current behavioral repertoire. Fourth, the Think Rules have intuitive appeal for use with the BI patient because they present ideas and plans for behavior that are concrete, easily understood, and skill-oriented as opposed to conceptually oriented or deficit-oriented. A brief description of each of the Think Rules follows, after which a case example is used to illustrate their application.

"Think behavior" suggests that problem situations and solutions to these problems must be described in terms of cognitive or overt behaviors or emotional responses, both for oneself and others. The patient is discouraged from thinking in terms of causal explanations, personality traits, or states or vague subjective feelings or attitudes. Instead, the patient is encouraged to think in behavioral terms and focus on questions that provide behavioral descriptions of the problem situation. For example, with Mr. P., his proclivity to constantly ask "Why" questions was challenged with the Think Behavior rule. In early sessions, he would often focus on questions such as: "Why do I get so angry and chase motorists?" and "Why do I always criticize myself so severely?" In using the Think Behavior rule, he was quickly encouraged to focus on how he could change chasing motorists and criticizing himself, and what he could do differently to assist this change in behavior. He was also helped to observe and describe his own cognitive, physical, and emotional responses throughout problem behavior sequences to assist in identifying response components that could first be described in terms of action and then targeted for change.

"Think solution" emphasizes that no problem situation is accurately understood by focusing solely on a description of difficulties. Problem description requires not only knowledge about the current state, but also of the situation that will be more desirable as a future end state and the means to reach it. In clinical use, assistance in generating possible solutions is provided by the therapist to interrupt automatic behavior sequences that focus on problem states and to encourage consideration of ways for changing behavior.

"Think positive" serves as a useful rule to encourage patients to monitor and direct their thinking toward perceiving positive features of a situation. It also helps patients to divert their attention away from negative aspects of their lives. Despite its apparent triteness, "Think positive" is a rule for behavior that helps the patient to focus on their strengths and personal resources and their potentials. It encourages realistic optimism as it reminds the patient to consider positive potentials of the current life situation as well as past achievements. When this rule is presented, patients will frequently indicate that they know how to think positively, and that this is not new or useful for them. In fact, most BI patients do *not* know how to regulate their moods or to direct their thoughts to create positive and optimistic moods. When these skills remain after injury, they are only rarely used. BI patients present a burden of sadness and dysphoria that relates to physical, cognitive, and interpersonal losses which have been sustained in relation to the brain injury (cf. Prigatano, 1991a). This behavioral rule is therefore particularly important to help the patient to redirect preoccupations away from the many negative and unchangeable aspects of their current life situation toward an optimistic and hopeful perspective. It also helps him to plan and then execute actions and ideas that utilize the cognitive skills and strengths which remain.

"Think small steps" recognizes the long tradition in the practice of behavior therapy that encourages patients to set limited goals for progressive steps (cf. Goldfried & Davison, 1976). This enhances the patient's perception of his ability to achieve goals and makes a problem situation appear more manageable. Use of this rule provides the patient with subgoals and helps to specify particular actions which are needed. The use of the "Think small steps" rule also accommodates the dynamic and recursive nature of the treatment process by allowing consideration of change after each small step depending on the outcome of that step. In working with BI patients, "Think small steps" is especially useful because it requires the splitting of a task into a number of component parts. Steps are then developed to deal with one component at a time. This procedure reduces the information processing load on the BI patient and facilitates selective attention to single issues. The application of this rule is illustrated by the clinician's challenging of the patient with the question "What is the least that you can do to alter this situation?" The focus on minimal goals recognizes that a combination of specific, concrete, and realistic goals that can be achieved in the near future has greater motivational value than long-term and difficult outcomes.

"Think flexible" is an especially important rule to teach BI patients because the orbital frontal lesions that occur following brain injury often leave these individuals with rigid, stereotyped, and perseverative behavior sequences which do not accommodate the need for backup plans or the anticipation of unforeseen events. Patients are actively assisted in preparing backups for important action sequences. An illustration of this with Mr. P., following a recent success experience, was the therapist saying, "It's great that when you monitored your S.U.D.S. level you ended up stopping and you didn't chase the motorist. But what else could you do if that doesn't work next time?" With "Think flexible," the patient is therefore helped to recognize that there may be many different paths to reach a goal and that it is important not to give up efforts to change if one plan is unsuccessful.

"Think future" is based on recognition of the human proclivity to ruminate about past events and seek causal explanations for behavior in the past. For BI patients, it is an important strategy for use to discourage rumination about the accident and other details of the injury that led to the cognitive impairments and the current problem situation. The patient is taught that dwelling on the past is insufficient preparation for dealing with the future. Although an understanding of the factors that surround the current problem situation is important, this understanding must relate to future actions and outcomes. In using the "Think future" rule, the clinician emphasizes the importance of planning and anticipating possible outcomes. The systematic use of this rule is especially important for BI patients because the impulsive and frequently immature nature of their behavior often precludes anticipation of future events. The clinical use of "Think future" therefore not only encourages the patient to stop ruminating about past negative events but also helps the patient prepare for new situations by anticipating future events and outcomes. The application of the "Think future" rule is extended as therapy progresses by helping the patient to prepare for the future use of a newly acquired skill and for its generalization to different contexts in the future.

Table 9.2 has been reproduced from the memory notebook of a severely impaired BI patient to illustrate the application of the six Think Rules.

Mr. Q is a 26-year-old single White male who sustained a brain injury secondary to a

TABLE 9.2.
The Six Think Rules for a Severely Impaired BI Patient

1. Think Behavior:	Do not think general things like "My life is worthless.	Think about specific behaviors, like doing the things on the checklist, which make you feel good about yourself.
2. Think solution:	Do not think only about your problems, like not being able to write very well.	Think about what you can do, like type on your word processor.
3. Think positive:	Do not think about negative things too much, like people who have died.	Think about pleasant things, like people who are alive and care about you.
4. Think small steps:	Do not think about things that are impossible, like going on a vacation to another planet.	Think about small things you can do to get out of the apartment, like going to a movie.
5. Think flexible:	Do not get stuck on one idea and give up if it doesn't work.	Have a Plan "A" and also a Plan "B" for backup, like if you can't get a ride to the National Head Injury Foundation meeting, you could call ACCESS.
6. Think future:	Do not think about what has happened to you in the past, like your accident.	Think about what you plan to do in the future, like perhaps how to live more independently.

motor vehicle accident when he was 4 years of age. He was seen in an outpatient rehabilitation center for treatment of a number of disabling behavioral, cognitive, and emotional responses, including poor frustration tolerance, dysfunctional social skills, and ineffective problem solving. A referral was made by the patient's case manager, who was attempting to provide independent living arrangements for him.

Neuropsychological examination revealed a poorly groomed and behaviorally disinhibited young man who alternated between use of a walker and wheelchair for ambulation. His gait was broad-based and unstable; motor problems included ataxia, apraxia, agraphia, and severely labored speech with dysarthria. There were signs of frequent frustration with his behavioral limitations, and there was a long history related to problems with anxiety and depression. Neuropsychological test performance revealed uniformly defective functioning across cognitive areas including new learning, recent memory, visuoperception, and simple visual planning. Overall intellectual functioning level was in the defective range.

This patient is similar to many BI patients who present with severe impairments that impact on their cognitive, emotional, and behavioral effectiveness. Table 9.2 briefly illustrates the main emphasis taken in treatment for assisting Mr. Q to understand, gradually learn, and incorporate each of the six Think Rules into his daily life. The frequent use of repetition, role play, and experientially based rehearsal techniques and the memory notebook were essential for building a skill-based (procedural memory) incorporation of the six Think Rules into Mr. Q's behavioral repertoire.

Goal and Value Clarification

Even neurologically normal patients who seek psychotherapy often describe their goals vaguely, such as a desire to be healthy, problem free, and happy. Of course, patients are never able to achieve such vague goals. The difficulty of this situation is greatly intensified for the clinician who treats BI patients, especially because of the significant problems with self-awareness that these patients present (Cicerone, 1989; Prigatano, 1991b; Stuss, 1991). Accurate self-appraisals in relationship to goals and values are consequently most difficult for BI individuals.

The goal and value clarification process addresses the patient's important concern that is often expressed by the question "Why should I?" The process is intended to clarify the patient's major goals, to assist a realistic appraisal of these goals in relationship to capacities and limitations, and to help the patient to create a clear image of what his life would be like if he were able to be satisfied. Implicit in this process is the necessity for helping the patient gradually recognize his cognitive and behavioral limitations and begin to generate goal options that are consistent with personal resources. The examination of various goal options in relationship to the patient's cognitive and emotional limitations helps one to focus attention on the assessment of behaviors, feelings, events, and situations that are relevant to adaptive behavior change. Patient involvement in this process increases the general level of treatment participation and is linked to later goal involvement (Evans, 1984). It also has a motivational effect because the devotion of time and energy to definition of goals enhances the attractiveness of these goals, and makes them appear less distant and unattainable (cf. Hart, 1978).

A final characteristic of the goal and value clarification procedures is that they help to clarify what particular incentives may be useful for motivating behavior change for the individual patient. These incentives represent events that have reinforcement value and that can be used for shaping individual behavior patterns. For example, for Mr. P., a passing grade on a computer science examination would be such a reinforcer. The problem, of course, is that his cognitive limitations may not permit passing computer science graduate-level program courses. In this situation, the task for the clinician becomes one of identifying alternative options that represent the values reflected in pursuit of the unattainable reinforcer, which was a computer science master's degree, in Mr. P.'s case. These values for Mr. P. included achievement, professional advancement, intellectual stimulation, and demonstration of personal competence. In effect, the goal and value clarification process helps the patient to identify and prioritize his values and it lays a groundwork for exploration of alternative goal options and associated reinforcers that are consistent with these values and the patient's abilities. In this situation, goal and value clarification led to identification of less intellectually ambitious but related goals which yielded similar satisfaction for Mr. P. They involved pursuit of training in computer programming in an associate degree program of a local technical college.

An important assumption of our self-regulation therapy model is that a person should never be asked to act against his or her own self-interest (Kanfer & Schefft, 1988). It is especially true that in the treatment of BI patients, the clinician must help the patient to have a clear understanding of what can be achieved in therapy, the effort that must necessarily be invested, and the outcomes that can be reasonably anticipated. In working with BI patients, it is critical for the clinician to assume the patient's perspective and to attempt to answer a number of critical questions that are vital to assuring patient cooperation and motivation. The clinician must clearly appraise the extent to which the patient's expectations can be met in relation to what we have called "the client's five basic questions."

The first of these questions is, *"What will it be like if I change?"* To a brain-injured patient, imagining that he or she will never be able to engage in productive independent living activities, to maintain employment in some area of work that yields personal satisfaction, or to engage in intellectual activities that provide challenge and stimulation does not make change a joyful prospect. At the same time, distorted and otherwise unrealistic self-images also clearly have a negative impact on treatment. Therefore, the patient must be helped to recognize what a complete daily routine might be like, within the limits of his or her abilities, rather than simply being presented with an unrealistically pessimistic or optimistic picture of what life might be like. The picture of the patient's future life needs to be developed jointly by the patient and therapist with a full accommodation of the image of what the client finds acceptable as well as the outcomes which could be supported by his cognitive, emotional, and behavioral resources. Imagery and related techniques can be used to help the patient to perceive alternative images that would be possible with behavioral change.

The second basic question we have identified is, *"How will I be better off if I change?"* It is, of course, relatively easy for the patient to imagine that his life will be better if he is no longer acutely anxious or depressed, but it is more difficult to help the patient to understand that he might be better off if he no longer strove toward goals that are impossible to attain. Assisting the BI patient to conduct a careful examination of the personal consequences of failed goal-related efforts can be a very useful therapeutic strategy that can help the BI patient to evaluate the positive effects of selecting more realistic goal options. Usually this assessment also involves a recognition of the need to give up the short-term benefits associated with the injury, such as financial compensations, sympathy, and the like. In the case of Mr. P., in-session exercises and between-session assignments focused on helping him to identify and then to examine negative emotional responses that were related to his self-criticism, which in turn helped him accept some of the beneficial effects of lowering his academic and intellectual achievement goals. Subsequent to this step, the clinician's therapeutic task lies in helping the patient to realize and to develop confidence that adaptive behavior change (in this example, reduction in magnitude of goals) will result in a better final outcome.

The patient's third basic question is, *"Can I change?"* Questions about capacity to change are quite frequent even among neurologically normal patients. As the BI patient develops a clearer sense of cognitive and behavioral options and activities that are within his range of potential mastery, there comes a related understanding of one's cognitive limitations and physical difficulties. This increased understanding of realistic limitations naturally precipitates doubts about personal competence and the capacity to reach meaningful goals. The clinician's task is to carefully evaluate the patient's capacity to carry out behavioral changes that are in line with the identified realistic goals. The patient's capacity to meet these goals must be tested in successive small steps that have been made as manageable and attainable as possible. The adaptive behavior change program should be carefully controlled by the therapist so that it is individualized to the patient's needs through arrangement of particular subgoals, rate of progress, and the use of supportive devices so that attainment of therapeutic objectives is facilitated. The therapeutic goals must be carefully monitored in relation to the success of patient efforts. It is critical for the clinician to reevaluate and help the patient to reformulate his goal level when there is evidence that he will not reach his objectives.

A fourth basic question for the patient is, *"What will it cost to change?"* The primary focus of this question is on the time, energy, effort, and sacrifice necessary for the patient to achieve adaptive behavior change. Giving up the pursuit of highly valued but personally unattainable goals is certainly one such cost that Mr. P. had to be carefully assisted to evaluate. His ambition to hold a master's degree in computer science and to work as a computer science engineer was one of the single greatest motivating, albeit dysfunctional, factors in his life. Factors such as these and others must be realistically confronted and worked through with the patient in order to prevent the possibility that the patient will drop out of treatment because he views the effort of change as not worth the cost.

The final basic question of the patient is, *"Can I trust this therapist and setting to help me get there?"* The methods used for helping the patient to answer this question affirmatively chiefly draw on procedures for developing the therapeutic alliance. Setting conditions which create favorable expectations for change, enhance therapist credibility, decrease demoralization, and strengthen expectations that positive outcomes will result from treatment are all conditions which strengthen the therapeutic alliance and facilitate the patient's affirmative answer to this question (cf. Kanfer & Schefft, 1987).

To the extent that the goal and value clarification process results in assisting the patient to realistically and affirmatively answer the five basic questions we have outlined, the patient is then in a position to clearly and appropriately address the central motivational issue; namely, "Why should I invest maximum effort in therapy?" The product of the goal and value clarification process is a specification of realistic goal states that are clearly in line with the patient's values, beliefs, and interests and consequently will have motivational value. More importantly, with the BI patient, the goals have to be mutually negotiated and accepted by the patient, yet they must also lie within the limitations that have been created by the patient's cognitive, emotional, and behavioral impairments.

Goals and potential end states that are negotiated with BI patients must typically involve a consideration of reduced capacity for sustained attention and concentration, complex problem solving, efficiency of information processing, effectiveness of new verbal learning, and decreased frustration tolerance which are so commonly displayed as neurobehavioral sequelae of BI patients (Levin et al., 1982; Levin, Goldstein, Williams, & Eisenberg, 1991; Lovell & Starratt, 1992). The difficult but critical task of the clinician involves facilitation of the patient's acceptance of goals and therapeutic strivings that acknowledge these limitations. Indeed, patient acceptance of goals and life activities that are within the limitations that have been created by their cognitive impairments has been identified by Diller (1994) as one of the most effective predictors of positive outcomes in neuropsychological rehabilitation with BI patients.

Future Directions

Is Psychotherapy Effective? A challenging issue that faces the empirically and theoretically minded clinician is whether or not psychotherapy is effective with BI patients. There is evidence that BI patients' unmanaged problems worsen over time, particularly with regard to the patient becoming more withdrawn and depressed (Prigatano, 1992). There is not as yet much available objective evidence that supports the effectiveness of psychotherapy for BI patients. There are published case reports that describe a particular form of psychotherapy and its success with an individual BI patient (e.g., Ball, 1988; Lewis & Rosenberg, 1990), and there are studies of treatment outcome of rehabilitation programs in which psychotherapy is but one of the many treatment components being provided to the BI patient (e.g., Prigatano et al., 1984). However, there are as yet no controlled, randomized trial studies of the effectiveness of psychotherapy per se with BI patients.

Research is needed to establish whether psychotherapy can make a positive impact not only on the patient's rehabilitation outcome, but also on the long-term maintenance and generalization of adaptive behavior. Because the patients and their families often have lifelong adaptive behavior problems with which to contend, there is a need to evaluate psychotherapy's ability to effect improvement in the many environments in which the patient currently functions (e.g., work, home), the durability of these improvements over time, and the impact of treatment on future problem solving. It may be the case, for example, that more return trips to treatment or "booster sessions" are required with this type of patient population because of the often enduring and troublesome cognitive impairments that these patients sustain after BI.

Using Premorbid Competencies to Accomplish Treatment Goals. The literature on treatment of BI patients typically focuses on the patient's deficits. One area that has received little systematic attention concerns their premorbid competencies. Clearly, BI can cause impairment in many areas leading to disability in cognitive, emotional, and social functioning. There can be automatic, maladaptive behaviors that predate the injury and persist afterward, such as the abuse of substances in response to emotional stress. There can also be maladaptive behaviors that develop after the injury which become automatic, such as physically striking out at others when frustrated. However, there may still be residual adaptive skills that can be demonstrated by the BI patient after injury which were also overlearned and automatic before onset of the brain injury. When these residual adaptive skills can be identified during the assessment, they can be used by the clinician to facilitate coping and change.

Because new learning can often be affected after a brain injury, identifying these well-established adaptive skills can reduce the overall burden of demands placed on the patient in the change process. This approach also provides a treatment perspective for balancing the ever-present temptation to mourn cognitive and behavioral losses after BI rather than maximizing use of positive aspects of premorbid personality that remain intact after the injury. Although this is more possible with persons of high premorbid functioning and less severe brain injury, there can still be a preservation of automatic and well-learned adaptive skills in more severely impaired BI patients that can be used in treatment.

Three cases are presented here to illustrate how BI patients with varying levels of cognitive and emotional abilities can still demonstrate premorbid adaptive behavior that can be used to facilitate treatment effects. The first is Mr. J., who sustained a severe BI and had such significant physical and cognitive deficits postinjury that he was placed in a long-term care facility. He was consistently disoriented, was only able to learn simple new information gradually with constant repetition, and was noncompliant with most aspects of daily care and medical treatment. Although many different treatment interventions were implemented in order to bring about improved treatment compliance and behavioral control in this individual, a significant change was noted in his behavior when staff identified and used one aspect of his adaptive premorbid behavioral repertoire to aid treatment efforts. Prior to injury, Mr. J. was a nurturing individual who enjoyed helping others who were less fortunate than himself. Consequently, he was paired with another patient who was also significantly noncompliant but who had even greater disabilities. Mr. J. was given the responsibility of attending treatment sessions with this other patient and encouraging this person in his therapy exercises. Mr. J. did this with great enthusiasm and showed a noticeable improvement in mood, positive social interactions with staff, and compliance with some aspects of his morning routine. For example, he now had to get out of bed at a reasonable hour in the morning so that he could be ready to take his "charge" to his first therapy appointment. This was not a solution to all of his problems, but it did give the staff and the patient reason to hope that his behavior and his situation in the facility could improve.

The second patient, Mr. B, also sustained a severe brain injury (with a Glasgow Coma Scale of 3 on admission to the emergency room) but experienced some neurological recovery postinjury. He was able to return home to his family, even though he could not return to work. He sustained permanent deficits in motor functioning, which included right hemiparesis, and permanent deficits in cognitive function, which included attentional, memorial, and spatial reasoning impairments. Emotional lability compounded this deficit picture. Psychotherapy was initiated approximately 3 years after the injury, and issues addressed included acceptance of his life situation, improvement of his marital relationship, and control of the emotional lability. Of these treatment goals, Mr. B. was most concerned about the lability. Premorbidly, he had prided himself on his stoicism and had been the member of his family on which others relied for calm problem resolution. His lability resulted in him becoming tearful or rageful in response to mild provocation, and this embarrassed him. Others' reactions to him ranged from surprise and alarm to encouraging the lability based on the false belief that he needed to vent his feelings to reduce the occurrence of future labile episodes.

A preserved and adaptive premorbid skill that was identified in the assessment was his capacity to meditate. He had learned how to meditate as a young adult in order to manage a significant trauma at that time in his life. Even though he had not used this skill in recent years, there was reason to believe that he retained sufficient competence with it to help him to control his lability.

During treatment, he was initially encouraged just to practice this skill again. The realization that he could still have some control over his emotional reactions helped him to combat his demoralization and gave him renewed hope that he still had positive and useful cognitive capabilities after his brain injury. He was encouraged by his early success, and he became motivated to utilize his meditation to interrupt and manage emotional lability. Mr. B.'s regular practice of meditation gave his day more structure and also helped reduce his general level of emotional arousal.

Of course, there were new skills that needed to be learned to assist Mr. B. to optimally use these premorbid skills to achieve therapeutic gains. For example, it was necessary for him to learn which situations were more likely to elicit his lability and to monitor physical signs that he was becoming emotionally aroused. His family's involvement and support was also centrally important to his progress. However, the fact that Mr. B. could identify something that he could still do competently after the injury provided a significant boost to his self-esteem and to his willingness to try other treatment strategies.

The third patient, Mr. M., sustained a mild brain injury with a brief loss of consciousness and hospitalization. He received no outpatient therapies and resumed the management of his business. However, he experienced great distress over his difficulty in managing simultaneous inputs, such as the phone ringing, an employee being at his door, and a report that he had to complete. He felt that since his BI his "mental edge" was gone, and he was becoming increasingly depressed about this. Because Mr. M. had functioned at a high intellectual level premorbidly, easily handling the multiple stressors and demands of a challenging job, the therapist decided to examine the skills he previously used to cope with the feeling of being overwhelmed. Mr. M. could recall instances in which he had felt overwhelmed, and he was helped to identify a standard strategy that he used at these times. He would first tell others that he would have to get back to them later on a particular subject and he would then schedule a time to do this. With therapeutic support, he began to use this strategy at work. An immediate effect was that it allowed him some time to consider each problem in turn, but it also ensured that issues were addressed and that others did not feel disregarded by him. A related effect of this intervention was Mr. M.'s realization that although he felt overstimulated more frequently now, postinjury, this situation was not completely foreign to him. He was helped to rediscover that he had developed a coping mechanism in the past that could be used again effectively in the present.

As these cases illustrate, identification of premorbid competencies is important for several reasons. First, these competencies can be useful resources that can be used to maximize treatment gains. As we have suggested, the neuropsychological evaluation of BI patients should identify both strengths and weaknesses of the patients so that the therapist is aware of available assets that can be incorporated to reach treatment targets. Too often, the evaluation can focus exclusively on the patient's deficits. This can leave the therapist and the patient discouraged by the apparent enormity of the tasks that remain to be accomplished. Identification of premorbid competencies helps one keep perspectives balanced and assists the patient in feeling reduced demoralization and renewed hope for improvement. A corresponding effect is enhanced willingness to invest energy and effort into therapy. Finally, because learning capacity is often affected after BI, the identification of existing competencies can reduce the burden of learning demands on the patient in treatment. The BI patient will inevitably have to learn and use new behavior to cope adaptively, but the ability to immediately utilize well-preserved, automatic, and adaptive premorbid behaviors can reduce some of the demands for cognitive processing and facilitate early success in treatment.

SUMMARY AND CONCLUSIONS

In this chapter, we have reviewed factors that can affect the self-regulatory processes of BI patients. These include neurological factors such as the nature and foci of central nervous system damage, physical factors such as gait disturbance and pain, and psychological factors such as depression, anxiety, and the individual's level of self-esteem. A distinction was made between an impairment of a cognitive process, such as memory, and the possible resulting disabilities and handicaps. Not all impairments lead to disability, because the person may be able to use his or her self-regulatory processes to compensate for the impairment.

Several methods of evaluating patients were then discussed. As a method of assessment, the Mayo–Portland Adaptability Inventory was presented because it provides a meaningful profile of BI-related impairments and disabilities and can be used to gather information from the patient and others. A thorough understanding of different perspectives including the patient, family, and staff can be especially helpful for planning treatment and in maximizing the involvement of all concerned.

Types of psychological interventions currently used with BI patients were then reviewed. These interventions vary in the extent to which they attempt to directly alter the self-regulatory processes of the BI patient. Typically, those interventions that do not directly modify the patient's self-regulatory processes, such as behavior modification and psychotropic medications, can be used with the broadest range of patients. The patient's active involvement is not required, and thus patient characteristics are relatively less important in determining who can be treated by these methods. Self-regulation therapy, however, requires the active involvement and participation of the patient. As a result, the patient's relative strengths and limitations assume greater importance in determining suitability of this treatment methodology. We noted that therapy is being extended to persons with greater cognitive impairment and thus the conception of suitability and corresponding criteria also are being expanded. In one sense, the BI patient has represented a common denominator for diverse forms of psychotherapy and the modifications recommended by these approaches for treatment of the BI patient are remarkably similar.

A model and related clinical strategies for self-regulation therapy with the BI patient were then presented. The focus of this approach is on creating the conditions that favor adaptive behavior change and assisting the patient to actively participate and share responsibility for the treatment process. A formulation of dysfunctional behavior was described as a vehicle for conceptualizing problematic behavior sequences and for identifying behavioral intervention targets. A therapeutic model that sequentially orders a series of phases and related subgoals in the treatment process was then presented and its clinical application was illustrated with several clinical case examples. The process of change was described as one in which automatic dysfunctional behavior sequences are replaced by more adaptive response patterns that are gradually integrated into the BI patient's daily life. Self-regulation therapy was conceptualized as a dynamic and recursive approach that is implemented in a problem-solving fashion with continued assessment of the patient's response to treatment efforts and corresponding adjustment of therapeutic goals and techniques. Specific techniques for instigation of change were reviewed and procedures for use in the goal and value clarification process were discussed. Patient motivation, response generalization, and posttreatment maintenance were described as key issues in therapeutic change using the self-regulation approach.

Although there has been new interest in extending therapy approaches to BI patients, there still is not strong evidence that their application significantly enhances the patient's quality of life or meaningfully effects future cognitive-behavioral outcomes. This will be an important, although difficult, area to empirically examine because it will be difficult to match patients on level of injury severity and resulting cognitive disability. It is necessary to investigate the effectiveness of various approaches in order to identify the nature and timing of therapeutic strategies and techniques that are most useful for treatment of patients with different types of deficit syndromes. Expanding the empirical knowledge base to enhance posttreatment maintenance and generalization will be critical to furthering the contributions that have been made by psychological therapy for the BI patient. Although the potential role of self-regulation therapy for the treatment of the BI patient is now beginning to emerge, careful empirical work remains to be done before its utility can be fully evaluated and its application can be documented for broad clinical use.

MAYO PORTLAND ADAPTABILITY INVENTORY

NAME________________ CLINIC NO: ______________ DATE: ________ TOTAL SCORE: _______

PHYSICAL/MEDICAL ________

1. MOBILITY
- 0 No impairment
- 1 Gait deviations or balance disturbances evident on clinical exam but do not interfere with independent mobility
- 2 Gait deviations or balance disturbances are significant enough that gait aid or wheelchair is required for independent mobility
- 3 Manual assistance required for mobility with gait aid or wheelchair

2. USE OF HANDS
- 0 No impairment of either hand
- 1 Impairment of either hand on clinical exam but does not interfere with everyday functioning
- 2 Impairment of either hand interferes with everyday functioning
- 3 Minimal or no use of both hands

3. AUDITION (score with corrective device if used)
- 0 No impairment
- 1 Impaired on clinical exam but does not interfere with everyday functioning
- 2 Impairment interferes with everyday functioning
- 3 Minimal to no hearing

4. VISION (score with corrective device if used)
- 0 No impairment
- 1 Impaired on clinical exam but does not interfere with everyday functioning
- 2 Impairment interferes with everyday functioning
- 3 Minimal or no vision

5. MOTOR SPEECH
- 0 No impairment
- 1 Impaired on clinical exam but does not interfere with everyday communication
- 2 Impairment interferes with everyday communication
- 3 Minimal speech or no speech

6. PAIN
- 0 None
- 1 Current problem *but does not interfere with everyday functioning
- 2 Pain behavior interferes with everyday functioning
- 3 Pain behavior is totally or almost totally disabling

COGNITION ________

7. COMMUNICATION
- 0 No impairment
- 1 Impaired on clinical exam but does not interfere with everyday communication
- 2 Impairment interferes with everyday communication or is significant enough to require the use of an alternative mode of communication
- 3 Minimal communication ability with or without the use of an alternative mode of communication; or no communication ability

8. MEMORY
- 0 No impairment
- 1 Impaired on clinical exam but does not interfere with everyday functioning
- 2 Impairment interferes with everyday functioning
- 3 Minimal or no memory

9. ATTENTION/CONCENTRATION
- 0 No impairment
- 1 Impaired on clinical exam but does not interfere with everyday functioning
- 2 Impairment interferes with everyday functioning
- 3 Extremely distractible; minimal or no ability to sustain attention

10. NOVEL PROBLEM SOLVING
- 0 No impairment
- 1 Impaired on clinical exam but does not interfere with everyday functioning
- 2 Impairment interferes with everyday functioning
- 3 Extremely concrete thinking; minimal or no ability to abstract or to anticipate possible outcomes

11. VISUOSPATIAL ABILITIES
- 0 No impairment
- 1 Impaired on clinical exam but does not interfere with everyday functioning
- 2 Impairment interferes with everyday functioning
- 3 Minimal or no route-finding or other visuospatial abilities

12. FUND OF INFORMATION (common knowledge)
- 0 Average for educational/vocational history
- 1 Low average for educational/vocational history
- 2 Significant gaps in fund of information
- 3 Extremely limited fund of information

EMOTION ________

13. IRRITABILITY TO AGGRESSION
- 0 Socially appropriate
- 1 Reported by patient or significant other; not observed
- 2 Verbal aggression observed
- 3 Physically aggressive or threatening behavior observed

14. ANXIETY TO AGITATION
- 0 Socially appropriate
- 1 Current problem* but does not interfere with everyday functioning
- 2 Interferes with everyday functioning
- 3 Severe problem that requires inpatient or residential management

15. DEPRESSION
- 0 Socially appropriate
- 1 Current problem* but does not interfere with everyday functioning
- 2 Interferes with everyday functioning
- 3 Severe problem that requires inpatient or residential management

EVERYDAY ACTIVITIES ______________

16. RESIDENCE
0 Independent living, handles own finances
1 Independent living, cannot handle own finances
2 Supported living (eg, half-way house, with attendant, supervised apartment)
3 Residence with full-time supervision or no regular place of residence

17. SELF-CARES (eating, dressing, hygiene)
0 Independent and safe in self cares
1 Generally independent in self-cares, but slow to initiate or complete or requires assistive device; or minor safety concerns expressed by patient or significant other
2 Requires intermittent assistance or supervision in self cares
3 Dependent or requires full-time supervision in self cares

18. WORK/SCHOOL
0 Competitive work, school, or homemaking with no restrictions or supports
1 Competitive work, school, or homemaking with injury-related restrictions but without supports or assistance
2 Sheltered, supported, or assisted work, school, or homemaking
3 Not working, in school or homemaking

19. LEISURE ACTIVITIES
0 Normal initiation of and participation in leisure activities
1 Some deficits in initiating leisure activities, but adequate participation
2 No or minimal initiation of leisure activities, but adequate participation
3 No or minimal participation in leisure activities

20. DRIVING
0 Drives with no problems; or does not drive for reasons unrelated to injury
1 Concern about driving safety reported by patient or significant other
2 History of motor vehicle accident(s) or law violation(s) after injury
3 License suspended or revoked; or cannot drive

SOCIAL BEHAVIOR ______________

21. FAMILY/SIGNIFICANT RELATIONSHIPS
0 Normal
1 Dissatisfactions; mildly to moderately disturbed
2 Very disrupted or deteriorated
3 No family or significant relationships

22. SOCIAL CONTACT (beyond family and professional contacts)
0 Normal initiation of social activities and adequate social support
1 Some deficits in initiation of social activities, but has adequate network of social support
2 No or minimal initiation of social activities, but has adequate network of social support
3 Inadequate network of social support

---

*Current problem includes problem for which patient is receiving treatment even if symptoms are not currently apparent

23. APPROPRIATE SOCIAL INTERACTION
0 Socially appropriate
1 Infrequent inappropriate social behavior
2 Frequent inappropriate social behavior (childish, silly, out of place)
3 Practically complete lack of social awareness

BEHAVIOR ______________

24. INDIFFERENCE
0 Identifies disabilities and their impact in specific daily activities
1 Identifies disabilities, but not their impact in specific daily activities
2 Identifies problems in general, but no consistent identification of specific disabilities
3 Denies existence of problems or unable to comprehend them

25. DELUSIONS AND HALLUCINATIONS
0 None
1 Current problem* but does not interfere with everyday functioning
2 Interferes with everyday functioning
3 Severe problem that requires inpatient or residential management

26. PARANOIA
0 None
1 Current problem* but does not interfere with everyday functioning
2 Interferes with everyday functioning
3 Severe problem that requires inpatient or residential management

27. INITIATION
0 Normal
1 Initiation problems present (eg, in conversation, activity) but do not interfere with everyday functioning
2 Initiation problems interfere with everyday functioning
3 Initiates no conversation or activity without cueing, prompting, or or other stimulation

28. LAW VIOLATIONS
0 None
1 Misdemeanor(s)
2 Felony conviction
3 Repeat felony conviction(s)

29. ALCOHOL USE
0 Nonuser or occasional use
1 Concerns about alcohol use reported by patient or significant other but does not interfere with everyday functioning
2 Interferes with everyday functioning
3 Interferes greatly with everyday functioning; results in neglect of some responsibilities

30. DRUG USE
0 Nonuse
1 Concern about drug use reported by patient or significant other but does not interfere with everyday functioning
2 Interferes with everyday functioning
3 Interferes greatly with everyday functioning; results in neglect of some responsibilities

REFERENCES

Ball, J. D. (1988). Psychotherapy with head-injured patients. *Medical Psychotherapy, 1,* 15–22.

Basso, M. R., Scheff t, B. K., & Hoffmann, R. G., (1994). Mood-moderating effects of affect intensity on cognition: Sometimes euphoria is not beneficial and dysphoria is not detrimental. *Journal of Personality and Social Psychology, 66,* 363–368.

Becker, M. C., Abrams, K. S., & Onder, J. (1974). Goal setting: A joint patient–staff methods. *Archives of Physical Medicine and Rehabilitation, 55,* 87–89.

Ben-Yishay, Y. & Lakin, P. (1989). Structured group treatment for brain-injury survivors. In D. W. Ellis & A. L. Christensen (Eds.), *Neuropsychological treatment after brain injury* (pp. 271–295). Boston: Kluwer.

Ben-Yishay, Y., & Prigatano, G. P. (1990). Cognitive remediation. In M. Rosenthal, E. R. Griffith, M. R. Bond, & J. D. Miller (Eds.), *Rehabilitation of the adult and child with traumatic brain injury* (2nd ed., pp. 393–409). Philadelphia: Davis.

Brooks, D. N. (Ed.). (1984). *Closed head injury: Psychological, social, and family consequences.* New York: Oxford University Press.

Brooks, D. N., & Aughton, M. E. (1979). Psychological consequences of blunt head injury. *International Rehabilitation Medicine, 1,* 160–165.

Brooks, N. (1989). Closed head trauma: Assessing the common cognitive problems. In M. D. Lezak (Ed.), *Assessment of the behavioral consequences of head trauma* (pp. 61–85). New York: A. Liss.

Brooks, N., Campsie, L., Symington, C., Beattie, A., & McKinlay, W. (1986). The five year outcome of severe blunt head injury: A relative's view. *Journal of Neurology, Neurosurgery, and Psychiatry, 49,* 764–770.

Calhoun, K. S., & Turner, S. M. (1981). Historical perspectives and current issues in behavior therapy. In S. M. Turner, K. S. Calhoun, & H. E. Adams (Eds.), *Handbook of clinical behavior therapy* (pp. 1–11). New York: Wiley.

Christensen, A. L., & Rosenberg, N. K. (1991). A critique of the role of psychotherapy in brain injury rehabilitation. *Journal of Head Trauma Rehabilitation, 6,* 56–61.

Cicerone, K. D. (1989). Psychotherapeutic interventions with traumatically brain-injured patients. *Rehabilitation Psychology, 34,* 105–114.

Cicerone, K. D., & Giacino, J. T. (1992). Remediation of executive function deficits after traumatic brain injury. *NeuroRehabilitation, 2,* 12–22.

Cohen, N. J., & Squire, L. R. (1980). Preserved learning and retention of pattern-analyzing skill in amnesia: Dissociation of "knowing how" and "knowing that." *Science, 210,* 207–209.

Cope, D. N., Cole, J. R., Hall, K. M., & Barkan, H. (1991). Brain injury: Analysis of outcome in a post-acute rehabilitation system. Part 2: Subanalyses. *Brain Injury, 5,* 127–139.

Costa, L. (1983). Clinical neuropsychology: A discipline in evolution. *Journal of Clinical Neuropsychology, 5,* 1–11.

Definition of mild traumatic brain injury. (1993). *Journal of Head Trauma Rehabilitation, 8,* 86–87.

DePompei, R., & Zarski, J. J. (1991). Assessment of the family. In J. M. Williams & T. Kay (Eds.), *Head injury: A family matter* (pp. 101–120). Baltimore: Paul H. Brookes.

Diller, L. (1994, February). *Neuropsychological rehabilitation.* Workshop presented at the Annual Meeting of the International Neuropsychological Society, Cincinnati, OH.

Eames, P., Haffey, W. J., & Cope, D. N. (1989). Treatment of behavioral disorders. In M. Rosenthal, E. R. Griffith, M. R. Bond, & J. D. Miller (Eds.), *Rehabilitation of the adult and child with traumatic brain injury* (pp. 179–192). Philadelphia: Davis.

Evans, H. M. (1984). Increasing patient involvement with therapy goals. *Journal of Clinical Psychology, 40,* 728–733.

Florian, V., Katz, S., & Lahav, V. (1989). Impact of traumatic brain damage on family dynamics and functioning: A review. *Brain Injury, 3,* 219–233.

Frank, J. D. (1985). Therapeutic components shared by all psychotherapists. In M. J. Mahoney & A. Freeman (Eds.), *Cognition and psychotherapy* (pp. 49–79). New York: Plenum.

Garfield, S. L., & Bergin, A. E. (Eds.). (1994). *Handbook of psychotherapy and behavior change: An empirical analysis* (3rd ed.). New York: Wiley.

Glisky, E. L., & Schachter, D. L. (1986). Remediation of organic memory disorders: Current status and future prospects. *Journal of Head Trauma Rehabilitation, 1,* 54–63.

Godfrey, H. P., Knight, R. G., & Bishara, S. N. (1991). The relationship between social skill and family problem-solving following very severe closed head injury. *Brain Injury, 5,* 207–211.

Godfrey, H.P.D., Partridge, F. M., Knight, R. G., & Bishara, S. (1993). Insight disorder and emotional dysfunction following closed-head injury: A controlled cross-sectional follow-up study. *Journal of Clinical and Experimental Neuropsychology, 15,* 503–515.

Goldberg, E., & Barr, W. D. (1992). Selective knowledge loss in activational and representational amnesias. In L. R. Squire & N. Butters (Eds.), *Neuropsychology of memory* (2nd ed., pp. 72–80). New York: Guilford.

Goldfried, M. R., & Davison, G. C. (1976). *Clinical behavior therapy.* New York: Holt, Rhinehart & Winston.

Gomes-Schwartz, B. (1978). Effective ingredients in psychotherapy: Prediction of outcome from process variables. *Journal of Consulting and Clinical Psychology, 46,* 1023–1035.

Grahame, L. (1991). The family system in acute care and acute rehabilitation. In J. W. Williams & T. Kay (Eds.), *Head injury: A family matter* (pp. 153–164). Baltimore: Paul H. Brookes.

Gualtieri, C. T. (1988). Pharmacotherapy and the neurobehavioral sequelae of traumatic brain injury. *Brain Injury, 2,* 101–129.

Guilford, J. P. (1967). *The nature of human intelligence.* New York: McGraw-Hill.

Hart, R. (1978). Therapeutic effectiveness of setting and monitoring goals. *Journal of Consulting and Clinical Psychology, 46,* 1242–1245.

Hollon, T. H. (1973). Behavior modification in a community hospital rehabilitation unit. *Archives of Physical Medicine and Rehabilitation, 54,* 65–72.

Horton, A. M., & Barrett, D. (1988). Neuropsychological assessment and behavior therapy: New directions in head trauma rehabilitation. *Journal of Head Trauma Rehabilitation, 3,* 57–64.

Jacobs, H. E. (1993). *Behavior analysis guidelines and brain injury rehabilitation.* Gaithersburg, MD: Aspen.

Kanfer, F. H. (1971). The maintenance of behavior by self-generated stimuli and reinforcement. In A. Jacobs & L. B. Sachs (Eds.), *The psychology of private events* (pp. 39–57). New York: Academic Press.

Kanfer, F. H. (1979). Self-management: Strategies and tactics. In A. P. Goldstein & F. H. Kanfer (Eds.), *Maximizing treatment gains: Transfer-enhancement in psychotherapy* (pp. 185–224). New York: Academic Press.

Kanfer, F. H. (1985). Target selection for clinical change programs. *Behavioral Assessment, 7,* 7–20.

Kanfer, F. H. (1986). Implications of a self-regulation model of therapy for treatment of addictive behavior. In W. R. Miller & N. Heather (Eds.), *Treating addictive behaviors: Processes of change* (pp. 29–47). New York: Plenum.

Kanfer, F. H., & Grimm, L. G. (1980). Managing clinical change: A process model of therapy. *Behavior Modification, 4,* 419–444.

Kanfer, F. H., & Schefft, B. K. (1987). Self-management therapy in clinical practice. In N. S. Jacobson (Ed.), *Psychotherapists in clinical practice: Cognitive and behavioral perspectives* (pp. 10–77). New York: Guilford.

Kanfer, F. H., & Schefft, B. K. (1988). *Guiding the process of therapeutic change.* Champaign, IL: Research Press.

Kay, T. (1993). Neuropsychological treatment of mild traumatic brain injury. *Journal of Head Trauma Rehabilitation, 8,* 74–85.

Kay, T., Newman, B., Cavallo, M., Ezrachi, O., & Resnick, M. (1992). Toward a neuropsychological model of functional disability after mild traumatic brain injury. *Neuropsychology, 6,* 371–384.

Kirschenbaum, D. S. (1987). Self-regulatory failure: A review with clinical implications. *Clinical Psychology Review, 7,* 77–104.

Klonoff, P. S., & Lage, G. A. (1991). Narcissistic injury in patients with traumatic brain injury. *Journal of Head Trauma Rehabilitation, 6,* 11–21.

Kolb, B., & Whishaw, I. Q. (1990). *Fundamentals of human neuropsychology* (3rd ed.). New York: Freeman.

LaBerge, D. (1981). Automatic information processing: A review. In J. Long & A. Baddely (Eds.), *Attention and performance* (Vol. 18, pp. 173–186), Hillsdale, NJ: Lawrence Erlbaum Associates.

Leichtman, M. (1992). Psychotherapeutic interventions with brain-injured children and their families: II. Psychotherapy. *Bulletin of the Menninger Clinic, 56,* 338–360.

Lehr, B. K., & Schefft, B. K. (1987, August). *Self-management therapy vs. cognitive-behavioral therapy in cardiac rehabilitation.* Paper presented at the 95th annual convention of the American Psychological Association, New York.

Levin, H. S., Benton, A. L., & Grossman, R. G. (1982). *Neurobehavioral consequences of closed head injury.* New York: Oxford University Press.

Levin, H. S., Goldstein, F. C., Williams, D. H., & Eisenberg, H. M. (1991). The contribution of frontal lobe lesions to the neurobehavioral outcome of closed head injury. In H. S. Levin, H. M. Eisenberg, & A. L. Benton (Eds.), *Frontal lobe function and dysfunction* (pp. 318–339). New York: Oxford University Press.

Lewis, L. (1991a). A framework for developing a psychotherapy treatment plan with brain-injured patients. *Journal of Head Trauma Rehabilitation, 6,* 22–29.

Lewis, L. (1991b). *Head injury: Issues in psychotherapy.* Topeka, KS: Menninger Video.

Lewis, L., & Rosenberg, S. J. (1990). Psychoanalytic psychotherapy with brain-injured adult psychiatric patients. *Journal of Nervous and Mental Disease, 178,* 69–77.

Lezak, M. D. (1978). Living with the characterologically altered brain injured patient. *Journal of Clinical Psychiatry, 39,* 592–598.

Lezak, M. D. (1983). *Neuropsychological assessment* (2nd ed.). New York: Oxford University Press.

Lezak, M. D. (1986). Psychological implications of traumatic brain damage for the patient's family. *Rehabilitation Psychology, 31,* 241–250.
Lezak, M. D. (1988). Brain damage is a family affair. *Journal of Clinical and Experimental Neuropsychology, 10,* 111–123.
Lira, F. T., Carne, W., & Masri, A. M. (1983). Treatment of anger and impulsivity in a brain damaged patient: A case study applying stress inoculation. *Clinical Neuropsychology, 5,* 159–160.
Livingston, M. G. (1987). Head injury: The relatives' response. *Brain Injury, 1,* 33–39.
Livingston, M. G. (1990). Effects on the family system. In M. Rosenthal, E. R. Griffith, M. R. Bond, & J. D. Miller (Eds.), *Rehabilitation of the adult and child with traumatic brain injury* (2nd. ed., pp. 225–235). Philadelphia: F. A. Davis.
Lovell, M. R., & Starrett, C. (1992). Cognitive rehabilitation and behavior therapy of neuropsychiatric disorders. In S. C. Yudofsky & R. E. Hales (Eds.), *Textbook of neuropsychiatry* (Vol. 2, pp. 741–754). Washington, DC: American Psychiatric Press.
Lowenfels, A. B., & Miller, T. T. (1984). Alcohol and trauma. *Annals of Emergency Medicine, 13,* 1056–1060.
Luria, A. R. (1973). *The working brain.* New York: Basic Books.
Malec, J. F. (1984). Training the brain-injured client in behavioral self-management skills. In B. A. Edelstein & E. T. Couture (Eds.), *Behavioral assessment and rehabilitation of the traumatically brain-damaged* (pp. 121–150). New York: Plenum.
Malec, J. F. (1990). The neuropsychological evaluation. In D. Corthell (Ed.), *Traumatic brain injury and vocational rehabilitation* (pp. 81–102). Menomonee: University of Wisconsin–Stout.
Malec, J. F., & Machulda, M. M. (1994). [Differing perceptions of impairment after brain injury among staff, survivors, and families]. Unpublished raw data.
Malec, J. F., Machulda, M. M., & Smigielski, J. S. (1993). Cluster analysis of neuropsychological test results among patients with traumatic brain injury (TBI): Implications for a model of TBI-related disability. *The Clinical Neuropsychologist, 7,* 48–58.
Malec, J. F., Schafer, D., & Jacket, M. (1992). Comprehensive-integrated postacute outpatient brain injury rehabilitation. *NeuroRehabilitation, 2,* 1–11.
Malec, J. F., Smigielski, J. S., & DePompolo, R. W. (1991). Goal attainment scaling and outcome measurement in postacute brain injury rehabilitation. *Archives of Physical Medicine and Rehabilitation, 72,* 138–143.
Malec, J. F., Smigielski, J. S., DePompolo, R. W., & Thompson, J. W. (1993). Outcome evaluation and prediction in a comprehensive-integrated postacute outpatient brain injury rehabilitation program. *Brain Injury, 7,* 15–29.
Malec, J. F., & Thompson, J. M. (1994). Relationship of the Mayo–Portland Adaptability Inventory to functional outcome and cognitive performance measures. *Journal of Head Trauma Rehabilitation, 9,* 1–15.
Marks, I. (1978). Behavioral psychotherapy of adult neurosis. In S. L. Garfield & A. E. Bergin (Eds.), *Handbook of psychotherapy and behavior change* (pp. 493–547). New York: Wiley.
Marlatt, G. A., & Gordon, J. R. (Eds.). (1985). *Relapse prevention: Maintenance strategies in the treatment of addictive behaviors.* New York: Guilford.
McGlynn, S. M., & Schacter, D. L. (1989). Unawareness of deficits in neuropsychological syndromes. *Journal of Clinical and Experimental Neuropsychology, 12,* 143–205.
McLaughlin, A. M., & Carey, J. L. (1993). The adversarial alliance: Developing therapeutic relationships between families and the team in brain injury rehabilitation. *Brain Injury, 7,* 45–51.
Meier, M. J., Benton, A. L., & Diller, L. (1987). *Neuropsychological rehabilitation.* New York: Guilford.
Miller, L. (1993). *Psychotherapy of the brain-injured patient: Reclaiming the shattered self.* New York: Norton.
Mishkin, M. (1993). Cerebral memory circuits. In T. A. Poggio & D. A. Glaser (Eds.), *Exploring brain functions: Models in neuroscience* (pp. 113–126). New York: Wiley.
Mishkin, M., Malamut, B., & Bachevalier, J. (1984). Memories and habits: Two neural systems. In G. Lynch, J. L. McGaugh, & N. M. Weinberger (Eds.), *Neurobiology of learning and memory* (pp. 65–77). New York: Guilford.
Mishkin, M., & Petri, H. L. (1984). Memories and habits: Some implications for the analysis of learning and retention. In L. R. Squire & N. Butters (Eds.), *Neuropsychology of memory* (pp. 287–296). New York: Guilford.
Moscovitch, M. (1992). A neuropsychological model of memory and consciousness. In L. R. Squire & N. Butters (Eds.), *Neuropsychology of memory* (2nd ed., pp. 5–22). New York: Guilford.
Muir, C. A., Rosenthal, M., & Diehl, L. N. (1990). Methods of family intervention. In M. Rosenthal, E. R. Griffith, M. R. Bond, & J. D. Miller (Eds.), *Rehabilitation of the adult and child with traumatic brain injury* (2nd. ed., pp. 433–448). Philadelphia: Davis.
Murphy, S. T. (1976). Effects of a token economy program on self-care behaviors of neurologically impaired patients. *Journal of Behavior Therapy and Experimental Psychiatry, 7,* 145–147.
National Head Injury Foundation (1988). *National Head Injury Foundation - Professional Council Substance Abuse Task Force white paper.* Southborough, MA: Author.

O'Hara, C. C., & Harrell, M. (1991). *Rehabilitation with brain injury survivors: An empowerment approach.* Gaithersburg, MD: Aspen.
O'Shanick, G. J. (1987). Clinical aspects of psychopharmacologic treatment in head injured patients. *Journal of Head Trauma Rehabilitation, 2,* 59–67.
O'Shanick, G. J. (1988). Psychotropic management of behavioral disorders after head trauma. *Psychiatric Medicine, 6,* 67–82.
Petri, H. L., & Mishkin, M. (1994). Behaviorism, cognitivism and the neuropsychology of memory. *American Scientist, 82,* 30–37.
Ponsford, J., & Kinsella, G. (1992). Attentional deficits following closed-head injury. *Journal of Clinical and Experimental Neuropsychology, 14,* 822–838.
Posner, M. I., & Snyder, C. R. (1975). Attention and cognitive control. In R. L. Solso (Ed.), *Information processing and cognition* (pp. 55–86). Hillsdale, NJ: Laurence Erlbaum Associates.
Prigatano, G. P., with Fordyce, D. J., Zeiner, H. K., Roueche, J. R., Pepping, M., & Wood, B. C. (1986). *Neuropsychological rehabilitation after brain injury.* Baltimore: Johns Hopkins University Press.
Prigatano, G. P. (1991a). Disordered mind, wounded soul: The emerging role of psychotherapy in rehabilitation after brain injury. *Journal of Head Trauma Rehabilitation, 6,* 1–10.
Prigatano, G. P. (1991b). The relationship of frontal lobe damage to diminished awareness: Studies in rehabilitation. In H. S. Levin, H. M., Eisenberg, & A. L. Benton, (Eds.), *Frontal lobe function and dysfunction* (pp. 381–397). New York: Oxford University Press.
Prigatano, G. P. (1992). Personality disturbances associated with traumatic brain injury. *Journal of Consulting and Clinical Psychology, 60,* 360–368.
Prigatano, G. P., Fordyce, D. J., Zeiner, H. K., Roueche, J. R., Pepping, M., & Wood, B. C. (1984). Neuropsychological rehabilitation after closed head injury in young adults. *Journal of Neurology, Neurosurgery, and Psychiatry, 47,* 505–513.
Prutting, A., & Kirchner, D. M. (1987). A clinical appraisal of the pragmatic aspects of language. *Journal of Speech and Hearing Disorders, 52,* 105–119.
Putnam, S. H., & DeLuca, J. W. (1990). The TCN professional practice survey: Part 1: General practices of neuropsychologists in primary employment and private practice settings. *The Clinical Neuropsychologist, 4,* 199–244.
Reitan, R. M., & Wolfson, D. (1986). *Traumatic brain injury. Volume I: Pathophysiology and neuropsychological evaluation.* Tucson, AZ: Neuropsychology Press.
Rimel, R. W. (1981). A prospective study of patients with central nervous system trauma. *Journal of Neurosurgical Nursing, 13,* 132–141.
Sachs, P. R. (1991). *Treating families of brain-injury survivors.* New York: Springer.
Saltzman, C., Luetgert, M. J., Roth, C. H., Creaser, J., & Howard, L. (1976). Formation of a therapeutic relationship: Experiences during the initial phase of psychotherapy as predictors of treatment duration and outcome. *Journal of Consulting and Clinical Psychology, 44,* 546–555.
Satz, P., & Fletcher, J. M. (1981). Emergent trends in neuropsychology: An overview. *Journal of Consulting and Clinical Psychology, 49,* 851–865.
Schefft, B. K., Backscheider, A., & O'Dell, M. (1996). The effects of self-regulatory procedures on recognition memory of traumatically brain-injured patients. *Journal of the International Neuropsychological Society, 2,* 17.
Schefft, B. K., & Basso, M. R. (1994). *Somatic and autonomic arousal effects of self-generated learning.* Unpublished manuscript.
Schefft, B. K., & Biederman, J. (1990). Emotional effects of self-generated behavior and the influence of resourcefulness and depressed mood. *Journal of Social and Clinical Psychology, 9,* 354–366.
Schefft, B. K., & Kanfer, F. H. (1986, November). *A process analysis of self-management, cognitive–behavioral, and relationship therapies.* Paper presented at the 20th annual convention of the Association for the Advancement of Behavior Therapy, Chicago, IL.
Schefft, B. K., & Kanfer, F. H. (1987). The utility of a process model in therapy: A comparative study of treatment effects. *Behavior Therapy, 18,* 113–134.
Schefft, B. K., & Lehr, B. K. (1985). A self-regulatory model of adjunctive behavior change. *Behavior Modification, 9,* 455–476.
Schefft, B. K., & Lehr, B. K. (1990). Psychological problems of older adults. In K. F. Ferraro (Ed.), *Gerontology: Perspectives and issues* (pp. 283–293). New York: Springer.
Schefft, B. K., & Lehr, B. K. (1994, November). *Memory and mood effects of self-generation in elderly rehabilitation patients.* Unpublished manuscript. Paper also presented at the 26th annual convention of the Association for the Advancement of Behavior Therapy, Boston, Massachusetts.
Schefft, B. K., Moses, J. A., Jr., & Schmidt, G. L. (1985). Neuropsychology and emotion: A self-regulatory model. *International Journal of Clinical Neuropsychology, 7,* 207–213.

Schefft, B. K., & Zueck, V. M. (1987, October). *The effects of self-management therapy on Alzheimer's disease patients.* Paper presented at the 7th annual meeting of the National Academy of Neuropsychologists, Chicago, IL.

Schneider, W., & Shiffrin, R. M. (1977). Controlled and automatic human information processing: I. Detection, search and attention. *Psychological Review, 84,* 1–66.

Sloane, R. B., Staples, F. R., Cristol, A. H., Yorkston, N. J., & Whipple, K. (1975). *Psychotherapy vs. behavior therapy.* Cambridge, MA: Harvard University Press.

Smigielski, J. S., Malec, J. F., Thompson, J . M., & DePompolo, R. W. (1992). Mayo Medical Center Brain Injury Outpatient Program: Treatment procedures and early outcome data. *Mayo Clinic Proceedings, 67,* 767–774.

Sohlberg, M. M., & Mateer, C. A. (1989a). *Cognitive rehabilitation: Theory and practice* [Introduction]. New York: Guilford.

Sohlberg, M. M., & Mateer, C. A. (1989b). Training use of compensatory memory books: A three-stage behavioral approach. *Journal of Clinical and Experimental Neuropsychology, 11,* 871–891.

Stern, J. M. (1985). The psychotherapeutic process with brain-injured patients: A dynamic approach. *Israel Journal of Psychiatry and Related Sciences, 22,* 83–87.

Stuss, D. T. (1991). Disturbance of self-awareness after frontal system damage. In G. P. Prigatano & D. L. Schachter (Eds.), *Awareness of deficit after brain injury: Clinical and theoretical issues* (pp. 63–83). New York: Oxford University Press.

Stuss, D. T., & Benson, D. F. (1986). *The frontal lobes.* New York: Raven.

Sullivan, T. E., Schefft, B. K., Warm, J. S., & Dember, W. N. (1994). Closed head injury assessment and research methodology. *Journal of Neuroscience Nursing, 26,* 24–29.

Sullivan, T. E., Schefft, B. K., Warm, J. S., Dember, W. N., O'Dell, M. W., & Peterson, S. J. (1995). Recent advances in the neuropsychology of human olfaction and anosmia. *Brain Injury, 19,* 641–646.

Turner, S. M., Calhoun, K. S., & Adams, H. (Eds.). (1981). *Handbook of clinical behavior therapy.* New York: Wiley.

Weddell, R., Oddy, M., & Jenkins, D. (1980). Social adjustment after rehabilitation: A two-year follow-up of patients with severe head injury. *Psychological Medicine, 10,* 257–263.

Wesolowski, M. D., & Burke, W. H. (1988). Behavior management techniques. In P. M. Deutsch & K. Fralish (Eds.), *Innovations in head injury rehabilitation* (Section 11.1–11.43). New York: Matthew Bender.

Williams, J. M., & Kay, T. (Eds.). (1991). *Head injury: A family matter.* Baltimore: Paul H. Brookes.

Wolpe, J. (1982). *The practice of behavior therapy.* New York: Pergamon.

World Health Organization. (1980). *International classification of impairments, disabilities, and handicaps.* Geneva: Author.

Yalom, I. D. (1983). *Inpatient group psychotherapy.* New York: Basic Books.

Zarski, J. J., & DePompei, K. (1991). Family therapy as applied to head injury. In J. M. Williams & T. Kay (Eds.), *Head injury: A family matter* (pp. 283–297). Baltimore: Paul H. Brookes.

Zasler, N. D. (1992). Advances in neuropharmacological rehabilitation for brain dysfunction. *Brain Injury, 6,* 1–14.

10

The Etiology of Mental Illness

Gerald Goldstein
Highland Drive VA Medical Center
and the *University of Pittsburgh*

THE BIOLOGICAL REVOLUTION

The history of the evolution of concepts of mental illness is a fascinating chapter in the general history of ideas. It impinges on such diverse areas as social philosophy, medicine, religion, and several of the social sciences. The more recent history appears to have evolved from a period of certainty about at least some mental disorders to an ongoing period of questioning and doubt. That period was probably ushered in by empirical science, and it reflected the emerging view that mental disorders could be studied in the manner of a laboratory science. When the methods of science were applied to the mental disorders, it soon became apparent that many beliefs originally based in superstition and later in clinical observation had to be discarded.

This transformation has been characterized in detail in Andreasen's (1984) *The Broken Brain*. It is a book about the biological revolution in psychiatry that illustrates how biological concepts concerning the various mental disorders have begun to dominate the field of psychopathology. This process has changed many beliefs and concepts.

A major change concerns thinking about etiology. It was assumed until recent times that certain mental disorders had an organic basis, whereas others were described as functional. The term *functional* was conservatively defined as having no known organic basis. There was a widespread belief that functional disorders were acquired through experience and interaction with the environment. The distinction between functional and organic disturbance has become increasingly vague, and a set of new beliefs have developed. They may be summarized as follows. Some mental disorders, previously thought to be based on experience and interaction with the environment, are now thought to be biological in nature, although definitive knowledge of the specific pathophysiology has not been established in most, if not all, cases. Some of these disorders are now thought to have a genetic component. A vulnerability or stress-diathesis model has been developed for some disorders in which a putatively genetic propensity for development of a disorder can be triggered into expression of the disorder itself by adverse environmental events. Therefore, individuals may now be viewed as at risk for, or vulnerable to, mental illness based on biological considerations, notably genetic endowment.

A highly pertinent example of these considerations is to be found in changes in thinking about the disorder called infantile autism. Autism was first described by Leo Kanner in 1943 based on the observation of 11 cases with symptoms of severe isolation, insistence on the preservation of sameness, and severe impairment of language, sometimes extending to mutism. Kanner believed that infantile autism is caused by a restricted early environment produced by aloof, obsessive parents who were popularly described as "refrigerator parents." Although Kanner's brilliant observations leading to the discovery of autism as a syndrome are still widely recognized, there is little if any belief that his views concerning etiology were correct. Extensive scientific investigation suggests that autism is a neurobiological disorder, with clear evidence of structural and functional brain abnormalities observable in at least some cases. New neuroimaging technologies and sophisticated neuropathological studies of the brains of deceased autistic individuals have made extensive contributions to the neurobiology of the disorder, although the specific causative factor is still unknown. However, the consequences of the biological revolution are seen remarkably clearly in the case of autism.

There has been significant interplay between the concept of the biological revolution and treatment of the mental disorders. It would probably be reasonable to mark the beginnings of the revolution with the early use of psychotropic drugs to treat schizophrenia and anxiety. The opinion that many mental disorders may have biological etiologies was clearly given impetus when it became apparent that these drugs reduced symptoms in patients with various mental disorders. Since that time, there has been a major interaction between the study of drug response and conceptualization concerning the etiologies of various disorders. This line of research has led to such major developments as the dopamine hypothesis of schizophrenia, an understanding of such neurotransmitters as serotonin in regard to depression, and the significance of dopamine for addiction. Various medications are now used not only as treatment agents but also as chemical challenges to assess various disorders. There is some ongoing debate as to whether drug response can be used for diagnostic purposes, but there seems little question that drugs can be used as research probes for the study of various disorders.

In summary, it is now commonly believed that most, if not all, mental disorders have biological bases. In some cases, the biological connection with expression of the illness is reasonably direct, whereas in others a vulnerability or stress-diathesis model seems more appropriate. A more detailed presentation of how these views are expressed in the modern classification of mental disorders is contained in chapter 14 of this volume. There, Csernansky and Faustman describe *DSM–III* (APA, 1980), *DSM–III–R* (APA, 1987), and *DSM–IV* (APA, 1993) systems for classification of disorders relevant to neuropsychology. I would only point out here that the changes contained in *DSM–IV* connote even more of an abandonment of the distinction between functional and organic disorders. Up until the development of the *DSM–III–R* criteria, a distinction was made between "Organic Mental Syndromes and Disorders" and the other disorders. That distinction is not abandoned in *DSM–IV*, but the terminology is modified in deference to the "biologizing" of psychiatry. The new terminology is "Delirium, Dementia, Amnestic and Other Cognitive Disorders." This modification connotes that although the functional versus organic distinction is obsolete, there is still a class of disorders, notably dementia, in which impairment of cognitive function is a cardinal symptom.

BIOLOGICAL PSYCHIATRY AND NEUROPSYCHOLOGY: A NEW ALLIANCE

There has been a revolution in neuropsychology as well as in psychiatry, albeit of lesser magnitude and pervasiveness. At least some neuropsychologists have become interested in psychopathology. Neuropsychologists with those interests either devote their entire professional activities to analysis of psychiatric disorders, or they share their interest in such disorders with the more traditional focus on patients with neurological disease. Historically, the refocusing probably began in the area of alcoholism, this being the first psychopathological entity extensively researched by modern neuropsychology. Some time after the early alcoholism studies were published, an interest developed in neuropsychological aspects of schizophrenia. More recently, neuropsychological research began to appear involving the mood disorders and a variety of individual disorders such as attention deficit hyperactivity disorder, autism, and obsessive–compulsive disorder. I consider these areas of inquiry in historical sequence.

Neuropsychological Models of Alcoholism and Other Addictions

The major early discovery in this area was that chronic alcoholic patients have neuropsychological deficits. This discovery was initially presented in a paper by Fitzhugh, Fitzhugh, and Reitan (1960), in which it was reported that alcoholic patients did significantly less well than controls on certain subtests of the Halstead–Reitan Neuropsychological Test Battery. Later studies by groups of investigators in Oklahoma City and Topeka, Kansas, replicated this finding. Although the view that excessive, long-term ingestion of alcohol can produce a dementia has been in the clinical folklore perhaps since antiquity, these studies demonstrated cognitive deficits using objective tests in patients who were sober at time of testing and who did not have apparent clinical signs of dementia. Furthermore, these patients demonstrated a cognitive profile characterized by impaired conceptual, psychomotor, and spatial abilities with preserved verbal intelligence and primary sensory and motor skills. Another group of investigators led by George Talland (1965) also began neuropsychological investigations of alcoholics, but initially restricted their interests to only a segment of the alcoholic population, that is, those patients with alcoholic Korsakoff's syndrome.

The original research groups studying alcoholism were subsequently joined by groups in Brooklyn, San Diego, St. Louis, and Toronto, all of which participated in the building of alternative neuropsychological models. They may be characterized as the *premature aging*, *right hemisphere* (Tarter & Edwards, 1985), *continuity hypothesis* (Butters & Granholm, 1987), and genetic models (Goodwin, 1979, 1992). I briefly discuss each of them here.

The premature aging model argues that alcoholism produces changes in the brain that would normally occur with advancing age, but accelerates the process (Ryan & Butters, 1980). In the "accelerated aging" version of the model, alcoholics exhibit deficits relative to nonalcoholics across the adult life span. In the "increased vulnerability" version, mainly older patients are affected, and differences between alcoholics and nonalcoholics increase in magnitude with age (Noonberg, Goldstein, & Page, 1985). In either case, the associated neuropathology is assumed to be generalized neuronal depletion. Supportive findings indicate that alcoholics perform on tests much like patients with nonalcoholic diffuse brain damage.

The right hemisphere model of alcoholic cognitive deficit takes note of the aforementioned cognitive profile (Tarter & Edwards, 1985). Typically, chronic alcoholics do relatively well on verbal tests and poorly on visual–spatial tasks such as the Wechsler Adult Intelligence Scale Block Design subtest (G. Goldstein, 1976). Because this pattern is often seen in patients with identifiable, structural right hemisphere brain damage, the analogy was made to alcoholism, and it was proposed that alcoholism selectively impairs right hemispheric functions.

The continuity hypothesis model is based on observation of alcoholic Korsakoff patients and chronic alcoholics (Butters & Granholm, 1987). It was proposed that alcoholism in general lies on a continuum of deficit with alcoholic Korsakoff's syndrome as the end state. The implication of this model is that the major neuropathology of alcoholism is in the same areas as it is relatively well established to be in the case of Korsakoff's syndrome. The diencephalon is the major site of the pathology with the mamillary bodies and the dorsomedial nucleus of the thalamus particularly involved.

The genetic models are better characterized as genetic-developmental models and can be divided into two types. One type is mainly developmental in nature and is based on the *antecedent predisposition hypothesis* (Tarter & Edwards, 1985). The theory is that at least some of the neuropsychological deficits found in chronic alcoholics were present prior to the onset of alcoholism, may in fact be detectable during childhood, and may be related to the acquisition of alcoholism. The theory is not specific about the etiology of the antecedent deficits. An early view was that they represented a predisposing personality trait known as *field dependence*, whereas more contemporary views suggest neurological etiology. The second type is a more straightforward genetic theory, postulating that a predisposition to alcoholism may be inherited (Goodwin, 1979, 1992). Indeed, substantial effort has been made to find the actual chromosomal abnormality. Neuropsychological studies related to this view have involved nonalcoholic children of alcoholics, full families with alcoholic members, and alcoholics with and without positive family histories.

Evidence is available for all of these models, but over the years some of them have fallen out of favor while others remain popular. The continuity hypothesis and right hemisphere models have been widely criticized and generally are not well accepted. With regard to the continuity hypothesis, numerous studies have shown that cognitive function in chronic alcoholics has quite different characteristics from what is seen in patients with Korsakoff's syndrome. The right hemisphere model of alcoholic cognitive deficit has not fared well, probably for several reasons. There is lack of anatomic evidence for the model, comparisons between patients with identifiable structural right hemisphere lesions did not demonstrate a cognitive profile comparable to what was found for chronic alcoholics, and alternative explanations for the difficulties alcoholics have with spatial-relation tasks have been convincing.

The premature aging theory remains viable but has been criticized, not because of the fact that there apparently is a progressive deterioration of brain function accompanying chronic alcoholism, but because of changes in thinking about the nature of age-associated changes in the brain. One commonly accepted view is that the brain does not deteriorate in equal steps during the presenile and senile periods of life; rather, the brain appears to remain relatively stable throughout that period and then degenerates rapidly during the last year of life. This view is known as the *terminal drop* hypothesis (Siegler, 1975). Therefore, alcoholic deterioration may resemble the process that was once thought to occur later in life with normal aging, but may not, in fact, occur.

The genetic–developmental models are very viable and are generating a great deal of research among neuropsychologists and members of allied disciplines. There has been productive interaction of neuropsychologists with geneticists in joint efforts to identify genetic variations that may be associated with vulnerability to alcoholism. The fact that having an alcoholic parent is an important risk factor for acquisition of alcoholism has become part of the common wisdom. Representative research designs have involved studies of children of alcoholics, comparing alcoholics and nonalcoholics with and without positive family histories, and longitudinal studies of children and adolescents at risk for alcoholism (Hill, Steinhauer, & Zubin, 1987). There is substantial interest in risk factors for alcoholism, with many ongoing studies of genetic, other biological, and psychosocial influences on acquisition of alcoholism and other substance use disorders. Among the more interesting findings from the standpoint of neuropsychology are the documentation of deficits in the children of alcoholics, and differences in cognitive functioning between nonalcoholics with and without positive family histories.

There is a growing literature on the neuropsychological consequences of other abused substances, notably cannabis, cocaine, and heroin. The findings in this area are preliminary and mixed, and do not yet permit postulation of a model or general conclusions (Grant & Reed, 1985). An important issue is obviously the nature of the substance itself with regard to its neurotoxicity. Another important consideration is whether the neuropsychological assessment is conducted while the individual is addicted or following recovery. This field is also made more complicated by the rather common comorbidity found in substance abusers involving both psychiatric and physical disorders (Alterman, 1985; Alterman, Erdlen, & Murphy, 1981). With regard to the latter, infection, malnutrition, and trauma commonly accompany addiction. From the standpoint of neuropsychology, the neurotoxicology would appear to be a crucial consideration, because some abused substances clearly destroy brain tissue, whereas others, such as heroin, were specifically synthesized to protect the body when analgesic therapy is needed.

Models of Schizophrenia

Introduction. Despite Herculean efforts, schizophrenia remains a disorder of unknown etiology. Its various presentations, course, and phenomenology have been thoroughly described, and treatments are available that may produce remarkable alleviation of symptoms of the disorder. However, because the specific cause of schizophrenia has not been identified, there is no definitive treatment and it cannot be "cured" as the term is usually used in medicine. In the absence of a definitive understanding of the disorder, we have a number of theoretical models of the syndrome, some of which are conflicting, but most if not all of which are based on some substantive evidence.

Schizophrenia research is a part of the biological revolution. Earlier views about a psychosocial etiology have largely been replaced by the view that schizophrenia is produced by an as yet unspecified neurobiological abnormality. Actually, there is a widely shared belief that the vulnerability or stress-diathesis concept is quite appropriate for schizophrenia (Zubin & Spring, 1977). That is, a biological predisposition only eventuates in acquisition of a schizophrenic illness under conditions of substantial life stress. Zubin has proposed a kind of sliding scale concept in which the strength of the predisposition is balanced off against the severity of stress (Day, Zubin, & Steinhauer, 1987). Therefore, an individual with a particularly strong disposition to develop the disorder may become ill with minimal stress, whereas the reverse would be true for an individual with less of a decompensatory predisposition.

The *dopamine hypothesis* is currently the most widely accepted doctrine concerning the neurochemical basis of schizophrenia. Put simply, it states that increased dopaminergic activity is the basis for the disorder. Apparently, there is not an increase in dopamine but rather an increased number of receptors in the brain for dopamine, more specifically referred to as the D-2 receptors, that is associated with the disorder. It is also widely accepted that the neurobiological anlage for schizophrenia develops early in life. Whether or not the disorder has a genetic component remains an open question, but there seems to be a general consensus that it is a neurodevelopmental disorder. In the discussion that follows, I pursue the various neuropsychological models for schizophrenia, and only touch on the controversies concerning its purported genetic and neurochemical bases as they relate to neuropsychology.

As a historical note, neuropsychologists who were then functioning as clinical psychologists originally entered the area of schizophrenia to determine whether or not cognitive aspects of schizophrenia could be distinguished from cognitive characteristics of patients with identifiable structural brain damage (G. Goldstein, 1978). At the time, this distinction was thought to reflect a problem in differential diagnosis. There was also a group of psychopathologists who were particularly interested in schizophrenic thought and language. Numerous efforts were made to characterize schizophrenic thinking through the use of sorting tests, tests of logical reasoning, and related procedures. The currently used Wisconsin Card Sorting Test (Heaton, 1980) is actually a descendant of the procedures that were used some time ago to study schizophrenic thinking.

Current thinking now regards schizophrenia as a neurobehavioral syndrome, and the focus of neuropsychological interest has become the identification of functional-structural relationships. There is also substantial interest in the effects of various medications and other treatments on neuropsychological test performance. The former interest is expressed in studies involving correlation of neuropsychological test findings with the results of various structural and functional neuroimaging procedures (T. E. Goldberg & Weinberger, 1988). The testing may be done online in the form of an activation procedure, or it may be done offline but close to the time that the neuroimaging procedure is conducted. Earlier studies demonstrated robust correlations between various neuropsychological test findings and radiological indices of neuronal depletion (reviewed in Weinberger & Wyatt, 1982). Current studies using activation and functional imaging techniques, notably positron emission tomography (PET), have produced more specific findings showing, in particular, impairment of frontal lobe function in schizophrenics during activation with appropriate measures, notably the Wisconsin Card Sorting Test (DeLisi, 1991; Weinberger, Berman, & Zec, 1986).

There have also been some studies in which neuropsychological test results were correlated with neurochemical data, particularly neurotransmitter metabolite levels. Treatment studies can be accomplished when it is possible to retest patients before and after treatment or when they are on and off medication. One of the first applications of neuropsychological testing to schizophrenic patients were the Greystone studies of lobotomy (Mettler, 1949), in which patients were administered a battery of cognitive tests before and after psychosurgery. Treatment studies may be made more sophisticated if medication blood levels are measured, and if some rating of symptomatology, such as the Brief Psychiatric Rating Scale (BPRS; Overall & Gorham, 1962) is administered in addition to the neuropsychological tests.

The neuropsychological models of schizophrenia have been largely concerned with the matter of localization. E. Goldberg and Seidman (1991), in their review, distinguished between frontal lobe and hemispheric specialization theories. G. Goldstein (1986) distinguished among "Front versus Back," "Right versus Left," and "Top versus Bottom" theories. Structures in the limbic system, notably the amygdala and hippocampus, are also thought to be important for the pathophysiology of schizophrenia. With regard to the hemispheric specialization group of theories, the preponderance of the evidence suggests that the left hemisphere is more involved in the pathophysiology of schizophrenia than the right hemisphere. The literature reflecting the debate about these localization issues has been extensively reviewed in numerous articles and chapters, and are not repeated here. Localization models are not the only viable neuropsychological models for schizophrenia, and I will go on to discuss other alternatives.

Vulnerability–Stress Diathesis Models. Localization- and lesion-oriented models of schizophrenia are probably more compatible with an earlier view of the disorder which reflects the belief that it is a degenerative illness, much like the dementias of the elderly. Indeed, schizophrenia was originally called "dementia praecox" (Kraepelin, 1925). This belief has been largely rejected based on numerous considerations including longitudinal studies, studies of elderly schizophrenic individuals, and the artifactual nature of the observations on which the belief about degeneration was made (Bleuler, 1978). Specifically, it was made on the basis of observation of patients who relapsed and had to be rehospitalized, to the neglect of patients who remained out of the hospital indefinitely following treatment. It is now widely accepted that schizophrenia is an episodic disorder marked by periods of acute psychosis intermixed with stable functioning either in the community or in minimally structured institutional settings, such as halfway houses. Indeed, the circumstances that produce relapse are currently undergoing extensive investigation (van Kammen, 1991). It is understood that noncompliance with medication schedules is an important factor, but there are apparently other physiological and environmental considerations involved. There is also a relatively recently developed view that there is a degenerative form of schizophrenia. It has been called "Kraepelinian schizophrenia," or poor outcome schizophrenia, and apparently does not constitute a large proportion of the schizophrenic population (Keefe et al., 1987). However, its course resembles the initial formulation of "dementia praecox" in that there is an inexorable deterioration much like what is seen in the presenile and senile dementias. The subtype is identified by the presence of a 5-year history of hospitalization or inability to maintain independent personal self-care.

The episodic nature of the course of at least most subtypes of schizophrenia provides difficulties for simple neuropsychological models because it introduces a state–trait dimension. The behavior of a schizophrenic patient when in an episode is quite different from the patient's mental status when the episode is over. This episodic course has obvious implications for neuropsychological test performance. However, even out of an episode, the schizophrenic patient is thought to still have the disorder. Whatever he or she shows at that point constitutes the trait component of schizophrenia. Therefore, investigators have recently been distinguishing between state and trait markers or indicators of schizophrenia. The term *marker* is probably less preferable because it connotes a genetic etiology, but it is nevertheless possible that some traits are, in fact, genetically determined.

Full studies utilizing this concept require testing the patient before, during, and after onset of an episode. A behavior that exists both before and after an episode is characterized as a trait indicator. A behavior that exists only during an episode is a state indicator. In more extensive studies utilizing this design, unaffected twins or other siblings may be included. If they also demonstrate the presence of the trait indicator, the possibility of a genetic etiology would bear further investigation. As an example of this strategy, smooth pursuit eye movements are generally found to be defective in schizophrenic patients in and out of episodes (Holzman, 1991). They also are often found to be defective in unaffected family members. Therefore, smooth pursuit eye movement defects may be viewed as a trait with a possible genetic etiology.

There is a complication involved in family studies in that family members, although not suffering from schizophrenia, may have a schizophrenic spectrum disorder such as schizotypal or paranoid personality disorder. Therefore, only family members with these disorders may have the trait whereas completely unaffected relatives might not. For example, Condray, Steinhauer, and Goldstein (1992) reported the presence of language comprehension abnormalities in schizophrenic probands and their brothers. However, only the brothers who met diagnostic criteria for a schizophrenic spectrum disorder actually showed the abnormal trait.

It has been suggested that behaviors identified as trait indicators may reflect the individual's propensity for developing a schizophrenic illness (Zubin & Spring, 1977). They have therefore been characterized as "vulnerability markers," indicating that the individual might be at risk for acquiring a schizophrenic illness in a manner conceptualized by the stress-diathesis concept. Within this framework, questions may be raised about neuropsychological tests. Are they state or trait indicators? Are they selectively distributed such that performance on specific tests is stable regardless of presence or absence of an episode, or transient, changing with onset or termination of an episode? Do family members perform in a manner characteristic of proband patients?

Neuropsychologists, by virtue of the manner in which they practice, rarely consider state–trait issues. It is difficult to test schizophrenic patients with standard neuropsychological tests while they are in episode. Even with testable patients, the reliability of the testing accomplished may be questionable and problems of practice effects from repeated testing become problematic (Chelune & Goldstein, 1991). The opportunity to test patients when they are not in an episode and out of the hospital is often not present unless there is continued treatment in an outpatient status. The termination of an episode is frequently mediated by stabilization on psychotropic drugs, and the effects of those drugs on test performance is also a consideration. Testing of relatives also typically is not feasible. Nevertheless, because of some provocative evidence coming from studies in which state–trait issues could be examined, it would be worthwhile to look at this matter with regard to neuropsychological assessment (Nuechterlein & Dawson, 1984). For example, the well-known evoked potential "P300" abnormality found in many schizophrenic patients (Friedman, 1991) has been shown to become reduced with pharmacological treatment. Whether P300 is a state indicator or sensitive to medication effects is unclear.

The vulnerability-stress diathesis model, if accurate, provides difficulties for the localization models because they appear to be derived from the traditional neuropsychological model in which associations are developed between behaviors and pathology of some specific brain lesion site. This model is exemplified in an extreme way by animal lesion studies in which behaviors are associated with specific brain lesion sites. Neuropsychological deficit in schizophrenia may not be of that nature, but rather it may be a more dynamic process associated with ongoing fluctuations in brain function status. If that is the case, it would be more probable that observed deficits are associated, at least to some extent, with a changing neurochemical milieu rather than with a stable, structural lesion. Actually, there may be a combination of structural and state changes, because many schizophrenics experience some frank neuronal depletion, as may be readily observed with the unaided eye through the use of CT or MRI scans.

Heterogeneity Models. In 1911, Bleuler (1911/1952) published a book called *Dementia Praecox or The Group of Schizophrenias*. The title suggests that even at that time, there was some belief that schizophrenia was not a single illness, but a group of related disorders. That issue remains with us as a problem to this day. It is commonly accepted that there are clinical subtypes of schizophrenia, but the generally employed typology system has changed over the years. An early typology classed schizophrenics into simple, hebephrenic, catatonic, and paranoid types. The catatonic and paranoid types have survived into *DSM–III–R* and *DSM–IV* with their original names. The hebephrenic type is now called the disorganized type, and the simple type has been abandoned. There are now also undifferentiated and residual types. The types are now viewed only as descriptive of clinical pictures, and it is understood that they may not be stable over time. That is, they have no established neurochemical, pharmacological, or neuropsychological significance.

Efforts have been made to establish neuropsychological differences between paranoid and nonparanoid schizophrenics, with mixed results. The commonly held view that paranoid patients are more intelligent than nonparanoid patients has not been well documented (G. Goldstein & Halperin, 1977). Other efforts to establish meaningful subtypes include the distinctions made between "process" and "reactive" schizophrenia (Herron, 1962), positive and negative schizophrenia (Andreasen & Olsen, 1982), schizophrenia with and without neuropsychological impairment (Silverstein & Zerwic, 1985), and classification made on the basis of response to medication, notably the separation out of poor drug responders, which has been called treatment-resistant schizophrenia (Kelley, Gilbertson, Mouton, & van Kammen, 1992). As indicated earlier, work is being done to delineate a deteriorating type, known as Kraepelinian schizophrenia. The distinction made by Crow and collaborators between Type I and Type II schizophrenia continues to attract much interest (Crow, Cross, Johnstone, & Owen, 1984). The acceptance of these subtypes have all had some difficulty, with many of the same considerations involved in all of them. The major issues are diagnostic reliability, stability, and presence of some neurobiological substrate for the differing clinical phenomenologies that are used to make the classification.

Examination of lengthy medical records often reveals that a variety of subtypes have been applied to the same patient. It is generally unclear as to whether the basis for the changes are alterations in the patient's condition or lack of reliability among the diagnosticians. The reforms of *DSM III* and the structured psychiatric interviews have alleviated the situation somewhat, but only in settings in which the criteria are strictly observed and the structured interviews are used. Alternatively, the diagnostic types may actually reflect stages in the course of the disorder, and one type may flow into another. Therefore, the clinical types may be state variables that lack stability. Clinicians sometimes find that patients that are "treatment resistant" at one point in time may be quite responsive to conventional medications at a later time.

The distinction between process and reactive schizophrenia has had an interesting fate. Basically, the developers of *DSM–III* determined that for a disorder to be called schizophrenia, there had to be at least a 6-month duration of illness. In recent-onset patients, the diagnosis of schizophrenia has to be deferred until the patient is ill for 6 months. Therefore, transient periods of psychosis of brief duration are no longer characterized as schizophrenia, but may be classified as a schizophreniform disorder or an atypical psychosis. It is likely that these are the cases that used to be described as having reactive schizophrenia.

Current thinking appears to reflect either a general discouragement about potential for finding meaningful subtypes or a continued interest in perhaps three potentially neurobiologically based subtypes. Rather than there being stable types, schizophrenia may represent a wide range of multiple deficits, perhaps in the manner of Pasamanick and Knobloch's (1966) concept of a "continuum of reproductive casualty." Subtypes may be transient clinical phenomena, with the patient demonstrating one subtype at some point in life and another subtype at another time. This apparently nihilistic but possibly correct view suggests that there is no "gene" for schizophrenia, no single etiology, and no stable typology. A multiplicity of genetic, developmental, metabolic, toxic, and neurochemical anomalies may eventuate in the disorder as a final common path. This possibility of multiple determination may aid in explaining the difficulty experienced in finding a definitive etiology for schizophrenia. It may also aid in explaining the extensive diversity of the disorder.

Those who find subtyping to be at least a heuristic aid are struck by the common observation that not all schizophrenic patients respond favorably to standard pharmacological treatment achieved through dopamine blockade. Drugs of the haloperidol type are typically effective, but not with all patients. The Crow group (Crow et al., 1984) has suggested that there are two types of schizophrenia; one of which is associated with excessive dopamine uptake, whereas the other may be produced by a viral agent. The latter, called Type II schizophrenia, is described as being resistant to medication. Ostensibly, the difficulty is not with dopamine; rather, it appears to be more associated with demonstrable, structural brain damage.

Another medication-response-related potential typology revolves around the drug clozapine. It has been widely reported that a subgroup of schizophrenic patients who did not respond well to extensive treatment efforts with haloperidol and related drugs were remarkably benefited by clozapine (Baldesarrini & Frankenburg, 1991). This experience has somewhat modified the practice of characterizing schizophrenic patients as treatment-resistant, and now there is the more hopeful view that effective treatment may be a matter of prescribing "the right drug for the right patient."

The other typology under serious consideration is the separating out of the "Kraepelinian" subgroup. These patients, despite the best efforts of clinicians, deteriorate much like patients with Alzheimer's disease and related disorders. They are characterized relative to non-Kraepelinian schizophrenics by fewer affective symptoms and more thought disorder and negative symptoms, greater risk for a schizophrenia spectrum disorder in first degree relatives, poor response to haloperidol, and more asymmetry of the lateral ventricles seen on CT scan. Silverstein and Zerwic (1985) also proposed a distinction between neuropsychologically impaired and intact schizophrenics. The intact patients putatively exhibit more positive symptoms and greater insight than the impaired patients. In summary, therefore, there appear to be three proposed typology systems that distinguish between schizophrenics with and without significant neuropsychological dysfunction and observable loss of brain tissue: the Crow group's distinction between Type I and Type II schizophrenia, the presence or absence of Kraepelinian or poor-outcome schizophrenia, and Silverstein and Zerwic's distinction between neuropsychologically impaired and intact schizophrenics.

Empirical Typologies. An alternative method of developing a typology is through the application of various statistical methods. These methods generate subtypes on the basis of similarity of subjects on sets of multivariate data. A variant of factor analysis called Q-Type factor analysis is sometimes used; also, a variety of versions of the technique called cluster analysis is available. Recently, other methods have also been applied to the classification of psychopathology; particularly, various taxometric methods that have been developed by Meehl (1993), which do not employ the concept of similarity. The major procedure is called "Coherent Cut Kinetics Method," one version of which uses mean differences around successive cut points; the other uses a covariance mixture formula.

There have been several studies in which cluster analysis was used to approach the problem of neuropsychological heterogeneity in schizophrenia. G. Goldstein and Shelly (1987) cluster analyzed the Halstead–Reitan Battery, the Luria–Nebraska Neuropsychological Battery, and the Wechsler Adult Intelligence Scale (WAIS), each of which was applied to the same sample of heterogeneous psychiatric patients (38% of whom were schizophrenic). Schear (1987) performed two cluster analyses of the WAIS and a modified Halstead–Reitan Battery with samples of 300 heterogeneous psychiatric patients. About 25% of his subjects were schizophrenic. Both studies achieved stable, internally reliable clustering solutions. Perhaps more interestingly, both studies found no relationship between psychiatric diagnosis and cluster membership. Some schizophrenics were found in each cluster. This latter finding also was noted by Townes et al. (1985) using a different classification method. Therefore, it would appear that these three studies impressively demonstrate the heterogeneous performance of schizophrenic patients on standard neuropsychological tests. One could draw the conclusion that these tests lack utility for assessment of schizophrenics because of their lack of specificity. The lack of sensitivity also has been documented because of the finding that some schizophrenic patients perform normally on these tests. The position taken by Townes et al. was that although neuropsychological tests may not identify schizophrenia, they may assess the schizophrenic's pattern and level of what they described as cognitive "competence."

In our own subsequent work, we assumed that the level and pattern of cognitive function is indeed heterogeneous in schizophrenia, but despite the fact that there is no single sensitive and specific schizophrenic cognitive deficit profile, it is nevertheless of interest to explore the diagnostic heterogeneity within schizophrenia. Schizophrenics with different cognitive profiles may have varying characteristics associated with those profiles. Therefore, the tests could potentially provide pertinent information about the patient that would not be obtainable from an interview based on clinical phenomenology.

G. Goldstein (1990) conducted a cluster analytic study that evaluated schizophrenic patients only, and concentrated on one domain of cognitive function, abstraction and problem-solving ability. There is abundant evidence that has accumulated over many years and in many settings that impairment of abstract reasoning is a core feature of schizophrenia. From the early clinical studies of K. Goldstein (1959) and Hanfmann and Kasanin (1942) with sorting tests, to the most recent investigations with the Wisconsin Card Sorting Test that was administered in association with sophisticated functional neuroimaging procedures (T. E. Goldberg & Weinberger, 1988; Weinberger et al., 1986), the practice of giving conceptual sorting tests to schizophrenics and noting their frequent failures has persisted.

In the G. Goldstein (1990) study, a battery was administered consisting of the Halstead Category and Tactual Performance Tests, the Wisconsin Card Sorting Test, and the Trail Making Test. Only data from Part B of the Trail Making Test were considered. Data from 136 male schizophrenic patients who received all of these tests were cluster analyzed, using a hierarchical agglomerative method (Ward's method), and squared Euclidean distance as the similarity measure. A five-cluster solution was proposed. Internal validity of the solution was evaluated by plotting the clusters in discriminant function space and inspecting for overlap. The five clusters appeared as clear separate entities, with minimal overlap. Therefore, heterogeneity among our schizophrenic subjects was clearly found, but it could be accounted for on a preliminary basis within the framework of five empirically derived subtypes. The pattern of heterogeneity obtained, although identifying five clusters, divided cases into what would really appear to be three performance level subgroups: one with generalized moderate impairment, one with relative absence of impairment and functioning that approaches normal, and one with dense impairment suggestive of significant deterioration. A fourth group resembles the first subgroup, but is somewhat more severely impaired. A fifth group also resembles the first subgroup, but has superior psychomotor speed capabilities and a lower prevalence of neurological comorbidity. Therefore, the clustering seems to have been based on a combination of schizophrenia-related and neurological comorbidity-related considerations. Neurological comorbidity was a substantial source of heterogeneity, but was far from being the sole determinant. Perhaps one of the most important findings of the G. Goldstein (1990) study was that the cognitive heterogeneity found, although influenced by demographic and other external considerations, was not entirely accounted for by them. I have speculated that current classification schemes, notably those proposed by the Crow group and the isolation of Kraepelinian schizophrenia as a separate syndrome, may constitute additional, schizophrenia-related influences.

As we view the matter, the major problem is that of relating neuropsychological heterogeneity to schizophrenia-related parameters. I have suggested the possibility that this additional heterogeneity can be understood in terms of some of the proposed neurobiological subtypes of schizophrenia. Thus far, I have speculated that severe deficit in a range consistent with the presence of dementia may appear in patients who would meet criteria for the Kraepelinian subtype. Patients with lesser degrees of impairment may fit into the Crow group's Type II schizophrenia, whereas patients with little in the way of cognitive deficit may be Crow group Type I patients. Admittedly, there are ambiguities here, because it is possible that patients with mild to moderate deficits might be evolving into Kraepelinian schizophrenia, whereas the relatively unimpaired patients may eventually acquire schizophrenia-related impairment. The types would not be permanent in that case, but would be developmental phenomena. We have already indicated that state–trait considerations may also have this temporal characteristic. Only longitudinal studies will answer these questions.

There are some data that suggest that heterogeneity will appear even among carefully diagnosed cases. It is reported that the Genain quadruplets (Rosenthal, 1963) exhibited heterogeneity on an attention task. Condray, Steinhauer, van Kammen, and Zubin (1992) studied a set of monozygotic twins who were concordant for paranoid schizophrenia, and who were diagnosed independently by two psychiatrists using structured psychiatric interviews. Neither twin had examinational evidence or a history of neurological comorbidity. Nevertheless, they showed striking differences on the Wisconsin Card Sorting, Trail Making, and other neuropsychological tests. Therefore, cognitive heterogeneity was found even in this exceptionally well-matched pair of subjects.

Models of Mood and Anxiety Disorders

Until quite recently, the mood and anxiety disorders stood as the last diagnostic entities that were viewed as largely functional or developed through interaction with the environment. It is probably true that these disorders have not become characterized as being neurobiological in origin in a manner comparable to schizophrenia. Nevertheless, the neurobiology of depression, mania, and anxiety have been extensively studied over the past several years. As in other areas, much of this research is connected to the development and testing of pharmacological agents, but there have been many basic scientific studies as well.

Perhaps more than would be the case for schizophrenia and alcoholism, there is a considerable state–trait question, particularly in the case of the mood disorders. If a patient is depressed and has cognitive deficits, do the deficits disappear with the depression, or do they remain stable? With regard to depression, there is a specialized area regarding depression in the elderly, primarily because of the common clinical observation that depression is often mistaken for Alzheimer's disease or a related form of senile dementia in elderly individuals. Indeed, the term *pseudodementia* was borrowed from its original application in hysteria and applied to elderly individuals who appeared to be demented, but who were actually depressed. The point was demonstrated by disappearance of the "dementia" following recovery from depression. A recent review by Lawson-Kerr, Smith, and Beck (1991) has called our attention to the particular problems of patients with organically based affective and mood disorders, such as stroke. Ruckdeschel-Hibbard, Gordon, and Diller (1986) provided an earlier review of this problem area.

There appear to be three major areas in which neuropsychologists have considered the mood disorders: depression in the elderly in relation to dementia, depression as a result of medical illness, and the mood disorders themselves. Because I am addressing here the area of psychopathology, and the mental illnesses as thought of traditionally, I will restrict my remarks to the mood disorders themselves. Specifically, I will focus on major depression of the single episode or recurrent type and bipolar disorder.

The Neuropsychology of Depression. The major neurobiological consideration in depression is thought to be an alteration of catecholamine metabolism in the brain, with norepinephrine and its metabolite MHPG being the first system studied. Platelet monoamine oxidase activity in interaction with MHPG was also widely studied. Additional neurochemicals, notably serotonin and dopamine, have been studied in relation to the mood disorders. Depue and Iacono (1989) have provided an elaborate model supporting the importance of the dopamine pathways in the ventral tegmental areas for the mood disorders. Modern medications for depression, such as fluoxytene, block uptake of serotonin.

More specifically, neuropsychological theories, as in the case of schizophrenia, involve functional system localization. Several theorists have suggested that the major dysfunction underlying depression is in the right hemisphere. Much of the evidence for this hypothesis comes from neuropsychological test data showing that depressed patients perform poorly at those tasks that are typically impaired in patients with structural right hemisphere brain damage (Flor-Henry, 1990). There is another line of evidence suggesting that the right hemisphere is predominantly responsible for the mediation of affect (Borod, 1992). An alternative view associated with laterality is that impairment of right hemisphere function is associated with denial, indifference, or euphoria, whereas left hemisphere dysfunction is associated with catastrophic reactions and depression (Silberman & Weingartner, 1986). The significant work of Robinson and collaborators (reviewed in Ruckdeschel-Hibbard et al., 1986) has made a strong case for the view that patients become depressed following left hemisphere brain damage far more often than is the case for right hemisphere brain damage.

Kluger and Goldberg (1990) argued against the right hemisphere theory of depression, indicating that the evidence for the hypothesis could just as well be interpreted in terms of bilateral/diffuse brain damage. They also pointed to numerous inconsistencies in the world literature as well as to Marin and Tucker's (1981) conclusion that there is no characteristic pattern of hemispheric dysfunction in the affective disorders. Some clarification of this debate may be made by referring to the distinctions among *emotion*, *affect*, and *mood*. The emotions are the basic feeling states such as fear or pleasure. The hypothalamus and related subcortical structures have a great deal to do with mediation of the emotions. Affect refers largely to the manner of expression of a feeling, as when we say the patient exhibited a blunted affect. Mood is a pervasive, prolonged emotional state, ranging from elation to depression.

The authors of the *DSM–III–R* changed the term *affective disorders* to *mood disorders* in recognition of the fact that these disorders involved sustained feeling states, rather than expression of those states. This distinction is critical for neuropsychology because neurological patients may have disturbances of emotion, affect, or mood. The patient with a hypothalamic lesion may sustain a basic dysregulation of emotion. The patient with right hemisphere brain damage may have a disturbance of affect as expressed in aprosodic speech or behavior, suggesting indifference if not euphoria. However, there may be no disturbance of underlying mood. Brain-damaged patients may also be genuinely depressed or manic and have a diagnosable mood disorder. Therefore, when we make reference to the neuropsychology of the mood disorders, we should properly restrict that term to those disorders characterized by sustained and pervasive feelings of depression or elation.

In view of these considerations, the ideal case for the study of the neuropsychology of mood disorder is the patient who meets *DSM–III–R* criteria for one of the diagnoses classified under the mood disorder category, who does not have other psychiatric or neurological diagnoses, and who is not in an age range that would make senile or presenile dementia a possibility. Studies of such patients, although reporting a variety of cognitive deficits, have focused largely on memory. Through the extensive and influential work of Weingartner and colleagues (e.g., Weingartner, 1986), it now seems clear that the distinction originally made by Hasher and Zacks (1979) between effortful and automatic remembering is quite pertinent for depression. Depressed individuals have difficulty with memory tasks that require active organization of material for optimal learning; however, they do not have difficulty with tasks not requiring such organization. Therefore, they may do poorly relative to controls on delayed recall of a lengthy list of words, but well on recognition or cued recall tasks.

In a review by Newman and Sweet (1992), the major neuropsychological deficits found to be associated with depression are in the areas of psychomotor function, memory and learning, and some little-studied areas including productive naming and qualitative aspects of vocabulary test performance. That review provides the reader with a more detailed account of neuropsychological aspects of depression than is possible here. An area that appears to have experienced little investigation is that of bipolar mood disorder. However, there has been substantial investigation of the effects of its major treatment agent, lithium carbonate, on cognitive function. The influence of lithium carbonate on memory and psychomotor function has been studied extensively, but apparently these studies rarely if ever were conceptualized within the cognitive context of the bipolar disorder patients that served as subjects. The results of the lithium studies have been mixed, with some reports of no effect, some of a detrimental effect, and some a beneficial effect of the drug on cognitive function (Joffe, MacDonald, & Kutcher, 1988; Williams & Goldstein, 1979). Clinically, the neuropsychological assessment of bipolar disorder is significantly impacted by state–trait considerations. Bipolar disorder is the ultimate state–trait disease, and it would seem apparent that test performance during a manic episode is likely to be quite different from performance during depression, or while the patient is stabilized on lithium carbonate.

With regard to state–trait considerations in the mood disorders in general, it does appear to be the case that improvement in cognitive function often occurs after resolution of the depression. However, Sackeim et al. (1992) reported that a performance IQ deficit is characteristic of depression regardless of state, and there are other lines of evidence such as brain electrical activity mapping (BEAM) for state-independent characteristics (Davidson, 1992). Much of the literature in this area is based on the testing of patients while they are depressed, and often while they are hospitalized, which generally connotes serious depression. Therefore, state–trait factors are often not considered. However, it appears that there is substantial recovery following lifting of depression in many patients.

There is also a heterogeneity consideration that may have implications for recovery. Massman, Delis, Butters, Dupont, and Gillin (1992) have identified a subtype of depressed patients whose performance on a number of verbal learning and memory tasks resembled that of a group of patients with Huntington's disease, a form of subcortical dementia. The other depressed patients were classified with normal controls. If this typology is successfully cross-validated, there may be a form of depressive illness that is associated with subcortical structural brain damage. The proposers of this "subcortical dysfunction hypothesis" are aware of the state-trait issue this distinction raises. They remarked:

> Longitudinal studies should be conducted to determine whether the learning and memory difficulties displayed by some depressives are a state or trait phenomenon. If these patients' deficits are associated with subcortical structural abnormalities, one would expect that they might have at least subtle memory problems even when they are not depressed." (p. 703)

It would appear that, as in the case of schizophrenia, observation of diversity and treatment of it with empirical classification methods may have substantial heuristic value.

The Neuropsychology of Anxiety Disorders. In the light of current developments, it is particularly interesting to reflect that the original conceptions of the anxiety disorders were based on the belief that they were organic illnesses. Indeed, the term for these disorders used to be *neurosis*, and the condition of anxiety continues to be popularly known as *nervousness*.

Terms such as *neurasthenia*, *anorexia nervosa*, and *hysteria* continue to persist to some extent in our technical vocabulary. Charcot, perhaps the earliest scientific investigator of the anxiety disorders, believed that hysteria was based on a hereditary predisposition (Abse, 1959). He had what might now be described as a stress-diathesis model in which an inherited constitutional factor interacts with what he described as an "occasional cause" producing symptom formation. These comments become particularly poignant in view of recent studies seeking a hereditary influence, not on hysteria, but on obsessive–compulsive disorder (OCD), another form of anxiety disorder.

OCD is a condition in which the individual becomes highly distressed by intrusive, recurrent thoughts, the compulsion to perform repetitive, stereotyped acts in response to an obsession, or both. There is now a widely held view that OCD has a biological basis, at least in the form of a predisposition to the disorder. This view has been based on the combined impact of family, pharmacological, and neuropsychological studies (Rapaport, 1989). Although OCD appears to run in families, definitive genetic studies have not yet separated hereditary from environmental etiological factors. Because OCD is a relatively rare disorder, twin studies are difficult to conduct, but a study of normal twins did suggest a heritability component of obsessive–compulsive characteristics as a personality trait. There is substantial evidence of an elevated incidence of psychopathology in general in families of OCD patients. Therefore, the genetic contribution might be nonspecific, but that is not clear as yet.

Defects in the serotonergic and noradrenergic neurotransmitter systems are felt to be a biological basis for OCD. Probably the most exciting ongoing pharmacological research utilizes the drug clomipramine, which acts on both serotonin and norepinephrine. It appears to be an effective treatment for OCD symptoms, probably through increasing the amount of available serotonin and perhaps norepinephrine. Focusing on the aspect of OCD that involves ritualistic motor behavior, Ananth (1985) stressed the role of dopamine, because dopamine supersensitivity appears to be the biochemical basis for disorders involving involuntary repetitive movements, including Tourette's syndrome, Huntington's disease, and tardive dyskinesia.

As in the case of the mood disorders, but less frequently, OCD—or at least some of its symptoms—may follow brain injury. However, a literature has recently appeared that indicates that patients with OCD and without structural brain damage may have neuropsychological deficits. In an early study, Flor-Henry, Yeudall, Koles, and Howarth (1979) proposed that the left frontal lobe was the area of major dysfunction. Utilizing Halstead–Reitan battery and other test data, they found that their OCD subjects did worse than the controls on the Halstead Category Test, the Tactual Performance Test, the Seashore Rhythm Test, the Purdue Pegboard, and Raven's Colored Progressive Matrices. Left hemisphere dysfunction in particular was suggested by poor performance relative to controls on the Wepman–Jones Aphasia Test and the WAIS Digit Span and Digit Symbol subtests.

Insel, Donnelly, Lalakea, Alterman, and Murphy (1983), using a similar battery, were unable to replicate the Flor-Henry findings, with the exception of those for the Tactual Performance Test. Insel et al. also found a substantially higher ($\geq$ 15 points) WAIS Verbal than Performance IQ in his obsessive–compulsive subjects. These findings were interpreted in terms of a relative weakness in spatial abilities. Several subsequent studies also implicated spatial but not verbal abilities as an area of deficiency in individuals with OCD. In other studies, frontal lobe function was implicated, because OCD patients were found to perform more poorly than controls on the Wisconsin Card Sorting Test and the Money Road Map Test, both of which require shifting of cognitive set (Behar et al., 1984). Whether spatial deficits or reduction of capacity to shift cognitive sets is the primary deficit is debatable.

OCD and anorexia nervosa, a related disorder, appear to be the only anxiety disorders that have undergone extensive neurobehavioral scrutiny. The neuropsychological findings are similar in both disorders. There is no definitive model established, but there is converging evidence that people with OCD have what appears as a combination of right hemisphere and frontal lobe dysfunction that manifests itself in the form of impairment of spatial abilities and cognitive flexibility, with sparing of language. To the best of our knowledge, the state–trait issue in OCD has not been examined. OCD is a very chronic disorder, but it would nevertheless be of value to evaluate the effects of successful behavioral treatment, pharmacological treatment, or both.

The Neuropsychology of Personality and Developmental Disorders. I have little to say here about the Axis II personality disorders, except in those cases in which the disorder is associated with some aspect of cognitive function. The *DSM–III*, *DSM–III–R*, and *DSM–IV* list the specific developmental disorders under Axis II, but they are not included in the present discussion, as the area of learning disability constitutes a separate specialty in neuropsychology and is typically not viewed as a "mental illness." The developmental disorders of particular interest to neuropsychologists are mental retardation, autistic disorder, and attention-deficit hyperactivity disorder. Mental retardation is not discussed here, because it is essentially an area separate from mental illness with a vast literature of its own. I do make some remarks about attention-deficit hyperactivity disorder and autism.

To the best of our knowledge, the major body of substantive neuropsychological research in the personality disorders concerns schizotypal personality disorder (SPD). Neuropsychological status is sometimes assessed in individuals with conduct or antisocial personality disorder, but the referral question typically involves the ruling out of an organic condition that might help in explaining an episode or pattern of violent or aggressive behavior. However, individuals with SPD have been reported to have neurocognitive deficits associated with the disorder itself. The *DSM–III–R* defines SPD as a condition marked by poor interpersonal relations and peculiarities in thinking and behavior. Symptoms of ideas of reference, social anxiety, magical thinking, illusions, and "oddness" in appearance, behavior, and speech may be present.

Gruzelier (1991) has reviewed many of the neuropsychological features of schizotypy, stressing those that relate to hemispheric imbalance. Many of these investigations involved visual field studies, with the general finding that there was an attenuation of the expected left hemisphere advantage for verbal stimuli. Auditory experiments utilizing individuals with schizoptypy as subjects and involving comparisons between monaural and binaural hearing and dichotic listening procedures showed right hemisphere superiority, which is opposite to the normal expectation. Several studies were reported to show that there are more leftward lateral eye movements in schizoptypic individuals, indicating greater right hemisphere activation. Gruzelier concluded that the weight of evidence supports the existence of a hemispheric imbalance in schizotypy, with most studies showing a right hemisphere functional advantage. That is, information that tends to be processed more accurately or rapidly by the left hemisphere in normal individuals is processed by individuals with schizotypy either better by the right hemisphere or without an advantage achieved by either hemisphere.

Our group in Pittsburgh has been conducting a long-term study of proband schizophrenic patients and their relatives. A substantial portion of the relatives were found to have schizophrenic-spectrum disorders, and many of them met diagnostic criteria for SPD. In one study (Condray & Steinhauer, 1992), these individuals with SPD were compared with subjects meeting criteria for SPD but without a family history of schizophrenia. These subjects were administered a continuous performance test, an event-related potential (ERP) procedure to assess the status of the P300 component, the Wisconsin Card Sorting Test, Trail Making, Part B, WAIS–R Information and Block Design, and the Relational Concepts factor scale from the Luria–Nebraska Battery. Performance on a measure of vigilance derived from the continuous performance test (*d′*) was significantly different between the two SPD and the normal control groups. The controls performed significantly better than the SPD groups with and without family histories of the disorder. No significant differences were found for the ERP procedure or for the other cognitive tests, with the exception of the Relational Concepts factorial measure. On this test, the SPD group with schizophrenic relatives performed significantly worse than did the SPD group without schizophrenic relatives and the controls.

The positive finding for the Relational Concepts factor scale led to an extended study in which the male schizophrenic probands were included, and brothers with a nonspectrum psychiatric disorder were separated out as a subgroup (Condray, Steinhauer, & Goldstein, 1992). It was particularly interesting to find that the worst mean score on Relational Concepts was found for the schizophrenic spectrum disorder brothers and not for the probands themselves. Statistically, they did not differ from each other. However, an overall significant difference was found among groups, with significantly more impairment in the probands and the brothers with spectrum disorders as compared to the unaffected brothers and controls. The results of this study would suggest that individuals with schizotypy may have subtle language deficits, and the risk for occurrence of this symptom complex appears to be greater for schizotypic individuals with schizophrenic relatives. This finding would be concordant with Gruzelier's left hemisphere deficit hypothesis, particularly because the same results were not found for Block Design or the Wisconsin Card Sorting Test.

Attention-Deficit Hyperactivity Disorder (ADHD)

ADHD represents a complex problem area for neuropsychology, particularly because it frequently does not appear as a pure syndrome and it may be associated with dyslexia and related learning disabilities, or conduct disorders. Originally, it was an area of interest primarily to child neuropsychologists, but it has been shown that the disorder may persist, sometimes in a residual form, into adulthood. The *DSM–III–R* criteria are child-oriented, which makes it problematic to diagnose the disorder in adults. The *DSM–IV* criteria improve this situation substantially. For example, the *DSM–III–R* item "has difficulty playing quietly" has been changed to "often has difficulty playing or engaging in leisure activities quietly."

Pennington (1991) provided an extensive consideration of ADHD from a neuropsychological standpoint. He places great weight on the role of executive function associated with dysfunction of the prefrontal lobe. The widely accepted view that at least some individuals with ADHD suffer from low CNS arousal is acknowledged; however, Pennington suggested, on the basis of findings involving reduced blood flow in the frontal areas, that this condition of so-called "hypofrontality" may explain the low arousal level of the autonomic component of the central nervous system. The role of reduced dopamine level in ADHD is widely accepted and provides the rationale for treatment with Ritalin, although the actual mode of action of this agent is not well understood.

Extensive efforts have been made to characterize the attentional disorder in ADHD utilizing behavioral, cognitive, and neuropsychological tests. Pennington (1991) outlined three major alternative models; the *voluntary motor control theory* of Conners, the *executive function theory* that Pennington himself advocates, and a *right hemisphere attentional systems* model based on Posner's work. Conners' model, as characterized by Pennington, stresses the role of hyperactivity and is based on observations of failures of motor inhibition. Pennington (1991) defined executive function as "the ability to maintain an appropriate problem-solving set for attainment of a future goal" (p. 13). His review of studies demonstrating contrasts between intact and preserved abilities in ADHD suggested that the underlying neurobehavioral deficit is not in a particular domain, but rather is a cross-domain regulatory ability that can be called executive function, as defined earlier. Application of the Posner (1987) theory of attention to ADHD in particular has not been accomplished, but application of that theory has been made to schizophrenia, a disorder also characterized by significant attentional dysfunction.

Mirsky and numerous collaborators have been studying attention for many years with various populations of normal individuals, neurological and psychiatric patient groups, and animals. This work has been conceptualized into a theory of attention based on a factor analysis of various measures of attention, such as cancellation tasks, the Stroop Test, and the continuous performance test (Mirsky, Anthony, Duncan, Ahearn, & Kellam, 1991). The analysis was based on an earlier attempt of Zubin (1975) to categorize attention. It divides attention into four elements; focusing, sustaining, encoding, and shifting. The four elements are hypothesized to be mediated by different brain structures. For example, encoding is thought to be mediated by the hippocampus and amygdala. Like the Posner theory, the Mirsky model has not yet been systematically applied to the problem of ADHD, but doing so would provide an attractive opportunity to incorporate existing literature with new studies in order to qualify the nature of the attention deficit in ADHD within a comprehensive conceptual framework.

Autism. Earlier in this chapter it was noted that the investigation of autism represented a particularly instructive example of changes in thinking about a specific disorder that occurred as a result of, and as a part of, the biological revolution in psychiatry. Here, more detailed information about models of autism is provided, particularly because it represents an area in which there has been intensive neuropsychological investigation during recent years.

Autism is described clinically as a pervasive developmental disorder, with cardinal symptoms of impaired social relations, poor communicative abilities, and a restricted range of interests and activities. Diagnostic difficulties are often present because of the wide range of severity of the disorder, particularly in the area of verbal communication. Some autistic individuals are mute, whereas others only show subtle impairments of language and language comprehension. Preoccupation with sameness or development of distress over apparently trivial changes is a well-known symptom of the disorder. Symptoms are generally observable during infancy. The disorder persists throughout life, but its clinical appearance generally changes, sometimes quite remarkably, over the years. There is always a delay in language development, but sometimes there is a notable improvement in language during the early school years.

Because of the wide range of severity of the disorder, it was found to be useful to distinguish between high- and low-functioning autism. The generally accepted cut-off point is an IQ of 70 (Schopler & Mesibov, 1992). There appears to be a widespread acceptance of Bartak and Rutter's (1976) view that IQ is the best index of the severity of autistic disorder. Although the matter remains somewhat controversial, there is some consensus that individuals with high-functioning and low-functioning autism suffer from the same disorder, and that their syndromes are not likely to have differing etiologies. The mental retardation often associated with autism is thought to be a part of the disorder, not a separate illness.

The opportunity to obtain reliable diagnoses of autism has been greatly expanded through the introduction of two structured instruments, the Autism Diagnostic Interview (ADI; LeCouteur et al., 1989) and the Autism Diagnostic Observation Schedule (ADOS; Lord et al., 1989). The ADI is a structured interview typically conducted with the mother. The ADOS is a set of structured tasks that the patient and interviewer role play. These procedures include algorithms to determine whether or not *DSM–III–R* criteria are met. The ADI and ADOS are compatible with the revised criteria for autistic disorder that appear in the *DSM–IV*. Highly satisfactory reliabilities have been established.

Models of Autism. Kanner's view that autism is produced by poor nurturing during early life by cold and rational ("refrigerator") parents has been abandoned. It is now thought that autism, although clearly a distinct syndrome, is a neurodevelopmental disorder. Evidence for its heritability is essentially negative, although it is more common in males than in females and incidence is increased in families in which there are autistic siblings. The actual etiology remains unknown, although the matter is currently under intensive study with preliminary findings coming from neurochemical, neuroimaging, and pathological investigations.

The investigation of the neurobiology of autism has become a controversial matter with several major competing theories. The theories differ both with regard to behavioral and neurological considerations. That is, each theory postulates that autism is characterized by some core cognitive deficit, purportedly based in some structure or system in the CNS. The earliest neurobiological investigations of autism were largely stimulated by observations of the abnormal sensory input observed in many autistic individuals. There may be a lack of responsiveness to sensation or an exaggerated response.

The DesLauriers–Carlson (DesLauriers & Carlson, 1969) hypothesis proposed that there was a central functional impairment in decoding the affective component of sensory experience. These observations clearly implicated brainstem arousal mechanisms in the etiology of autism and resulted in numerous laboratory studies of the brainstem in autism, including brainstem evoked potential, eye movement, and vestibular function studies (Ornitz, 1974). More recently, neuroanatomic evidence of subcortical pathology was produced, mainly involving the cerebellar vermis (Holttum, Minshew, Sanders, & Phillips, 1992). These findings were accompanied by increasingly sophisticated studies of visual, auditory, and brainstem evoked potentials and were conceptualized in terms of deficits in aspects of attention, notably selective and shifting attention.

There is now a major attentional theory of autism that postulates the presence of the major pathophysiology in brainstem and cerebellar structures (Courchesne, Yeung-Courchesne, Press, Hesselink, & Jernigan, 1988). Aside from the neuroanatomic findings, the basic evidence for this theory comes from cognitive evoked potential studies during which subjects perform various attentional tasks while electrophysiologic recordings are being made (Akshoomoff & Courchesne, 1992).

Other investigators have focused on an anatomic finding involving focal pathology of the hippocampus in autistic individuals, animal studies involving medial temporal–limbic ablation, and a group of studies of memory deficit in autism. The theory proposed was that autistic individuals, although not densely amnesic, may have an information-acquisition deficit associated with hippocampal dysfunction (Minshew & Goldstein, 1993). Other groups of investigators have developed theories proposing that the major autistic cognitive deficits found in autism are at the cortical network level, and are manifested either as a generalized information processing deficit or as a more specific deficit in executive function. These theories were based on neuropsychological assessment studies, primarily of high-functioning autistic individuals, and imagery studies including use of positron emission tomography (PET) and magnetic resonance spectroscopy (Minshew, Goldstein, Dombrowski, Panchaligam, & Pettegrew, 1993).

All of these theories are viable and continue to receive empirical support. Recently, this work has been summarized in a book by Bauman and Kemper (1994) that covers much of the imaging, psychophysiological, and neuropsychological work done in autistic syndrome analysis. Recent reconceptualizations of the various theories have led to some reconciliation of them, generally in a direction suggesting that autism does not have a focal etiology in the brain stem, cerebellum, hippocampus, or frontal lobes, but rather is based on a complex system dysfunction in which these structures may all be involved. On the behavioral side, it is currently generally accepted that autism is not a single deficit disorder, such as an amnesia or an attention deficit, but involves multiple deficits. Therefore, a multiple level, multiple-deficit general theory appears to be emerging, perhaps in the form of a neural network, but the exact system has not yet been described.

SUMMARY

This brief overview of neuropsychological aspects of the etiology of mental illness suggests the enormous complexity of this area. Most, if not all, of the specific etiologies of these disorders remain unknown, but there are important findings for all of them that should ultimately lead to basic syndrome analytic solutions. It is important to note that much of the recent work is driven by new technologies that were not available when the study of these disorders began. Each new technology appears to have provided new information, much of which is quite important. The discovery of brain atrophy in young schizophrenic patients, and the family/genetic studies of alcoholism, for example, approach the level of scientific breakthroughs. It would appear, however, that the flow of information coming from each new technology becomes exhausted before definitive solutions are found. It is therefore highly likely that we do not currently possess the technologies that are necessary for definitive etiologic analysis of the neurobehavioral deficits associated with psychiatric disorders.

Several major methodological considerations may provide heuristic aids in planning of future research. First, it appears that little progress will be made by adhering to simplistic models of brain function and naive concepts about how clinical syndrome entities may be represented in the brain. As long as we believe that schizophrenia lives in the left frontal lobe next to the Wisconsin Card Sorting Test, we will make little progress. As we have seen, for all of the disorders discussed, there are exceedingly complex pathophysiologies, involving neurochemical, neurophysiological, and structural processes at multiple neuroanatomic sites. Even within neurochemistry, it is becoming apparent that there probably are no single neurotransmitter disorders, and that all of the mental disorders that have a chemical basis probably involve interactions among multiple neurotransmitter systems. For example, although dopamine may be particularly important for schizophrenia, recent research also has demonstrated important roles for norepinephrine and serotonin, which interact with dopamine. It would be our view that the etiology of most, if not all, of the mental disorders will be at the systemic level, and will require such relatively new conceptual models as neural networks for further theoretical development. It now seems more than likely that the definitive biological factors may be at the level of dendritic coding or architecture, cell membrane metabolism, or complex genetic variations that are not of the single gene type. Indeed, intensive genetic investigation indicates that there is no "gene for schizophrenia," and the actual molecular genetics of the disorder, if they exist in a specific way, remain obscure. Very recently, there have been findings regarding distinct abnormalities of brain energy and membrane phospholipid metabolism in autistic and schizophrenic patients.

The second consideration involves state–trait considerations. The model of the static, focal lesion that has been so useful for classical neuropsychology does not appear to work for psychopathology. The mental illnesses have varying courses and outcomes. In some cases, state conditions fluctuate quickly and dramatically, the extreme case being the "rapid cycler" category of bipolar mood disorder. Schizophrenia is now thought to be mainly an episodic disorder marked by alternating periods of psychosis and relatively symptom-free status. Recurrent depression is manifested by sometimes unpredictable repetitions of severe depressive episodes. Therefore, an adequate neuropsychological model of these and other mental disorders has to imagine a condition of fluctuating brain function, sometimes giving rise to episodes of severe illness and sometimes allowing for relatively normal function. In bipolar disorder, allowance must be made for two kinds of disorder: mania and depression. In view of these considerations, it becomes particularly important to trace the clinical course of the various mental disorders, and to distinguish between state and trait indicators as one does so.

The major surprises coming from longitudinal investigation appear in the case of schizophrenia. Neuropsychologists typically assess schizophrenic patients, perhaps not when they are acutely psychotic, but when they are hospitalized and still symptomatic. The more recent longitudinal outcome studies, however, produce a more benign picture than was previously painted, finding that many authentically schizophrenic patients do well in the community over long time periods without relapse. We know very little about the neuropsychological status of these individuals, because they are stable community residents who are not in need of medical attention, except perhaps for medication management. It would be of particular interest to examine such individuals for trait indicators. In general, as we have already suggested, the ideal situation involves evaluating patients in and out of psychotic episodes, on and off medication, and during different phases of the disorder under study.

A final consideration has to do with symptomatic/diagnostic heterogeneity. As one reviews the contemporary literature, there appears to be an increase in concern with heterogeneity, and, in particular, with whether the various diagnostic categories represent homogeneous disorders. This question has been raised directly in the cases of schizophrenia, autism, alcoholism, and attention-deficit hyperactivity disorder. Perhaps a more basic question relates to the classification system itself. The broad categories of types of disorders, as well as the specific diagnoses contained in the various *DSM*s are based primarily on clinical and descriptive data; they do not necessarily relate to the underlying biologies of the mental disorders. For example, mania and depression are both classified as mood disorders, but it would be difficult to imagine that they both have the same neurobiology. On the other hand, biological links have been made between disorders across broad categories, such as the relationships that have been found among OCD, anorexia nervosa, and Tourette's syndrome. The work discussed earlier regarding the subcortical theory of depression suggests a link between some, but clearly not all, depressive disorders and the subcortical dementias. In essence, there appears to be a disparity in categorization between clinical description and underlying pathophysiology.

Some of the mental disorders appear to be inherently heterogeneous, the clearest case being schizophrenia. Although the reforms of the *DSM–III* clearly aided in defining and reliably diagnosing the disorder, heterogeneity still exists within the limits of the diagnostic criteria. It exists in numerous aspects including clinical phenomenology, course and outcome, level and pattern of cognitive function, neuroradiological and other laboratory findings, and response to treatment. Again, what appears to hold the diagnosis together as a viable scientific construct is the clinical phenomenology, and not necessarily the pathophysiology. Crow and collaborators (Crow et al., 1984) were careful to assert that their Type I and Type II categories were both schizophrenic syndromes, despite the possibility of there being different etiologies. They stated: "Although the two syndromes may represent separate dimensions of pathology, it is clear that they do not constitute separate diseases" (p. 218).

As an alternative to descriptive or rule-based classification systems, we have proposed the use of quantitative multivariate methods such as cluster analysis. Systems of numerical taxonomy (Sokal & Sneath, 1963) in neuropsychology and other disciplines have provided the opportunity to make classifications on the basis of diverse but relevant data that are objective and quantifiable. In neuropsychology, these methods have been particularly useful in the area of learning disability, particularly because they aided in describing clinically relevant subtypes (Rourke, 1985, 1991). Schear (1987), the Townes group, (Townes et al., 1985) and I (G. Goldstein, 1990) have done some preliminary work in the area of schizophrenia and other neuropsychiatric disorders. As described earlier, Meehl has been working for many years on development of empirical taxonomic systems for the classification of psychopathology that differ from cluster analysis.

The usual aims of the quantitative classification methods are to identify and describe taxons, or subtypes within a heterogeneous sample. If a successful typology is created from the mathematical standpoint, then there is hope of relating subtype membership to any number of explanatory variables. The process of forming these relationships, or establishing the "external validity" of the taxonomic system, could lead to significant discoveries regarding the basis for the clinical heterogeneity of the disorder. Within the realm of neuropsychology, these discoveries may cut across various diagnostic categories and provide an alternative paradigm for classifying patients. Thus far, in three independent studies utilizing the combination of quantitative classification methods, neuropsychological tests as the variables, and heterogeneous samples of psychiatric patients as subjects, no relationship has been found between empirically derived subtype membership and psychiatric diagnosis. That is, the actuarial classification systems that have been developed did not contain disproportionate numbers of patients with a particular diagnosis in any subtype. Therefore, the standard neuropsychological tests do not appear to be diagnostic of any particular common mental illness. The question then becomes one of determining the basis of the classification.

Townes et al. (1985) suggested that the tests evaluated the individual's level of "competence" regardless of his or her psychiatric diagnosis. What the results of actuarial classification studies may also suggest is clinically significant heterogeneity within various psychiatric groups, as in the case of the Massman et al. (1992) study in which some of the depressed subjects performed normally on tests, whereas others performed in a manner that did not distinguish them from patients with known subcortical dementias. Here, the neuropsychological tests might have been quite useful with regard to distinguishing between patients with the same clinical phenomenology, but possibly very different underlying pathophysiologies. The hope of discovering such potential neurobiological subtypes exists for many, if not all, of the mental disorders. Alternatively, the quantitative classification methods have the capability of determining that there is, in actuality, no meaningful typology, and that the variability within a group under study is best understood as a continuum. This contingency occurs when the mathematics of the methods used do not provide an interpretable dendogram or other form of disjoint subtype representation, or when no meaningful external validity criteria can be found.

Neuropsychology has, in recent years, become increasingly relevant to neurobehavioral analysis of most, if not all, of the mental disorders. Clinical neuropsychology has progressed from initial interests in whether a particular condition presented by a patient was "functional or organic," through a period of what retrospectively appears to be a naive attempt to "localize" the functional system basis of various mental disorders, to full participation as a neuroscience involved in state-of-the-art study of the pathophysiology and etiology of the various mental or neurobehavioral disorders. Neuropsychologists are now working in collaboration with neuroradiologists, neurochemists, research psychiatrists, geneticists, and other clinical neuroscientists. I have suggested that these interactions have produced a number of substantive findings and raised a number of methodological issues.

It now seems reasonably clear that most, if not all, of the mental disorders have some neurobiological foundations which appear to be at the functional system level. That is, they are not the product of single localized structures, although localized structures may be significantly involved in complex networks. Second, the mental disorders have varying courses and outcomes, and typically they have both state and trait characteristics. Some of these characteristics are modifiable by treatment, notably with various pharmacological agents that have cognitive effects. Third, many of the mental disorders are heterogeneous even when one only considers cases that meet strict diagnostic criteria. In some cases, the heterogeneity may be resolvable into meaningful diagnostic subtypes, but that may not always be possible.

There appears to be both diagnostic and neuropsychological heterogeneity within diagnostic groups. Diagnostic heterogeneity occurs when a diagnostic category itself includes more than one syndrome or disease; for example, the Crow group's Type I and Type II schizophrenia, or the possibility of subgroups of depressives with and without a subcortical pathophysiology. Neuropsychological heterogeneity occurs when there is extensive variability on neuropsychological tests within a diagnostic category. This phenomenon appears to occur most frequently in schizophrenia; however, it can be said with some assurance that there is no neuropsychological profile or test result that characterizes the full clinical spectrum of any of the mental disorders. This consideration, in combination with the replicated finding that there is no association between neuropsychologically based classification and psychiatric diagnosis, has dramatically altered the role of neuropsychological assessment in the field of psychopathology, taking it from an initial effort to diagnose the mental disorders toward an attempt to etiologically understand them.

ACKNOWLEDGMENT

Indebtedness is expressed to the Department of Veterans Affairs for support of this work.

REFERENCES

Abse, D. W. (1959). Hysteria. In S. Arieti (Ed.), *American handbook of psychiatry*, (Vol. 1, pp. 272–292). New York: Basic Books.

Akshoomoff, N. A., & Courchesne, E. (1992). A new role for the cerebellum in cognitive operations. *Behavioral Neuroscience, 106*, 731–738.

Alterman, A. I. (1985). Relationships between substance abuse and psychopathology: Overview. In A. I. Alterman (Ed.), *Substance abuse and psychopathology* (pp. 1–12). New York: Plenum.

Alterman, A. I., Erdlen, F. E., & Murphy, E. (1981). Alcohol abuse in the psychiatric population. *Addictive Behaviors, 6*, 69–73.

American Psychiatric Association. (1980). *Diagnostic and statistical manual of mental disorders* (3rd ed.), Washington, DC: Author.

American Psychiatric Association. (1987). *Diagnostic and statistical manual of mental disorders* (3rd ed., rev.). Washington, DC: Author.

American Psychiatric Association. (1994). *Diagnostic and statistical manual of mental disorders* (4th ed.). Washington DC: Author.

Ananth, J. (1985). Pharmacotherapy of obsessive–compulsive disorder. In M. Mavissakalian, S. M. Turner, & L. Michelson (Eds.), *Obessive–compulsive disorder: Psychological and pharmacological treatment* (pp. 167–211). New York: Plenum.

Andreasen, N. C. (1984). *The broken brain: The biological revolution in psychiatry*. New York: Harper & Row.

Andreasen, N. C., & Olsen, S. (1982). Negative versus positive schizophrenia: Definition and validity. *Archives of General Psychiatry, 39*, 789–794.

Baldesarrini, R. J., & Frankenburg, F. R. (1991). Clozapine, a novel antipsychotic agent. *New England Journal of Medicine, 324*, 746–754.

Bauman, M. L., & Kemper, T. L. (1994). *The neurobiology of autism*. Baltimore: Johns Hopkins University Press.

Bartak, L., & Rutter, M. (1976). Differences between mentally retarded and normally intelligent autistic children. *Journal of Autism and Childhood Schizophrenia, 126*, 127–145.

Behar, D., Rapoport, J. L., Berg, C. J., Denckla, M. B., Mann, L., Cox, C., Fedio, P., Zahn, T., & Wolfman, M. G. (1984). Computerized tomography and neuropsychological test measures in adolescents with obsessive–compulsive disorder. *American Journal of Psychiatry, 141*, 363–368.

Bleuler, E. (1952). *Dementia praecox or the group of schizophrenias*. New York: International Universities Press. (Original work published 1911)

Bleuler, M. (1978). *The schizophrenic disorders: Long-term patient and family studies*. (S. M. Clemens, Trans.) New Haven, CT: Yale University Press.

Borod, J. C. (1992). Interhemispheric and intrahemispheric control of emotion: A focus on unilateral brain damage. *Journal of Consulting and Clinical Psychology, 60*, 339–348.

Butters, N., & Granholm, E. (1987). The continuity hypothesis: Some conclusions and their implications for the etiology and neuropathology of alcoholic Korsakoff's syndrome. In O. A. Parsons, N. Butters, & P. E. Nathan (Eds.), *Neuropsychology of alcoholism: Implications for diagnosis and treatment* (pp. 176–206). New York: Guilford.

Chelune, G. J., & Goldstein, G. (1991, August). *Interpreting test–retest changes in neuropsychological practice.* Symposium presented at the annual meeting of the American Psychological Association, San Francisco, CA.

Condray, R., & Steinhauer, S. R. (1992). Schizotypal personality disorder in individuals with and without schizophrenic relatives: Similarities and contrasts in neurocognitive and clinical functioning. *Schizophrenia Research, 7*, 33–41

Condray, R., Steinhauer, S., & Goldstein, G. (1992). Language comprehension in schizophrenics and their brothers. *Biological Psychiatry, 32*, 790–802.

Condray, R., Steinhauer, S., van Kammen, D. P., & Zubin, J. (1992). Dissociation of neurocognitive deficits in a monozygotic twin pair concordant for schizophrenia. *Journal of Neuropsychiatry and Clinical Neuroscience, 4*, 449–453.

Courchesne, E., Yeung-Courchesne, R., Press, G. A., Hesselink, J. R., & Jernigan, T. L. (1988). Hypoplasia of cerebellar vermal lobules VI and VII in autism. *New England Journal of Medicine, 318*, 1349–1354.

Crow, T. J., Cross, A. J., Johnstone, E. C., & Owen, F. (1984). Two syndromes in schizophrenia and their pathogenesis. In F. A. Henn & H. A. Nasrallah (Eds.), *Schizophrenia as a brain disease* (pp. 196–234). New York: Oxford University Press.

Davidson, R. J. (1992). Brain asymmetry, the emotions, and mood disorders. *Harvard Mental Health Letter, 9*, 4–5.

Day, R., Zubin, J., & Steinhauer, S. R. (1987). Psychosocial factors in schizophrenia in light of vulnerability theory. In D. Magnusson & A. Ohmann (Eds.), *Psychopathology: An interactional perspective* (pp. 25–39). New York: Academic Press.

DeLisi, L. E. (1991). Brain imaging studies of cerebral morphology and activation in schizophrenia. In S. R. Steinhauer, J. H. Gruzelier, & J. Zubin (Eds.), *Handbook of schizophrenia: Vol. 5. Neuropsychology, psychophysiology and information processing* (pp. 147–160). London: Elsevier.

Depue, R. A., & Iacono, W. G. (1989). Neurobehavioral aspects of affective disorders. *Annual Review of Psychology, 40*, 457–492.

DesLauriers, A. M., & Carlson, C. F. (1969). *Your child is asleep: Early infantile autism.* Homewood, IL: Dorsey.

Fitzhugh, L., Fitzhugh, K., & Reitan, R. M. (1960). Adaptive abilities and intellectual functioning in hospitalized alcoholics. *Quarterly Journal of Studies on Alcohol, 21*, 414–423.

Flor-Henry, P. (1990). Neuropsychology and psychopathology: A progress report. *Neuropsychology Review, 1*, 103–123.

Flor-Henry, P., Yeudall, L. T., Koles, Z. J., & Howarth, B. J. (1979). Neuropsychological and power spectral EEG investigations of the obsessive-compulsive syndrome. *Second World Congress of Biological Psychiatry, 4*, 119–130.

Friedman, D. (1991). Endogenous scalp-recorded brain potentials in schizophrenia: A methodological review. In S. R. Steinhauer, J. H. Gruzelier, & J. Zubin (Eds.), *Handbook of schizophrenia: Vol. 5. Neuropsychology, psychophysiology and information processing* (pp. 91–127). London: Elsevier.

Goldberg, E., & Seidman, L. J. (1991). Higher cortical functions in normals and in schizophrenic: A selective review. In S. R. Steinhauer, J. H. Gruzelier, & J. Zubin (Eds.), *Handbook of schizophrenia: Vol. 5. Neuropsychology, psychophysiology and information processing* (pp. 553–597). London: Elsevier.

Goldberg, T. E., & Weinberger, D. R. (1988). Probing prefrontal function in schizophrenia with neuropsychological paradigms. *Schizophrenia Bulletin, 14*, 179–183.

Goldstein, G. (1976). Perceptual and cognitive deficit in alcoholics. In G. Goldstein & C. Neuringer (Eds.), *Empirical studies of alcoholism* (pp. 115–151). Cambridge, MA: Ballinger.

Goldstein, G. (1978). Cognitive and perceptual differences between schizophrenics and organics. *Schizophrenia Bulletin, 4*, 160–185.

Goldstein, G. (1986). The neuropsychology of schizophrenia. In I. Grant & K. Adams (Eds.), *Neuropsychological assessment of psychiatric disorders* (pp. 147–171). New York: Plenum.

Goldstein, G. (1990). Neuropsychological heterogeneity in schizophrenia: A consideration of abstraction and problem solving abilities. *Archives of Clinical Neuropsychology, 5*, 251–264.

Goldstein, G., & Halperin, K. M. (1977). Neuropsychological differences among subtypes of schizophrenia. *Journal of Abnormal Psychology, 86*, 34–40.

Goldstein, G., & Shelly, C. (1987) The classification of neuropsychological deficit. *Journal of Psychopathology and Behavioral Assessment, 9*, 183–202.

Goldstein, K. (1959). Concerning the concreteness in schizophrenia. *Journal of Abnormal and Social Psychology, 59*, 146.

Goodwin, D. W. (1979). Alcoholism and heredity: A review and hypothesis. *Archives of General Psychiatry, 36*, 57–61.

Goodwin, D. W. (1992). Genetics of alcoholism. In L. K. G. Hsu & M. Hersen (Eds.), *Research in psychiatry* (pp. 359–372). New York: Plenum.

Grant, I., & Reed, R. (1985). Neuropsychology of alcohol and drug abuse. In A. I. Alterman (Ed.), *Substance abuse and psychopathology* (pp. 289–341). New York: Plenum.

Gruzelier, J. H. (1991). Hemispheric imbalance: Syndromes of schizophrenia, premorbid personality, and neurodevelopmental influences. In S. R. Steinhauer, J. H. Gruzelier, & J. Zubin (Eds.), *Handbook of schizophrenia: Vol. 5. Neuropsychology, psychophysiology and information processing* (pp. 599–650). London: Elsevier.

Hanfmann, E., & Kasanin, J. (1942). Conceptual thinking in schizophrenia. *Nervous and Mental Disease Monographs*, No. *67*.

Hasher, L., & Zacks, R. T. (1979). Automatic and effortful processes in memory. *Journal of Experimental Psychology: General, 108*, 356–388.

Heaton, R. K. (1980). *A manual for the Wisconsin Card Sorting Test*. Odessa, FL: Psychological Assessment Resources.

Herron, W. G. (1962). The process-reactive classification of schizophrenia. *Psychological Bulletin, 59*, 329–343.

Hill, S. Y., Steinhauer, S. R., & Zubin, J. (1987). Biological markers for alcoholism: A vulnerability model conceptualization. In C. Rivers (Ed.), *Nebraska Symposium on Motivation: Vol. 34. Alcohol and addictive behavior* (pp. 207–256). Lincoln: University of Nebraska Press.

Holttum, J. R., Minshew, N. J., Sanders, R. S., & Phillips, N. E. (1992). Magnetic resonance imaging of the posterior fossa in autism. *Biological Psychiatry, 32*, 1091–1101.

Holzman, P. S. (1991). Eye movement dysfunctions in schizophrenia. In S. R. Steinhauer, J. H. Gruzelier, & J. Zubin (Eds.), *Handbook of schizophrenia: Vol. 5. Neuropsychology, psychophysiology and information processing* (pp. 129–145). London: Elsevier.

Insel, T. R., Donnelly, E. F., Lalakea, M. L., Alterman, I. S., & Murphy, D. L. (1983). Neurological and neuropsychological studies of patients with obsessive–compulsive disorder. *Biological Psychiatry, 18*, 741–751.

Joffe, R. T., MacDonald, C., & Kutcher, S. P. (1988). Lack of differential cognitive effects of lithium and carbamazepine in bipolar affective disorder. *Journal of Clinical Psychopharmacology, 8*, 425–428.

Kanner, L. (1943). Autistic disturbances of affective contact. *Nervous Child, 2*, 217–250.

Keefe, R. S. E., Mohs, R. C., Losonczy, M. F., Davidson, M., Silverman, J. M., Kendler, K. S., Horvath, T. B., Nora, N., & Davis, K. L. (1987). Characteristics of very poor outcome schizophrenia. *American Journal of Psychiatry, 144*, 889–895.

Kelley, M. E., Gilbertson, M., Mouton, A., & van Kammen, D. P. (1992). Deterioration in premorbid functioning in schizophrenia: A developmental model of negative symptoms in drug-free patients. *American Journal of Psychiatry, 149*, 1543–1548.

Kluger, A., & Goldberg, E. (1990). IQ patterns in affective disorder, lateralized and diffuse brain damage. *Journal of Clinical and Experimental Neuropsychology, 12*, 182–194.

Kraepelin, E. (1925). *Dementia praecox and paraphrenia*. Edinburgh: Livingston.

Lawson-Kerr, K., Smith, P., & Beck, D. (1991). Behavioral neuropsychology: Past, present, and future direction with organically based affect/mood disorders. *Neuropsychology Review, 2*, 65–107.

LeCouteur, A., Rutter, M., Lord, C., Rios, P., Robertson, S., Holdgrafer, M., & McLennan, J. (1989). Autism diagnostic interview: A standardized investigator-based instrument. *Journal of Autism and Developmental Disorders, 19*, 363–387.

Lord, C., Rutter, M., Goode, S., Heemsbergen, J., Jordan, H., Mawhood, L., & Schopler, E. (1989). Autism diagnostic observation schedule: A standardized observation of communicative and social behavior. *Journal of Autism and Developmental Disorders, 19*, 185–212.

Marin, R. S., & Tucker, G. J. (1981). Psychopathology and hemispheric dysfunction: A review. *Journal of Nervous and Mental Disease, 169*, 546–557.

Massman, P. J., Delis, D. C., Butters, N., Dupont, R. M., & Gillin, J. C. (1992). The subcortical dysfunction hypothesis of memory deficits in depression: Neuropsychological validation in a subgroup of patients. *Journal of Clinical and Experimental Psychology, 14*, 687–706.

Meehl, P. E. (October, 1993). *The problem of classification*. Joseph Zubin Award Address presented at the annual meeting of the Society for Research in Psychopathology, Chicago, IL.

Mettler, F. A. (Ed.). (1949). *Selective partial ablation of the frontal cortex*. New York: Hoeber

Minshew, N. J., & Goldstein, G. (1993). Is autism an amnesic disorder? *Neuropsychology, 7*, 209–216.

Minshew, N. J., Goldstein, G., Dombrowski, S. N., Panchaligam, K., & Pettegrew, J. W. (1993). A preliminary

^{31}p-NMR study of autism: Evidence for undersynthesis and increased degradation of brain membranes. *Biological Psychiatry, 33*, 762–773.
Mirsky, A. F., Anthony, B. J., Duncan, C. C., Ahearn, M. B., & Kellam, S. G. (1991). Analysis of the elements of attention: A neuropsychological approach. *Neuropsychology Review, 2*, 109–145.
Newman, P. J., & Sweet, J. J. (1992). Depressive disorders. In A. E. Puente & R. J. McCaffrey (Eds.), *Handbook of neuropsychological assessment: A biopsychosocial perspective* (pp. 263–307). New York: Plenum.
Noonberg, A., Goldstein, G., & Page, H. A. (1985). Premature aging in alcoholism: "Accelerated aging" or "Increased vulnerability?" *Alcoholism: Clinical and Experimental Research, 9*, 449–469.
Nuechterlein, K., & Dawson, M. E. (1984). Information processing and attentional functioning in the developmental course of schizophrenic disorders. *Schizophrenia Bulletin, 10*, 160–202.
Ornitz, E. M. (1974). The modulation of sensory input and motor output in autistic children. *Journal of Autism and Childhood Schizophrenia, 4*, 197–215.
Overall, J. E., & Gorham, J. R. (1962). The Brief Psychiatric Rating Scale. *Psychological Reports, 10*, 799–812.
Pasamanick, B., & Knobloch, H. (1966). Retrospective studies on the epidemiology of reproductive casualty: Old and new. *Merrill–Palmer Quarterly of Behavioural Development, 12*, 7–26.
Pennington, B. F. (1991). *Diagnosing learning disorders: A neuropsychological framework.* New York: Guilford.
Posner, M. I. (1987). Structures and function of selective attention. In T. Boll & B. K. Bryant (Eds.), *Clinical neuropsychology and brain function: Research, measurement, and practice* (pp. 169–202). Washington, DC: American Psychological Association.
Rapaport, J. L. (1989, March). The biology of obsessions and compulsions. *Scientific American*, 82–89.
Rosenthal, D. (Ed.). (1963). *The Genain quadruplets.* New York: Basic Books.
Rourke, B. P. (Ed.). (1985). *Neuropsychology of learning disabilities: Essentials of subtype analysis.* New York: Guilford.
Rourke, B. P. (Ed.). (1991). *Neuropsychological validation of learning disability subtypes.* New York: Guilford.
Ruckdeschel-Hibbard, M., Gordon, W. A., & Diller, L. (1986). Affective disturbances associated with brain damage. In S. B. Filskov & T. J. Boll (Eds.), *Handbook of clinical neuropsychology* (Vol. 2, pp. 305–337). New York: Wiley–Interscience.
Ryan, C., & Butters, N. (1980). Learning and memory impairments in young and old alcoholics: Evidence for the premature-aging hypothesis. *Alcoholism: Clinical and Experimental Research, 4*, 288–293.
Sackeim, H. A., Freeman, J., McElhiney, M., Coleman, E., Prudic, J., & Devanand, D. P. (1992). Effects of major depression on estimates of intelligence. *Journal of Clinical and Experimental Psychology, 14*, 268–288.
Schear, J. M. (1987). Utility of cluster analysis in classification of mixed neuropsychiatric patients. *Archives of Clinical Neuropsychology, 2*, 329–341.
Schopler, E., & Mesibov, G. B. (Eds.). (1992). *High-functioning individuals with autism.* New York: Plenum.
Siegler, I. C. (1975). The terminal drop hypothesis: Fact or artifact? *Experimental Aging Research, 1*, 169–185.
Silberman, E. K., & Weingartner, H. (1986). Hemispheric lateralization of functions related to emotion. *Brain and Cognition, 5*, 322–353.
Silverstein, M. L., & Zerwic, M. J. (1985). Clinical psychopathological symptoms in neuropsychologically impaired and intact schizophrenics. *Journal of Consulting and Clinical Psychology, 53*, 267–268.
Sokal, R., & Sneath, P. (1963). *Principles of numerical taxonomy.* San Francisco: Freeman.
Talland, G. A. (1965). *Deranged memory.* New York: Academic Press.
Tarter, R. E., & Edwards, K. L. (1985). Neuropsychology of alcoholism. In R. E. Tarter & D. H. Van Thiel (Eds.), *Alcohol and the brain* (pp. 217–242). New York: Plenum.
Townes, B. D., Martin, D. C., Nelson, D., Prosser, R., Pepping, M., Maxwell, J., & Peel, J. (1985). Neurobehavioral approach to classification of psychiatric patients using a competency model. *Journal of Consulting and Clinical Psychology, 53*, 33–42.
van Kammen, D. P. (1991). The biochemical basis of relapse and drug response in schizophrenia: Review and hypothesis. *Psychological Medicine, 21*, 881–895.
Weinberger, D., Berman, K., & Zec, R. (1986). Physiological dysfunction of dorsolateral prefrontal cortex in schizophrenia: I. Regional cerebral blood flow evidence. *Archives of General Psychiatry, 43*, 114–125.
Weinberger, D. R., & Wyatt, R. J. (1982). Brain morphology in schizophrenia: In vivo studies. In F. A. Henn & H. A. Nasrallah (Eds.), *Schizophrenia as a brain disease* (pp. 148–175). New York: Oxford University Press.
Weingartner, H. (1986). Automatic and effort-demanding cognitive processes in depression. In L. W. Poon (Ed.), *Clinical memory assessment of older adults* (pp. 218–226). Washington, DC: American Psychological Association.

Williams, K. H., & Goldstein, G. (1979). Cognitive and affective responses to lithium in patients with organic brain syndrome. *American Journal of Psychiatry*, *136*, 800–803.
Zubin, J. (1975). Problem of attention in schizophrenia. In M. L. Kietzman, S. Sutton, & J. Zubin (Eds.), *Experimental approaches to psychopathology* (pp. 139–166). New York: Academic Press.
Zubin J., & Spring, B. (1977). Vulnerability—A new view of schizophrenia. *Journal of Abnormal Psychology*, *86*, 103–126.

11

The Interface Between Standard Psychiatric and Neuropsychological Diagnosis

John G. Csernansky
Kevin J. Black
Washington University School of Medicine
William O. Faustman
Veterans Affairs Palo Alto Health Care System and Stanford University School of Medicine

The goal of this chapter is to provide an overview of the use of the *Diagnostic and Statistical Manual for Mental Disorders* (e.g., *DSM–III–R, DSM–IV;* American Psychiatric Association, 1987, 1994) as they relate to the diagnosis and understanding of mental disorders whose hallmarks include significant cognitive deficits. Considerable discussion is provided regarding changes in prevailing notions regarding the term "organic" in the *DSM–IV.* Distinctions made by the *DSM* constructs of delirium and dementia are outlined and a review of recent neuropsychological findings in selected neuropsychiatric forms of classical dementias (e.g., Alzheimer's disease, vascular dementia) is provided.

The range of disorders and syndromes covered by standard psychiatric diagnostic manuals and that involve elements of cognitive impairment is extremely broad, and it encompasses dementias due to degenerative processes or vascular disease, idiopathic psychiatric disorders of unknown causes, and mimics of idiopathic psychiatric disorders due to metabolic or structural brain disease. Accordingly, it is beyond the scope of this chapter to provide an exhaustive review of the characteristics of all disorders where cognitive impairment is present. With regard to the major forms of dementia, we focus on two (e.g., Alzheimer's disease, vascular dementia) that are among the most commonly encountered in neuropsychiatric settings and in which the DSM is frequently employed. In addition, the role of underlying medical conditions in psychiatric diagnosis is reviewed.

MODERN PSYCHIATRIC NOSOLOGY

History of Psychiatric Nosology in General

In order to explain, treat, and predict the outcome of illness, clinicians have traditionally relied on *diagnosis*—the process of categorizing a collection of symptoms and signs as similar to those of other patients. The advent of modern pathology in the 1800s helped to validate the purely clinical diagnostic criteria for many illnesses (such as pneumonia) and led to further diagnostic subcategories (such as streptococcal pneumonia). These new, pathology-verified diagnoses enjoyed great success simply because they were superior to the purely clinical diagnoses in the three functions mentioned earlier: (a) explaining illness, (b) suggesting treatment, and (c) predicting outcome.

Nineteenth-century psychiatrists eagerly applied these elements of medical science to disorders of cognition and behavior, and enjoyed some important successes, such as the clinical–pathological correlation of general paresis of the insane (neurosyphilis) and Alzheimer's disease. In those exciting years for medical psychiatry, mental illnesses were generally presumed to be due to some alteration in brain function. When the structure of the brain was visibly affected at autopsy, one spoke of "organic" illness; otherwise, changes in the physiological function of the brain were assumed, and one spoke of "functional" illness. A neurological substrate was originally presumed in both categories of illness.

However, the increased knowledge about neuroanatomy demonstrated that some patients had neurological symptoms or signs that did not correspond to known anatomy—conversion symptoms, in modern terms. A neurologist, Sigmund Freud, developed a special interest in these cases, and eventually developed a broad theory of human behavior that did not depend on altered brain function to explain abnormal behavior. In the early and mid-20th century, American psychiatry turned almost wholly to psychoanalysis, and by and large abandoned its former interest in "organic" illnesses such as pellagra, epilepsy, and neurosyphilis.

The past 20 years have seen psychiatry worldwide renew its interest in biology. The availability of more powerful research tools has shown that whether or not one can associate a given illness with pathology depends largely on the sensitivity and specificity of one's research methods. This paradigm shift has fostered new, atheoretical psychiatric nosologies, and, conversely, reliable research criteria have proven essential for biological investigations of mental illnesses.

Prominent milestones in modern psychiatric nosology include the development of the Washington University Criteria (Feighner et al., 1972), the Research Diagnostic Criteria (Spitzer, Endicott, & Robins, 1975), and the *DSM–III, DSM–III–R,* and *DSM–IV.* The main virtue of such classifications is reliability. This allows etiologic, therapeutic, and prognostic studies to have relevance across different sites of investigation and different study populations. Reliability has been further enhanced by gathering diagnostic information in structured interviews, well-known examples of which include the Structured Clinical Interview for *DSM–III–R* (SCID) and the Present State Examination (PSE).

The other desired virtue of a diagnostic classification is validity, or the extent to which patients with the same diagnosis turn out to have the same "disease," with identical causes and outcomes. Reliability is an essential prerequisite to validity, but reliability alone is inadequate for etiologic research. Criteria for the validation of psychiatric illness were suggested in 1970 by Robins and Guze. However, the *DSM–III* revisions have been aimed primarily at clinical rather than research utility, so validation of new diagnoses has been inadequately studied. In fact, Cloninger (1989) lamented that in the 20 years since development of the so-called Feighner criteria for 15 psychiatric illnesses, no further diagnoses have been satisfactorily validated.

Nosology of "Organic" Mental Disorders

As noted earlier, psychiatric disorders have traditionally been dichotomized as "organic" and "functional," depending on the degree to which each is associated with obvious brain pathology. The term "organic" has been applied to a broad spectrum of cognitive and behavioral disorders, which we propose to divide into separate classes. Among those syndromes classically defined as "organic" are those most likely to demonstrate neuropsychological impairment.

For the purposes of the following discussion, all mental disorders with some element of inherent cognitive impairment may be divided into five "classes" (see Table 11.1). Class I disorders have been classically associated with brain damage. These include global cerebral disorders such as mental retardation (although traditionally classified outside the "organic mental disorders"; Spitzer et al., 1992), dementias, and delirium (Lipowski, 1989); circumscribed deficits such as aphasia, amnesia, abulia, and pathological laughing and weeping (Ironside, 1956); and partial complex seizures with ictal abnormalities of behavior (Cummings, 1985). The neuropsychological characteristics of Class I disorders are reviewed later in this chapter.

Class II disorders would include psychiatric symptoms associated with psychotropic drug use, such as alcohol intoxication, amphetamine or PCP psychosis, and delirium tremens. These disorders would very likely demonstrate a broad range of both acute and chronic cognitive impairments. They are not reviewed in detail in this chapter.

Class III disorders include disorders where a classic psychiatric syndrome arises in association with another medical illness known to affect the brain, often in a setting atypical for the idiopathic illness. An example would be a first episode of mania accompanying hyperthyroidism at age 65, with no prior depression. These "biological phenocopies" of classically functional syndromes were called "organic mental disorders" in the *DSM–III–R* and include, among others: Tourette's syndrome and obsessive–compulsive disorder with encephalitis lethargica (Sacks, 1989), reserpine-induced melancholia (Goodwin, Ebert, & Bunney, 1972), and schizophrenia-like psychosis with metachromatic leukodystrophy or Wilson's disease (Cummings, 1986). A detailed discussion of these disorders follows the review of classical dementia and delirium syndromes in this chapter.

Class IV disorders have no consistent clinical–pathological correlational findings, but because of associated sensory or motor signs, these disorders are usually considered nonpsychiatric. Examples include classic migraine, idiopathic dystonias, and tic disorders. These disorders are not reviewed in detail in this chapter.

Finally, Class V disorders include the most severe "functional" disorders, but are now considered by many psychiatrists to be caused by abnormalities of brain development and anatomy. These illnesses are associated with high heritability, therapeutic response to psychotropic medications, low placebo response rates, neurological "soft signs," abnormalities on brain morphometric or functional brain imaging studies (or any combination thereof), or electrophysiological studies (Rush et al., 1991). Examples include autism, schizophrenia,

TABLE 11.1
Classes of "Organic" Disorders of Behavior, Emotion, or Cognition

Class I. Traditionally seen as neurologically based
Class II. Psychotropic substance induced
Class III. Classic psychiatric syndromes following known brain insults
Class IV. No consistent pathology but traditionally seen by neurologists
Class V. The most severe psychiatric illnesses

bipolar disorder, and panic disorder. Cognitive impairment in some of these disorders is considered in other chapters of this volume.

From the viewpoint of nosology, Class I syndromes tend not to generate debate. Mental symptoms in these syndromes are almost universally viewed as being directly caused by the brain pathology. Diagnostic questions tend to be threshold rather than categorical in nature. Most of these are grouped as "cognitive" and "amnesic" disorders in *DSM–IV* (Caine, 1993; Tucker et al., 1992). Similarly, Class II syndromes cause little controversy. Symptoms are generally thought to originate from pharmacologic substance effects. Nevertheless, in some cases the etiology of substance-related psychological symptoms is unclear; for instance, depression in alcoholics may derive from pharmacological, genetic, or psychosocial causes. Syndromes from classes IV and V generally are not included in discussions of organic mental disorders, and we follow that convention here.

However, it has been harder to satisfactorily categorize the Class III disorders. A stride forward was made in *DSM–III*, where the concept of "organicity" was broadened so that neuropsychological impairment was not required to recognize mood, psychotic, and personality disorders as "organic." *DSM–III–R* added the category of Organic Anxiety Disorder. *DSM–IV* offers a more substantial revision of nosological thinking that will resolve two problems associated with the *DSM–III* organic mental disorders criteria. First, calling Class III disorders "organic" strengthened the unfortunate impression that Class V or other mental disorders have no basis in brain dysfunction (Popkin & Tucker, 1992; Spitzer et al., 1992; Tucker, 1991). Therefore, although the organic/nonorganic distinction was essentially maintained (Spitzer et al., 1992), as proposed by Lipowski (1990a, 1990b, 1991), the term *organic* was discarded in favor of *secondary* and *drug-induced.* This approach emphasizes the stereotypical nature of the syndromes (whether arising spontaneously or with medical illness), but notes the probable difference in etiology and potential differences in treatment and prognosis. Second, *DSM–IV* groups secondary anxiety disorders with primary anxiety disorders rather than with the other organic disorders. This change emphasizes the similarities of psychiatric syndromes arising in the presence or absence of certain known physical illnesses. It is meant not only to be useful clinically (Spitzer et al., 1992; Spitzer, Williams, First, & Kendler, 1989; Tucker, 1991), but also to stimulate research. For instance, nearly all secondary cases of obsessive–compulsive disorder (OCD) arise in illnesses affecting the basal ganglia, which in turn may help to validate and interpret findings of blood flow abnormalities in the basal ganglia in idiopathic OCD. *DSM–IV* also introduces new "secondary" categories for catatonia and dissociative syndromes.

Despite these advances, the *DSM–III* through *DSM–IV* classifications of organic mental disorders still engender substantial debate. The most serious criticism is that *DSM–III* requires the clinician to judge whether or not the mental illness is caused by a physical illness, although in most cases such definitive attribution is impossible (Roth, 1981). This flaw has continued to the present in *DSM–IV.* For example, "the clinician must decide whether depressive syndromes in the medically ill are reactions to the experience and impact of physical illness or whether they are manifestations of the intrinsic pathologic process" (Popkin & Tucker, 1992, p. 370), even though "what suffices to establish that a mood disorder is *due to* a medical illness remains unresolved" (p. 374). The framers of *DSM–IV* explicitly recognized that this clinical distinction is "sometimes impossible" (Spitzer et al., 1992, p. 243), rendering these diagnoses less useful for research purposes (Fava, 1992), but they felt the distinction had to be left to clinical judgment because it is "treatment-relevant" (Spitzer et al., 1992, p. 243). This abandonment of reliability in favor of clinical utility has major implications for the validity of the *DSM–III* and *–IV* classification of organic mental disorders.

One way to circumvent the impossibility of assigning causality was the approach of

Feighner et al. (1972) to diagnosing depression in the medically ill. First, these investigators defined attribution to a medical illness at the symptom, not syndrome, level so that individual "symptoms [were] *not* scored positive if they can be explained by a known medical disease of the patient" (p. 58). This symptom distinction is arguably easier to make than the analogous etiologic distinction (Black, 1995). Second, these investigators defined the diagnosis of "secondary" depression on a strictly temporal basis. Here, the primary diagnosis would be "a life-threatening or incapacitating medical illness which precedes and parallels the symptoms of depression" (Feighner et al., 1972, p. 59; see also Robins & Guze, 1972). Krauthammer and Klerman (1978) dealt similarly with secondary mania, with a typical manic syndrome "following or in association with medical and pharmacological conditions" (p. 1334) but excluding "a clear history of manic–depressive or other affective disease" (p. 1335) and concurrent confusional states. This requirement for temporal precedence was abandoned by the *DSM–III* and subsequent revisions in favor of clinical judgment, after considering all relevant factors (Fava, 1992; Spitzer & First, 1992).

Another way around the difficulty of assigning causality to medical illness would have been to exploit the multiaxial diagnostic system introduced by *DSM–III* by simply naming the syndrome (e.g., "manic syndrome") rather than supposing an etiology ("bipolar disorder, manic" or "organic mood disorder"), and then listing potentially relevant illnesses (e.g., "Axis III. hyperthyroidism"; Fogel, 1990). Unfortunately, this descriptive approach was rejected by the *DSM–IV* committee (Spitzer et al., 1992).

Why Seek to Classify the "Organic Mental Disorders" (Class III)?

Sometimes emotional symptoms appear after brain injury without meeting clinical criteria for a traditional psychiatric disorder. One could interpret this trend as evidence that these are different conditions which should not be forced into categories invented to describe psychiatric patients without gross brain pathology. However, there are several other reasonable interpretations. Clinical differences in the brain-injured population could equally well be ascribed to: (a) partial syndromes or *formes frustes* of classic psychiatric disorders, (b) altered clinical presentation of typical psychiatric disorders due to cognitive or neurological deficits (Black, 1995), or (c) simple association (medically ill patients with "the same" major depressive illness as otherwise healthy depressives will have a poorer outcome).

The aforementioned distinction is important, because if these patients are seen as having true phenocopies of classic psychiatric disorders, then traditional neurological lesion analysis may help to reveal the pathological anatomy of idiopathic disorders. For this purpose, standard diagnostic criteria are essential (Black, 1995). However, diagnosis serves various purposes, and a nosology useful for research on etiology and pathophysiology may not necessarily be as helpful clinically in addressing a particular distressing symptom; treatment response and prognostication in "organic" mental disorders requires separate study.

NEUROPSYCHOLOGICAL AND BIOLOGICAL FINDINGS IN CLASSICAL ORGANIC MENTAL DISORDERS (CLASS I AND II)

The *DSM–III–R* and the *DSM–IV* provide extensive coverage of disorders of primary neuropsychological impairment. The *DSM–III–R* (American Psychiatric Association, 1987) groups these disorders into a general heading of "organic mental syndromes and disorders." Disorders under this heading may take on a wide scope, ranging from chronic degenerative conditions (e.g., Alzheimer's disease) to acute and fully reversible changes in consciousness and mental function (e.g., alcohol intoxication).

TABLE 11.2
DSM–III–R Criteria for Dementia

A. Demonstrable evidence of impairment in short- and long-term memory. Impairment in short-term memory (inability to learn new information) may be indicated by inability to remember three objects after 5 minutes. Long-term memory impairment (inability to remember information that was known in the past) may be indicated by inability to remember past personal information (e.g., what happened yesterday, birthplace, occupation) or facts of common knowledge (e.g., past presidents, well-known dates).
B. At least one of the following:
   (1) impairment in abstract thinking, as indicated by inability to find similarities and differences between related words, difficulty in defining words and concepts, and other similar tasks
   (2) impaired judgment, as indicated by inability to make reasonable plans to deal with interpersonal, family, and job-related problems and issues
   (3) other disturbances of higher cortical function, such as aphasia (disorder of language), apraxia (inability to carry our motor activities despite intact comprehension and motor function), agnosia (failure to recognize or identify objects despite intact sensory function), and "constructional difficulty" (e.g., inability to copy three-dimensional figures, assemble blocks, or arrange sticks in specific designs)
   (4) personality change, i.e., alteration or accentuation of premorbid traits
C. The disturbance in A and B significantly interferes with work or usual social activities or relationships with others.
D. Not occuring exclusively during the course of Delirium.
E. Either (1) or (2):
   (1) there is evidence from the history, physical examination, or laboratory tests of a specific organic factor (or factors) judged to be etiologically related to the disturbance
   (2) in the absence of such evidence, an etiologic organic factor can be presumed if the disturbance cannot be accounted for by any nonorganic mental disorder, e.g., Major Depression accounting for cognitive impairment

Note. From American Psychiatric Association (1987). © 1987 by American Psychiatric Association. Reprinted with permission.

TABLE 11.3
DSM–III–R Criteria for Delirium

A. Reduced ability to maintain attention to external stimuli (e.g., questions must be repeated because attention wanders) and to appropriately shift attention to new external stimuli (e.g., perseverates answer to a previous question).
B. Disorganized thinking, as indicated by rambling, irrelevant, or incoherent speech.
C. At least two of the following:
   (1) reduced level of consciousness (e.g., difficulty keeping awake during examination)
   (2) perceptual disturbances: misinterpretations, illusions, or hallucinations
   (3) disturbance of sleep–wake cycle with insomnia or daytime sleepiness
   (4) increased or decreased psychomotor activity
   (5) disorientation to time, place, or person
   (6) memory impairment, e.g., inability to learn new material, such as the names of several unrelated objects after 5 minutes, or to remember past events, such as history of current episode of illness
D. Clinical features develop over a short period of time (usually hours to days) and tend to fluctuate over the course of a day.
E. Either (1) or (2):
   (1) evidence from the history, physical examination, or laboratory tests of a specific organic factor (or factors) judged to be etiologically related to the disturbance
   (2) in the absence of such evidence, an etiologic organic factor can be presumed if the disturbance cannot be accounted for by any nonorganic mental disorder (e.g., Manic Episode accounting for agitation and sleep disturbance)

Note. From American Psychiatric Association (1987). © 1987 by American Psychiatric Association. Reprinted with permission.

TABLE 11.4
DSM–IV Criteria for Delirium Due to a General Medical Condition

A. Disturbance of consciousness (i.e., reduced clarity of awareness of the environment) with reduced ability to focus, sustain, or shift attention.
B. A change in cognition (such as memory deficit, disorientation, language disturbance, perceptual disturbance) or the development of a perceptual disturbance that is not better accounted for by a preexisting, established, or evolving dementia.
C. The disturbance develops over a short period of time (usually hours to days) and tends to fluctuate during the course of the day.
D. There is evidence from the history, physical examination, or laboratory findings that the disturbance is caused by the direct physiological consequences of a general medical condition.

Note. From American Psychiatric Association (1994).

The *DSM–IV* uses somewhat different general nomenclature and diagnostic schemas. The term "organic mental disorder" is not continued in the *DSM–IV.* Recent research in major psychiatric disorders (e.g., schizophrenia) suggests that such disorders have major biological underpinnings. In prior years, such disorders were viewed as "functional," and the term *organic mental disorders* was reserved for disorders such as degenerative dementia. The *DSM–IV* takes steps to avoid giving the impression that such disorders (e.g., schizophrenia) are "functional," thus not having a biologic or organic basis. Disorders such as delirium and dementia are grouped in terms of *cognitive disorders.* Forms of dementia due to recognized medical conditions form an additional grouping under *DSM–IV.*

The *DSM–III–R* and *DSM–IV* make significant distinctions between delirium and dementia. Although both conditions may evidence cognitive impairment such as memory problems, delirium requires a disturbance in consciousness that develops over a short period of time (e.g., hours to days; American Psychiatric Association, 1987). Dementia typically reflects a more enduring syndrome in which persistent areas of cognitive impairment are present. The *DSM–III–R* definitions of dementia and delirium appear in Tables 11.2 and 11.3, respectively. The wording of the diagnosis of delirium differs somewhat in the *DSM–IV,* although the general intention of the diagnosis of an acute disturbance of consciousness remains the same. The *DSM–IV* offers specific diagnostic categories such as substance-induced delirium, delirium due to a general medical condition, and delirium due to multiple etiologies (American Psychiatric Association, 1994). An example of the criteria for the diagnosis of delirium due to a general medical condition is offered in Table 11.4.

Alzheimer's Disease—Introduction to DSM and Other Diagnostic Criteria

Alzheimer's disease (AD) is separately listed in *DSM–III–R* and *DSM–IV,* and represents one of the most common forms of dementia seen in clinical neuropsychological practice. The distribution of forms of dementia is strongly related to age (Amaducci & Lippi, 1992), with AD representing a major cause of dementia in middle-to-late life and other conditions (e.g., HIV-related cognitive impairments) being more common in younger populations.

Although AD has characteristic histopathological features that are found at autopsy (e.g., neurofibrillary tangles and neuritic plaques), the diagnosis of AD in life typically remains dependent on behavioral criteria in association with a thorough medical, neurologic, and psychological evaluation. The *DSM–III–R* and *DSM–IV* offer criteria for the diagnosis of AD (see Table 11.5) and represents only one of many diagnostic systems that have been produced. *DSM–III–R* defines AD based on the presence of dementia with an "insidious onset with a generally progressive deteriorating course" (American Psychiatric Association,

1987, p. 121). Deficits in both cognitive and behavioral domains (e.g., changes in vocational functioning) are required to make the diagnosis. Similarly, the *DSM–IV* criteria (see Table 11.5) state that the illness has a "course characterized by a gradual onset and continuing cognitive decline" (American Psychiatric Association, 1994, p. 142). Similar to the *DSM–III–R,* the *DSM–IV* criteria require the presence of cognitive deficits in multiple domains (e.g., memory impairment in addition to aphasia, apraxia, agnosia, or executive functioning) in addition to diminished social or occupational functioning (American Psychiatric Association, 1994). A differentiation is made between early (age 65 or below) and late onset AD (after age 65). Compared to the *DSM–III–R* criteria, *DSM–IV* criteria are more specific in terms of differential diagnoses that must be excluded. The criteria also allow for the diagnostic coding of numerous behavioral disturbances and clinical features (e.g., delusions) that are often present in the disorder (American Psychiatric Association, 1994).

As noted previously, the DSM criteria represent only one of several available diagnostic criteria for AD. An alternative and widely used diagnostic system for AD was produced through a collaborative project conducted by the National Institute of Neurological Disorders and Stroke (NINDS) and the Alzheimer's Disease and Related Disorders Association (ADRDA; McKhann et al., 1984). Known as the NINDS–ADRDA criteria, this system allows for the judgment of "probable" and "possible" AD based on the presence or absence of symptoms judged to be both typical or atypical. This system allows for a diagnosis of definite AD when histopathological analysis provides confirmation of findings consistent with AD. Other work (Eisdorfer & Cohen, 1980) has offered a diagnostic system for AD that

TABLE 11.5
DSM–III–R Criteria for Primary Degenerative Dementia of the Alzheimer Type and *DSM–IV* Criteria for Dementia of the Alzheimer's Type

DSM–III–R Criteria for Primary Degenerative Dementia of the Alzheimer Type

A. Dementia (as outlined in Table 11.2).
B. Insidious onset with a generally progressive deteriorating course.
C. Exclusion of all other specific causes of Dementia by history, physical examination, and laboratory tests.

DSM–IV Criteria for Dementia of the Alzheimer's Type

A. The development of multiple cognitive deficits manifested by both:
    (1) memory impairment (inability to learn new information and to recall previously learned information)
    (2) one (or more) of the following cognitive disturbances:
        (a) aphasia (language disturbance)
        (b) apraxia (impaired ability to carry out motor activities despite intact motor function)
        (c) agnosia (failure to recognize or identify objects despite intact sensory function)
        (d) disturbance in executive functioning (i.e., planning, organizing, sequencing, abstracting)
B. The cognitive deficits in criteria A1 and A2 each cause significant impairment in social or occupational functioning and represent a significant decline from a previous level of functioning.
C. The course is characterized by gradual onset and continuing cognitive decline.
D. The cognitive deficits in criteria A1 and A2 are not due to any of the following:
    (1) other central nervous system conditions that cause progressive deficits in memory and cognition (e.g., cerebrovascular disease, Parkinson's disease, Huntington's disease, subdural hematoma, normal pressure hydrocephalus, brain tumor)
    (2) systemic conditions that are known to cause dementia (e.g., hypothyroidism, vitamin B12 or folic acid deficiency, niacin deficiency, hypercalcemia, neurosyphilis, HIV infection)
    (3) substance-induced conditions
E. The deficits do not occur exclusively during the course of a Delirium.
F. The disturbance is not better accounted for by another Axis I disorder (e.g., Major Depressive Disorder, Schizophrenia)

Note. From American Psychiatric Association (1987, 1994).

includes the psychometric documentation of cognitive impairment (e.g., WAIS, Mini-Mental State) in association with psychosocial deficits.

Accuracy of Behavioral Criteria for the Diagnosis of AD

Even though neuritic plaques and neurofibrillary tangles may be found as a feature of normal aging, the presence of such histopathological findings in combination with a dementing process is a postmortem confirmatory technique for the behaviorally based diagnosis of AD. Accordingly, one may use these histopathological data to evaluate the efficiency of behavioral criteria that are applied to patients earlier in the course of their illness. Such studies suggest a fairly high degree of variance in the accuracy of diagnostic systems. Studies employing standardized criteria, such as those of the *DSM–III,* can yield a misdiagnosis rate of approximately 15%–30% when postmortem histological data are used for diagnostic confirmation (Nielsen et al., 1991; see Burns, 1991, for a review). Some data (Morris, McKeel, Fulling, Torack, & Berg, 1988) suggest that the NINDS–ADRDA criteria can yield quite high rates of diagnostic accuracy.

Several recent works have specifically addressed the strengths and limitations of *DSM–III–R* diagnoses for dementia. These studies (Fratiglioni, Grut, Forsell, Viitanen, & Winblad, 1992; Kukull et al., 1990) suggest moderate levels of reliability for dementia diagnoses. Fratiglioni et al. used a population survey technique to evaluate interrater diagnostic agreements using the *DSM–III–R*. Moderate levels of interrater agreement were found, and an analysis of reasons for disagreement suggested that allowing for a "questionable dementia" category improved overall reliability. Other work (Nussbaum, Treves, & Korczyn, 1992) has suggested that the *DSM–III–R* criteria exclude a large percentage of patients from both the primary degenerative dementia (AD) and multi-infarct diagnoses. Patients with a stepwise deteriorating course (a multi-infarct dementia criteria) were found to often have an insidious onset (an AD criterion). Nussbaum et al. noted that the *DSM–III–R* criteria do not provide for a suitable differential diagnostic classification for such patients.

In sum, *DSM–III–R* and *DSM–IV* criteria provide one set of fairly reliable diagnostic criteria for classification of major forms of degenerative dementia such as AD. Similar to any other diagnostic system, such criteria will continue to evolve based on further studies of the reliability and validity of the criteria.

Historical Perspectives and Cellular Pathology of AD

The most valid diagnosis of Alzheimer's disease is made at autopsy, based on the presence of characteristic and specific neuropathological findings. The association of the name "Alzheimer's disease" with Alois Alzheimer is based on a 1907 publication (see Wilkins & Brody, 1969, for an English translation). This paper describes a case study of a 51-year-old woman with progressive dementia, psychosis, and postmortem findings of cortical cellular pathology (e.g., tangles and degenerating nerve endings). Berrios (1990) noted that although some of the findings observed by Alzheimer were not new, the description of the combination of syndrome findings was a new contribution.

The notion that AD was synonymous with presenile dementia (i.e., relatively early age of onset) was consistent with the original case study of Alzheimer and persisted until relatively recently (Amaducci et al., 1986). Neuropathological studies suggested that the histopathological features described by Alzheimer also were present in patients who had onset of dementia at significantly older ages. The neuropathological findings that were originally noted by Alzheimer continue to serve as postmortem markers for diagnostic confirmation of the disorder. Important elements of cellular pathology in AD now are known as neurofibrillary tangles and senile neuritic plaques. Katzman (1986) described the tangles as "abnormal neurons in which the cytoplasm is filled with bundles of submicroscopic filamentous structures that are wound around each other in a helical"; neuritic plaques are described as consisting of a group of "degenerating nerve terminals, both dendritic and axonal, with a core that contains extracellular arrays of filaments that have the histochemical and ultrastructural characteristics of amyloid protein" (p. 967).

AD is typified by pathology in brain areas such as the entorhinal cortex, hippocampus, and amygdala (Koo & Price, 1993). Naturally, such areas are important in memorial functions (a pathognomic finding in the disorder) as well as in cortical/subcortical pathway connections. Recent work by Berg, McKeel, Miller, Baty, and Morris (1993) has demonstrated that the density of neurofibrillary tangles is associated with the degree of dementia at a time near death in an older population of AD patients. Similar correlations between tangle densities and the general severity of dementia also have been found by other groups (e.g., McKee, Kosik, & Kowall, 1991).

One of the most active lines of biological AD research has focused on the presence of beta amyloid protein in neuritic plaques. Beta amyloid protein is a substance formed from amyloid precursor protein (Clark & Goate, 1993). The possibility exists that this deposition of beta amyloid protein is a core feature in the pathology of the disorder. A wide range of molecular biology and genetic linkage studies have started to focus on the role of amyloid pathology. The degree to which this pathology is a core feature of AD or represents an artifactual phenomenon may be clarified in the near future.

Risk Factors for AD

Studies have sought to demonstrate a wide range of risk factors for the development of AD (see Amaducci & Lippi, 1992, for a review). Rates of AD correlate positively with increasing age. Prior head injury has been suggested to be a predisposing risk factor (Mortimer, French, Hutton, & Schuman, 1985), as rates of head injury with loss of consciousness were nearly twice as frequent in AD patients as among matched controls. Some (Amaducci et al., 1986; Cohen, Eisdorfer, & Leverenz, 1982) but not all (Corkin, Growdon, & Rasmussen, 1983) data have suggested late maternal age of the patient's mother as a risk factor. A recent work (Bidaut-Russell & Grossberg, 1991) noted that the prior alcohol drinking patterns of AD patients were similar to those of the general population. A nonsignificant trend was found for shorter survival in AD patients with a history of alcohol abuse. Crapper, Krishman, and Dalton (1973) provided evidence of elevated aluminum levels in the brains of AD patients, and thus created extensive concern that environmental hazards (e.g., cooking utensils) may be an AD risk factor. Some work (see Amaducci & Lippi, 1992, for a review) has not been able to link such risks with the disease and the possibility has been suggested that elevated brain aluminum levels are the result of some secondary neuropathological process.

In addition to increasing age, perhaps the most replicated risk factor for AD is the presence of a relative who has had the disorder (see Li, Silverman, & Mohs, 1991, for a review). Various studies have strongly implicated genetic factors in the expression of AD (Amaducci et al., 1986; Heston, Mastri, Anderson, & White, 1981). A form of AD appears to exist that has a fairly high penetrance with an early age of onset. These observations of early-onset familial AD have been taken to suggest that early onset is related to a more strongly familial form of the disorder. Transmission patterns in some of these families have suggested an autosomal dominant form of transmission (Li et al., 1991). It should be noted that these cases of AD represent a small subset of the total number of patients with the disorder, although it has been noted that such families have obvious research advantages (e.g., simultaneous access to multiple affected and unaffected family members). Some recent data (Luchins et al., 1992) failed to find age of onset differences between patients who were deemed to be either familial or nonfamilial cases. Other findings (Mohs, Breitner, Silverman, & Davis, 1987) suggest a fairly strong genetic component in AD with a later age of onset. Mohs et al. used a well-diagnosed sample of older probands (mean age = 68.8 years) and evaluated the risk of the disorder in first-degree relatives. An elevated risk of approximately four times the control group was found in first-degree relatives. The cumulative incidence of the disorder was found to approach 50% by the age of 90 years.

Important advances in genetic linkage studies have been made in recent years (see Clark & Goate, 1993, for a review). Several studies have applied molecular biology linkage techniques to high-penetrance families in which an early onset of AD was common. Several works (Chartier-Harlan et al., 1991; Murrell, Farlow, Ghetti, & Benson, 1991) have performed linkage studies suggesting a locus on chromosome 21 for selected pedigrees. These works implicate an abnormality in gene coding of amyloid precursor protein, which is an important finding given the widely replicated finding of beta amyloid protein in senile plaques of AD patients. Other work (Schellenberg et al., 1992) has found linkage on chromosome 14 in families with a high rate of early-onset AD. The exact meaning of these findings (e.g., implications for the genetic heterogeneity of the disorder) in early onset syndromes of the disorder remains to be clarified. It should also be noted that these genetic linkage findings in early-onset patients are likely to be representative of only a small portion of the AD population.

Exciting recent work (Corder et al., 1993) has suggested genetic linkage on chromosome 19 in late-onset familial and sporadic forms of AD. This novel work has focused on linkage on chromosome 19 at a site thought to code for apolipoprotein E. The exact mechanism by which this gene could account for the observed pathology of AD remains to be clarified. However, these early findings are extremely encouraging for future biological AD research given that they represent the strongest genetic evidence to date for the more common, late-onset forms of AD.

Behavioral Disturbances in AD

Behavioral and psychiatric disturbances are not essential features of major diagnostic systems for AD. However, such disturbances in AD at times may be even more disturbing than the core cognitive features or dementia. Behavioral changes noted in AD can include personality changes, psychosis, and violence or aggression (see Deutsch & Rovner, 1991, for a review). A common personality change associated with AD is an increase in passivity and a decrease in spontaneity (Rubin et al., 1987). Recent work (Chatterjee, Strauss, Smyth, & Whitehouse, 1992) surveyed caregivers for AD patients and noted a variety of personality changes associated with the disorder. Compared to premorbid estimates, patients were viewed as more neurotic (e.g., more anxious, depressed), less extroverted (e.g., less active and assertive), and less conscientious.

The development of psychotic symptoms (e.g., hallucinations, delusions) in AD is fairly common, although estimates about the frequency of occurrence of these symptoms show considerable variability. Recent work (Jeste, Wragg, Salmon, Harris, & Thal, 1992) noted that estimates for the presence of psychosis in AD have ranged between 10% and 73%. Burns, Jacoby, and Levy (1990) observed an overall rate of delusions of 16% and noted that sampling techniques (e.g., epidemiological catchment studies vs. research clinic samples) may account for some of the variance in estimates of symptom frequency. Several other recent studies (Deutsch, Bylsma, Rovner, Steele, & Folstein, 1991; Jeste et al., 1992) have estimated that delusions are evident in approximately 30%–40% of AD patients. Fairly consistent findings (Burns et al., 1990; Deutsch et al., 1991; Flynn, Cummings, & Gornbein, 1991; Jeste et al., 1992) suggest that persecutory and suspicious delusions are commonly observed. Such delusions may take the nature of thoughts of theft, infidelity, or people "hiding things" (Burns et al., 1990; Jeste et al., 1992). Several studies (Deutsch et al., 1991; Jeste et al., 1992; Lopez et al., 1991) have noted that delusions may be associated with hostility and aggression.

Multiple works have attempted to correlate the presence of psychosis with the degree of cognitive impairment in AD. Several (Cooper, Mungas, & Weiler, 1990; Jeste et al., 1992; Lopez et al., 1991) studies have suggested that the severity of cognitive impairment is positively associated with the presence of psychosis. In addition, some data (Lopez et al., 1991) have been interpreted to suggest that the presence of psychosis is associated with a more rapidly deteriorating course of the disorder.

Neurochemistry

The cholinergic neurotransmitter system has received the greatest interest in AD research (see McDonald & Nemeroff, 1991, for a review). A variety of evidence has implicated the importance of cholinergic function in AD. This evidence includes observations of degeneration of cholinergic neurons in the nucleus basalis of Meynert (Whitehouse et al., 1982). Anticholinergic agents such as atropine can exacerbate cognitive impairments in AD (Inzelberg, Shapira, & Korczyn, 1990). Pharmacological treatments for AD (e.g., tetrahydroamino-acridine, also known as Tacrine) have been directed towards increasing cholinergic functions through anticholinesterase activity (Small, 1992). Such agents may be able to produce mild improvements in some AD patients. It should be noted that AD is an illness that clearly affects multiple neurotransmitter systems other than cholinergic systems (Markesbery, 1992). Accordingly, the neurochemical substrates of AD are likely to be quite complex and drugs directed at single neurotransmitter systems probably will be of limited efficacy. Upcoming work may focus on pharmaceutical agents that are directed at diminishing amyloid deposition in neurons.

The Nature of Cognitive Impairment in AD

Because it is highly desirable to make a specific dementia diagnosis prior to death, the use of neuropsychological testing continues to be a key element in the diagnostic assessment of AD and other forms of dementia. Although technological advances (e.g., MRI scanning to detect infarcts in some forms of vascular dementia) have become integral in identifying lesions that may be important in the diagnostic process, only neuropsychological testing has the ability to assess directly the cognitive consequences of dementing illnesses and to monitor cognitive improvement or decline. Cognitive testing may be used to correlate with behavioral disturbances that are problematic for care givers of patients with AD (Jeste et al., 1992). In addition, neuropsychological assessment may be vital for the determination of residual functional capacities that would be required for the correct placement in both psychotherapeutic and vocational settings.

The selection of tests for the evaluation of AD may be dependent on both the goals of the testing (e.g., initial diagnosis, research purposes, documentation of cognitive decline) and the current status of the patient. Obviously, tests should be selected that tap a range of cognitive functions. Multiple studies (e.g., Hill, Storandt, & LaBarge, 1992) have detailed that patients with even mild to moderate dementia severity can "bottom out" (i.e., perform so poorly as to yield no useful information) on a range of cognitive tests. Accordingly, issues of general test difficulty (e.g., inclusion of very simple tasks) may be as important as the breadth of cognitive domains sampled by the tests selected for administration.

The research literature in the cognitive assessment of AD is somewhat hampered by studies typically employing only a few tests that tap limited domains of cognitive functioning. Studies employing a broad battery approach with patients who are capable of offering valid results are relatively rare. When a broad range of tests (e.g., Halstead–Reitan Battery) were administered to a large sample of AD patients (Hom, 1992) the results suggested impairments across a broad range of general and specific neuropsychological functions. Accordingly, one should cautiously view studies that administer single measures and subsequently promote such tests as selective and sensitive for the detection of AD.

The diagnosis of AD typically is based on the impairment of multiple cognitive domains. Memorial and linguistic deficits, which may overlap each other in terms of functional pathology, have received the most attention in AD research. In considering memorial functions it should be noted that the establishment of a firm theoretical framework for the precise classification of memorial phenomena is the continued source of debate (Bondi & Kaszniak, 1991). A full review of memory schemas is beyond the scope of the present review. Traditional distinctions between "short-term" memory (e.g. limited capacity storage for incoming information, often assessed with span of apprehension type tests) and long-term memory (consolidated information in long-term storage) continue to be applicable in approaching the body of research on AD.

A recent classification schema for memory that has particular implications for AD research is the division of memory functions into semantic and episodic memory. In a recent review on AD research, Nebes (1989) defined semantic memory as "an organized body of knowledge involving words, concepts, their meanings and associations, and the rules for manipulating these symbols and concepts" (p. 377). Such information is thought to be organized on a conceptual basis and is vital for the understanding and production of words and language (Hodges, Salmon, & Butters, 1992). Episodic memory has been viewed as a "record of unique events in an individual's experience encoded in relation to a spatial–temporal context" (Nebes, 1989, p. 377). Whereas semantic memory may be evaluated by tasks such as picture or object naming, tests of episodic memory may take the form of novel learning paradigms, such as list learning. One should note that this and other divisions of memorial functions remain the subject of ongoing research and theoretical evolution. Although some reports suggest that semantic memory is disproportionately diminished in AD (see Nebes, 1989, for a review), other data (Randolph, 1991) have noted that measures reputed to reflect a range of memory functions may in fact be intercorrelated and may decline in parallel in AD.

Memory impairments represent a hallmark neuropsychological finding in AD. The measurement of these impairments has included a broad range of testing approaches. Numerous studies have demonstrated impairments during novel learning tasks (e.g., Bernard, Wilson, & Gilley, 1992; Bigler, Rosa, Schultz, Hall, & Harris, 1989; Bondi & Kasziak, 1991; Kopelman, 1985) that employ both immediate and delayed recall designs. Deficits have frequently been elicited with common tasks such as verbal list learning (e.g., Rey Auditory Verbal Learning Test). A recent work (Huff, Protetch, Saxton, & Becker, 1989) provided a detailed analysis about specific features of verbal list learning that were the most effective in discriminating AD patients from normal controls. Delayed recall was one of several measures that was most effective in discriminating between the groups. Measures of total words learned across all trials and recent memory of the first trial items were also effective discriminators between groups.

Although explicit memory (e.g., list learning tasks) may be reduced in both AD and a variety of other forms of dementia, patients with AD often demonstrate additional significant deficits in semantic memory (Nebes, 1989). Measures of semantic memory have included tests of verbal fluency and confrontation naming. Several studies have utilized a fairly broad range of semantic measures in assessing AD. Cummings, Benson, Hill, and Read (1985) administered a battery of speech and language tests and concluded that all of their 30 AD patients studied had some form of linguistic deficit. Price et al. (1993) studied 20 autopsy-conformed AD patients and noted a fairly consistent level of anomic aphasia during the illness progression. Other work (Kontiola, Laaksonen, Sulkava, & Erkinjuntti, 1990) employed a wide variety of Luria-based measures of expressive and receptive speech to note deficits in both AD and patients with multi-infarct dementia. The language problems in multi-infarct dementia were viewed as being more elementary (e.g., simple and basic language abilities), whereas AD patients showed deficits in functions such as understanding and constructing complex grammatical structure.

Simple measures of verbal fluency have been shown to be impaired in all phases of AD. Fluency typically is measured by asking a patient to produce words either that fit a specified category or that start with a given letter. Butters, Granholm, Salmon, and Grant (1987) provided data that suggest that although category and letter fluency were both impaired in AD, these patients evidenced relatively greater deficits in category fluency. More recent work (Monsch et al., 1992) compared various verbal fluency tasks to discriminate AD patients from normal controls. Category fluency (e.g., produce words that are animals, fruits) demonstrated the greatest degree of discrimination between AD patients and controls, whereas letter fluency was the least accurate measure. The authors noted that the use of category fluency may tap the structure of semantic knowledge which may be diminished even in early phases of AD.

Confrontation naming tasks represent another major approach in the evaluation of linguistic/semantic deficits in AD. The Boston Naming Test (BNT) has been shown to be sensitive for cognitive deficit in AD, even when these patients are in early phases of the illness (Williams, Mack, & Henderson, 1989). Margolin, Pate, Friedrich, and Elia (1990) found that BNT performance in AD was even more abnormal than that found in anomic aphasic stroke patients. The authors noted that the AD deficits are likely to represent a semantic deficit, whereas the anomic aphasic patients possess lexical–phonological deficits, articulatory deficits, or both.

Several studies have attempted to examine the clinical significance of semantic deficits in AD. Knesevich, LaBarge, and Edwards (1986) suggested that BNT deficits are correlated with a more rapidly progressive course of the illness. Grosse, Gilley, and Wilson (1991) have argued that late-onset (age 68 or older) AD patients have relatively greater semantic memory deficits than AD patients with an earlier age of onset. However, other work (Selnes, Carson, Rovner, & Gordon, 1988) has failed to find language differences between early- and late-onset patients.

An interesting question raised by the pervasiveness of semantic memory deficits in AD is whether these deficits are due to a lack of access to retained verbal knowledge or whether they are caused by an actual loss of the knowledge itself. Prior work (Martin & Fedio, 1983) using category fluency tasks has suggested that impairments in language function in AD follows a pattern in which patients show a lack of categorical exemplars (naming of specific items in a category) and an excess of superordinate categorical naming (i.e., major category titles). Therefore, significant categorical features may be retained although examples within the categories are lost. This pattern could be interpreted as a loss of specific semantic knowledge. An interesting recent study (Hodges et al., 1992) administered a range of semantic memory tests in an experimental design in which the same target items were carried across tests. A relative preservation was noted on sorting and definition tasks. A further analysis of errors made by each patient across different tests suggested a consistency of deficits across the measures. The authors persuasively argued that such a pattern offers evidence that deficits in semantic memory are caused by primary storage degradation (i.e., loss of semantic information; Hodges et al., 1992).

Results From Selected Testing Approaches

Wechsler Adult Intelligence Scale. The Wechsler Adult Intelligence Scale (WAIS) or its revised version (WAIS–R; Weschler, 1981) represents one of the most widely administered measures in psychometric assessment. This scale may have utility as a portion of a more extended standardized battery (e.g., Halstead–Reitan Neuropsychological Battery) or as a facet of a more flexible testing approach. The Wechsler scales yield valid, widely accepted, and reliable estimates of social and adaptive intellectual functioning. Approximately 10 years ago, Fuld (1984) outlined a profile of WAIS subtest performance that was reported to have good specificity and sensitivity for AD. The general formula employed in this work took advantage of a hypothesized preservation of overlearned verbal skills (e.g., Vocabulary subtest) in association with relative deficits in more conceptually based tests (e.g., Block Design subtest). Demonstration of a consistent and unique WAIS test profile clearly would have important implications for the psychometric detection of AD.

The validity of the AD profile proposed by Fuld (1984) has received mixed support in recent research studies. Gfeller and Rankin (1991) sought to determine whether the "Fuld profile" could distinguish between samples of patients with AD and multi-infarct dementia. Only small numbers (e.g., 12%–15%) of patients fit the "Fuld profile" and it could not discriminate between the two diagnostic groups. Logsdon, Teri, Williams, Vitello, and Prinz (1989) used the *WAIS–R* to compare groups of AD patients, nondemented geriatric patients, nondemented depressed patients, and normal controls. Once again, the profile suggested by Fuld could not differentiate the various groups. A recent metanalysis (Christensen & MacKinnon, 1992) of WAIS studies in healthy elderly and AD patients noted that the profiles of the two groups tended to be different on all WAIS subscales to an approximately equal and parallel degree. Therefore, no subtest shows a uniquely poorer performance in AD, and verbal tests that are often thought to be spared measures may show clear impairments in AD.

Visual–Spatial Measures. There has been a moderate amount of interest in the performance of AD patients on measures of visual–spatial functions. This line of research represents a logical extension of clinical observations that AD patients frequently become spatially disoriented, even in familiar surroundings. Accordingly, studies in this area can assess the degree to which such problems are related to central deficits in visual–spatial integration. Some work (Henderson, Mack, & Williams, 1989) noted that the tendency for AD patients to "get lost" represents a central problem for caregivers. These authors specifically studied the neuropsychological and disease process predictors of spatial disorientation in a sample of AD patients. Patients were administered a variety of cognitive and behavioral measures. Stepwise regression analysis revealed that both a memory measure (e.g., delayed recall) and measures of visuoconstructive performance were significant predictors of spatial disorientation in patients. Overall, dementia severity (e.g., performance on the Mini-Mental State) did not predict spatial disorientation. This work is of practical interest because it used neuropsychological measures to predict a common behavioral problem (e.g., wandering), thus demonstrating the ecological behavioral validity of the measures.

Other works have directly assessed the nature of visual–spatial deficits in AD. One recent work (Ska, Poissant, & Joanette, 1990) administered the Benton Judgment of Line Orientation Test (Benton, Varney, & Hamsher, 1978), a visuospatial task thought to reflect right hemisphere functions, to a large group of normal controls ranging in age from 55 to 84. No effect of normal aging was found in line orientation performance. However, a group of AD patients were found to be significantly impaired on this task relative to the normal controls. Kirk and Kertesz (1991) performed a qualitative analysis of the drawings of AD patients that were obtained from administration of the Western Aphasia Battery. The authors concluded that the drawings of AD patients are suggestive of both left and right hemisphere pathology. Interestingly, there were no correlations between scores of overall drawing impairment and either Weschler Memory Scale scores or language measures. Other work (Storandt, 1990) has noted that the Bender–Gestalt Test was not useful in differentiating very mild or mild AD from normal aging effects.

Olfactory Deficits. Perceptual tests of olfactory identification have been studied as a potential early marker of AD. Olfactory functions may have a neurochemical basis in cholinergic function, which is an observation that is of importance given the interest in cholinergic pathology in AD. A series of studies (Peabody & Tinklenberg, 1985; Warner, Peabody, Flattery, & Tinklenberg, 1986) suggest that olfactory deficits (e.g., multiple choice identification of smells) may represent an early form of pathology in AD.

Frontal Lobe Functions. An interest in frontal lobe function has been evidenced in the investigations of neuropsychiatric disorders, especially in schizophrenia research. A majority of such studies infer frontal lobe function from tests (e.g., Wisconsin Card Sorting Test—WCST) that are thought to be sensitive to frontal lobe dysfunction. However, it should be noted that some work (e.g., Anderson, Damasio, Jones, & Tranel, 1991) suggests that measures such as the WCST may have relatively poor specificity, as nonfrontal and diffuse cortical insult can produce levels of impairment that are similar to those associated with specific frontal lobe lesions. Bhutani, Montaldi, Brooks, and McCulloch (1992) administered several tests (e.g., WCST, delayed alternation) to a sample of controls and AD patients. The AD patients showed relative impairment on several of these tests. These results are interpreted as suggesting frontal involvement even in the early stages of the disease. Other work in AD has utilized the Stroop Color–Word test, a brief instrument that is also thought to tap some aspects of frontal lobe functioning. Fisher, Freed, and Corkin (1990) noted that AD patients exhibit significant color confusion in performing this task. The authors urged caution in the use of this test in AD because color confusion may alter the validity of the measure in this population.

Perception of Affect. The recognition of affect (e.g., recognition of facial expressions of emotion) may represent a right hemisphere dominant phenomenon (Lezak, 1983). Albert, Cohen, and Koff (1991) noted that little work on affective recognition has been done in AD. They administered a battery of standardized tests and measures of affective perception to a sample of AD patients. In an initial analysis the AD patients could be significantly differentiated from controls; however, after performing analysis of covariance to adjust for the presence of other cognitive deficits in the patients, the tests of affective recognition generally failed to differentiate the groups. Therefore, observed impairments in affective recognition in AD may well be secondary to generalized cognitive impairment.

Mental Calculation. Mental calculation can tap a range of cognitive abilities (Lezak, 1983). Parlato et al. (1992) noted that mental arithmetic per se has received little attention in AD research. A serial seven subtraction task and WAIS-derived calculation item were administered to mildly demented AD patients and controls. The measures were found to significantly differ between the two groups. The WAIS item was found to correlate with other measures of attention and visuospatial skills, whereas serial seven performance correlated with the Mini-Mental State Examination and a measure of receptive language skills derived from the Western Aphasia Battery. The authors suggested that mental calculation impairments may be an early sign of AD.

Motor Skills. Motoric tasks represent commonly administered measures that may be relatively free of some mental functions that may be impaired in AD (e.g., language skills). Recent work (Müller, Weisbrod, & Klingberg, 1991) administered several finger tapping tasks to mildly impaired AD patients (mean age = 54 years). AD patients performed finger tapping tasks both more slowly and less accurately than control subjects. No other tasks of higher cortical functions were administered, which did not allow for a determination of the degree to which motoric deficits are related to a range of other functions.

Relationships Between the Stage of AD and Cognitive Impairment

A growing literature has sought to determine the relationship between neuropsychological test performance and the stage (i.e., global level of severity) of AD. The identification of a form of cognitive impairment that was linked to the initial onset of the disorder would be useful for early disorder screening, identification, and potential treatment. Moreover, as the AD syndrome progresses one could speculate that there could be a differential pattern of cognitive sparing and loss. Such a pattern could help to elucidate the pathological process related to the progression of the disorder.

Some reports (Welsh, Butters, Hughes, Mohs, & Heyman, 1992) have suggested that tests of delayed recall are particularly sensitive and specific to early cognitive impairment in AD. Welsh et al. (1992) noted that a combination of measures of verbal fluency, praxis, and recognition memory was the most successful battery for discriminating stages of AD based on overall dementia severity. The authors stressed that delayed recall measures may bottom out quickly with disease progression, and thus be of little use for quantifying the severity of cognitive deficit in the disorder beyond its early stages. However, delayed recall was by far the most effective measure in detecting early aspects of AD. Other work (Moss, Albert, Butters, & Payne, 1986) adds further support for the sensitivity and specificity of a delayed interval in discriminating performances of patients with AD from those with Huntington's disease, alcoholic Korsakoff's syndrome, and normal controls. In a 2-minute verbal condition the AD patients lost a significantly greater amount of information that the other groups. Other work (Salmon, Granholm, McCullough, Butters, & Grant, 1989) used similar tasks to demonstrate poor performance in AD patients during a 2-minute recall task.

Further work (Hill, Storandt et al., 1992; Storandt & Hill, 1989) that focused on the relationship between the staging of AD and neuropsychological testing has examined the differentiation of normal controls from AD patients with very mild, mild, and moderate global dementia severity ratings. Measures of memory (e.g., Weschler Memory Scale), psychomotor speed (e.g., Trail Making test) and language (e.g., Boston Naming Test) were diminished in both the very mildly and mildly impaired stages of dementia. However, the performance of patients who were deemed to be very mildly ill was found to significantly overlap with that of controls (Storandt & Hill, 1989). Comparisons between patients classified as moderately and mildly demented showed significant impairments on a range of measures (e.g., Boston Naming, Weschler Memory Scale; Hill et al., 1992). The authors suggest that memory dysfunction continues to make a major contribution to the differentiation of AD patients. Other work (Youngjohn, Larrabee, & Crook, 1992) has noted that individuals with memory decline suggestive of age-associated memory impairment generally could be discriminated from AD patients.

In sum, delayed recall tasks may be useful for detection of deficits in patients who are at the early stage of AD. Additional measures of verbal fluency and praxis also may be useful (Welsh et al., 1992). Performance patterns at the very early stage of the illness may overlap with normal controls (Storandt & Hill, 1989), but by the moderate stage of disease severity patients may have bottomed out on a range of tests that are routinely used in clinical practice (Hill, Stoudemire, et al., 1992).

Longitudinal studies of cognitive functioning can supplement data that are obtained in cross-sectional studies that evaluate patients at different stages of the illness. In one recent study (Rebok, Brandt, & Folstein, 1990) the investigators administered a short battery (e.g., Boston Naming Test, Benton Visual Retention Test, Token Test, Category Fluency Test) to 51 AD patients at 6-month intervals over a 2-year period. All patients were deemed to be at the early to middle stage of illness at initial assessment. Though declines were observed on all tests across the study period, relatively greater declines were noted on tests of semantic/lexical processing and comprehension of syntactic relationships. Other work (Haxby, Raffaele, Gillette, Schapiro, & Rapoport, 1992) studied patients approximately yearly over a period of 2.7 to 6.8 years from initial testing. A plateau phase, with little change in cognitive functioning (e.g., WAIS, Dementia Rating Scale), was observed in approximately one third of the sample. Declines in cognitive functioning appeared to be fairly consistent within patients but rates of decline varied across patients.

Vascular Dementia, Multi-Infarct Dementia, and Other Dementias

Diagnostic Considerations. A portion of older dementia patients have a dementing process that is etiologically based in vascular brain pathology. Several diagnostic terms (e.g., vascular dementia, multi-infarct dementia,) have been applied to this form of dementia. The use of these terms depends somewhat on the emphasis of multiple ischemic changes versus other substrates (e.g., white matter changes) of the disorder. Neuropathological observations (e.g., Tomlinson, Blessed, & Roth, 1970) suggest that vascular or multi-infarct dementia (MID) makes up the second most common form of dementia in older populations. These works noted a subset of patients in which the degree of infarcted brain tissue corresponded to the general severity of dementia. The exact prevalence of vascular pathology remains somewhat unclear, as vascular pathology can be noted in patients with AD. Some estimates suggest that a vascular form of dementia accounts for approximately 15–30% of dementia in elderly populations (Erkinjuntti & Sulkava, 1991).

Vascular dementia represents a quite heterogeneous disorder that can have a variety of pathologic origins and clinical presentations. Erkinjuntti and Sulkava (1991) summarized the nature of MID by noting: "Multi-infarct dementia is a spectrum with primary cortical involvement at one end and chiefly white matter changes at the other, but in most cases diagnosed both clinically and neuropathologically a combination of changes is observed" (pp. 112–113). A recent review (Marshall, 1993) of the nature of vascular dementia concludes that the principal cause of dementia in such syndromes is infarction-induced loss of brain parenchyma. Another recent review (Munoz, 1991) has attempted to classify the types of tissue changes noted in MID. These changes were noted to include the following: (a) macroscopic infarcts producing cavitation and gliosis near a large vessel, (b) cortical microinfarcts, (c) lacunes consisting of small cavity infarcts often found in the white matter, and (d) disorders of white matter pathology such as that found in Binswanger's disease.

Some (McGonigal, McQuade, Thomas, & Whalley, 1992) data suggest that MID may have a shorter survival time (i.e., time from symptom onset to death) than AD. A major risk factor for the development of vascular dementia is hypertension (see Starr & Whalley, 1992, for a review). Behavioral pathology (e.g., psychosis) similar to that viewed in AD may be present in MID (Mahler & Cummings, 1991).

The *DSM–III–R* clinical criteria for MID are displayed in Table 11.6. The *DSM–III–R* suggests several factors for the differentiation of MID from other forms of dementia such as AD. Although not a formal diagnostic criterion, the *DSM–III–R* suggests that MID typically has an abrupt onset rather than the insidious onset which is often seen in AD. Second, diagnostic criteria note that MID has a stepwise progression unlike the generally progressive course thought to be more typical of AD. These general distinctions have been the subject of some controversy (Erkinjuntti & Sukava, 1991). It has been suggested that MID can have an apparent insidious onset and that a stepwise deteriorating course may not always be present. Other authors have noted that the clinical description of MID offered by the *DSM–III–R* may result in generally low diagnostic accuracies when postmortem verification is used as the diagnostic standard.

Neuroimaging may be of some assistance in refining the diagnosis of vascular dementia. Although gross measures of pathology (e.g., lateral ventricle enlargement) may be present in all forms of dementia, specific ischemic changes may be visualized in some MID patients (Erkinjuntti & Sulkava, 1991). Some work (Jayakumar, Taly, Shanmugam, Nagaraja, & Arya, 1989) noted that CT scans could reveal infarcts in nearly all their sample of MID patients. Elevated rates of white matter low attenuation were also noted in MID patients. Schmidt (1992) compared MRI scans in groups of patients with AD, vascular dementia, and normal controls. Vascular disease patients had significantly more thromboembolic infarcts and white matter hyperintensities than AD patients. Other recent work (Liu et al., 1992) used MRI to study the nature of pathology that produces dementia in patients with a history of stroke. Such work can provide information on the nature of vascular pathology that produces

TABLE 11.6
DSM–III–R Criteria for Multi-Infarct Dementia and *DSM–IV* Criteria for Vascular Dementia

DSM–III–R Criteria for Multi-infarct Dementia

A. Dementia (as defined in Table 11.2).
B. Stepwise deteriorating course with "patchy" distribution of deficits (i.e., affecting some functions, but not others) early in the course.
C. Focal neurologic signs and symptoms (e.g., exaggeration of deep tendon reflexes, extensor plantar response, pseudobulbar palsy, gait abnormalities, weakness of an extremity, etc.)
D. Evidence from history, physical examination, or laboratory tests of significant cerebrovascular disease (recorded on Axis III) that is judged to be etiologically related to the disturbance.

DSM–IV Criteria for Vascular Dementia

A. The development of multiple cognitive deficits manifested by both:
   (1) memory impairment (impaired ability to learn new information or to recall previously learned information)
   (2) one (or more) of the following cognitive disturbances:
      (a) aphasia (language disturbance)
      (b) apraxia (impaired ability to carry out motor activities despite intact motor function)
      (c) agnosia (failure to recognize or identify objects despite intact sensory function)
      (d) disturbance in executive functioning (i.e., planning, organizing, sequencing, abstracting)
B. The cognitive deficits in criteria A1 and A2 each cause significant impairment in social or occupational functioning and represent a significant decline from a previous level of functioning.
C. Focal neurological signs and symptoms (e.g., exaggeration of deep tendon reflexes, extensor plantar response, pseudobulbar palsy, gait abnormalities, weakness of an extremity) or laboratory evidence indicative of cerebral vascular disease (e.g., multiple infarctions involving cortex and underlying white matter) that are judged to be etiologically related to the disturbance.
D. The deficits do not occur exclusively during the course of Delirium.

Note. From American Psychiatric Association (1987, 1994).

measurable dementia. Separate groups of MRI-verified stroke patients were studied with the groups differing in the presence or absence of dementia. Cortical infarcts and a greater infarction area were more common in the demented group. The demented group also had far greater infarction of the left hemisphere.

A recent review (Erkinjuntti & Sulkava, 1991) has summarized a breadth of findings to offer suggestions for the improvement of *DSM–III–R* MID criteria. These authors have suggested emphasizing clear evidence of infarcts from history/clinical observation, brain imaging findings, or both (e.g., CT or MRI evidence of multiple vascular lesions). The authors noted that such criteria, when added to data for the presence of dementia and the absence of other pathology (e.g., tumors), could improve the diagnostic accuracy of MID.

DSM–IV criteria (see Table 11.6) note a shift from a *DSM–III–R* diagnostic entity of "multi-infarct dementia" to a *DSM–IV* diagnosis of "vascular dementia." Similar to the Alzheimer's disease criteria, the vascular dementia criteria allow for the diagnosis to include information on qualitative psychiatric aspects of the illness that may be present (e.g., delusions, depressed mood, hallucinations). *DSM–IV* criteria requires evidence of neurological signs typical of ischemia (e.g., gait disturbance) or laboratory evidence indicative of cerebral vascular disease (e.g., neuroimaging documentation of multiple infarctions). The suggestion of a stepwise progression contained in the *DSM–III–R* diagnosis of MID was removed from the *DSM–IV* construct of vascular dementia.

Neuropsychological Findings in Multi-Infarct Dementia and Vascular Dementia

The neuropsychology of *DSM–III–R* MID or *DSM–IV* vascular dementia is not as widely studied as AD. A recent review (Mahler & Cummings, 1991) of the behavioral neurology of MID stresses the broad heterogeneity and clinical pathology of the disorder. Therefore, attempts to develop a specific pattern of deficits indicative of vascular dementia would seem rather difficult. However, several works have either attempted to typify vascular dementia or compare such patients to patients with AD.

Several studies have compared speech and language functions in AD and MID patients. Kontiola et al. (1990) administered receptive and expressive speech measures derived from the work of Luria. The MID patients were impaired in simple and basic language skills (i.e., a dysphasia syndrome secondary to major infarcts). The AD patients demonstrated difficulties in understanding and constructing complex grammatical structures. Powell, Cummings, Hill, and Benson (1988) noted that MID patients showed more problems in the motor aspects of speech, whereas AD patients had a relative sparing of motor speech functions. The information content of speech and confrontation naming were more impaired in AD.

A recent work of Mendez and Ashla-Mendez (1991) examined separate groups of AD and MID patients who were administered both structured (e.g., Boston Naming Test, California Verbal Learning Test, Trail Making Test) and unstructured (e.g., Lezak Tinker Toy Test, Lezak, 1983) cognitive measures. The AD and MID patients were generally similar on the structured tasks with the exception of several California Verbal Learning Test measures in which the AD patients showed more impairment. The MID patients demonstrated relatively poorer performance on both unstructured cognitive measures. The authors suggested that the unstructured tasks may preferentially tap frontal–subcortical pathways that are disturbed in MID. Given these novel findings and the small sample size ($N = 18$ per group), replication of this finding would be required. Other work (Fisher, Gatterer, Marterer, & Danielczyk, 1988) also has suggested that AD and MID patients have generally similar impairment of semantic memory.

Bernard, Wilson, and Gilley (1992) studied patients with Binswanger's disease that was diagnosed by both clinical and radiological criteria. Binswanger's disease is a form of progressive subcortical vascular dementia that commonly is characterized by deep white matter ischemic lesions (Marshall, 1993). A battery of semantic and explicit memory tests (e.g., word learning lists, letter and category fluency) were administered to groups of AD patients, Binswanger's disease patients, and normal controls. The AD patients showed significantly greater deficits on measures of explicit memory, but the AD and Binswanger's disease patients demonstrated similar impairments in semantic memory. The authors noted that a subcortical dementia such as Biswanger's disease can create impairments similar to those that occur in the cortical pathology of AD.

In summary, vascular dementia can present with a broad array of cognitive impairment syndromes that may be difficult to distinguish from other degenerative dementias. Although some patients may show an abrupt onset and a step-wise deterioration with concurrent ischemic neurologic events, such findings may not always be present. Documentation of ischemic pathology that is associated with the dementia may facilitate diagnostic accuracy.

Dementias Due to Other General Medical Conditions

The *DSM–IV* includes a variety of diagnoses that fall under the heading "Dementias Due to Other General Medical Conditions." Clinicians use Axis III of the DSM system to code the specific medical condition that is associated with each form of dementia. The general medical conditions include HIV disease, head trauma, Parkinson's disease, Creutzfeld–Jacob disease, Huntington's disease, and Pick's disease (American Psychiatric Association, 1994). The use of separate coding numbers for each of these conditions in *DSM–IV* represents a small change from *DSM–III–R,* which grouped some of these conditions under a diagnosis of "Presenile Dementia Not Otherwise Specified" (American Psychiatric Association, 1987).

Addition of a Specific Diagnosis for Dementia Due to HIV Disease

The inclusion of a diagnostic category for human immunodeficiency virus (HIV) related dementia represents a new addition to the *DSM–IV.* This addition seems important given the fact that in some geographical regions HIV-related cognitive impairments are the leading cause of dementia and death in males under the age of 40. Since the original syndromic formulation of acquired immune deficiency syndrome (AIDS), it has been noted that some patients with AIDS can show both acute and chronic neuropsychiatric impairment. However, it was only in recent years that the nature of cognitive deficits in HIV infection have become clear. Several studies now suggest that asymptomatic HIV positive individuals generally show little or no evidence for neuropsychological impairment. Individuals in the later stages of HIV infection of the CNS may show evidence of mental slowness, concentration difficulties, and memory impairment (Egan, 1992). In some cases these cognitive deficits may be quite significant.

The exact nomenclature for use with cognitive impairment resulting from HIV infection continues to evolve. Some prior work has utilized the term *AIDS dementia complex.* However, as recently noted (Egan, 1992), this title has limitations because dementia may be present in HIV seropositive individuals who do not have AIDS. In addition, minor forms of cognitive impairment found in many HIV seropositive individuals lack the severity to be classified as symptoms of dementia. Recent work ("Report of a Working Group," 1991) has used a general term of *HIV-1-associated cognitive/motor complex* that may then be further divided into more specific clinical entities. More severe manifestations are grouped under *HIV-1-associated dementia complex,* whereas milder forms of impairment fall under a title of *HIV-1-associated minor cognitive/motor disorder* ("Report of a Working Group," 1991).

Two major studies (Navia, Cho, Petito, & Price, 1986; Navia, Jordan & Price, 1986) provided important early details of the cognitive and neuropathological sequelae of dementia in 70 individuals who had died of AIDS. Psychomotor slowing and memory impairment were common during the later stages of AIDS. In addition, behavioral changes (e.g., apathy, withdrawal) and motoric deficits were also frequently noted. Neuropathological changes included involvement of the white matter and subcortical structures. Other early work (Grant et al., 1987) suggested a fairly high rate of cognitive abnormalities in all stages of HIV progression, including individuals who were asymptomatic. More recent work (e.g., Stern & Marder, 1991) has noted that this study used a quite small sample and may have defined abnormality in too liberal terms.

More recent studies have detailed the relationship between the stage of HIV infection and cognitive functioning. Janssen et al. (1989) performed cognitive assessments of individuals in a broad range of HIV stages. Individuals with AIDS-related complex performed significantly worse on neuropsychological measures than an HIV seronegative group. However, subjects with generalized lymphadenopathy and seropositive subjects with no signs of HIV-related infection showed neuropsychological profiles that were similar to HIV seronegative individuals. More recent work (Poutiainen et al., 1993) obtained generally similar results noting that individuals in early stages of HIV infection showed only slight cognitive impairments. Subjects with AIDS or AIDS-related complex tended to have deficits in cognitive speed and memory functions, whereas individuals in early stages of HIV infection showed only slight cognitive impairments. Other work (Goethe et al., 1989; McArthur et al., 1989) has failed to find differences in neuropsychological status between groups of asymptomatic seropositive HIV and seronegative subjects. The mild cognitive impairments seen in some asymptomatic seropositive individuals are not likely to be due to concurrent depression (Bornstein et al., 1993).

In sum, the inclusion of a DSM diagnosis of "dementia due to HIV disease" provides for a diagnostic description of a syndrome that is of growing recognition in clinical neuropsychology. Further research into the breadth and utility of diagnostic criteria for HIV related impairments is warranted.

DSM–III–R and *DSM–IV* Amnestic Disorders

The *DSM–III–R* and the *DSM–IV* both include diagnostic criteria for amnestic conditions. The defining characteristic of these disorders is an impairment in memorial function of either learning new information or recalling previously learned information. Criteria for *DSM–III–R* amnestic syndrome and *DSM–IV* substance-induced persisting amnestic disorder are listed in Table 11.7. The *DSM–IV* criteria include a division into different types of the disorder based on whether it is judged to be due to a general medical condition or it is substance induced. The *DSM–III–R* criteria include a "dementia associated with alcoholism" category. As noted in these diagnostic criteria, the diagnoses are for use in evaluation of patients who demonstrate specific deficits in memorial functions in the absence of other forms of significant cognitive impairment.

Korsakoff's syndrome represents one form of amnestic syndrome and has been thought to be associated with thiamine deficiency in patients who chronically abuse alcohol. However, some recent work has questioned aspects of this syndrome. Jacobson, Acker, and Lishman (1990) noted deficits in cognitive functions other than memorial functions in a sample of 38 patients with alcoholic Korsakoff's syndrome. The authors speculated that direct alcohol neurotoxicity may play a role in the development of amnesia in these patients. A recent review (Lishman, 1990) notes that patients may vary in their susceptibility to the toxic effects of both alcohol and thiamine deficiency, which creates a range of possible syndromic out-

TABLE 11.7
DSM–III–R Criteria for Amnestic Syndrome and *DSM–IV* Criteria for Substance Induced Persisting Amnestic Disorder

DSM–III–R Criteria for Amnestic Syndrome

A. Demonstratable evidence of impairment in both short- and long-term memory; with regard to long-term memory, very remote events are remembered better than more recent events. Impairment in short-term memory (inability to learn new information) may be indicated by inability to remember three objects after 5 minutes. Long-term memory impairment (inability to remember information that was known in the past) may be indicated by inability to remember past personal information (e.g., what happened yesterday, birthplace, occupation) or facts of common knowledge (e.g., past Presidents, well known dates).

B. Not occuring exclusively during the course of Delirium, and does not meet the criteria for Dementia (i.e., no impairment in abstract thinking or judgment, no other disturbances of higher cortical function, and no personality change).

C. There is evidence from the history, physical examination, or laboratory tests of a specific organic factor (or factors) judged to be etiologically related to the disturbance.

DSM–IV Criteria for Substance-Induced Persisting Amnestic Disorder

A. The development of memory impairment as manifested by impairment in the ability to learn new information or the inability to recall previously learned information.

B. The memory disturbance causes significant impairment in social or occupational functioning and represents a significant decline from a previous level of functioning.

C. The memory disturbance does not occur exclusively during the course of delirium or dementia and persists beyond the usual duration of Substance Intoxication or Withdrawal.

D. There is evidence from the history, physical examination, or laboratory findings that the memory disturbance is etiologically related to the persisting effects of substance use (e.g., a drug of abuse, a medication).

Note. From American Psychiatric Association (1987, 1994).

comes that can be found in patients with chronic alcohol use and poor nutrition. Other work (Solomon & Malloy, 1992) has pointed out that rates of head injury, much of which may be unreported, are quite high in alcoholics. In summary, amnestic syndromes may occur in some patients with significant chronic alcohol use histories, although the exact etiology of these syndromes (e.g., thiamine deficiency vs. alcohol toxicity) may require further clarification.

"SECONDARY" ORGANIC MENTAL DISORDERS AND UNDERLYING CONDITIONS

There is a disappointing lack of neuropsychological data for most of the Class III ("secondary") organic mental disorders, as defined in the first section of this chapter. This is not entirely surprising, given the apparent rarity of some conditions (e.g., secondary mania), the relative recency of accepted diagnostic criteria for these organic mental disorders, and the near impossibility of using standardized neuropsychological tests in some patients (e.g., during catatonic episodes in secondary catatonia). Additionally, psychiatrists and neuropsychologists often study these patients separately, so that published reports usually lack either neuropsychological data or psychiatric diagnoses. Some reviews of neuropsychological function (without psychiatric diagnosis) in various systemic or neurological conditions can be found (Csernansky, Liederman, Mandabach, & Moses, 1990; Gutierrez, Atkinson, & Grant, 1993; Lishman, 1987; Peyser, Rao, LaRocca, & Kaplan, 1990). In addition, few studies directly compare patients with primary psychiatric disorders and patients with the corresponding secondary psychiatric disorders on neuropsychological test performance.

A key question that remains largely unanswered is to what extent the "secondary" psychiatric disorders can have consistent clinical and neuropsychological findings despite different underlying primary diseases (e.g., stroke, seizures). One might hope for some such consistency if the secondary disorders are truly caused by the underlying primary disorders, rather than simply occurring together with them by chance. Unfortunately, the *DSM* (*–III* and following) classifications of organic mental disorders confuse this issue somewhat.

Taking secondary depression as an example, the *DSM* criteria give the impression that *any* medical condition can cause depression (Fava, 1992). In fact, although depression has been reported to be "caused by" numerous illnesses, from colon cancer to renal failure, "few studies have distinguished those psychiatric syndromes caused by the physical illness from those arising in response to the illness or merely coincident with it" (Popkin & Tucker, 1992, p. 375). For instance, there is little proof for most of these diseases that depression occurs more frequently with them than with illness in general or other life stresses. For this reason, the reader is referred elsewhere for encyclopedic reports of psychiatric symptoms attributed to various somatic illnesses or treatments (Cummings, 1988; Exstein & Gold, 1986; Gelenberg, 1976; Pascualy & Veith, 1989; Soreff & McNeil, 1987; Yudofsky & Hales, 1992; Whitlock, 1982).

On the other hand, examining those conditions that do seem to have a robust connection with secondary depression can give useful hints about the pathophysiology of idiopathic

TABLE 11.8
Etiologies Linked to Secondary Mental Disorders

Secondary depression	
Stroke (especially anterior left hemisphere)	HIV infection
Parkinson's disease	Reserpine or alpha-methyl-dopa
Huntington's disease	Cushing's disease
Wilson's disease	Addison's disease
Multiple sclerosis (temporal lobe plaque predominance)	
Secondary mania	
Adrenergic agonists	Right orbitofrontal brain injury
Corticosteroids	Encephalitides
Hyperthyroidism	Orbitofrontal and brainstem tumors
Secondary anxiety	
As a symptom	*Obsessive–compulsive disorder:*
Hypoglycemia	Manganese poisoning
Hypoxia	Carbon monoxide poisoning
Hyperthyroidism	Postencephalitis lethargica
Caffeine	Sydenham's chorea
Adrenergic agonists	
Alcohol/sedative withdrawal	
Secondary psychosis	
Strokes (subcortical and right parietal cortex)	Dopamine agonist intoxication
Metachromatic leukodystrophy	LSD and other hallucinogen use
Wilson's disease	Phencyclidine (PCP) intoxication
Epilepsy (limbic epilepsy especially)	
Secondary catatonia	
Bilateral anterior cerebral artery infarction	Neuroleptic toxicity
Brainstem and globus pallidus infarcts	Phencyclidine (PCP) intoxication
Hypothalamic tumors	
Secondary personality change	
Focal head injury (frontal and temporal lobe)	Diffuse head injury
Dementia of the Alzheimer's type	Epilepsy (limbic epilepsy especially)
General paresis (neurosyphilis)	

major depression (Drevets et al., 1992; Fava, 1992; Morris, Robinson, & Raphael, 1992), and the same should obtain for the other secondary disorders. Therefore, for each of the *DSM–IV* secondary psychiatric syndromes (except for secondary dissociative disorder and secondary sleep disorders), Table 11.8 lists several possible "primary," or underlying, conditions. Later we discuss each secondary syndrome briefly, including (a) pathophysiological similarities among the primary conditions, and (b) neuropsychological studies, especially comparisons between primary and secondary psychiatric syndromes, when data are available.

Secondary Depression

Conditions that appear to cause depression give support to recent anatomical and pharmacological findings in primary major depression. Depression in stroke patients without a personal or family history of affective illness is more frequent following left anterior lesions than following strokes elsewhere (Morris et al., 1992). Cortical and subcortical lesions are similar in this regard (Robinson, Kubos, Starr, Rao, & Price, 1984). Similarly, depression is common in illnesses affecting the basal ganglia, such as Parkinson's disease and Huntington's chorea. In Parkinson's disease, apathy correlates with time-dependent tasks and appears more related to dopamine function, whereas major depression in Parkinson's patients is associated with altered serotonin metabolism (Cummings, 1992; Starkstein, Mayberg, Preziosi et al., 1992). Case reports from the behavioral neurology literature implicate the medial frontal lobes in the regulation of volition versus anhedonia and apathy (Damasio & Van Hoesen, 1983). These brain regions coincide with neuroanatomical circuits that are known to be related to idiopathic unipolar depression (Coffey, 1993; Drevets & Raichle, 1992; Drevets et al., 1992). Similarly, systemic conditions strongly associated with depression include those which produce altered function of the hypothalamic–pituitary axis or lowered monoamine activity, consistent with findings in primary major depression (Drevets & Raichle, 1992; Rush et al., 1991).

Numerous studies have examined neuropsychological testing in patients with primary depression (see Cassens, Wolfe, & Zola, 1990, and Weingartner & Silberman, 1984, for reviews). However, there is surprising variability in the outcome of these works, which makes it difficult to test hypotheses about cognitive differences between primary and secondary depression. Cognitive testing profiles range from minimal attentional problems to significant impairments in multiple cognitive domains in patients with primary depression (Cassens et al., 1990). Some recent work (Richards & Ruff, 1989) has suggested that depression is related to visuospatial memory and verbal learning deficits that are not attributable to motivational factors. Unfortunately, many of these studies have employed nonstandardized tests of unknown reliability and validity in psychiatric samples. In addition, many studies fail to sample large groups of unmedicated patients. One recent work (Miller, Faustman, Moses, & Csernansky, 1991) used a standardized battery (the Luria–Nebraska Neuropsychological Battery) in a fairly large sample of unmediated depressed patients and matched controls. Few, if any, differences were noted between patients and control samples and there was no association of cognitive performance level to depression severity. In sum, a diverse set of findings have been found using cognitive testing in patients diagnosed with primary depression. These studies noted that this subgroup of depressed patients may show a range from significant cognitive deficits to little or no impairment. As noted by Cassens et al. (1990), this wide range of cognitive status may represent a useful classification variable for design of future studies into the neurobiology of primary depression.

Several studies have examined depression secondary to dementia. One work (Harper, Chacko, Kotic-Harper, & Kirby, 1992) compared geriatric inpatients with primary depression alone to those with depression and dementia. The results suggested that the groups could be discriminated reasonably well using several screening tasks for dementia. Total correct responses on the Boston Naming Test predicted dementia with depression versus depression with no, or reversible, cognitive deficit (Hill, Stoudemire et al., 1992). Therefore, primary depression manifests less cognitive impairment than depression with dementia. However, this difference should be specifically attributed to the added diagnosis of dementia rather than to general differences between primary and secondary depression. Evidence for this conclusion derives from a longitudinal study that found no additional cognitive deficits due to depression in patients with probable Alzheimer's disease (Lopez, Boller, Becker, Miller, & Reynolds, 1990).

A less complicated question is whether demented patients without depression have a different neuropsychological profile than depressed patients without dementia. This distinction may be relatively clear in Alzheimer's disease of at least mild degree (Hart, Kwentus, Wade, & Hamer, 1987; King, Caine, Conwell, & Cox, 1991; Rubin et al., 1987), but one careful study noted that neuropsychological tests were unable to distinguish depression-only geriatric patients from those with very mild dementia of the Alzheimer's type (Ruben, Kinscherf, Grant, & Storandt, 1991).

There is a good deal of data on cognitive impairment and psychiatric symptoms (e.g., depression) in multiple sclerosis (MS; see Lishman, 1987, for a review of earlier work). Several more recent studies are potentially relevant but did not use standard psychiatric diagnostic criteria (Arias Bal, Vásquez-Barquero, Peña, Miro, & Berciao, 1991; Clark et al., 1992; Feinstein, Kartsounis, Miller, Youl, & Ron, 1992; Rabins et al., 1986). Generally, although recent memory and abstract reasoning are impaired in MS patients (Peyser et al., 1990), this cognitive impairment appears not to have an obvious correlation with the presence of depressed mood.

In Parkinson's disease, major depression may characterize a poor-prognosis group in both clinical and cognitive domains (Starkstein, Bolduc, Preziosi, & Robinson, 1989; Starkstein, Mayberg, Leiguarda, Preziosi, & Robinson, 1992). In patients with left (but not right) hemisphere stroke, a diagnosis of major depression makes neuropsychological abnormalities more likely, even after controlling for demographic variables and lesion volume and location (Johnson, 1991; Starkstein, 1993).

Other Secondary Disorders

Mania. There have been relatively few well-documented cases of secondary mania (Cummings, 1986; Krauthammer & Klerman, 1978; Stasiek & Zetin, 1985). Nevertheless, these cases suggest common threads of ventral brain injury (brainstem and right orbitofrontal cortex) or of elevated monoamine levels. Neuropsychological testing in this population would be difficult during acute illness even if the condition were more common.

Anxiety Disorders. Anxiety as a symptom has been reported in numerous illnesses and in certain metabolic states (e.g., hypoxia, hypoglycemia). Furthermore, anxiogenic effects of certain drugs (see Table 11.8) have suggested a pharmacology of anxiety as a *symptom*. However, the *syndromes* of panic disorder or generalized anxiety may be less frequently mimicked. Specific studies of secondary panic or generalized anxiety have either not excluded coincidence or preexisting anxiety, have not included medical controls (Lustman, Griffith, Clouse, & Cryer, 1986), or have reported no striking excess of anxiety (Starkman, Cameron, Nesse, & Zelnik, 1990).

For obsessive–compulsive disorder, however, cases secondary to neurological illness suggest a fairly consistent anatomical picture that again supports findings in idiopathic OCD

(Cummings, 1993). Conditions that have produced obsessions and compulsions involve the orbital frontal lobe or subcortical structures anatomically linked to it (see Table 11.8). We are unaware of systematic neuropsychological studies in secondary OCD.

Psychosis. Certain neurological lesions produce delusions so commonly and specifically that psychiatric or neuropsychological evaluation is rarely sought (e.g., the alien hand syndrome after right parietal stroke, or denial of blindness after occipital infarcts). Furthermore, stereotyped hallucinations are common in classic migraine (visual), after amputation (tactile), or as ictal phenomena of partial seizures (varied).

More interesting are cases that bear a closer resemblance to the idiopathic psychoses. A substantial, but somewhat controversial, literature links the development of delusions and thought disorder in patients with epilepsy to seizure foci in limbic areas (Cummings, 1985; Lishman, 1987). Although the literature outside of epilepsy is largely anecdotal, subcortical grey matter and limbic areas are often involved in reports of secondary delusions (Popkin & Tucker, 1992). Pharmacologically induced psychosis without delirium points especially to glutamatergic (PCP) and monoaminergic (e.g., L-DOPA, amphetamines, LSD) pathways, although a host of other drugs have been implicated in case reports.

The psychiatrist Emil Kraepelin used the term *dementia praecox* to describe patients we would now call schizophrenic. As the term suggests, many investigators have noted abnormal neuropsychological function in patients with schizophrenia. In fact, Heaton and Crowley (1981) concluded that on the whole, neuropsychological tests were unable to distinguish chronic schizophrenic patients from "organic" patients with known brain disease. Flor-Henry (1983) added that dominant temporal lobe tests did worst at discriminating the two groups. However, these authors pointed out that the studies on which these conclusions were based were complicated by numerous methodological errors. In fact, more sophisticated studies were more likely to find differences, and certain subtests or test items that were performed adequately (Sawicki & Golden, 1984).

Against this background, Goldstein and Halperin (1977) tried to distinguish primary schizophrenia from secondary schizophrenia (due to "known brain disorders") in chronic psychiatric patients. They found that neuropsychological dysfunction was more a function of chronicity and severity of the schizophrenic syndrome than of the presence of known anatomic brain disease. In patients with limbic epilepsy, circumstantiality of speech and depressive and anxious symptoms were correlated with Luria–Nebraska global impairment (Csernansky et al., 1990).

Catatonia. Numerous apparently unrelated factors have been claimed to cause the catatonic syndrome. Among these, conditions affecting dopamine pathways or the basal ganglia are more easily understood as causing this movement disorder. Abulia, or akinetic mutism, bears some resemblance to idiopathic catatonia and follows bilateral medial frontal damage. Injury to the hypothalamus has produced an unfortunate syndrome reminiscent of lethal catatonia, with manic symptoms, agitation, fever, and death. We are unaware of systematic neuropsychological studies in this population.

Personality Change. Despite the descriptive breadth of the label "secondary personality change," one recent paper (Popkin & Tucker, 1992) noted "there can be little question that structural CNS injury (epilepsy aside) can and will give rise to alterations and disturbances of personality" (p. 382). Personality changes are classically associated with injury to frontal and temporal lobe structures, and there are some suggestions of even further anatomic specificity. For instance, orbitofrontal lesions are often associated with disinhibition, facetiousness, poor judgment, and euphoria (Lishman, 1987). Similarly, philosophical, humorless, and overinclusive traits are traditionally sought in patients with longstanding temporal lobe epilepsy (TLE). However, prospective studies in patients with epilepsy have found it difficult to substantiate this clinical impression; diminished libido may be the only consistent psychological symptom in TLE. Similarly, personality changes are seen with regularity in Alzheimer's disease, closed head injury, and other diffuse brain insults, as well as with focal injuries outside the frontal and temporal lobes.

In general, such personality changes are thought to correlate with demonstrable neuropsychological dysfunction. As these changes often do not fit well with traditional psychiatric nomenclature, neuropsychological investigations have generally not used the *DSM–III* (and subsequent) category of "organic personality disorder."

Lack of Neuropsychological Data for Class III Disorders

Neuropsychological studies have often not addressed the primary–secondary distinction using standard psychiatric diagnostic criteria. Available evidence suggests that secondary illnesses have generally similar neuropsychological profiles to the corresponding primary illnesses.

SUMMARY AND FUTURE DIRECTIONS

The use of neuropsychological testing in the psychiatric diagnostic process has demonstrated an evolution over the past 15 years. There has been a growth in data supportive of the biological basis of schizophrenia and major mood disorders. Traditional differential diagnostic questions of "functional versus organic," which were common in the 1970s, are now viewed as largely irrelevant. Diagnostic systems such as the *DSM–IV* have evolved to reflect some of these paradigm shifts. The concept of functional disorders has diminished and the notion of cognitive deficit disorders has developed.

Neuropsychiatric disorders such as schizophrenia are likely to have complicated etiologies. Genetic and environmental (e.g., obstetric complications, prenatal viral exposure) factors may contribute independently or may interact among each other in the etiology of the disorder. It is likely that other psychiatric conditions are similar to schizophrenia in this regard with disorders having a genetic version as well as an "environmentally" produced (e.g., head injuries, neurodevelopmental insults) variant of the disorder also possible. Therefore, nongenetic phenocopies of certain psychiatric conditions may be fairly common. Genetic studies that are directed at obtaining chromosomal linkage for such disorders may be confounded by this complex etiology. Biological measures that were capable of discriminating genetic forms of a disorder from nongenetic phenocopies would be of great importance in increasing the sensitivity of genetic studies. Neuropsychological measures represent a potential source of such indices. As noted in this review, some psychiatric disorders show a heterogeneous pattern of cognitive impairment and sparing. Such a pattern could well be due to the concurrent presence of genetic and nongenetic phenocopies with different patterns and absolute levels of cognitive performance. Clearly, more research is needed to clarify these issues.

The pressures of the current crisis in American health care delivery will likely force a further examination of the efficiency and utility of all aspects of psychiatric diagnosis and treatment. Clinical diagnosis remains an inexact science for the many illnesses which lack a specific laboratory test, such as the DNA test for Huntington's disease. Unfortunately, the most common psychiatric disorders fall in this category. The use of cognitive testing in a range of disorders remains one of the most highly reliable sources of information that is available to objectify the diagnostic and treatment process. Such testing continues to be one of the few types of measures that can contribute quantified, objective data to the understanding of the functional capacities of a patient. In addition, neuropsychological testing represents the most reliable and valid means for tracking the progression of impairments found in many neuropsychiatric disorders.

ACKNOWLEDGMENTS

The preparation of this chapter was supported in part by the Department of Veterans Affairs and Grant No. MH–30854 to the Stanford/VA Mental Health Clinical Research Center. Thanks are offered to Ms. Pamela Elliott for administrative assistance, gathering of materials, and manuscript preparation.

REFERENCES

Albert, M. S., Cohen, C., & Koff, E. (1991). Perception of affect in patients with dementia of the Alzheimer type. *Archives of Neurology, 48,* 791–795.

Amaducci, L., & Lippi, A. (1992). Risk factors for Alzheimer's disease. *International Journal of Geriatric Psychiatry, 7,* 383–388.

Amaducci, L. A., Fratiglioni, L., Rocca, W. A., Fieschi, C., Livrea, P., Pedone, D., Bracco, L., Lippi, A., Gandolfo, C., Bino, G., Prencipe, M., Bonatti, M. L., Girotti, F., Carella, F., Tacolato, B., Ferla, S., Lenzi, G. L., Carolei, A., Gambi, A., Grigoletto, F., & Schoenberg, B. S. (1986). Risk factors for clinically diagnosed Alzheimer's disease: A case-control study of an Italian population. *Neurology, 36,* 922–931.

American Psychiatric Association. (1987). *Diagnostic and statistical manual of mental disorders* (3rd ed., rev.). Washington, DC: Author.

American Psychiatric Association. (1994). *Diagnostic and statistical manual of mental disorders* (4th ed.). Washington, DC: Author.

Anderson, S. W., Damasio, H., Jones, R. D., & Tranel, D. (1991). Wisconsin Card Sorting Test performance as a measure of frontal lobe damage. *Journal of Clinical and Experimental Neuropsychology, 13,* 909–922.

Arias Bal, M. A., Vásquez-Barquero, J. L., Peña, C., Miro, J., & Berciao, J. A. (1991). Psychiatric aspects of multiple sclerosis. *Acta Psychiatrica Scandinavica, 83,* 292–296.

Benton, A. L., Varney, N. R., & Hamsher, K. de S. (1978). Visuospatial judgment. A clinical test. *Archives of Neurology, 35,* 364–367.

Berg, L., McKeel, D. W., Miller, J. P., Baty, J., & Morris, J. C. (1993). Neuropathological indexes of Alzheimer's disease in demented and nondemented persons aged 80 years and older. *Archives of Neurology, 50,* 349–358.

Bernard, B. A., Wilson, R. S., & Gilley, D. W. (1992). Memory failure in Binswanger's disease and Alzheimer disease. *The Clinical Neuropsychologist, 6,* 230–240.

Berrios, G. E. (1990). Alzheimer's disease: A conceptual history. *International Journal of Geriatric Psychiatry, 5,* 355–365.

Bhutani, G. E., Montaldi, D., Brooks, D. N., & McCulloch, J. (1992). A neuropsychological investigation into frontal lobe involvement in dementia of the Alzheimer type. *Neuropsychology, 6,* 211–224

Bidaut-Russell, M., & Grossberg, G. T. (1991). Relationship between alcohol intake, age of onset and duration of Alzheimer's disease: A pilot survey of 84 autopsy-confirmed cases. *International Journal of Geriatric Psychiatry, 6,* 797–800.

Bigler, E. D., Rosa, L., Schultz, F., Hall, S., & Harris, J. (1989). Rey–Auditory Verbal Learning and Rey–Osterrieth Complex Figure Design performance in Alzheimer's disease and closed head injury. *Journal of Clinical Psychology, 45,* 277–280.

Black, K. J. (1995). Diagnosing depression after stroke. *Southern Medical Journal, 88,* 699–708.

Bondi, M. W., & Kaszniak, A. W. (1991). Implicit and explicit memory in Alzheimer's disease and Parkinson's disease. *Journal of Clinical and Experimental Neuropsychology, 13,* 339–358.

Bornstein, R. A., Pace, P., Rosenberger, P., Nasrallah, H. A., Para, M. F., Whitacre, C. C., & Fass, R. J. (1993). Depression and neuropsychological performance in asymptomatic HIV infection. *American Journal of Psychiatry, 150,* 922–927.

Burns, A. (1991). Clinical diagnosis of Alzheimer's disease. *Dementia, 2,* 186–194.

Burns, A., Jacoby, R., & Levy, R. (1990). Psychiatric phenomena in Alzheimer's disease. I: Disorders of thought content. *British Journal of Psychiatry, 157,* 72–76.

Butters, N., Granholm, E., Salmon, D. P., & Grant, I. (1987). Episodic and semantic memory: A comparison of amnestic and demented patients. *Journal of Clinical and Experimental Neuropsychology, 5,* 479–497.

Caine, E. D. (1993). Amnesic disorders. *Journal of Neuropsychiatry and Clinical Neurosciences, 5,* 6–8.

Cassens, G., Wolfe, L., & Zola, M. (1990). The neuropsychology of depressions. *Journal of Neuropsychiatry and Clinical Neurosciences, 2,* 202–213.

Chartier-Harlin, M. C., Crawford, F., Houlden, H., Warren, A., Hughes, D., Fidani, L., Goate, A., Ressor, M., Roques, P., Hardy, J., & Mullan, M. (1991). Early-onset Alzheimer's disease caused by mutations at codon 717 of the beta-amyloid precursor protein gene. *Nature, 353,* 844–846.

Chatterjee, A., Strauss, M. E., Smyth, K. A., & Whitehouse, P. J. (1992). Personality changes in Alzheimer's disease. *Archives of Neurology, 49,* 486–491.

Christensen, H., & MacKinnon, A. (1992). Wechsler Intelligence Scales profiles in Alzheimer type dementia and healthy aging. *International Journal of Geriatric Psychiatry, 7,* 241–246.

Clark, C. M., James, G., Li, D., Oger, J., Paty, D., & Klonoff, H. (1992). Ventricular size, cognitive function and depression in patients with multiple sclerosis. *Canadian Journal of Neurological Sciences, 19,* 352–356.

Clark, R. F., & Goate, A. M. (1993). Molecular genetics of Alzheimer's disease. *Archives of Neurology, 50,* 1164–1171.

Cloninger, C. R. (1989). Establishment of diagnostic validity in psychiatric illness: Robins and Guze's method revisited. In L. N. Robins & J. E. Barrett (Eds.), *The validity of psychiatric diagnosis* (pp. 9–18). New York: Raven.

Coffey, C. E. (1993). Structural brain imaging and ECT. In C.E. Coffey (Ed.), *The clinical science of electroconvulsive therapy* (pp. 73–92). New York: American Psychiatric Press.

Cohen, D., Eisdorfer, C., & Leverenz, J. (1982). Alzheimer's disease and maternal age. *Journal of the American Geriatrics Society, 30,* 656–659.

Cooper, J. K., Mungas, D., & Weiler, P. G. (1990). Relation of cognitive status and abnormal behaviors in Alzheimer's disease. *Journal of the American Geriatrics Society, 38,* 867–870.

Corder, E. H., Saunders, A. M., Strittmatter, W. J., Schmechel, D. E., Gaskell, P. C., Small, G. W., Roses, A. D., Haines, J. L., & Pericak-Vance, A. (1993). Gene dose of apolipoprotein E type 4 allele and the risk of Alzheimer's disease in late onset families. *Science, 261,* 921–923.

Corkin, S., Growdon, J. H., Rasmussen, S. L. (1983). Paternal age as a risk factor in Alzheimer's disease, *Annals of Neurology, 13,* 674–676.

Crapper, D. R., Krishman, S. S., & Dalton, A. J. (1973). Brain aluminum distribution in Alzheimer's disease and experimental neurofibrillary degeneration. *Science, 180,* 511–513.

Csernansky, J. G., Leiderman, D. B., Mandabach, M., & Moses, J. A., Jr. (1990). Psychopathology and limbic epilepsy: Relationship to seizure variables and neuropsychological function. *Epilepsia, 31,* 275–280.

Cummings, J. L. (1985). Epilepsy: Ictal and interictal behavioral alterations. In J. L. Cummings (Ed.), *Clinical neuropsychiatry* (pp. 95–116). Orlando, FL: Grune & Stratton.

Cummings, J. L. (1986). Organic psychoses: delusional disorders and secondary mania. *Psychiatric Clinics of North America, 9,* 293–312.

Cummings, J. L. (1988). Organic psychosis. *Psychosomatics, 29,* 16–26.

Cummings, J. L. (1992). Depression and Parkinson's disease: A review. *American Journal of Psychiatry, 149,* 443–454.

Cummings, J. L. (1993, May). *The neurology of obsessive–compulsive disorder.* Paper presented at the annual meeting of the American Psychiatric Association, San Francisco, CA.

Cummings, J. L., Benson, F., Hill, M. A., & Read, S. (1985). Aphasia in dementia of the Alzheimer type. *Neurology, 35,* 394–397.

Damasio, A. R., & Van Hoesen, G. W. (1983). Emotional disturbances associated with focal lesions of the limbic frontal lobe. In K. M. Heilman, & P. Satz (Eds.), *Neuropsychology of human emotion* (pp. 85–110). New York: Guilford.

Deutsch, L. H., & Rovner, B. W. (1991). Agitation and other noncognitive abnormalities in Alzheimer's disease. *The Psychiatric Clinics of North America, 14,* 341–351.

Deutsch, L. H., Bylsma, F. W., Rovner, B. W., Steele, C., & Folstein, M. (1991). Psychosis and physical aggression in probable Alzheimer's disease. *American Journal of Psychiatry, 148,* 1159–1163.

Drevets, W. C., & Raichle, M. E. (1992). Neuroanatomical circuits in depression: Implications for treatment mechanisms. *Psychopharmacol Bulletin, 28,* 261–274.

Drevets, W. C., Videen, T. O., Price, J. L., Preskorn, S. H., Carmichael, S. T., & Raichle, M. E. (1992). A functional anatomical study of unipolar depression. *Journal of Neuroscience, 12,* 3628–3641.

Egan, V. (1992). Neuropsychological aspects of HIV infection. *AIDS Care, 4,* 3–10.

Eisdorfer, C., & Cohen, D. (1980). Diagnostic criteria for primary neuronal degeneration of the Alzheimer's type. *Journal of Family Practice, 11*, 553–557.

Erkinjuntti, T., & Sulkava, R. (1991). Diagnosis of multi-infarct dementia. *Alzheimer Disease and Associated Disorders, 5*, 112–121.

Exstein, I., & Gold, M. S. (Eds.). (1986). *Medical mimics of psychiatric disorders*. Washington, DC: American Psychiatric Press.

Fava, G. A. (1992). Comments on the proposal to eliminate the organic mental disorders category in DSM–IV. *American Journal of Psychiatry, 149*, 429–430.

Feighner, J. P., Robins, E., Guze, S. B., Woodruff, R. A., Jr., Winokur, G., & Munoz, R. (1972). Diagnostic criteria for use in psychiatric research. *Archives of General Psychiatry, 26*, 57–63.

Feinstein, A., Kartsounis, L. D., Miller, D. H., Youl, B. D., & Ron, M. A. (1992). Clinically isolated lesions of the type seen in multiple sclerosis: A cognitive, psychiatric, and MRI follow up study. *Journal of Neurology, Neurosurgery, and Psychiatry, 55*, 869–876.

Fisher, L. M., Freed, D. M., & Corkin, S. (1990). Stroop Color–Word Test performance in patients with Alzheimer's disease. *Journal of Clinical and Experimental Neuropsychology, 12*, 745–758.

Fisher, P., Gatterer, G., Marterer, A., & Danielczyk, W. (1988). Nonspecificity of semantic impairment in dementia of Alzheimer's type. *Archives of Neurology, 45*, 1341–1343.

Flor-Henry, P. (1983). Neuropsychological studies in patients with psychiatric disorders. In K. M. Heilman & P. Satz (Eds.), *Neuropsychology of human emotion* (pp. 193–220). New York: Guilford.

Flynn, F. G., Cummings, J. L., & Gornbein, J. (1991). Delusions in dementia syndromes: Investigation of behavioral and neuropsychological correlates. *The Journal of Neuropsychiatry and Clinical Neurosciences, 3*, 364–370.

Fogel, G. S. (1990). Major depression versus organic mood disorder: A questionable distinction. *Journal of Clinical Psychiatry, 51*, 53–56.

Fratiglioni, L., Grut, M., Forsell, Y., Viitanen, M., & Winblad, B. (1992). Clinical diagnosis of Alzheimer's disease and other dementias in a population survey. *Archives of Neurology, 49*, 927–932.

Fuld, P. A. (1984). Test profile of cholinergic dysfunction and of Alzheimer-type dementia. *Journal of Clinical Neuropsychology, 6*, 380–392.

Gelenberg, A. J. (1976). The catatonic syndrome. *Lancet, 1*, 1339–1341.

Gfeller, J. D., & Rankin, E. J. (1991). The WAIS–R profile as a cognitive marker of Alzheimer's disease: A misguided venture? *Journal of Clinical and Experimental Neuropsychology, 13*, 629–636.

Goethe, C. E., Mitchell, J. E., Marshall, D. W., Brey, R. L., Cahill, W. T., Leger, G. D., Hoy, L. J., & Boswell, R. N. (1989). Neuropsychological and neurological function of human immunodeficiency virus seropositive asymptomatic individuals. *Archives of Neurology, 46*, 129–133.

Goldstein, G., & Halperin, K. M. (1977). Neuropsychological differences among subtypes of schizophrenia. *Journal of Abnormal Psychology, 86*, 34–40.

Goodwin, F. K., Ebert, M. H., & Bunney, W. E. (1972). Mental effects of reserpine in man: A review. In R. I. Shader (Ed.), *Psychiatric complications of medical drugs* (pp. 73–101). New York: Raven.

Grant, I., Atkinson, J. H., Hesselink, J. R., Kennedy, C. J., Richman, D. D., Spector, S. A., & McCutchan, J. A. (1987). Evidence for early central nervous system involvement in the acquired immunodeficiency syndrome (AIDS) and other human immunodeficiency virus (HIV) infections. *Annals of Internal Medicine, 107*, 828–836.

Grosse, D. A., Gilley, D. W., & Wilson, R. S. (1991). Episodic and semantic memory in early versus late onset Alzheimer's disease. *Brain and Language, 41*, 531–537.

Gutierrez, R., Atkinson, J. H., & Grant, I. (1993). Mild neurocognitive disorder: Needed addition to the nosology of cognitive impairment (organic mental) disorders. *Journal of Neuropsychiatry and Clinical Neurosciences, 5*, 161–177.

Harper, R. G., Chacko, R. C., Kotic-Harper, D., & Kirby, H. B. (1992). Comparison of two cognitive screening measures for efficacy in differentiating dementia from depression in a geriatric inpatient population. *Journal of Neuropsychiatry and Clinical Neurosciences, 4*, 179–184.

Hart, R. P., Kwentus, J. A., Wade, J. B., & Hamer, R. M. (1987). Digit symbol performance and mild dementia and depression. *Journal of Consulting and Clinical Psychology, 55*, 236–238.

Haxby, J. V., Raffaele, K., Gillette, J., Schapiro, M. B., & Rapoport, S. I. (1992). Individual trajectories of cognitive decline in patients with dementia of the Alzheimer type. *Journal of Clinical and Experimental Neuropsychology, 14*, 575–592.

Heaton, R. K., & Crowley, T. J. (1981). Effects of psychiatric disorders and their somatic treatments on neuropsychological test results. In S. B. Filsko & T. J. Boll (Eds.), *Handbook of clinical neuropsychology* (pp. 481–525). New York: Wiley.

Henderson, V. W., Mack, W., & Williams, B. W. (1989). Spatial disorientation in Alzheimer's disease. *Archives of Neurology, 46*, 391–394.

Heston, L. L., Mastri, A. R., Anderson, E., & White, J. (1981). Dementia of the Alzheimer's type: Clinical genetics, natural history, and associated conditions. *Archives of General Psychiatry, 38,* 1085–1090.

Hill, C. D., Stoudemire, A., Morris, R., Martino-Saltzman, D., Markwalter, H. R., & Lewison, B. J. (1992). Dysnomia in the differential diagnosis of major depression, depression-related cognitive dysfunction, and dementia. *Journal of Neuropsychiatry and Clinical Neurosciences, 4,* 64–69.

Hill, R. D., Storandt, M., & LaBarge, E. (1992). Psychometric discrimination of moderate senile dementia of the Alzheimer type. *Archives of Neurology, 49,* 377–380.

Hodges, J. R., Salmon, D. P., & Butters, N. (1992). Semantic memory impairment in Alzheimer's disease: Failure of access or degraded knowledge? *Neuropsychologia, 30,* 301–314.

Hom, J. (1992). General and specific cognitive dysfunctions in patients with Alzheimer's disease. *Archives of Clinical Neuropsychology, 7,* 121–133.

Huff, F. J., Protetch, J., Saxton, J., & Becker, J. T. (1989). A comparison of measures of memory impairment for use in the diagnosis of Alzheimer's disease. *Neuropsychology, 3,* 29–40.

Inzelberg, R., Shapira, T., & Korczyn, A. D. (1990). Effects of atropine on learning and memory functions in dementia. *Clinical Neuropharmacology, 13,* 241–247.

Ironside, R. (1956). Disorders of laughter due to brain lesions. *Brain, 79,* 589–609.

Jacobson, R. R., Acker, C. F., & Lishman, W. A. (1990). Patterns of neuropsychological deficit in alcoholic Korsakoff's syndrome. *Psychological Medicine, 20,* 321–334.

Janssen, R. S., Saykin, A. J., Cannon, L., Campbell, J., Pinsky, P. F., Hessol, N. A., O'Malley, P. M., Lifson, A. R., Doll, L. S., Rutherford, G. W., & Kaplan, J. E. (1989). Neurological and neuropsychological manifestations of HIV-1 infection: Association with AIDS-related complex but not asymptomatic HIV-1 infection. *Annals of Neurology, 26,* 592–600.

Jayakumar, P. N., Taly, A. B., Shanmugam, V., Nagaraja, D., & Arya, B.Y.T. (1989). Multi-infarct dementia: A computed tomographic study. *Acta Neurologica Scandinavica, 73,* 292–295.

Jeste, D. V., Wragg, R. E., Salmon, D. P., Harris, M. J., & Thal, L. J. (1992). Cognitive deficits of patients with Alzheimer's disease with and without delusions. *American Journal of Psychiatry, 149,* 184–189.

Johnson, G. A. (1991). Research into psychiatric disorder after stroke: The need for further studies. *Australia and New Zealand Journal of Psychiatry, 25,* 385–370.

Katzman, R. (1986). Alzheimer's disease. *The New England Journal of Medicine, 314,* 964–973.

King, D. A., Caine, E. D., Conwell, Y., & Cox, C. (1991). The neuropsychology of depression in the elderly: A comparative study of normal aging and Alzheimer's disease. *Journal of Neuropsychiatry and Clinical Neuroscience, 3,* 163–168.

Kirk, A., & Kertesz, A. (1991). On drawing impairment in Alzheimer's disease. *Archives of Neurology, 48,* 73–77.

Knesevich, J. W., LaBarge, E., & Edwards, D. (1986). Predictive value of the Boston Naming Test in mild senile dementia of the Alzheimer type. *Psychiatry Research, 19,* 155–161.

Kontiola, P., Laaksonen, R., Sulkava, R., & Erkinjuntti, T. (1990). Pattern of language impairment is different in Alzheimer's disease and multi-infarct dementia. *Brain and Language, 38,* 364–383.

Koo, E. H., & Price, D. L. (1993). The neurobiology of dementia. In P. J. Whitehouse (Ed.), *Dementia* (pp. 55–91). Philadelphia: Davis.

Kopelman, M. D. (1985). Multiple memory deficits in Alzheimer-type dementia: Implications for pharmacotherapy. *Psychological Medicine, 15,* 527–541.

Krauthammer, C., & Klerman, G. L. (1978). Secondary mania: Manic syndromes associated with antecedent physical illness or drugs. *Archives of General Psychiatry, 35,* 1333–1339.

Kukull, W. A., Larson, E. B., Reifler, B. V., Lampe, T. H., Yerby, M., & Hughes, J. (1990). Interrater reliability of Alzheimer's disease diagnosis. *Neurology, 40,* 257–260.

Lezak, M. D. (1983). *Neuropsychological assessment.* New York: Oxford University Press.

Li, G., Silverman, J. M., & Mohs, R. C. (1991). Clinical genetic studies of Alzheimer's disease. *The Psychiatric Clinics of North America, 14,* 267–286.

Lipowski, Z. J. (1989). Delirium in the elderly patient. *New England Journal of Medicine, 32,* 578–581.

Lipowski, Z. J. (1990a). Is "organic" obsolete? *Psychosomatics, 31,* 342–344.

Lipowski, Z. J. (1990b). Organic mental disorders and DSM–IV. *American Journal of Psychiatry, 147,* 947.

Lipowski, Z. J. (1991). Reply to R. L. Spitzer, M. First, G. Tucker. Organic mental disorders and DSM–IV [letter]. *American Journal of Psychiatry, 148,* 396.

Lishman, W. A. (1987). *Organic psychiatry: The psychological consequences of cerebral disorder* (2nd ed.). Boston: Blackwell.

Lishman, W. A. (1990). Alcohol and the brain. *British Journal of Psychiatry, 156,* 635–644.

Liu, C. K., Miller, B. L., Cummings, J. L., Mehringer, C. M., Goldberg, M. A., Howng, S. L., & Benson, D. F. (1992). A quantitative MRI study of vascular dementia. *Neurology, 42,* 138–143.

Loewenstein, D. A., & Rubert, M. P. (1992). The NINCSD–ADRDA neuropsychological criteria for the assessment of dementia: Limitations of current diagnostic guidelines. *Behavior, Health, and Aging, 2,* 113–121.

Logsdon, R. G., Teri, L., Williams, D. E., Vitello, M. V., & Prinz, P. N. (1989). The WAIS–R profile: A diagnostic tool for Alzheimer's disease? *Journal of Clinical and Experimental Neuropsychology, 11,* 892–898.

Lopez, O. L., Becker, J. T., Brenner, R. P., Rosen, J., Bajulaiye, O. I., & Reynolds, C. F. (1991). Alzheimer's disease with delusions and hallucinations: Neuropsychological and electroencephalographic correlates. *Neurology, 41,* 906–912.

Lopez, O. L., Boller, F., Becker, J. T., Miller, M., & Reynolds, C. F., III. (1990). Alzheimer's disease and depression: Neuropsychological impairment and progression of the illness. *American Journal of Psychiatry, 147,* 855–860.

Luchins, D. J., Cohen, D., Hanrahan, P., Eisdorfer, C., Paveza, G., Ashford, J. W., Gorelick, P., Hirschman, R., Freels, S., Levy, P., Semla, T., & Shaw, H. (1992). Are there clinical differences between familial and nonfamilial Alzheimer's disease? *American Journal of Psychiatry, 149,* 1023–1027.

Lustman, P. J., Griffith, L. S., Clouse, R. E., & Cryer, P. E. (1986). Psychiatric illness in diabetes mellitus: Relationship to symptoms and glucose control. *Journal of Nervous and Mental Disease, 174,* 736–742.

Mahler, M. E., & Cummings, J. L. (1991). Behavioral neurology of multi-infarct dementia. *Alzheimer Disease and Associated Disorders, 5,* 122–130.

Margolin, D. I., Pate, D. S., Friedrich, F. J., & Elia, E. (1990). Dysnomia in dementia and in stroke patients: Different underlying cognitive deficits. *Journal of Clinical and Experimental Neuropsychology, 12,* 597–612.

Markesbery, W. R. (1992). Alzheimer's disease. In A. K. Asbury, G. M. McKhann, & W. I. McDonald (Eds.), *Diseases of the nervous system: Clinical neurobiology* (2nd ed., pp. 795–803). Philadelphia: Saunders.

Marshall, J. (1993). Vascular dementia. In P. J. Whitehouse (Ed.), *Dementia* (pp. 215–236), Philadelphia: Davis.

Martin, A., & Fedio, P. (1983). Word production and comprehension in Alzheimer's disease: The breakdown of semantic knowledge. *Brain and Language, 19,* 124–141.

McArthur, J. C., Cohen, B. A., Selnes, O. A., Kumar, A. J., Cooper, K., McArthur, J. H., Soucy, G., Cornblath, D. R., Chmiel, J. S., Wang, M. C., Starkey, D. L., Ginzburg, H., Ostrow, D. G., Johnson, R. T., Phair, J. P., & Polk, B. F. (1989). Low prevalence of neurological and neuropsychological abnormalities in otherwise healthy HIV-1-infected individuals: Results for the multicenter AIDS cohort study. *Annals of Neurology, 26,* 601–611.

McDonald, W. M., & Nemeroff, C. B. (1991). Neurotransmitters and neuropeptides in Alzheimer's disease. *The Psychiatric Clinics of North America, 14,* 421–442.

McGonigal, G., McQuade, C. A., Thomas, B. M., & Whalley, L. J. (1992). Survival in presenile Alzheimer's and multi-infarct dementias. *Neuroepidemiology, 11,* 121–126.

McKee, A. C., Kosik, K. S., & Kowall, N. W. (1991). Neuritic pathology and dementia in Alzheimer's disease. *Annals of Neurology, 30,* 156–165.

McKhann, G., Drachman, D., Folstein, M., Katzman, R., Price, D., & Stadlan, E. M. (1984). Clinical diagnosis of Alzheimer's disease: Report of the NINCDS–ADRDA Work Group under the auspices of Department of Health and Human Services Task Force on Alzheimer's Disease. *Neurology, 34,* 939–944.

Mendez, M. F., & Ashla-Mendez, M. (1991). Differences between multi-infarct dementia and Alzheimer's disease on unstructured neuropsychological tasks. *Journal of Clinical and Experimental Neuropsychology, 13,* 923–932.

Miller, L. S., Faustman, W. O., Moses, J. A., Jr., & Csernansky, J. G. (1991). Evaluating cognitive impairment in depression with the Luria–Nebraska Neuropsychological Battery: Severity correlates and comparisons with nonpsychiatric controls. *Psychiatry Research, 37,* 219–227.

Mohs, R. C., Breitner, J.C.S., Silverman, J. M., & Davis, K. L. (1987). Alzheimer's disease: Morbid risk among first-degree relatives approximates 50% by 90 years of age. *Archives of General Psychiatry, 44,* 405–408.

Monsch, A. U., Bondi, M. W., Butters, N., Salmon, D. P., Katzman, R., & Thal, L. J. (1992). Comparisons of verbal fluency tasks in the detection of dementia of the Alzheimer type. *Archives of Neurology, 49,* 1253–1258.

Morris, J. C., McKeel, D. W., Fulling, K., Torack, R. M., & Berg, L. (1988). Validation of clinical diagnostic criteria for Alzheimer's disease. *Annals of Neurology, 24,* 17–22.

Morris, P.L.P., Robinson, R. G., & Raphael, B. (1992). Lesion location and depression in hospitalized stroke patients: Evidence supporting a specific relationship in the left hemisphere. *Neuropsychiatry, Neuropsychology, and Behavioral Neurology, 5,* 75–82.

Mortimer, J. A., French, L. R., Hutton, T. J., & Schuman, L. M. (1985). Head injury as a risk factor for Alzheimer's disease. *Neurology, 35,* 264–267.

Moss, M. B., Albert, M. S., Butters, N., & Payne, M. (1986). Differential patterns of memory loss among patients with Alzheimer's disease, Huntington's disease, and alcoholic Korsakoff's syndrome. *Archives of Neurology, 43,* 239–246.

Müller, G., Weisbrod, S., & Klingberg, F. (1991). Finger tapping frequency and accuracy are decreased in early stage primary degenerative dementia. *Dementia, 2,* 169–172.

Munoz, D. G. (1991). The pathological basis of multi-infarct dementia. *Alzheimer Disease and Associated Disorders, 5,* 77–90.

Murrell, J., Farlow, M., Ghetti, B., & Benson, M. D. (1991). A mutation in the amyloid precursor protein associated with hereditary Alzheimer's disease. *Science, 254,* 97–99.

Navia, B. A., Cho, E. S., Petito, C. K., & Price, R. W. (1986). The AIDS dementia complex: II. Neuropathology. *Annals of Neurology, 19,* 525–535.

Navia, B. A., Jordan, B. D., & Price, R. W. (1986). The AIDS dementia complex: I. Clinical features. *Annals of Neurology, 19,* 517–524.

Nebes, R. D. (1989). Semantic memory in Alzheimer's disease. *Psychological Bulletin, 106,* 377–394.

Nielsen, H., Lolk, A., Pedersen, I., Autzen, M., Sennef, C., & Kragh-Sørensen, P. (1991). The accuracy of early diagnosis and predictors of death in Alzheimer's disease and vascular dementia—A follow-up study. *Acta Psychiatrica Scandinavica, 84,* 277–282.

Nussbaum, M., Treves, T. A., & Korczyn, A. D. (1992). DSM–III criteria for primary degenerative dementia and multi-infarct dementia. *Alzheimer Disease and Associated Disorders, 6,* 111–118.

Parlato, V., Lopes, O. L., Panisset, M., Iavarone, A., Grafman, J., & Boller, F. (1992). Mental calculation in mild Alzheimer's disease: A pilot study. *International Journal of Geriatric Psychiatry, 7,* 599–602.

Pascualy, M., & Veith, R. C. (1989). Depression as an adverse drug reaction. In R. G. Robinson & P. V. Rabins (Eds.), *Depression and coexisting disease* (pp. 132–151). New York: Igaku-Shoin.

Peabody, C. A., & Tinklenberg, J. R. (1985). Olfactory deficits and primary degenerative dementia. *American Journal of Psychiatry, 142,* 524–525.

Peyser, J. M., Rao, S. M., LaRocca, N. G., & Kaplan, E. (1990). Guidelines for neuropsychological research in multiple sclerosis. *Archives of Neurology, 47,* 94–97.

Popkin, M. K., & Tucker, G. J. (1992). "Secondary" and drug-induced mood, anxiety, psychotic, catatonic and personality disorders: A review of the literature. *Journal of Neuropsychiatry and Clinical Neurosciences, 4,* 369–385.

Poutiainen, E., Elovaara, I., Raininko, R., Hokkanen, L., Valle, S.-L., Lähdevirta, J., & Iivanainen, M. (1993). Cognitive performance in HIV-1 infection: Relationship to severity of disease and brain atrophy. *Acta Neurologica Scandinavica, 87,* 88–94.

Powell, A. L., Cummings, J. L., Hill, M. A., & Benson, D. F. (1988). Speech and language alterations in multi-infarct dementia. *Neurology, 38,* 717–719.

Price, B. H., Gurvit, H., Weintraub, S., Geula, C., Leimkuhler, E., & Mesulam, M. (1993). Neuropsychological patterns and language deficits in 20 consecutive cases of autopsy-confirmed Alzheimer disease. *Archives of Neurology, 50,* 931–937.

Rabins, P. V., Brooks, B. R., O'Donnell, P., Pearlson, G. D., Moberg, P., Jubelt, B., Coyle, P., Dalos, N., & Folstein, M. F. (1986). Structural brain correlates of emotional disorder in multiple sclerosis. *Brain, 109,* 585–597.

Randolph, C. (1991). Implicit, explicit, and semantic memory functions in Alzheimer's disease and Huntington's disease. *Journal of Clinical and Experimental Neuropsychology, 4,* 479–494.

Rebok, G., Brandt, J., & Folstein, M. (1990). Longitudinal cognitive decline in patients with Alzheimer's disease. *Journal of Geriatric Psychiatry and Neurology, 3,* 91–97.

Report of a Working Group of the American Academy of Neurology AIDS Task Force. (1991). Nomenclature and research case definitions for neurologic manifestations of human immunodeficiency virus-type 1 (HIV-1) infection. *Neurology, 41,* 778–785.

Richards, P. M., & Ruff, R. M. (1989). Motivational effects on neuropsychological functioning: Comparison of depressed versus nondepressed individuals. *Journal of Consulting and Clinical Psychology, 57,* 396–402.

Robins, E., & Guze, S. B. (1970). Establishment of diagnostic validity in psychiatric illness: Its application to schizophrenia. *American Journal of Psychiatry, 126,* 983–987.

Robins, E., & Guze, S. B. (1972). Classification of affective disorders—The primary–secondary, the endogenous–reactive and the neurotic–psychotic. In T. A. Williams, M. M. Katz, & J. A. Shield (Eds.), *Recent advances in the psychobiology of the depressive illnesses* (pp. 283–293). Washington, DC: U.S. Government Printing Office.

Robinson, R. G., Kubos, K. L., Starr, L. B., Rao, K., & Price, T. R. (1984). Mood disorders in stroke patients: Importance of location of lesion. *Brain, 107,* 81–93.

Roth, M. (1981). Discussion of "Classification of late life organic states and the DSM–III" by Clayton P. J., & Martin, R. In N. E. Miller & G. D. Cohen (Eds.), *Clinical aspects of Alzheimer's disease and senile dementia* (pp. 56–57). New York: Raven.

Rubin, E. H., Kinscherf, D. A., Grant, E. A., & Storandt, M. (1991). The influence of major depression on clinical and psychometric assessment of senile dementia of the Alzheimer type. *American Journal of Psychiatry, 148,* 1164–1171.

Rubin, E. H., Storandt, M., Miller, J. P., Grant, E. A., Kinscherf, D. A., Morris, J. C., & Berg, L. (1987).

Influence of age on clinical and psychometric assessment of subjects with very mild or mild dementia of the Alzheimer type. *Archives of Neurology, 50*, 380–383.

Rush, A. J., Cain, J. W., Raese, J., Stewart, R. S., Walker, D. A., & Debus, J. R. (1991). Neurobiological bases for psychiatric disorders. In R. N. Rosenberg (Ed.), *Comprehensive neurology* (pp. 555–603). New York: Raven.

Sacks, O. W. (1989). Neuropsychiatry and Tourette's. In J. Mueller (Ed.), *Neurology and psychiatry: A meeting of minds* (pp. 156–174). Basel, Switzerland: Karger.

Salmon, D. P., Granholm, E., McCullough, D., Butters, N., & Grant, I. (1989). Recognition memory span in mildly and moderately demented patients with Alzheimer's disease. *Journal of Clinical and Experimental Neuropsychology, 11*, 429–443.

Sawicki, R. F., & Golden, C. J. (1984). Examination of two decision rules for the global interpretation of the Luria–Nebraska Neuropsychological Battery summary profile. *International Journal of Neurosciences, 22*, 209–220.

Schellenberg, G. D., Bird, T. D., Wijsman, E. M., Orr, H. T., Anderson, L., Nemens, E., White, J. A., Bonnycastle, L., Weber, J. L., Alonso, M. E., Potter, H., Heston, L. L., & Martin, G. M. (1992). Genetic linkage evidence for a familial Alzheimer's disease locus on chromosome 14. *Science, 258*, 668–671.

Schmidt, R. (1992). Comparison of magnetic resonance imaging in Alzheimer's disease, vascular dementia, and normal aging. *European Neurology, 32*, 164–169.

Selnes, O. A., Carson, K., Rovner, B., & Gordon, B. (1988). Language dysfunction in early- and late-onset possible Alzheimer disease. *Neurology, 38*, 1053–1056.

Ska, B., Poissant, A., & Joanette, Y. (1990). Line orientation judgment in normal elderly and subjects with dementia of the Alzheimer's type. *Journal of Clinical and Experimental Neuropsychology, 5*, 695–702.

Small, G. W. (1992). Tacrine for treating Alzheimer's disease. *Journal of the American Medical Association, 268*, 2564–2565.

Solomon, D. A., & Malloy, P. F. (1992). Alcohol, head injury, and neuropsychological function. *Neuropsychology Review, 3*, 249–280.

Soreff, S. M., & McNeil, G. N. (1987). *Handbook of psychiatric differential diagnosis*. Littleton, MA: PSG Publishing.

Spitzer, R. L., Endicott, J., & Robins, E. (1975). *Research diagnostic criteria for a selected group of functional disorders* (2nd ed.). New York: New York State Psychiatric Institute.

Spitzer, R. L., & First, M. B. (1992). Dr. Spitzer and Dr. First reply. *American Journal of Psychiatry, 149*, 430.

Spitzer, R. L., First, M. B., Williams, J.B.W., Kendler, K., Pincus, H. A., & Tucker, G. (1992). Now is the time to retire the term "organic mental disorders." *American Journal of Psychiatry, 149*, 240–244.

Spitzer, R. L., Williams, J.B.W., First, M. B., & Kendler, K. (1989). A proposal for DSM–IV: Solving the organic–non-organic problem. *Journal of Neuropsychiatry and Clinical Neurosciences, 1*, 126–127.

Starkman, M. N., Cameron, O. G., Nesse, R. M., & Zelnik, T. (1990). Peripheral catecholamine levels and the symptoms of anxiety: Studies in patients with and without pheochromocytoma. *Psychosomatic Medicine, 52*, 129–142.

Starkstein, S. E. (1993). Dementia of depression in patients with neurologic disease. In S. E. Starkstein & R. G. Robinson (Eds.), *Depression in neurologic disease* (pp. 217–235). Baltimore: Johns Hopkins University Press.

Starkstein, S. E., Bolduc, P. L., Preziosi, T. J., & Robinson, R. G. (1989). Cognitive impairments in different stages of Parkinson's disease. *Journal of Neuropsychiatry and Clinical Neurosciences, 1*, 243–248.

Starkstein, S. E., Mayberg, H. S., Leiguarda, R., Preziosi, T. J., & Robinson, R. G. (1992). A prospective longitudinal study of depression, cognitive decline, and physical impairments in patients with Parkinson's disease. *Journal of Neurology, Neurosurgery, and Psychiatry, 55*, 377–382.

Starkstein, S. E., Mayberg, H. S., Preziosi, T. J., Andrezejewski, P., Leiguarda, R., & Robinson, R. G. (1992). Reliability, validity, and clinical correlates of apathy in Parkinson's disease. *Journal of Neuropsychiatry and Clinical Neurosciences, 4*, 134–139.

Starr, J. M., & Whalley, L. J. (1992). Senile hypertension and cognitive impairment: An overview. *Journal of Hypertension, 10* (Suppl. 2), S31–S42.

Stasiek, C., & Zetin, M. (1985). Organic manic disorders. *Psychosomatics, 26*, 394–402.

Stern, Y., & Marder, K. (1991). The neurology and neuropsychology of HIV infection. In F. Boller & J. Grafman (Eds.), *Handbook of neuropsychology, Vol. 5* (pp. 265–284). Amsterdam: Elsevier.

Storandt, M. (1990). Bender–Gestalt test performance in senile dementia of the Alzheimer type. *Psychology and Aging, 5*, 604–606.

Storandt, M., & Hill, R. D. (1989). Very mild senile dementia of the Alzheimer type II. Psychometric test performance. *Archives of Neurology, 46*, 383–386.

Tomlinson, B. E., Blessed, G., & Roth, M. (1970). Observations of the brains of demented old people. *Journal of Neurological Sciences, 11*, 205–242.

Tucker, G. J. (1991). DSM–IV: Proposals for revision of diagnostic criteria for delirium. *International Psychogeriatrics, 3*, 197–208.

Tucker, G. J., Caine, E. D., Folstein, M. F., Grant, I. G., Liptzin, B., & Popkin, M. K. (1992). Introduction to background papers for the suggested changes to DSM–IV: Cognitive disorders. *Journal of Neuropsychiatry and Clinical Neurosciences, 4,* 360–368.

Warner, M. D., Peabody, C. A., Flattery, J. J., & Tinklenberg, J. R. (1986). Olfactory deficits and Alzheimer's disease. *Biological Psychiatry, 21,* 116–118.

Wechsler, D. (1981). *WAIS–R manual.* New York: Psychological Corporation.

Weingartner, H., & Silberman, E. (1984). Cognitive changes in depression. In R. M. Post & J. C. Ballenger (Eds.), *Neurobiology of mood disorders* (pp. 121–135). Baltimore: Williams & Wilkins.

Welsh, K. A., Butters, N., Hughes, J. P., Mohs, R. C., & Heyman, A. (1992). Detection and staging of dementia in Alzheimer's disease: Use of neuropsychological measures developed for the consortium to establish a registry for Alzheimer's disease. *Archives of Neurology, 49,* 448–452.

Whitehouse, P. J., Price, D. L., Struble, R. G., Clark, A. W., Coyle, J. T., & DeLong, M. R. (1982). Alzheimer's disease and senile dementia: Loss of neurons in the basal forebrain. *Science, 215,* 1237–1239.

Whitlock, F. A. (1982). *Symptomatic affective disorders.* Sydney: Academic Press.

Wilkins, R. H., & Brody, I. A. (1969). Alzheimer's disease. *Archives of Neurology, 21,* 109–110.

Williams, B. W., Mack, W., & Henderson, V. W. (1989). Boston Naming Test in Alzheimer's disease. *Neuropsychologia, 27,* 1073–1079.

Youngjohn, J. R., Larrabee, G. L., & Crook, T. H. (1992). Discriminating age-associated memory impairment from Alzheimer's disease. *Psychological Assessment, 4,* 54–59.

Yudofsky, S. C., & Hales, R. E. (1992). *The American Psychiatric Press textbook of neuropsychiatry* (2nd ed.). Washington, DC: American Psychiatric Press.

12

Development of Neuropsychological Measures

Cecil R. Reynolds
Elizabeth Murdoch James
Texas A & M University

Diagnosis of neuropsychological deficits has, until recently, mostly depended on the depth and breadth of clinical experience of the neuropsychologist (Reynolds, 1989). Traditional neuropsychological assessment instruments frequently had little or no published psychometric information or norm tables. Those that did include psychometric information or norms of some description were often basing that information on so small a sample as to make it statistically unstable and unreliable, and therefore unusable for the population at large. The feeling among neuropsychologists was apparently that new clinicians eventually would come to know what a deviant score was simply from experience and from "developing" personal norm tables in their heads.

As recently as 1989 Franzen wrote, "It is true that the use of standardized psychometric instruments is not preferred over the use of instruments that require intuitive interpretation or instruments that are scored qualitatively" (p. 5). Reitan's fabled answer to the question of how to become a good neuropsychologist was, "Work in the field for 30 years" (Reynolds, 1989). Although this approach likely would have worked well for the few clinicians who had the chance to work with Dr. Reitan and to observe his legendary diagnostic abilities, it was not practical advice for the many inexperienced neuropsychologists entering a growing field. Certainly, clinical acumen is an important part of any neuropsychological assessment. However, psychometric methods need to be applied to established and newly published tests to enable those without extensive prior clinical neuropsychological experience to become effective neuropsychologists. Even neurologists and neuroradiologists are moving toward more quantitative methods than ever before.

There are several plausible reasons why psychometric methods generally have not been applied to neuropsychological instruments. Neuropsychology is a young field that, until recently, had a small number of practicing clinicians. Their numbers were so few that assessment instruments specific to neuropsychology were not widely used, reported, or taught. Established neuropsychologists could teach interested newcomers their methods in an apprentice-type relationship. The internalized norms of the established clinician would be passed on to the newer clinician through direct experience and mentoring.

If a neuropsychologist was experienced with a certain population, and knew what loss of skills might be expected in that population, it was possible that an assessment instrument of some kind would be developed to assess those skills in that population. Beginning in the 1940s and continuing into the 1960s, tests were developed by psychologists, psychiatrists, and neurologists seeking to differentiate organically induced difficulties from psychiatrically induced difficulties. There was not a unified view of brain damage at that time, so many tests were developed in order to satisfy various views and test highly specific populations. Many of those tests and tasks are still in use today. Currently, hundreds of different tests, tasks, and assessment instruments used with the infant, child, adult, and elderly populations are mentioned in the literature (La Rue, 1992; Lezak, 1983). Many of these instruments are familiar (e.g., WAIS–R, Halstead–Reitan Neuropsychological Test Battery, Wisconsin Card Sorting Test); many have acceptable standardization data; and many are population- and function-specific without acceptable standardization data. Holding neuropsychologists accountable for using only psychometrically sound tests would severely limit the pool of tests from which they could choose, and would thereby limit experienced clinicians' use of their internalized norms, often to the detriment of the examinees' well-being.

To run standardization studies for an assessment instrument requires a large amount of time, money, and people. Because the earliest neuropsychological instruments were designed with localization of function and lesion in mind, the population on which the tests were used consisted of individuals with a history of brain damage. To administer these instruments to a large enough population of individuals with and without brain damage so as to garner acceptable psychometric data would have been a task for which most clinicians would have had little enthusiasm (and likely even less funding). Given that initially most neuropsychologists had a greater interest and background in the medical and physiological rather than psychological aspects of neuropsychology, it is likely that they did not appreciate the need nor have the knowledge and skills required to design and complete standardization of their instruments.

TYPES OF NEUROPSYCHOLOGICAL INSTRUMENTS

Neuropsychology is often described as a bridge between neurology and psychology. Its earliest roots are in the field of neurology (Golden, Zillmer, & Spiers, 1992). Early tests of neuropsychological abilities were developed with localization of specific functions in mind, reflecting the influence of such early neuroanatomists as Franz Joseph Gall, Johann Spurzheim, Paul Broca, and Carl Wernicke (Golden et al., 1992; Luria, 1980). In the 1820s, Pierre Flourens set out to disprove Gall's localization theories and reported his belief in an integrated brain system. Forty years later John Hughlings Jackson put forth a theory of integration and brain organization that was incompatible with a strictly localizationist approach. Beginning in the 1950s and 1960s, and continuing into the 1980s, Aleksandr Luria, the Russian pioneer of modern clinical neuropsychology, whose background was in psychology and medicine, argued for an approach that emphasized the integrative nature of the brain and nervous system without dismissing the value of the work of earlier localizationists (Luria, 1980).

In the 1970s the instruments most frequently used as part of a neuropsychological battery included tests more commonly associated with psychology than neurology, such as the Rorschach Inkblot Test (Rorschach, 1966), Wechsler Scales, Thematic Apperception Test (Murray, 1943), Bender–Gestalt Test (Koppitz, 1963), Minnesota Multiphasic Personality Inventory (Hathaway & McKinley, 1943), and human figure drawings (Chelune, Ferguson, & Moehle, 1986; Goldstein, 1992). Today neuropsychological assessment makes greater use of tests of specific abilities and general abilities, utilizing brief tests and more comprehensive batteries. Information gathered from any and all of these instruments, if used properly, can be helpful to the neuropsychologist.

BRIEF MEASURES OF FUNCTIONING AND SPECIFIC ABILITIES TESTS

Brief measures of levels of performance may be appropriate as screening instruments and adjunct tests to a more comprehensive battery of tests. Often these instruments simply assess the presence or absence of a function by the use of cutoff scores. Neurological functioning exists along a continuum. Rarely is it the case that a function is completely lost. More often an individual will have lost *some degree* of function. Cutoff scores do not assess the degree of loss; rather, they seek only to indicate whether an individual's performance is normal or abnormal. False positive and false negative diagnoses are quite possible, depending on the level of the cutoff score (Lezak, 1983). Additionally, because cutoff scores do not indicate the depth and breadth of abnormal functioning, tests using this scoring method are not good at discriminating between organic and psychiatric patients, indicating the need for further, more comprehensive testing to arrive at a correct diagnosis.

Some brief measures of functioning available for use by the neuropsychologist are those that test specific abilities, such as sensory-motor, psycholinguistic, and sensory-perceptual abilities. Examples of such tests include the Bender–Gestalt Test, Token Test (DeRenzi & Vignolo, 1962), and Speech Sounds Perception Test (Reitan & Davison, 1974). Almost any test with a name reflecting only one specific aspect of neurological functioning (Beck Depression Inventory—Beck, Ward, Mendelson, Mock, & Erbaugh, 1961—Blessed Dementia Rating Scale—Blessed, Tomlinson, & Roth, 1968) can be included here. In addition to the problems stated previously, the danger of using *only* tests of specific abilities is the lack of breadth of coverage of neuropsychological functioning. Given that current theory stresses the integrative nature of brain functioning, the use of only brief measures of functioning increases the likelihood that something will be "missed."

GENERAL ABILITIES TESTS AND TEST BATTERIES

Assessment of more general abilities may include tests of learning ability, memory, intelligence, attention, academic achievement, personality, emotional stability, and abilities believed to be associated with a certain area of the brain, such as executive functions (frontal lobe). Such tests as the Wechsler Memory Scale–Revised (Wechsler, 1987), the various Wechsler Intelligence Scales (Wechsler, 1974, 1981), Wisconsin Card Sorting Test (Berg, 1948), Kaufman Test of Educational Achievement (Kaufman & Kaufman, 1985), and Rorschach Inkblot Test are often used in neuropsychological assessment as tests of general abilities. The Behavior Assessment System for Children (BASC; Reynolds & Kamphaus, 1992), although not developed specifically as a neuropsychological measure, may be used to assess social, emotional, and psychological fitness in children aged 4–18, and helps to round out the neuropsychological evaluation with careful, structured ratings of behavior and self-reports. Tests of general abilities provide the diagnostician with a broader picture of how the individual is functioning. Some tests, such as the various Wechsler Intelligence Scales, allow the diagnostician to refine a hypothesis regarding an individual's functioning through identification of patterns of scores.

Another means of assessing neuropsychological functioning is through the use of fixed test batteries such as the Halstead–Reitan Neuropsychological Test Battery (Reitan & Wolfson, 1985) and Luria–Nebraska Neuropsychological Battery (Hammeke, Golden, & Purisch, 1978). Although the prepackaged, all-in-one look of this type of instrument has appeal, there are both advantages and disadvantages to their use.

Chief advantages to the use of a fixed standard battery include the broad coverage of assessment, ease with which a diagnostic pattern of scores can be identified, and opportunity to gather information for longitudinal research and development of standards (Rourke, Bakker, Fisk, & Strang, 1983).

One disadvantage to the use of these batteries is the time involved in administration. Golden et al. (1992) wrote that because such a great amount of time is needed to administer these batteries, a technician is often the administrator rather than the neuropsychologist. This limits the amount of direct interaction the neuropsychologist has with the examinee and may prevent discovery of important clues to conditions that can be revealed through direct observation during testing. Additional disadvantages of relying solely on such batteries include the possibility of a poor choice of tests being included in the battery relative to a particular individual (a factor affecting validity), the inability to tailor the test and procedure to the specific needs of the individual, the possibility that, even with a broad spectrum of tests, something may be overlooked, and the lack of standardization and satisfactory norms. A battery of this type may appear to be easiest to administer, but it is a case of "one size fits all" and still requires a great deal of clinical experience, ability, and expertise to interpret correctly the results.

Perhaps the most effective and direct way to assess neuropsychological functioning is the use of an individualized, personalized test battery. Although it is possibly more time consuming, the flexible battery approach allows the neuropsychologist to tailor the testing to the individual examinee. Tests are chosen for breadth and depth of coverage of functions, and are augmented with specific ability tests that the clinician feels are warranted by the historical information, personal interview, and examination completed during intake procedures (Lezak, 1983), as well as by the individual's early test performance. Tests chosen for this type of battery will usually include measures of cognitive abilities and personality (Incagnoli, 1986) in combination with tests designed to confirm or rule out suspected dysfunction (Lezak, 1983). Lezak included tests administered by the neuropsychologist as well as paper-and-pencil tests that are, in part, self-administered and, in part, administered by staff. Seventeen basic measures are included.

The content of an individualized battery will be different depending on the orientation, training, and experience of the administrator, on examinee characteristics, and on assessment purposes and goals. The trick is to balance the need for efficient use of time (for the comfort of both diagnostician and examinee) with sufficient breadth and depth of coverage to ensure that all reasonable hypotheses regarding the individual's dysfunction have been tested. Care needs to be taken to ensure that the choice of tests in the flexible battery does not become a process of confirmation of the clinician's opinion (Golden, 1981).

Choice of tests will depend to a large extent on the goals of the assessment. Individuals for whom one of the goals of assessment is development of a hospital/clinic-based therapy/rehabilitative program will require testing that helps facilitate such programming in that setting. Testing for individuals who will receive services through the public school system necessarily needs to provide information that leads to the development of a treatment plan that can be implemented in a school setting.

All of the aforementioned hold true when *developing* a test of neuropsychological abilities. A test should be broad enough to cover the stated objectives, and specific enough to be of use. It should cover an aspect of neuropsychological functioning that is important and for which a new or improved instrument is called. Information gathered from the test should be of utility in assisting neuropsychologists to formulate diagnoses, prognoses, and rehabilitative recommendations for the examinee. Administration time should be efficient, taking into account examinee comfort and administration costs. The cost of purchasing the test should be kept to within a reasonable and competitive price range.

Construction of such an instrument will require a sound grounding in previously completed research regarding brain–behavior relationships, effects of closed head injury, and psychometrics. If a need exists for a test that measures frontal lobe functioning, the test developer who undertakes such a task would be well advised to study what is known about frontal lobe functioning, frontal lesions, behaviors resulting from frontal lobe trauma, and so on. It would be very unwise to attempt to develop a test claiming to measure abilities associated with frontal lobe functioning without first researching behavioral correlates of frontal lobe functioning, established tests of frontal lobe function, literature on frontal lobe trauma, and possible outcomes resulting from frontal lobe trauma.

Once a test developer has put together a test that is based soundly in known theory and research, the new test can then be field tested to determine if it does in fact measure what the developer had intended. One way of accomplishing this is to administer the new test along with an established test of the same neuropsychological function. By administering the two (or more) tests to the same group of people, the developer may submit both sets of scores to statistical analyses to determine the validity of the new test compared to the established instrument. Various other kinds of analysis can be completed to assist the examiner in refining the quality of items on the test.

GUIDING BASES AND CONSIDERATIONS FOR NEUROPSYCHOLOGICAL TEST DEVELOPMENT

The abnormal functioning that results from damage to the central nervous system is reflected in abnormal behaviors of some kind—emotional, academic, vocational, social, or any combination thereof (Lezak, 1983). Neuropsychology is concerned with identification and remediation of an individual's functional deficits. Tests are developed to achieve better such identification and to aid the neuropsychologist in developing a plan of remediation.

Development of an effective neuropsychological test is a task that requires grounding in and extensive knowledge of certain basics of psychology, neuropsychology, and psychometrics/test construction. The choice of items, breadth of coverage, "look" of the test, and extent to which it is standardized will reflect the biases of the test developer.

Ideally, the test developer should be aware of existing tests that measure the function the new test will attempt to measure. Any reported studies on such tests should be reviewed. Previous experience with assessing the function in question will be valuable when developing test items/tasks. The test developer should have extensive knowledge of normal development and behavior and how dysfunction may affect them. Items chosen for a test should be sensitive to subtle changes in normal performance. Item analyses should be conducted to select only the best items from a larger pool of potential items. An appropriate and understandable scoring system should be devised. For these scores to be useful to clinicians with varied experience in the field, standardization procedures should be implemented. The cost in time and money to develop and standardize an effective and psychometrically sound test is considerable. Costs should be ascertained, and a timeline for development and completion delineated and agreed on (with the publisher) before construction is begun.

IMPORTANT CONSIDERATIONS FOR TEST STANDARDIZATION: SELECTION OF TEST STIMULI

Test standardization is a complicated and lengthy process, involving every aspect of the test from item choice to wording of oral directions. Choice and type of test stimuli/items will depend on the test's target population (e.g., elderly), functions to be assessed, and the previous clinical and testing experience of the developer. Items sensitive to temporal lobe functioning will not be as sensitive to frontal lobe functioning. Similarly, items chosen to test overall cognitive abilities will differ from items assessing psychological health. The test developer must have determined what is to be assessed by the new test in order to choose appropriate items. Individual test items must be sensitive enough to specific central nervous system damage for that damage to be registered by the item, whereas the final group of items that comprise the entire test assess a wide enough range of subfunctions to "cover the territory."

The way in which test stimuli are presented to the examinee will vary, depending on individual abilities and on what is being assessed. Items requiring an oral response differ from paper-and-pencil items. Multiple-choice items differ from hands-on items wherein the examinee manipulates puzzle pieces. How appropriately the stimulus measures the target function is determined through item analyses conducted as part of the standardization procedures. Allen and Yen (1979) discussed four commonly used methods of item analysis: "(a) item difficulties and item-discrimination indices or item/total-test-score point-biserial correlations, (b) item-reliability and item-validity indices, (c) item-characteristic curves, and (d) factor analysis" (p. 119). (Reliability and validity issues are discussed more extensively in the sections subtitled "Reliability Considerations and Methods" and "Validity Considerations and Methods.")

Initially, a large pool of items should be developed; at a minimum, twice as many items should be written as are desired for the final version of the test. Through item analysis the best items will be identified and the items that do not measure the function well can be discarded or revised during the multiple tryouts that typically precede a national standardization.

OBJECTIVE SCORING

The use of objective scores in neuropsychological testing can be very helpful provided a complete neuropsychological assessment includes observation of the individual in question, personal interview, patient history, and the application of the clinical knowledge of the examiner. An objective scoring system is essential for proper test development. Without such a system, standardization of scores and development of norm tables are meaningless.

A test is objectively scored if a patient's performance can be quantified without subjective input from the examiner, and if experts in the field are in agreement on correct and incorrect responses. Items completed successfully according to the standards set up by the test developer will receive a predetermined amount of credit, whereas items not completed successfully will receive no credit. The individual receives a score based on actual performance, not on an interpretation of that performance. The personality and biases of the examiner will not enter into the examinee's earned score on a test with an objective scoring system, and, therefore, interrater reliability should be high for such a test.

How does a test developer know where to set the lower limit of normal functioning and the upper limit of abnormal functioning? Again, these limits are determined through the standardization procedure. A test developer administers a large pool of potential items to a substantial number of demographically representative individuals, including individuals with and without neuropsychological deficits. From the answers given, normative data can be derived that indicate the mean, median, and mode of the distribution of scores. These measurements can then be used to determine the standard deviation of the scores, thereby allowing the test developer to ascertain what a "normal" score is on those items, and what constitutes a deviant score. Subtest or item scores can then be transformed to standard scores (e.g., *z* scores, *T* scores) that are universally understood. The use of standard scores increases ease of communication among diagnosticians, some of whom may not be familiar with the test in question but are able to understand the meaning of the reported standard score. It also allows comparison of an individual's score with other scores within a test battery, and between the individual's scores and scores of others.

Many neuropsychological tests in use today do not have adequate normative data and do not use standard scores. These tests often use a nominal scoring procedure (cutoff scores) wherein the examinee passes or fails an item, indicating only the presence or absence of function and leaving no room for ascertainment of *degree* of functional loss or integrity. (Lezak, 1983, reported that a middle score of "fair" is sometimes used with scores of "pass" and "fail" in an attempt to "grade" items.) Scores can then be summed across items, subtests, or both for a summary score. The meaning of this score is dependent on the individual test given.

Again, it is important to remember that test scores are only a part of the data used to determine the state of an individual. Qualitative data *must* be incorporated *with* test data in order to arrive at a more complete picture of the individual and degree of dysfunction.

DIFFERENT FORMS OF TEST ADMINISTRATION: STANDARDIZATION AND COMPARABILITY

With the advent of easy access computer technology some test developers have sought to replicate existing paper-and-pencil tests to a computerized form. This increases the ease with which a test can be administered and scored, although there is cause for concern about test validity and loss of qualitative data when an examinee interacts with a computer program rather than with an examiner (Incagnoli, 1986). The MMPI and Rey–Osterreith Complex Figure Test (Osterreith, 1944) are two examples of tests that exist in both formats.

Standardization procedures for developing two psychometrically comparable forms of the same test will involve administration of both forms of the test to the same normative group, preferably administered within a very short period of time to avoid uncontrolled intervening effects (Franzen, 1989), and in a full counterbalanced design. The observed scores on both tests will then be correlated through the use of an alternate test forms reliability estimate. This correlation will reflect the reliability of the tests and the degree to which they are parallel (Allen & Yen, 1979). If equivalent, the covariance of the scores should be linear (Franzen, 1989). Separate norms should then be developed for each form of the test, as should standardized administration guidelines and directions.

Real problems exist in the development and standardization of alternate forms of the same test when the method of administration differs (e.g., pencil-and-paper vs. computer). Care must be taken to ensure to the greatest extent possible that both forms of the test are in fact measuring the same function. One would assume that the computer administration of the Rey–Osterreith Complex Figure, which uses a light pen, is measuring the same skill as if the pencil-and-paper form was used. Computer administration is frequently silent and usually requires the examinee to receive visual input. Such a form of administration would not be considered a parallel form of a test that requires verbal input, nonvisual input, or both.

Difficulties in determining the equality or parallelness of tests when different or modified forms are used also include questions about the efficacy of equating scores derived from nonrandom, preselected groups, and about how to interpret scores on a modified test (i.e., Does the modified test measure the same thing and to the same extent as the original test?; Staff, 1993). Scores derived from nonrandom groups cannot be equated, because the groups' individual differences before testing cannot be equated. If members of one group are impaired and members in the other group are not, the untested differences that will impact test performance will be so far reaching and pervasive that any correlation between groups will be meaningless. It will not be possible to attribute differences between these two groups to differences in the tests themselves. Test results and correlational studies will be confounded.

"Modifying tests for individuals with disabilities logically could alter both the construct and the predictive validity of the test for a given application" (Staff, 1993, p. 1). Altering the administration, form, directions, or response expectations of a test will make such an administration nonstandard, and may likely alter what the test is measuring, making construct validity meaningless. This set of circumstances would preclude the altered test from being considered a parallel form of the unaltered test. Test scores would take on a different meaning, as would the predictive validity of the test. The small amount of research that has been done in this area has shown both over and under prediction when modified forms of tests are given, depending on the type of disability of the group members.

CONSIDERATIONS FOR SELECTION OF THE NORMATIVE GROUP

The systematic development and presentation of normative data have not been of sufficient concern in the development and use of neuropsychological assessment instruments. Perhaps this is due to the tedious and mundane nature of such tasks, but the lack of sound normative data in neuropsychology is a distinct handicap to the field. Reports of normative data in the literature are typically based on inappropriately small sample sizes, do not employ normally functioning individuals, or both. Providing diagnosticians with norms developed from an inappropriate sample population is worse than providing no norms at all. If a test developer attempts to standardize a test on a poorly chosen normative group, the subsequent psychometric information will be misleading and erroneous and could be detrimental to the individual whose diagnostician is attempting to interpret test results from faulty data. Selecting a representative, balanced, demographically sound, and sufficient group on which to standardize an instrument is of the utmost importance.

Many neuropsychological measures report norms based on extremely small samples of neuropsychologically dysfunctional subjects, ignoring the need for stratified, demographically sound, wide-band samples that include primarily normal (i.e., nondiagnosed, nonimpaired) individuals drawn through the technique of population proportionate sampling. This serves to limit the neuropsychologist's ability accurately to interpret scores and results for individuals with "less than massive neurological trauma," and does not take into account the influence of such demographic factors as age, race, and gender on functional abilities. Often, neuropsychologists ignore such factors during test interpretation or believe that because brain function is being evaluated, demographic variables may be irrelevant. Although it has not been fashionable to note the existence of gender and racial differences in test performance, studies have been conducted that report systematic effects of many demographic variables on numerous tasks such as Coding and Digit Symbol (some of the most sensitive of all the Wechsler tasks to neurological trauma) from the Wechsler Scales where females (Black and White) consistently outscore males. Ignorance of such findings could easily lead a clinician to faulty interpretation. The failure to provide good, stratified samples in the development and standardization of neuropsychological tests has been a major stumbling block in efforts to understand demographic influences.

Reynolds (1989) discussed three reasons for careful selection of a standardization sample:

> Good standardization samples provide a reliable standard against which to judge the performance of others and have additional benefits including at least the following: (1) communications between researchers, (2) training of clinical neuropsychologists, and (3) the deflation and exposure of a variety of clinical myths. (p. 149)

The development of scaled scores for neuropsychological tests based on good normative reference samples would greatly ease the task of comparing the performance of research samples. Interpretation of research results would be greatly simplified and researchers would be able to communicate their results to others more easily and efficiently. Communicating to those in training would also be facilitated. It is not uncommon for neuropsychologists to use their experience to develop norms in their own minds, because several widely used neuropsychological tests (including the Halstead–Reitan Neuropsychological Battery and the Luria–Nebraska Neuropsychological Battery) have poor, inadequate, or missing normative data. This is not an optimal way to teach others about uses and interpretation of assessment instruments in an efficient and reliable fashion. The transmission of the knowledge and the clinical skills of neuropsychology thus could be greatly enhanced by the presence of accurate, high-quality normative data.

Norms also have the advantage of allowing neuropsychologists to evaluate certain aspects of the "clinical mythology" of assessment. For many years, statistically significant Verbal-Performance IQ differences on the Wechsler Scales were believed to be indicative of brain damage, neurological dysfunction, or learning disabilities in children. A difference of 15 points was considered clinically significant in documenting the presence of a learning disability. In a study by Kaufman (1976), in which he analyzed Verbal-Performance IQ differences in 2,200 normally functioning children from the WISC–R standardization sample, it was found that the average difference was 9 points, with 12-point differences found in one in three normally functioning children ($p = .05$), and 15-point differences found in one in four such children ($p = .01$), thus doing considerable damage to an oft-believed myth. Without a good standardization sample, this study could not have been done.

In deciding who is to be considered part of the normative sample several factors need to be considered. How large a sample size is needed to get reliable data? For what specific population is the test being developed? How many sets of norms will need to be developed (taking into consideration factors such as age, race, gender, and patient status)?

Decisions about sample sizes are often made with economic considerations in mind. Certainly a large test-publishing firm will be able to sustain more easily a large-scale nationwide standardization procedure with a large sample population than a smaller, less-well-financed publishing house. Considering the enormous effect of sample size on the reliability and validity of a test, it is well worth the money to invest in a large-scale study. The larger the sample size, the lower the sampling error and the more stable parameter estimates become, and the more accurate the scores will be as a reflection of the function within the general population, provided stratified demographic procedures have been followed. A very small sample will yield scores with a large amount of error so that population parameters are more difficult to estimate, contain too much error, and make interpretation of scores tenuous at best.

The intended clinical population for use of the test should be a consideration when choosing a normative sample. If norms are to be a reflection of the level of memory function in the general population, then individuals *with and without* deficits in memory function need to be included in order to get an accurate representation. If a small standardization sample is chosen, including only individuals with varying degrees of memory *dysfunction,* the resulting norms will be highly skewed (i.e., not representative of normal functioning) and useless when attempting to establish degrees of difference in memory functioning between brain-damaged and non-brain-damaged individuals. Conversely, it makes no sense to norm such a test on only individuals with normal memory function if the purpose is to establish degree of dysfunction for rehabilitative purposes.

Age presents a special problem. La Rue (1992) reported that most tests are not appropriate for adults 80 years and older due to lack of age-appropriate norms. The elderly population is extremely heterogeneous, so she believes that even within that limited population different sets of norms may need to be developed for different subgroups (e.g., based on level of education). Age studies using the Halstead–Reitan Neuropsychological Battery have shown that, among subjects aged 15–81 years, age accounted for "20% to 35%" of the variance in scores from the Category Test, Tactual Performance Test, and Trail Making Test" (p. 81).

Individuals may perform differently depending on their status (e.g., inpatient, outpatient). For this reason, too, separate sets of norms may be needed. If, for instance, a subgroup of inpatient subjects performs significantly differently (Golden et al., 1992, cautioned that "statistically reliable" is not as important as "clinically reliable") from a subgroup of outpatient subjects, separate norms may be warranted. The Behavior Assessment System for Children (BASC; Reynolds & Kamphaus, 1992) provides the diagnostician with "Clinical" norms derived from samples of children who were diagnosed with emotional or behavioral problems "extreme in comparison with the general youth population" (p. 9). The authors explained that these separate norms were developed because children with significant emotional and behavior problems score so much higher on the BASC "that ceiling effects are encountered when General norms are used" (p. 9), thus preventing the diagnostician from getting an accurate score. Score distributions for this subpopulation also differ in the dispersion of scores and shape of the distribution. (The BASC also provides age-stratified norms for each gender due to similar reasons).

It is desirable to have a standardization sample that is demographically reflective of the population with whom the test will be used. This is called *population proportionate sampling,* is a costly procedure, and is used by most of the large test publishers (e.g., American Guidance Service, The Psychological Corporation) when they conduct standardization studies and develop norms for their tests. If a test is to be used in the population at large, across age, gender, race, geographical location, and so on, then the standardization sample should be representative of that general population. For example, if Latino boys make up 5% of the school-aged population, and a test publisher is developing a test for school-aged children, then 5% of the standardization sample should be made up of Latino boys. The large test-publishing houses use population proportionate sampling for several reasons, among them:

(a) they do not want to be accused of having a test biased against an incorrectly represented group, and (b) their tests are typically for broad, often nationwide, use, and should a group not be represented accurately in the norming sample, the norms may be inadequate and inappropriate for a particular group in a particular part of the country, possibly leading to faulty interpretations of test scores. As discussed earlier, demographic variables play a part in level of performance on certain tasks and, as such, need to be taken into serious account when developing norms for assessment instruments.

RELIABILITY CONSIDERATIONS AND METHODS

Aspects of reliability and validity have been mentioned throughout this chapter. A more in-depth discussion follows, but it is beyond the scope of this work to deal with reliability and validity in their entirety. For a more complete treatment of these subjects with specific reference to neuropsychology the reader is referred to Franzen (1989).

Reliability may be the single most influential psychometric concept because of its relationship to all other psychometric characteristics. It is the foundation of validity, and classical psychometric theory is known as reliability theory. Reliability influences the likelihood that any experimental or treatment effects can and will be identified. The problem of reliability, especially of internal consistency reliability, has not been well attended in clinical neuropsychology, and this has been recognized as an area of special need (e.g., see Parsons & Prigatano, 1978; Reynolds, 1982). Two widely used neuropsychological instruments demonstrate this need. The HRNB reports no reliability information at all, and the LNNB reports reliability information gathered in a study so poorly designed that reliabilities are most likely spuriously inflated. How, then, can these instruments, and many others like them, be considered reliable and valid measurements of neuropsychological functioning? A discussion of the nature of reliability and ways of achieving it will further clarify why the lack of reliability information is of such concern.

In classical test theory, an observed score is equal to a true score plus an error score. The degree to which a test can be said to be reliable is the degree to which the observed score is free from error and therefore reflective of an individual's true score. Error can be random or nonrandom. It can be due to many things, including how a test is developed and used, stability of the function being measured, procedural discrepancies, level of skill, place of testing, rapport between the examinee and test administrator, the emotional and physical state of the examinee, and temporal elements. Because an error-free test (and therefore a perfect measurement) is not possible, estimates of how close a test comes to being error free are reflected in reliability coefficients (Franzen, 1989). These coefficients are correlations between two sets of scores that indicate the extent to which the sets of scores covary. To obtain reliability coefficients a test developer may want to look at test–retest, parallel forms/alternate forms, split-half, internal consistency, interrater reliabilities, or any combination thereof. The type of reliability that is important to the test developer will depend on the test and on what the developer is seeking to know through the reliability study.

Another way to view reliability is as a way of estimating the stability of an individual's scores across time. Franzen (1989) pointed out that this is potentially problematic in neuropsychological assessment where a diagnostician may not necessarily expect an individual's functioning to remain stable over a period of time. If an individual had recently sustained brain damage due to a blow to the head, a neuropsychologist would expect to see an increase in functioning over a period of time—the individual's scores would be expected to change.

This situation would not affect the reliability of the test itself, however, because sustaining an injury and subsequent recovery would be considered outside sources of error.

The correlation coefficient most widely used to express test–retest and alternate form reliability is the Pearson product–moment correlation coefficient (*r*), which produces a number with a value ranging from -1.0 to $+1.0$. A value of 0 indicates that no linear relationship exists between the two sets of data; a value of $+1.0$ indicates a perfectly linear relationship exists, and a value of -1.0 indicates an inverse linear relationship exists.

Use of the Pearson correlation coefficient is dependent on several assumptions, and is best used when data are on a continuous, interval scale with a high level of variability. Using this measure of correlation with nominal or ordinal data with a low level of variability will yield a correlation coefficient that is misleading. When situations arise in which use of the Pearson correlation coefficient would be ill-advised, the phi coefficient, point-biserial coefficient, or tetrachoric coefficient may be appropriate. The phi coefficient is appropriately used when the variables being considered are both dichotomous. Point-biserial coefficients are used when the relationship between a dichotomous variable and a continuous variable is being measured. The tetrachoric coefficient is used when two artificially dichotomized variables with a bivariate normal distribution are being considered. Other calculations useful with ordinal data are the Kendall tau and the Spearman rank-order coefficient (Franzen, 1989).

Test–retest reliability is used to assess the stability of a test over time. The same measure is given to the same individuals on two separate occasions. Scores are then correlated to determine the degree to which they are the same. Allen and Yen (1979) recommended that only a short period of time intervene between test administrations to limit the effects of other variables. Other factors that may contribute to an increase in error include practice effects, an increase in an individual's information about what the test measures, a change in attitude toward the test or administrator, and examinee memory resulting in repetition of answers given in the first test.

Mitigation of some of the aforementioned effects may be accomplished through administration of a parallel or alternate form of the test in the second testing session. To determine the equivalence of the alternate test forms, both tests should be administered to the same individuals on two different test occasions. Again, a minimal amount of time should separate the two sessions to attempt to control other effects. Franzen (1989) remarked that in order for the resulting coefficient of equivalence to be meaningful, "the two forms must have the same format, level of difficulty, length, and psychometric properties" (p. 22). The resulting coefficient of equivalence will reflect the amount of linear covariance between the two forms as well as the reliability of either form.

Test reliability can be estimated through the calculation of internal consistency reliability using the split-half method. Split-half reliability is an indication of the degree to which a test is internally reliable. The test is given as a whole test in one sitting and is later divided into two parts (e.g., odd/even numbered items). These parts should be as parallel as possible. The Spearman–Brown formula can then be used to determine the degree to which the subtests covary. This formula allows the test developer to estimate the reliability of the whole test from the reliability of the two parallel parts. If the two parts are not parallel, Cronbach's alpha will need to be used to get an estimation of the whole test coefficient. Alpha is most often preferred because it is the mean of all possible split-halves of a test and is considered a "best estimate" of the correlation between true alternate forms of a test. Alpha and other measures of internal consistency indicate the relative precision or accuracy of a test score with regard to errors of domain sampling in the choice of items for the test. Tests requiring a speed element, and tests such as the Rorschach whose stimuli and scores are not amenable to "splitting," cannot be analyzed using split-half approaches, and internal consistency reliability (a measure dependent on the homogeneity of the content and the completeness of the content sample) should be determined using the Kuder–Richardson 20/21 formulas or their more general form, coefficient alpha.

Interrater reliability coefficients represent the degree to which a test is consistent across administrators or those assigning scores to performance. The coefficient is an indication of agreement when individual differences between raters are partialed and should always be reported when examiner judgment is required in test scoring.

VALIDITY CONSIDERATIONS AND METHODS

The extent to which a test can be said to be valid is the extent to which it measures what it purports to measure. A test is not valid or invalid by itself; it is valid for a purpose. That is, if the test is useful in assessing the function it claims to assess and provides information of clinical utility to the diagnostician, it can be said to be a valid measure of that function. Therefore, it is the inference drawn from performance on a test that possesses validity (or not) rather than the test itself (for a detailed discussion of this concept, see Messick, 1989). The Wechsler intelligence scales are accepted as valid measures of cognitive ability not only because of statistical studies confirming their satisfactory degrees of validity, but because clinicians using these scales accept that they do measure aspects of a construct we call "intelligence."

As with reliability, there are different types of validity, chief among them being content, criterion-related, and construct validity (Allen & Yen, 1979; Barnett & Macmann, 1990; Messick, 1989). Other types are subsumed under these general headings.

Content validity is concerned with how well the items on a test assess the function in question. Knowledge of functional behaviors and the theoretical base in which the test is grounded, as well as breadth of coverage of test items and generalizability of results, are of utmost concern when dealing with the content of a test. Some methods of determining content validity use logical subjectivity and not statistical methods of validity. When this is the case, content validity is more prone to error than other forms of validity (Allen & Yen, 1979).

Allen and Yen included face validity and logical/sampling validity as two types of content validity. The face validity of an item can be established when an individual looking at it determines that it does measure the function in question. Sawicki (1989) pointed out that face validity is an important consideration for the examinee, in that an examinee is more likely to cooperate and put forth good effort if he or she can determine that the test being given is measuring that with which they are concerned. Logical/sampling validity takes face validity a step further by systematizing the item selection process to ensure inclusion of items representative of the entire range of behaviors reflective of the functions and subfunctions being assessed.

Sawicki (1989) mentioned error analysis as another way of establishing content validity in neuropsychological assessment. If error patterns can be observed in individuals of known dysfunction, then certain items may be valid indications of specific lesions.

Criterion-related validity indicates the degree to which a test is correlated with an outside variable. Included are concurrent validity and predictive validity, which are derived in a statistical manner and expressed as correlation coefficients. Concurrent validity estimates the degree of correlation between two measures of related functions taken at the same time. The developer of a test of frontal lobe functioning may want to give it and a neuroanatomical measure (e.g., CAT scan) to the same population at the same time to determine the degree of correlation between these two methods. (Sawicki, 1989, pp. 44–45, discussed three considerations for the neuropsychologist interested in establishing concurrent validity between a test and neurophysiological measures—expense, target population, and clinical usefulness—and noted the need for development of "instruments that have been validated against behavioral criteria," as an alternative). Predictive validity estimates the correlation between current test scores and future behavior. A test developer interested in predicting achievement from intelligence test scores would administer the intelligence test, wait for a predetermined period of time, obtain achievement test scores, and correlate the two to determine the predictive validity of the intelligence test.

Construct validity reflects the degree to which a test measures aspects of the underlying construct that it was designed to measure. This should be of central concern to a test developer. It would be a waste of time and money to attempt to develop a test that measures visual–spatial abilities, for example, without having a good idea of what those abilities might be and how they would manifest themselves. Using a more abstract example, it would be virtually impossible to measure intelligence without a working definition of what constitutes intelligence. Two methods of establishing construct validity are the multitrait–multimethod correlation matrix and factor analysis.

The multitrait–multimethod method of determining construct validity was developed by Campbell and Fiske (1959) and may be used when two or more constructs are being measured by two or more methods. Two types of construct validity are the result of this method: convergent validity and discriminant validity. For a test to be construct valid it should correlate highly with tests that measure the same construct (convergent validity), and correlate poorly with tests measuring different constructs (discriminant validity).

Factor analysis attempts to establish factorial validity through various statistical analyses of the interrelationships between items "in order to reveal the major dimensions that underlie a set of items" (Barnett & Macmann, 1990, p. 39). Factor analysis typically is conducted by analyzing the matrix of correlations within a test but can be accomplished as well by correlating scores on a new test with scores from tests already known to measure highly specific factors. The new test should correlate highly with tests known to measure the same factors and should correlate poorly with tests known to measure different factors (demonstrating convergent and discriminant validity, as well). Factor analysis can evaluate the pattern of these relationships and determine, quantitatively, if the pattern of interrelationships among the new and old variable fits a predicted pattern.

QUANTIFICATION OF QUALITATIVE DATA

Neuropsychological assessment involves the gathering and consideration of two kinds of information—that which can be expressed numerically (quantitative data), and that which is expressed in a descriptive, narrative form (qualitative data). Quantitative data are more descriptive of the end product of a test, whereas qualitative data are observations made by the diagnostician that can be used to detail the individual's behaviors during the process of taking the test. The decision to express data quantitatively or qualitatively depends on the type of data and its purpose. If a diagnostician is interested in comparing an individual's ability to copy correctly abstract figures with that of others the same age, quantitative data would be more efficient and specific. If, on the other hand, a diagnostician is interested in *how* the examinee drew the figure—which lines were drawn first, did the examinee rotate the paper, was the examinee's attention focused on the task, what did the examinee say while drawing—qualitative data is indicated. Lezak (1983) discussed two types of qualitative test behavior to which neuropsychologists should pay attention: behavior that is different from what would normally be expected, and unsolicited comments the examinee makes during testing. Ideally, a complete assessment should include both qualitative and quantitative data.

In order for qualitative data to be useful to the diagnostician, some standard against which individual performance can be measured needs to be available. Lezak (1983) noted that this standard is often the set of internalized norms a diagnostician develops after years of experience with neurologically impaired individuals. Such experience will hopefully result in knowledge of which behaviors to look for, which are important, which are diagnostic, which are possibly transient, which are intentional or unintentional and due to the deficit, and which suggest areas for further assessment. Although diagnostic experience is a valuable resource, experience and internal standards can vary among clinicians, and the inexperienced practitioner needs more immediate assistance in understanding the potential importance of certain qualitative information. Unfortunately, this is another area in which neuropsychological assessment is lacking. Fennell and Bauer (1989) noted that the usefulness of qualitative data in assessment is dependent on "carefully documented empirical data relating qualitative aspects of performance to normal and abnormal development, which are still not widely available to clinical practitioners" (p. 174). Published charts and tables of normal development may be of some assistance in this area.

Russell (1986) pointed out that qualitative data can be transformed into quantitative nominal data and measured through frequency of occurrence and degrees of difference from normal performance. He uses as an example the Halstead–Reitan Battery's scoring system for the Greek cross that transformed qualitative information regarding degree of dysfunction measured through visual analysis of an individual's performance into quantitative information that was developed into a "scale of severity of impairment" (p. 57). A significant problem inherent in this sort of quantification of qualitative data is the amount of information that is lost by reducing an individual's performance to a number on a scale, especially a nominal scale, the lowest level of measurement.

In deciding which scale to use, the test developer must choose one that most accurately and appropriately communicates the underlying qualitative meaning of a raw score. Raw scores in and of themselves are generally of little use when comparisons need to be made between tasks, tests, or both, or when communicating with other professionals inexperienced with the test from which the raw score is taken. In such cases, simply reporting a numerical score communicates *neither* adequate qualitative nor quantitative information from which diagnostic conclusions may be drawn. Transforming raw scores to standardized scores (e.g., *T*-scores, *z* scores) helps to alleviate those problems. (Unfortunately, many tests report age and grade equivalent scores as standard scores. These scores are inappropriate and have serious limitations and deficiencies; Reynolds, 1989).

The scaling of neuropsychological tests has been undertaken in an attempt to transform what is essentially qualitative data into quantitative nominal data. Such scaling has been sporadic, with some tests scaled well, some poorly, and a significant number not at all. The LNNB provides standardized scaled scores in the form of *T*-scores (mean = 50, standard deviation = 10), although the scaling is questionable due to the shape of the distributions obtained and the sample used in their derivation. Tests are scaled to a variety of metrics. If reliability of tests are reasonably comparable and norm groups are comparable as well, Table 12.1 can be used to help equate scores across tests when different metrics have been employed, the choice of metric often being arbitrary or by convention.

Although not wrong, it is best not to use raw scores as a means of comparison for many reasons, chief among them being the lack of comparability of the raw score distributions among the tasks of the battery and for any one task across age. Using raw scores correctly is typically superior to the use of inaccurate score transformations however, but requires extensive work and numerous calculations on the part of the person interpreting the test scores.

TABLE 12.1
Conversion of Standard Scores Based on Several Scales to a Commonly Expressed Metric

$\bar{X} = 0$ S.D. = 1	$\bar{X} = 100$ S.D. = 15	$\bar{X} = 100$ S.D. = 16	$\bar{X} = 100$ S.D. = 20	$\bar{X} = 500$ S.D. = 100	$\bar{X} = 50$ S.D. = 10	$\bar{X} = 50$ S.D. = 15	$\bar{X} = 36$ S.D. = 6	$\bar{X} = 10$ S.D. = 3	Percentile rank
2.6	139	142	152	760	76	89	52	18	>99
2.4	136	138	148	740	74	86	51	17	99
2.2	133	135	144	720	72	83	49	17	99
2.0	130	132	140	700	70	80	48	16	98
1.8	127	129	136	680	68	77	47	15	96
1.6	124	126	132	660	66	74	46	15	95
1.4	121	122	128	640	64	71	44	14	92
1.2	118	119	124	620	62	68	43	14	88
1.0	115	116	120	600	60	65	42	13	84
0.8	112	113	116	580	58	62	41	12	79
0.6	109	110	112	560	56	59	40	12	73
0.4	106	106	108	540	54	56	38	11	66
0.2	103	103	104	520	52	53	37	11	58
0.0	100	100	100	500	50	50	36	10	50
−0.2	97	97	96	480	48	47	35	9	42
−0.4	94	94	92	460	46	44	34	9	34
−0.6	91	90	88	440	44	41	33	8	27
−0.8	88	87	84	420	42	38	31	8	21
−1.0	85	84	80	400	40	35	30	7	16
−1.2	82	81	76	380	38	32	29	6	12
−1.4	79	78	72	360	36	29	28	6	8
−1.6	76	74	68	340	34	26	26	5	5
−1.8	73	71	64	320	32	23	25	5	4
−2.0	70	68	60	300	30	20	24	4	2
−2.2	67	65	56	280	28	17	23	3	1
−2.4	64	62	52	260	26	14	21	3	1
−2.6	61	58	48	240	24	11	20	2	<1

DETERMINATION OF CLASSIFICATION ACCURACY

Accuracy of classification is an important consideration for a developer of neuropsychological tests. Classification of individuals into diagnostic categories can help to facilitate communication between professionals concerned with their care and rehabilitation. (It is also a necessary consideration when dealing with insurance companies). Misclassification due to inadequate assessment instruments, faulty scoring systems (inaccurate cutoff scores), misinterpretation of assessment data, or any combination thereof is an unfortunate possibility.

Determination of criteria (scores) for a specific classification (diagnostic category) utilizes actuarial principles of *hit rates* and *base rates*. A hit rate is the number of correct classifications a score or pattern of scores can achieve. Good hit rates are dependent on the test developer's knowledge and consideration of the incidence of a disorder in the general population, known as the base rate. A good assessment instrument should improve on the hit rate that could be inferred from the base rate alone (Willis, 1984). Reschly and Gresham (1989) pointed out that base rates (especially when diagnosing a condition such as learning disabilities) should be of concern to neuropsychologists because:

> Many of the characteristics interpreted as clinically significant . . . occur frequently in the general population . . . [e.g.,] hemispheric asymmetry, differential integrity of anterior and posterior parts of the brain, and differences in left- and right-brain subareas such as left and right temporal lobes. (p. 512)

Willis (1984) noted that it is seldom the case that base rates are taken into account when classification criteria are established in neuropsychological assessment, and that often instruments believed to be successful at classification actually have hit rates that are the same as (or sometimes worse than) base rates in the population. His investigation and analysis of reported hit rates in light of base rate considerations found that in 65% of instances reported "hit rates exceeded base rates, reducing prediction errors by amounts ranging from 21% to 62%" (p. 568). However, 34% of instances reported found insignificant differences between base rates and hit rates or found that base rates exceeded hit rates "indicating that the use of the actuarial rule resulted in significantly more errors than in relying on base rates alone" (p. 569). He suggested that consideration of base rates in neuropsychological assessment will improve accuracy in diagnostic classification.

Differential diagnosis is of particular importance in clinical neuropsychology, with many instruments designed to differentiate between brain-injured and neurologically intact individuals. Further identification of the brain-injured individuals into subgroups according to location of injury, cause, time of onset, and prognosis is also desirable. The use of tests for these purposes brings out another problem with methodological and statistical procedures in clinical neuropsychology. In differential diagnosis, rather than being naive about the underlying psychometrics or scaling, the tendency has been to perform analyses that are too sophisticated for the data.

Researchers have, over the last decade, brought to bear the most sophisticated statistical methodologies directly on the problem of diagnosis and classification of mental disorders in the form of various multivariate analytical techniques, which have proven to be very powerful when used for determining group membership. When performing a neuropsychological assessment to determine diagnosis of an examinee's condition, it is typical to assess a wide range of behaviors using several instruments. When using such a large set of variables it is crucial to have a large number of subjects to rule out classification on the basis of random or chance variation that takes maximum advantage of correlated error variances. However, in the study of clinical disorders, the researcher is frequently limited to small sample sizes. Although most researchers acknowledge this difficulty, few realize the devastating effects of subject/variable ratios approaching 1:1 on the generalizability of studies of differential diagnosis. Large N studies of clinical populations are the exception, not the rule. Willson and Reynolds (1982; Reynolds, 1989) evaluated the effects of small samples on the validity of research attempting to discriminate among clinical disorders on the basis of neuropsychological test performance and have reported on many of the statistical problems that seem to plague the area.

In predicting group membership from a set of variables (e.g., neuropsychological test scores), there are several considerations. First, procedures that use *samples* of the target populations involve sampling error in the estimation of the relationships being examined. Results are expected to fluctuate from sample to sample due to random differences inherent in the samples. The squared multiple correlation (R^2) is used as the measure of prediction. In applying results of a particular sample to a second sample, R is expected to decrease because R^2 was made as big as possible for the first sample capitalizing on correlated error variances whenever possible. It is unlikely that the same fit of the data will occur in a second sample. Therefore, rules for classification derived from a particular sample cannot necessarily be expected to generalize to any other sample without a cross-validation effort to demonstrate that such a generalization is warranted.

When a prediction uses a strategy for selecting a small number of variables from a much larger initial set of variables, some correlations underestimate and some overestimate the population value. When stepwise regression or discriminant procedures and related multivariate methods are used, the overestimates are always chosen. When a large number of predictors is available, stepwise procedures maximize the chance of selecting random or near-random predictors. These variables predict poorly in the general population, but do correlate well with the outcome in the particular sample being used.

The degree of decrease in R^2 from sample to population can be estimated. The most commonly used estimate is from Wherry (1932) and is

$$R_\rho^2 = 1 - (1 - R^2)(N - 1)/(N - K - 1) \tag{1}$$

N is the number of observations, K the number of predictors, R^2 the observed squared multiple correlation between outcome and predictors and R_ρ^2 the population squared multiple correlation. This formula holds for either multiple regression or discriminant analysis.

Equation 1 has been widely cited. A review by Cattin (1980) suggested that for small N and large K, another approximation should be used:

$$\hat{R}^2 = \frac{(N - K - 3)\,\rho^4 + \rho^2}{(N - 2K - 2)\,\rho^2 + K} \tag{2}$$

where

$$\rho^2 = 1 - \frac{N - 3}{N - K - 1}(1 - R^2)\left[1 + \frac{2(1 - R^2)}{N - K - 1} + \frac{8(1 - R^2)^2}{(N - K - 1)(N - K + 3)}\right]$$

Although $R^2$is biased, the amount of bias is on the order of .01–0.02 for $N = 60$ and $K = 50$.

In some cases, there are more predictors than people, and then there is no unique solution to a best prediction. When using discriminant analysis this situation may result in perfect classification entirely at random by the predictors. Mathematically, this results from having more parameters to estimate than data points. In that case the researcher must make enough additional conditions to constrain the solution or must accept the solution which results from a particular order of entering predictors. As it is mathematically impossible to estimate all regression coefficients, there will be different solutions that would provide perfect classification but would not generalize to any other samples. It is also advisable, when using a large number of tests, to offset the small sample size so frequently seen in neuropsychological studies, because even when there are fewer predictors than subjects, the shrunken R^2 estimate will rapidly approach zero as the number of predictors becomes a significant proportion of the number of subjects.

When using two or more groups (e.g., brain-injured vs. neurologically intact individuals), discriminant analysis must be used instead of multiple regression. In discriminant analysis a canonical correlation—the R of relationship between predictor and between group distance—is computed for each discriminant function. The squared sum of the Rs is the maximum possible R^2.

For two groups, multiple regression and discriminant analysis yield the same results. For more than two groups, the canonical R^2 is still useful as an approximation to a multiple regression R^2. Although multiple group discriminant analysis is rarely used in neuropsychological research, it can be quite useful in many kinds of differential diagnosis.

To illustrate the problems that can be created by these statistical considerations, Willson and Reynolds (1982) examined all articles in three journals (*Psychology in the Schools, Journal of Consulting and Clinical Psychology,* and *Clinical Neuropsychology*) for the years 1979–1981. They selected studies that used test batteries, socioeconomic or demographic variables, or a combination of these variables to predict clinical group membership and that could help illustrate the difficulties on such work. Summaries of the relevant information in

TABLE 12.2
Summaries of Prediction Studies From Three Special Population Journals

Study		*Sample size*	*Total number of predictors*	*Number of predictors used*	R_F^2 *(reported)*	$\hat{R}_T^2$	$\hat{R}_F^2$
Dean (1978)		120	14	4	0.25*	0.09	0.21*
Selz & Reitan (1979)[a]		75	37	37	0.57	0.57	0.57
Wallbrown, Vance, & Pritchard (1979)		200	8	3	0.19*	0.13	0.17*
Purisch, Golden, & Hammeke (1979)	(a)	100	282	40	1.00*	0[b]	0[b]
	(b)	100	14	14	0.88*	0.84*	0.84*
Taylor & Imivey (1980)	(a)	30	16	5	0.44*	0.00	0.26
	(b)	30	3	1	0.08	0.00	0.05
	(c)	30	16	5	0.30	0.00	0.10
	(d)	30	3	1	0.14*	0.02	0.12
	(e)	30	16	2	0.25*	0.00	0.22*
	(f)	30	2	1	0.11	0.03	0.09
Dunleavy, Hansen, & Baade (1981)		24	37	3	0.82*	0[b]	0.79*
Fuller & Goh (1981)		80	22	12	0.38*	0.05	0.19
Golden, Moses, Graber, & Berg (1981)	(a)	60	11	2	0.55*	0.37*	0.54*
	(b)	120	11	2	0.68*	0.62*	0.68*
Malloy & Webster (1981)[c]	(a)	36	14	14	0.57	0.57	0.57
	(b)	36	14	14	0.94*[d]	0.94*	0.94*

[a] Trinomial classification table was reported; it was converted to a binomial (normal versus brain-damaged or LD) and the tetrachoric corrlation computed, which was squared to obtain R_F^2. Because it was based on a prediction equation from another study, no shrinkage was expected.

[b] An R^2 of 0.00 is expected in an overdetermined system, in which there are more predictors than subjects. Prefect classification is always possible.

[c] Binomial classification was reported. The tetrachoric correlation was computed as in footnote *a*.

[d] The R^2 values were estimated from a misclassification rate of 20% with 36 subjects. Although actual study was trinomial, the R^2 represents the equivalent for binomial classification for ease of computing.

*$p < 0.05$.

TABLE 12.3
Expected Misclassifications from Nine Studies

		t-equivalent for		*Estimated effect[a] size for two populations for*		*Two-population % misclassification for*	
		$\hat{R}^2_F$	$\hat{R}^2_T$	$\hat{R}^2_F$	$\hat{R}^2_T$	$\hat{R}^2_F$	$\hat{R}^2_T$
Dean (1978)		2.76	0.86	0.50	0.16	39%	47%
Purisch, Golden, & Hammeke (1979)	(a)	0	0	0	0	50%	50%
	(b)	6.27	6.27	1.25	1.25	27%	27%
Selz & Reitan (1979)[b]		1.15	1.15	0.27	0.27	45%	45%
Wallbrown, Vance, & Pritchard (1979)		3.12	1.89	0.44	0.27	41%	45%
Taylor & Imivey (1980)	(a)	1.69[c]	0.00	0.62	0.00	38%	50%
	(b)	1.21[c]	0.00	0.44	0.00	41%	50%
	(c)	0.73[c]	0.00	0.27	0.00	45%	50%
	(d)	1.95[c]	0.42	0.71	0.15	36%	47%
	(e)	2.84[c]	0.00	0.73	0.00	36%	50%
	(f)	1.76[c]	0.65	0.64	0.24	37%	45%
Dunleavy, Hansen, & Baade (1981)		5.01	0	2.05	0	16%	50%
Fuller & Goh (1981)		1.14	0.37	0.25	0.06	45%	49%
Golden, Moses, Graber, & Berg (1981)	(a)	5.78	1.61	1.49	0.42	23%	42%
	(b)	11.15	4.00	2.04	0.73	15%	36%
Malloy & Webster (1981)[b]	(a)	1.19	1.19	0.40	0.40	42%	42%
	(b)	5.04	5.04	1.68	1.68	20%	20%
Mean		3.11	1.38	0.81	0.33	35%	44%

[a]Effect = $t(1/n_1 + 1/n_2)^{1/2}$ (Glass, 1978).
[b]No shrinkage occurred.
[c]Single group statistics: effects were computed as if for two groups. Single group results are smaller than reported here.
From Willson and Reynolds 1982. © 1982 by Melnic Press. Reprinted with permission.

the nine studies they found are listed in Table 12.2. Several of the statistics listed represent the estimated values of R^2_ρ and their significance via their associated F-statistic. The statistic R^2_T represents the estimated R shrunken by Equation 1 to account for all the predictors originally considered. Because in no study was the overall R^2_T reported for all predictors, it was necessary to use the R^2_F based on the final regression. Therefore, R^2_T underestimated the shrunken R^2_ρ to some degree. Its upper bound is given by R^2_F, the shrunken estimate based on the number of predictors actually used. This is an *overestimate* of the actual shrunken R^2_ρ.

A second set of statistics was calculated from the nine studies to estimate loss of classification power due to shrinkage and is presented in Table 12.3. For the reported R^2_F and the R^2_T the t statistic equivalent was computed according to

$$t = \left[\frac{R^2/K}{(1 - R^2)/(N - K - 1)} \right]^{1/2} \tag{3}$$

Although most studies had only two groups, in Selz and Reitan (1979) the t statistic was based on reduction of the three groups to two (normal vs. abnormal). Then, an effect size was computed,

$$\in = t\,(1/n_1 + 1/n_2)^{1/2} \tag{4}$$

as defined by formula (4). This statistic is the number of standard deviations separating the two groups. Finally, the percentile point under the normal curve for *half* the effect is presented. This is the point that minimizes misclassification assuming equal cost for either false-positive or false-negative errors, and the equal population base rates.

The chance variation that can appear on the surface to be reliable discrimination with powerful multivariate techniques can be considerable. The importance of large subject/variable ratios and proper cross-validation becomes obvious in considering results summarized in Tables 12.2 and 12.3. Professionals concerned with predictive power of tests must consider the prediction rules generated from studies where R drops to nonsignificance.

In examining the misclassification rates (see Table 12.3), there is a change from about one third expected in the original studies (35%) to almost half (44%) using the corrected values. It is not surprising that the chance rates are very unimpressive when compared to the base rates in referral populations, when the considerable decline in effect size is taken into account.

The shrunken estimate of R^2 and the expected misclassification rate are the result of cross-validation. Cross-validation requires two independent samples, ideally drawn from the same population. When a single sample is split, regression is computed on one sample and weights applied to the scores of the second population to predict the outcome or group membership. The R^2 is a one-sample estimate of the R^2 in the nonvalidation sample, but it is not nearly so convincing because (a) it is a statistic that may vary, and (b) is uses information from only one sample, which is not as good as using information from two samples. In an effort to circumvent these problems, and to avoid the problem of splitting what is already most likely a very small N, a two-sample, cross-validation study drawn from the same population can be run.

Cross-validation studies take time that is well spent. Although a researcher/test developer may wish to publish results immediately, it is more likely that more accurate and useable results will be provided through cross-validation. Generalizability to other populations is not guaranteed by cross-validation results from two other samples, and therefore using any test for predicting outcomes with another group would require additional studies. Having the results of a study published in a reputable professional journal is not a guarantee that such results are correct, and practicing clinical neuropsychologists would be well advised to be aware of the pitfalls of using any actuarial rules for differential diagnosis that have not been submitted to cross-validation.

LIMITATIONS OF NEUROPSYCHOLOGICAL TESTS

The human central nervous system (CNS) is an extremely complex network of which we have only a rudimentary understanding. Neuropsychological assessment typically involves an attempt to piece together bits of information gathered during testing and interviews into a larger picture of what has gone wrong with an individual's CNS. Because our knowledge of the brain is so elementary, tests used to measure brain functioning give only rough ideas of CNS functioning. The complexity and intricate networking inside the brain means that focal lesions may have long-reaching effects of which we have limited or no knowledge, and tests that indicate the existence and location of such lesions may be inaccurate. Our knowledge of the effects of brain trauma and subsequent prognoses based on an individual's history, type of damage, etc. is growing constantly, but is still quite limited. To suppose a test measures with complete accuracy that which we know so little about is naive.

Tests alone will not provide the big picture, nor should they be expected to do so. Other types of assessment (e.g., medical, electrophysiological) should be used in an attempt to develop the clearest picture possible. All that aside, neuropsychological tests have limitations in and of themselves.

Due to many shortcomings in the development of most neuropsychological tests, it is not always certain that what these tests purport to measure is in fact what is being measured.

Lack of reliability, validity, standardization data, and small sample size may leave the knowledgeable clinician reluctant to use or rely on a test's results. Because good standardization information is the exception and not the rule, a test may be used for purposes for which it is unsuited, with the result of generating faulty hypotheses and diagnoses that may negatively impact an examinee. Certainly this will be true if a test is developed whose hit rate is less than the known base rate—and such tests are in use (Willis, 1984).

SUMMARY AND FUTURE DIRECTIONS

Development of assessment instruments to aid in diagnosis of neuropsychological dysfunction is a complicated, time-consuming, and expensive procedure. Most neuropsychological assessment instruments currently in use have some serious limitations. In many cases, standardized information is poor, inaccurate, or not available. This impedes the neuropsychologist's ability to train new neuropsychologists, communicate efficiently and effectively with other diagnosticians in related fields, and feel confident about the accuracy of a diagnosis and about the appropriateness of a patient's program of rehabilitation.

When planning a complete neuropsychological assessment the diagnostician should consider the presenting complaint of the individual, the individual's history, possible rehabilitation options, and time needed for completion of the assessment. Instruments should be chosen with an eye toward their stated purpose, psychometric soundness, standardization population, and hit rate versus base rate. Awareness of one's own clinical experience and acumen should be considered when deciding how broad an assessment is needed. Observations of the examinee are critical and should always be included as part of a neuropsychological assessment.

Although minimal attention has been paid to the standardization of neuropsychological instruments in the past, a stronger emphasis and keener focus on the need for such standardization has been seen in recent years (Franzen, 1989; Reynolds, 1989). With the high cost of collecting enough data to run a good standardization study in mind, ideas of how to collect data cheaply have been put forward. Data banks to which a collective of neuropsychologists contribute has been discussed and put into operation (Costa, 1988). Such operations are not without their problems, but the efficiency of data collection and the subsequent research possibilities make them a very attractive alternative. However, developmental norms are being collected for a variety of neurophysiological measures, including the EEG (e.g., Harmony, 1989) and quantitative MRI (Bigler, personal communication, 1995).

Computers will continue to have an impact on neuropsychological testing through the development of studies wherein electroencephalography (EEG), magnetic resonance imaging (MRI), and positron emission tomography (PET) are used. If, when an individual is performing tasks in a testing situation, their neurological activity can be monitored concurrently, this will give the neuropsychologist additional information that can be used to guide further assessment, diagnosis, prognosis, and rehabilitation. Research conducted in such situations will hopefully end in more finely tuned instruments yielding more specific results. These methods could be used to determine the validity of claims made for tests by their developers regarding particular neurological functions measured. Neurophysiological methods certainly will further our understanding of the workings of the human central nervous system.

ACKNOWLEDGMENT

Portions of this chapter are adapted from "Measurement and Statistical Problems in Neuropsychological Assessment of Children" by C. R. Reynolds, 1989, in C. R. Reynolds and E.

Fletcher-Janzen (Eds.), *Handbook of Clinical Child Neuropsychology,* New York: Plenum. Copyright © 1989 by Plenum Press. Adapted by permission.

REFERENCES

Allen, M. J., & Yen, W. M. (1979). *Introduction to measurement theory.* Monterey, CA: Brooks/Cole.

Barnett, D. W., & Macmann, G. M. (1990). Personality assessment: Critical issues for research and practice. In C. R. Reynolds & R. W. Kamphaus (Eds.), *Handbook of psychological and educational assessment of children* (pp. 30–51). New York: Guilford.

Beck, A. T., Ward, C. H., Mendelson, M., Mock, J., & Erbaugh, J. (1961). An inventory for measuring depression. *Archives of General Psychiatry, 4,* 561–571.

Berg, E. A. (1948). Simple objective technique for measuring flexibility in thinking. *Journal of General Psychology, 39,* 15–22.

Blessed, G., Tomlinson, B. E., & Roth, M. (1968). The association between quantitative measures of dementia and of senile change in the cerebral grey matter of elderly subjects. *British Journal of Psychiatry, 114,* 797–811.

Campbell, D. T., & Fiske, D. W. (1959). Convergent and discriminant validation by the multitrait–multimethod matrix. *Psychological Bulletin, 56,* 81–105.

Cattin, P. (1980). Note on the estimation of the squared cross-validated multiple correlation of a regression model. *Psychological Bulletin, 87,* 63–65.

Chelune, G. J., Ferguson, W., & Moehle, K. (1986). The role of standard cognitive and personality tests in neuropsychological assessment. In T. Incagnoli, G. Goldstein, & C. J. Golden (Eds.), *Clinical application of neuropsychological test batteries* (pp. 75–119). New York: Plenum.

Costa, L. (1988). Clinical neuropsychology: Prospects and problems. *The clinical neuropsychologist, 2*(1), 3–11.

Dean, R. S. (1978). Distinguishing learning-disabled and emotionally disturbed children on the WISC–R. *Journal of Consulting and Clinical Psychology, 46,* 381–382.

DeRenzi, E., & Vignolo, L. (1962). The Token Test: A sensitive test to detect receptive disturbances in aphasics. *Brain, 85,* 665–668.

Dunleavy, R. A., Hansen, J. L., & Baade, L. E. (1981). Discriminating powers of Halstead Battery tests in assessment of 9- to 14-year-old severely asthmatic children. *Clinical Neuropsychology, 3,* 9–12.

Fennell, E. B., & Bauer, R. M. (1989). Models of inference in evaluating brain–behavior relationships in children. In C. R. Reynolds & E. Fletcher-Janzen (Eds.), *Handbook of clinical child neuropsychology* (pp. 167–177). New York: Plenum.

Franzen, M. D. (1989). *Reliability and validity in neuropsychological assessment.* New York: Plenum.

Fuller, G. B., & Goh, D. S. (1981). Intelligence, achievement, and visual–motor performance among learning disabled and emotionally impaired children. *Psychology in the Schools, 18,* 262–268.

Golden, C. J. (1981). *Diagnosis and rehabilitation in clinical neuropsychology.* Springfield, IL: Charles Thomas.

Golden, C. J., Moses, J. A., Jr., Graber, B., & Berg, T. (1981). Objective clinical rules for interpreting the Luria–Nebraska Neuropsychological Battery: Derivation, effectiveness, and validation. *Journal of Consulting and Clinical Psychology, 49,* 616–618.

Golden, C. J., Zillmer, E., & Spiers, M. (1992). *Neuropsychological assessment and intervention.* Springfield, IL: Charles Thomas.

Goldstein, G. (1992). Historical perspectives. In A. E. Puente & R. J. McCaffrey (Eds.) *Handbook of neuropsychological assessment: A biopsychosocial perspective* (pp. 1–12). New York: Plenum.

Hammeke, T. A., Golden, C. J., Purisch, A. D. (1978). A standardized, short, and comprehensive neuropsychological test battery based on the Luria Neuropsychological Evaluation. *International Journal of Neuroscience, 8,* 135–141.

Harmony, T. (1989). Psychophysiological evaluation of children's neuropsychological disorders. In C. R. Reynolds & E. Fletcher-Janzen (Eds.), *Handbook of clinical child neuropsychology* (pp. 285–290). New York: Plenum.

Hathaway, S. R., & McKinley, J. C. (1943). *The Minnesota Multiphasic Personality Inventory manual.* Minneapolis: University of Minnesota Press.

Incagnoli, T. (1986). Current directions and future trends in clinical neuropsychology. In T. Incagnoli, G. Goldstein, & C. J. Golden (Eds.), *Clinical application of neuropsychological test batteries* (pp. 1–44). New York: Plenum.

Kaufman, A. S. (1976). A new approach to the interpretation of test scatter on the WISC–R. *Journal of Learning Disabilities, 9,* 160–167.

Kaufman, A., & Kaufman, N. (1985). *Kaufman test of educational achievement.* Circle Pines, MN: American Guidance Service.

Koppitz, E. M. (1963). *The Bender–Gestalt test for young children.* New York: Grune & Stratton.

La Rue, A. (1992). *Aging and neuropsychological assessment.* New York: Plenum.

Lezak, M. D. (1983). *Neuropsychological assessment* (2nd ed.). New York: Oxford University Press.

Luria, A. R. (1980). *Higher cortical functions in man* (2nd ed.). New York: Basic Books.

Malloy, P. F., & Webster, J. S. (1981). Detecting mild brain impairment using the Luria–Nebraska Neuropsychological Battery. *Journal of Consulting and Clinical Psychology, 49,* 768–770.

Messick, S. A. (1989). Validity. In R. Linn (Ed.), *Educational measurement* (3rd ed., pp. 13–103). Washington, DC: American Council on Education.

Murray, H. A. (1943). *The Thematic Apperception Test.* Cambridge, MA: Harvard University Press.

Osterreith, P. A. (1944). Le test de copie d'une figure complexe. *Archives de Psychologie, 30,* 206–356.

Parsons, O. A., & Prigatano, G. P. (1978). Methodological considerations in clinical neuropsychological research. *Journal of Consulting and Clinical Psychology, 46,* 608–619.

Purisch, A. D., Golden, C. J., & Hammeke, T. A. (1979). Discrimination of schizophrenic and brain injured patients by a standardized version of Luria's neuropsychological tests. *Clinical Neuropsychology, 1,* 53–59.

Reitan, R., & Davison, L. A. (Eds.). (1974). *Clinical neuropsychology: Current status and applications.* Washington, DC: Winston.

Reitan, R., & Wolfson, D. (1985). *The Halstead–Reitan neuropsychological test battery.* Tempe, AZ: Neuropsychology Press.

Reynolds, C. R. (1982). The importance of norms and other traditional psychometric concepts to assessment in clinical neuropsychology. In R. N. Malatesha & L. C. Hartlage (Eds.), *Neuropsychology and cognition* (Vol. II, pp. 55–76). The Hague: Nijhoff.

Reynolds, C. R. (1989). Measurement and statistical problems in neuropsychological assessment of children. In C. R. Reynolds & E. Fletcher-Janzen (Eds.), *Handbook of clinical child neuropsychology* (pp. 147–166). New York: Plenum.

Reynolds, C. R., & Kamphaus, R. W. (1992). *Behavior assessment system for children: Manual.* Circle Pines, MN: American Guidance.

Reschly, D. J., & Gresham, F. M. (1989). Current neuropsychological diagnosis of learning problems: A leap of faith. In C. R. Reynolds & E. Fletcher-Janzen (Eds.), *Handbook of clinical child neuropsychology* (pp. 503–519). New York: Plenum.

Rorschach, H. (1966). *Rorschach Ink Blot Technique.* New York: Grune & Stratton.

Rourke, B. P., Bakker, D. J., Fisk, J. L., & Strang, J. D. (1983). *Child neuropsychology: An introduction to theory, research, and clinical practice.* New York: Guilford.

Russell, E. W. (1986). The psychometric foundation of clinical neuropsychology. In S. B. Fiskov & T. J. Boll (Eds.), *Handbook of clinical neuropsychology* (Vol. 2, pp. 45–80). New York: Wiley.

Sawicki, R. F. (1989). Validity as applied to neuropsychological assessment. In M. D. Franzen (Ed.), *Reliability and validity in neuropsychological assessment* (pp. 37–51). New York: Plenum.

Selz, M., & Reitan, R. M. (1979). Rules for neuropsychological diagnosis: Classification of brain functions in older children. *Journal of Consulting and Clinical Psychology, 47,* 258–264.

Staff. (1993, January). Psychometric and assessment issues raised by the Americans with Disabilities Act (ADA). *The Score, 15*(4), 1–15.

Taylor, R. L., & Imivey, J. K. (1980). Diagnostic use of the WISC–R and McCarthy Scales: A regression analysis approach to learning disabilities. *Psychology in the Schools, 17,* 327–330.

Wallbrown, F. H., Vance, H., & Pritchard, K. K. (1979). Discriminating between attitudes expressed by normal and disabled readers. *Psychology in the Schools, 4,* 472–477.

Wechsler, D. (1974). *Wechsler Intelligence Scale for Children–Revised.* New York: Psychological Corporation.

Wechsler, D. (1981). *Wechsler Adult Intelligence Scale–Revised.* New York: Psychological Corporation.

Wechsler, D. (1987). *Wechsler Memory Scale–Revised.* New York: Psychological Corporation.

Wherry, R. J., Sr. (1932). A new formula for predicting the shrinkage of the coefficient for multiple correlation. *Annals of Mathematical Statistics, 2,* 404–457.

Willis, W. G. (1984). Reanalysis of an actuarial approach to neuropsychological diagnosis in consideration of base rates. *Journal of consulting and clinical psychology, 52*(4), 567–569.

Willson, V. L., & Reynolds, C. R. (1982). Methodological and statistical problems in determining membership in clinical populations. *Clinical Neuropsychology, 4,* 134–138.

13

Problems in Neuropsychological Research Methodology

Kevin R. Krull
University of Chicago
Russell L. Adams
University of Oklahoma Health Sciences Center

Unlike many subfields of psychology, neuropsychology is believed to offer the researcher the opportunity to study well-defined brain lesions. Vague diagnostic entities such as "schizophrenia" are rather nonspecific, and consequently the reliability of diagnosis is somewhat low. Brain lesions, on the other hand, may be more precisely localized and understood. Study of a more well-defined brain lesion group is likely to yield more meaningful results, especially if reliable and valid neuropsychological tests are used. Unfortunately, neuropsychology is plagued with numerous methodological problems which are inherent to the neurological groups that are studied. Patient groups are not always so "well defined." The purpose of this chapter is to delineate some of the research problems unique to neuropsychology.

In a review conducted over 14 years ago, Parsons and Prigatano (1978) outlined three criteria they believed to be important experiences to obtain prior to engaging in research in clinical neuropsychology. Specifically, they recommended that investigators have a working knowledge of psychometrics, neuroanatomy, and exposure to clinical neurology. In view of the many advances that have occurred since this review (i.e., increased use of advanced neuroimaging methods such as PET, SPECT, MRI, etc.), these experiences are likely to be of even greater importance to today's neuropsychological researcher than those that Parsons and Prigatano originally addressed.

This chapter explores a series of problems or issues that may be encountered when attempting to conduct a neuropsychological research investigation, or when reading the research of others. It is written on the premise that the reader already has a basic understanding of biostatistics and research methodology. Therefore, no attempt is made to explain basic statistical tools or basic research methodological paradigms. Instead, the focus is on research problems and issues as related specifically to conducting and evaluating neuropsychological research.

This chapter is organized in much the same way as a research paper is organized (i.e., introduction, statement of hypothesis, sample selection, procedural methodology, analysis of results, interpretation of results, and conclusions drawn from the data). Within each of these sections problems and issues are discussed. It is hoped that this organization will be easily followed by the reader. Toward the end of the chapter, a list is included that presents a series of "issues" and "questions" one may use as a guide when evaluating a specific neuropsychological research study.

PROBLEMS IN HYPOTHESIS GENERATION

As with most research, two general types of approaches to conducting neuropsychological research can be employed: exploratory and confirmatory. Confirmatory analyses require that all outcomes be anticipated, that results be viewed within a theoretical framework, that error rates be properly chosen, and that appropriate statistics be used (Lezak & Gray, 1984). On the other hand, exploratory analyses typically take a discovery approach, where new patterns in performance or new processes are investigated. A theoretical model is not vital to an exploratory investigation. Exploratory studies are often new investigations into areas that have previously received little or no attention.

In most instances confirmatory analysis can be attempted, because the field of neuropsychology has reached a level where reasonable hypotheses can be developed for many topics. Clearly, work that issues from some type of theoretical model or hypothesis is more desirable and provides for results that are more readily tested. However, when exploratory analyses are conducted, cross validation should always be performed prior to acceptance of new findings. Frequently this step is lacking, making results of such investigations difficult if not impossible to interpret.

METHODOLOGICAL ISSUES

A common and accessible data resource to clinical practitioners who engage in neuropsychological research are groups of patients who become available during the course of clinical practice, either through the sampling of records from files of patients who have been seen over a number of years or the use of successive referrals of patients in specific diagnostic groups. Although this type of research is extremely important and often of greatest relevance to clinical practice, it poses numerous problems for both the beginning and experienced clinician. These problems include, but are not limited to, issues related to sample selection and modifying variables. This section addresses these problems and attempts to offer viable solutions for design of research that is conducted in the clinical setting.

Problems in Sample Selection

The selection of samples for neuropsychological investigations carries with it numerous problems. These problems include low base rates that often are present in specific neuropsychological disorders, the vast number of variables that frequently are involved in the analysis, the extreme variability in performance processes measured, and incomplete records due to an inability to engage in specific types of test tasks (Lezak & Gray, 1984). Lack of sufficient reliability and validity data to establish clinical diagnoses of disorders or localization of lesions also limits precision of investigations.

Whereas certain neurological diseases are common, others occur infrequently. For example, recurrent seizures are very common, with 6 out of every 1,000 people being affected (Kaufman, 1990). On the hand, pediatric tumors are relatively rare, with a base rate of 2.4 per 100,000 (Cohen & Duffner, 1989). Common diseases may have infrequent presentations in specific populations. For example, multiple sclerosis is one of the most common neurologic diseases in adults, with a base rate of 50 per 100,000. However, its occurrence is relatively infrequent in children, with only 1 in 100,000 being affected in adolescence and 2 in 1,000,000 being affected prior to the age of 10 years (Fishman, 1989). With low base rates, one is left with the choice of using a small sample size, and thus a limited number of variables, increasing the heterogeneity of their sample, or unreasonably prolonging the time of data collection until a sufficient number of cases can be obtained. Obtaining a reasonable sample of children with pineal area tumors might require several years.

Numerous demographic variables have been found to influence performance on neuropsychological measures (e.g., age, education, sex, handedness). Therefore, matching on these variables is strongly recommended. However, given the already low base rates with certain disorders, restricting samples to predefined combinations of variables is often difficult if not impossible to achieve.

Even in relatively common disorders such as alcoholism, the proper control for demographic variables reduces the size of samples to the point of concern. Familial history of alcoholism has been shown to be associated with increased likelihood of alcohol abuse (Dawson, Harford, & Grant, 1992). It has also been shown to effect cognitive performance in nonabusing subjects (Hegedus, Alterman, & Tarter, 1984). Therefore, when designing a study to examine the consequences of alcohol abuse, one should control for familial history. The problem arises when attempting to match subjects on age, education, and sex, as well as familial history. Finding alcohol-abusing subjects with a negative family history is much more difficult than finding those with a positive family history. Similarly, locating nonabusing controls with a positive family history is more difficult than finding similar cases with a negative family history. When additional requirements for matching on other variables (such as education, occupation, and age) are included, subject selection becomes even more difficult.

In addition to reduction of cell size, matching on all available demographics can have a negative affect on generalizibility as well. Forcing subjects into comparison or clinical groups can produce a sample that is quite unlike the majority of patients in the population. Therefore, matching should be performed on demographic variables that are reasonable to control, without changing the clinical or demographic representativeness of the sample of interest. It is more often the case that relevant variables are not controlled.

Sample Sizes

Generalization from samples to populations can be constrained with either small or very large sample sizes. Small samples are frequently not representative of the population of interest, and may describe unique processes related to the sample itself. Although this pattern is unlikely with very large samples obtained from different research centers, other problems with generalization exist. When statistically significant differences exist between two very large samples, one must also examine the amount of explained variance. Larger sample sizes, by definition, have greater statistical power and therefore are conducive to finding statistically significant differences with small group deviations. However, because such a small proportion of the variance is explained, clinical relevance of such artificially "significant" findings is low. Therefore, generalization from results of the clinical investigation to a population of clinic patients may be inappropriate on an individual case basis.

Due to the vast number of dependent variables that often are created by neuropsychological tests in relation to the number of subjects available for a typical study, proper multivariate analyses often cannot be accomplished. Multivariate analysis of variance (MANOVA) requires anywhere from 5 to 10 subjects per variable, depending on the strength of the independent variable (Stevens, 1986). Typically, 10 subjects per variable is the recommended number for these multivariate analyses. With strong effect sizes, such as is found with brain injury cases, fewer subjects may be required. Using the Wisconsin Card Sorting Test as an example, to include all variables generated by this single test (categories achieved, total errors, perseverative errors, percent perseverative errors, nonperseverative errors, perseverative responses, trials to first category, percent conceptual level, learning to learn, and failure to maintain set) at least 100 subjects would be required in a discriminant function or factor analysis.

Instead of the multivariate statistical approach, many researchers elect to employ univariate statistical analysis. However, without correction of the Type I (alpha) significance level for the repeated analyses, the likelihood of Type I errors is vastly inflated. Proper corrections such as the Bonferroni method are acceptable, although they often tend to be overly conservative. An additional alternative is to employ composite or summary variables or factors in the multivariate design (e.g., using Verbal or Performance IQs as factor scores instead of each individual intelligence subtest). This technique will reduce the requirements of sample size and still allow for a meaningful analysis. Composite variables also reduce error variance in individual measures if they are properly chosen. However, minor differences in subtest pattern of performance, or specific subtest-related deficits, may be overlooked by this approach.

Data from samples of patients that are employed in neuropsychological research often form distributions that do not meet the assumptions of statistical normality. For example, the performance of aphasic patients on the Boston Diagnostic Aphasia Examination is likely to be positively skewed. This occurrence does not prevent proper statistical analysis. Such skewed distributions can be analyzed by converting raw scores into cutoffs, and then using nonparametric statistics (e.g., Fischer's exact probability test; Lezak & Gray, 1984), or by statistical transformation of raw scores into *z* scores.

Heterogeneity

Group heterogeneity or within-group variability in symptoms or deficits can mask intergroup differences. Within-group performance heterogeneity increases the within-group (error) variance and requires larger between group differences for statistical significance. Analysis of cognitive deficits in multiple sclerosis is an example of this problem. The location in the central nervous system in which the sclerotic plaques have congregated determine, in part, the symptom constellation (e.g., optic neuritis). Symptomatic homogeneity can be increased with proper subgroup identification and assessment techniques. Establishment of the reliability and validity of diagnoses is the essential first step in conducting research with clinical populations. Diagnostic criteria should be specified prior to subject selection. Furthermore, these criteria should be consistent with those that are commonly employed in the clinical setting (e.g., *DSM–IV*). Even with these requirements, however, some diagnoses are much more difficult to establish. For example, Alzheimer's disease cannot be definitively diagnosed until autopsy.

The choice of assessment devices will influence group homogeneity. Assessment techniques employed can be valid only if they are reliable. Reliability of performance on psychological measures is affected by (a) group homogeneity, (b) time limits employed in testing, and (c) test length (Crocker & Algina, 1986). Reliability of neuropsychological tests is also dependent on the characteristics of the groups for which they are employed. For example, test–retest reliability of the Halstead–Reitan Impairment Index was found to be .83 in non-brain-damaged patients, .82 in brain-damaged patients, and .63 in schizophrenic patients (Matarazzo, Matarazzo, Weins, Gallo, & Klonoff, 1976).

Heterogeneity also exists in samples of individuals with the same neurological process. Take, for example, Alzheimer's disease. Although it is true that individuals with this disease suffer from a disorder with the same etiology, the stage of decline in cognitive functioning or the progression of the disease can differ greatly. Patients with Alzheimer's disease can range from those with a mild decline in functioning, who frequently forget common objects or events but are capable of maintaining employment, to those who are essentially bedridden and require constant supervision. If such a range of patients were grouped together and contrasted to normal controls in an investigation of cognitive functioning, it is highly likely that the variability with the patient group would overshadow the differences between groups. Neurofibrillary tangles and senile plaques are present in different brain structures for different patients. Some patients can present with lateralized symptoms involving the right hemisphere, whereas others can present with a greater concentration of plaques and tangles in the left hemisphere.

Methods used to determine the presence or extent of brain damage vary in sensitivity and, as a result, can be problematic when they are used to select patients for group inclusion. Consistency in selection of methods is essential. For example, MRI is generally more sensitive in identifying lesions than CT scans (Walsh, 1987). Variability between the use of MRI and CT scans within or between groups will contribute to error variance. The use of EEGs as an assessment device poses additional problems. Given the high rate of false negatives, a normal EEG should never be used as proof of a nonbrain damaged condition. The absence of lesion evidence is not evidence of lesion absence. On the other hand, an EEG that clearly displays epileptic activity could serve as an indicator of electrical brain dysfunction.

Lateralization and localization of brain damage is an important determination in subject identification. Clinically significant closed head injuries often result in multiple lesion sites. On the other hand, anoxia and toxicity often result in diffuse cerebral damage. Furthermore, anoxia often is present after severe head injury. Localization of injuries is difficult to establish in these conditions. Even strokes and tumors pose problems in localization. Not all right lateralized cerebral hemispheric strokes are alike. For example, vascular lesions may involve anterior, middle, or posterior cerebral arteries, or may involve different branches of one of these arteries. Tumors are not limited to arbitrary landmark divisions in structures; they may involve multiple lobes or both cortical and subcortical sites. In addition, the effects of medical treatment of the condition are often overlooked. For example, is the patient receiving medication that would alter brain functioning? Whenever possible, localization and lateralization of brain trauma should be established. Without such evaluation, group homogeneity is compromised. However, studies that claim to have separated groups into explicit lesion sites should be viewed with some degree of skepticism. Such discrete localizations are extremely difficult, if not impossible, to achieve.

Moderator Variables

Patient-related or attribute variables are often overlooked or experimentally uncontrolled such that within-group variance is unnecessarily increased. Demographic variables that have been shown to be related to functioning on neuropsychological tests include age, education, occupation, socioeconomic status, sex, and ethnicity. Vega and Parsons (1967) found the correlations between age and performance on the Halstead Category Test to be +.63. Age has also been found to be correlated with cognitive performance level in samples of brain-damaged and non-brain-damaged subjects for the Category Test and the Tactual Performance Test, but only in non-brain-damaged subjects for Seashore Rhythm Test, Speech Sounds Perception Test, and Tapping Test (Prigatano & Parsons, 1976). In a large sample of normal nonclinical subjects, Heaton, Grant, and Matthews (1986) found a correlation of +.56 between age and −.39 between education and performance on the Category Test. Furthermore, the correlation between education and performance on the Halstead–Reitan Battery was less for individuals over 60 years of age compared with younger subjects. For younger individuals, the effects of age were greater for less educated subjects. Sex has also been found to contribute to neuropsychological performance differences. Dodrill (1979) and Heaton and colleagues (1986) reported lower performance on hand dynamometer and finger tapping in females.

Heaton, Grant, and Matthews (1986) reported a significant contribution of age, educational level, and sex to performance on the HRB, and they recently developed a regression-based formula for the correction of performance on the HRB based on these various demographic variables (1991). In fact, 48 and 24% of the variance in performance on the various HRB tests have been attributed to age and education, respectively. Although this correction process is a good first step toward establishing appropriate reference points, it too has problems that need to be addressed. In their correction process, Heaton and colleagues employed a regression-based approach to determine *T*-scores based on age, sex, and education. However, on the extreme ends of the distribution data points are lacking, and thus the slope of the regression line cannot be adequately assessed. Cross-validation of their formula should help address this problem, although to date this has not been accomplished.

In an earlier attempt to control for the influences of these demographic variables, Seidenberg et al. (1984) conducted a multiple-regression analysis of Halstead–Reitan Battery performance. With age, education, sex, socioeconomic status, and handedness as predictor variables, they found that 54% of the variance in grip strength was attributable to these variables. However, less than 2% of the variance in TPT was explained. Education appeared to have the greatest influence; alone, it accounted for 12% of the variance in the Halstead Impairment Index. These findings are surprising in light of the fact that these investigators used a sample of 288 seizure-disordered patients. In a sample of normal controls, the relationship between demographic variables and HRB performance would be expected to be much larger, because the *range* of the variables would likely be larger.

Although it has received relatively little attention to date, ethnicity may also be linked to performance differences. In a recent investigation conducted in the laboratory at the University of Oklahoma Health Sciences Center, we found significant differences in performance on the Halstead–Reitan Battery due to this variable. In this study, the performance of groups of African American and Anglo-American brain-damaged patients were compared with the performance of non-brain-damaged patients on the Halstead–Reitan Battery and the Wechsler Memory Scale. Groups were equated on age, education, sex, ethnicity, and Full Scale IQ. Standard scores were computed using the Heaton et al. (1991) comprehensive norms for age and education, which do not include data for ethnicity. A MANOVA indicated that African Americans scored below Anglo-Americans on the TPT, regardless of neurological status. Furthermore, the overall level of performance for both brain-damaged and non-brain-damaged African Americans was in the "impaired" range, based on the suggested *T*-score cutoff of 40. Therefore, using these norms for African Americans would be problematic.

Actuarial estimation of premorbid cognitive functioning level also should be attempted. Without such control, neuropsychological performance level differences could result from variations in the premorbid level of functioning. Education, socioeconomic status, and occupational level are variables of interest in such analyses. Formulas for the estimation of premorbid intelligence have also been developed. These methods include the prediction of premorbid intelligence from demographic data (Barona, Reynolds, & Chastain, 1984), the best current performance measure on subtests of the WAIS–R (Lezak, 1983), and the measurement of processes that are believed to be relatively insensitive to cognitive decline, such as reading level or vocabulary (Alekoumbides, Charter, Adkins, & Seacat, 1987; Nelson, 1982). Regression formulas for the prediction of premorbid intelligence are based on demographic data such as age, sex, race, education level, occupation, region of country, and urban or rural residence (Barona et al., 1984; Wilson et al., 1978). These methods have been criticized for producing a restricted range of estimated IQs, as well as for their poor performance in correctly discriminating normal and cerebrally compromised individuals (Eppinger, Craig, Adams, & Parsons, 1987; Silverstein, 1987; Sweet, Moberg, & Tovian, 1990).

A premorbid IQ-prediction formula based on the National Adult Reading Test–Revised (NART–R) has also been developed. This procedure uses reading and pronunciation of irregular words that violate the usual phonetic rules; therefore, it is dependent on previous familiarity. The NART–R has been recently criticized, however, for its decreased predictive ability at the high (above 120) and low (below 89) ends of the IQ distribution (Bryan, Wiens, & Crossen, 1992).

We have recently developed a formula based on both demographic and individual WAIS–R subtest performance (Krull, Scott, & Sherer, 1995). The Vocabulary and Picture Completion subtests from the WAIS–R were chosen for inclusion into the formula because of their demonstrated reliability (Sattler, 1988) and relative resistance to neurological insult (Alekoumbides et al., 1987). Furthermore, these two WAIS–R subtests are generally representative of both verbal and nonverbal cognitive performance levels (Sattler, 1988). When combined with selected demographic information, this formula provides more accurate estimates of intelligence in non-brain-damaged subjects without severely restricting the range of variability (Krull, Scott, et al., 1995; Krull, Sherer, & Adams, 1995). Recent studies attest to the usefulness of this approach for brain-damaged samples as well (Scott, Krull, Williamson, Iverson, & Adams, 1995).

Attribute variables are not limited to demographics. Tupper and Rosenblood (1984) listed common attribute variables as including sex, age, education, neurological status, laterality of lesion, cause of lesion, site of lesion, severity of lesion, time since lesion onset, handedness, socioeconomic status, and condition at time of testing. Furthermore, they made the point that these attributes may not be dimensionally independent of each other (i.e., nonorthogonal), and thus they cannot be randomly assigned (e.g., cause of lesion and severity).

Matching on too many attributes can give rise to research employing overly restrictive criteria and may lead to a sample that is not representative of the population in general. Furthermore, matching of attributes is not a random assignment of these conditions, and thus causal directionality may be ambiguous. In these situations, covariate procedures may be more appropriate.

Neglect of Various Groups

In order for generalization of results to more adequately occur, diversity in populations studied must be employed. However, all too often studies are repeatedly conducted using subject groups with little diversity in demographic makeup. In the examples used in the preceding discussion (familial history of alcoholism), the vast majority of research has been conducted with an Anglo-American population. In order to generalize these findings widely, further investigations, especially involving female and minority populations, are required. However, these studies are underrepresented in the recent literature. In a content analysis of six APA journals, Graham (1992) found a recent decline in studies on African Americans.

Furthermore, the existing studies were reported to lack control of variables such as socioeconomic status. In their new "comprehensive norms," Heaton et al. (1991) did not include ethnicity in the regression formula, although recent investigations suggest that they should have done so. If they did include such a correction, the differences between Anglo-Americans and African Americans on HRB tests described earlier could have been eliminated through the actuarial correction process. Clearly, a large and widely representative group of African American subjects would be needed for such a study.

The use of patient controls as comparison groups for assessment of neuropsychological deficits in neurologically compromised individuals has been extensively employed in clinical research. These controls have been referred to as pseudoneurologic (Matthews, Shaw, & Kløve, 1966), non-brain-damaged patients, and so on. On the one hand, these controls seem like the most logical choice as a comparison group, because the combined groups comprise common referrals to clinical neuropsychologists. However, prior to using these subjects as controls, their neuropsychological functioning must be fully understood and not merely assumed to be normal based on the absence of positive clinical findings. Many neuropsychological studies test patients in a hospital inpatient setting. Health status variables that lead to hospitalization for any reason can affect the neuropsychological findings of non-neurologically impaired control subjects.

Numerous difficulties exist in employing medical or psychiatric patients as controls, some of which are common to brain-damaged groups as well. Heaton, Baade, and Johnson (1978) summarized some of these problems. They noted proper identification of the patient population, use of standard neurological or medical (or both) tests to rule out brain damage, use of specific diagnostic criteria, and a common time when diagnosis is established (e.g., at admission or discharge). In addition to these variables, the demographic variables discussed earlier should also be experimentally controlled.

Although most investigators would not include patients with obvious symptoms of psychosis in control groups, depression may be more difficult to identify. Depression often occurs along with neurological insult, and therefore may influence performance on neuropsychological measures beyond that attributable to the brain injury. Mayeux, Williams, Stern, and Cote (1984) found that 40%–50% of Parkinson's patients display significant symptoms of depression. Starkstein and Robinson (1989) found 50% of acute stroke patients and 30% of post-acute patients to be diagnosably depressed. Wragg and Jeste (1989) found 40%–50% of Alzheimer's patients to display depressed mood, with 10%–20% of them being clinically depressed. Therefore, depression may add uncontrolled variance to the clinical group's performance level. Furthermore, one would expect the degree of depression to be related to the length of time since diagnosis. If testing occurs shortly after diagnosis, the influence of depression may be quite high.

Newman and Sweet (1992) examined the role of depression in neurological compromised patients and found the *presence* of depression rather than the *degree* of depression to be related to deficits on neuropsychological tests of attention, memory, and processing speed. They concluded that the use of depression inventories such as those of Hamilton and the Beck were not as effective as a detailed clinical history. In a recent summary, Sweet, Newman, and Bell (1992) suggested several steps to control for the influence of depression. First, neuropsychological tests that assess domains which discriminate between depression and brain damage should be used. Second, the use of depression inventories as the only criterion for depression diagnosis should be avoided. Interviews with collaterals should supplement the inventories. Third, to reduce fatigue and thereby to provide more reliable estimates, testing across multiple sessions is warranted. Finally, brain dysfunction should be diagnosed using processes that are not related to depression, such as visual neglect or aphasia.

Problems in Experimental Design and Procedure

The environment and procedures employed in conducting neuropsychological investigations are also important in influencing the reliability, validity, and generalizibility of the results. The average full neuropsychological evaluation requires between 6 and 8 hours to complete. Often this evaluation is conducted on one day. Motivation and fatigue will obviously fluctuate during the course of testing, which will contribute to variability in performance and may cause certain tests to remain uncompleted. The order in which the tests are administered also may contribute to the performance variability. For example, administering tests that are sensitive to attention and concentration (e.g., memory, problem solving) late in the day may cause scores to be lowered. Tests of sensory and motor functioning typically are less susceptible to this fatigue.

The effects of order of testing may even be specific to patient populations. Individuals with neurological insults may fatigue easier and sooner than control subjects, and may show more performance difficulty on measures of attention and memory. Therefore, in certain instances statistically significant differences on measures of memory may be attributed to differences in stamina and not to memory processes per se. When we consider the effect of these combined influences, the end result often is an incomplete data record, which reduces the likelihood that the requirements of parametric statistical analysis will be met (Lezak, 1983).

The length of time since onset of the brain lesion is another important factor in determining group homogeneity. The length of time since onset of symptomology and testing will influence results in different neurologic syndromes. For example, an individual who experienced a cerebral vascular accident or a closed head injury may be expected to regain some abilities during the recovery process following the injury. On the other hand, if one were conducting a study of a degenerative neurologic process such as progressive dementia or multiple sclerosis, one would expect further decline in the intervening interval from onset to the time of testing. Control and consistency with this interval between lesion onset and test administration are essential.

ANALYSIS AND INTERPRETATION OF RESULTS

With the popularization and increased power of personal computers, the ability to store, manage, and analyze large data files has moved into the clinical environment. Sophisticated computer programs have been simplified with pull-down menus and a variety of default options. However, this simplification is accompanied by numerous areas of possible subject selection problems. The researcher should never rely solely on the computer for the selection of options. Such computerized statistical analysis programs may permit violations of important statistical assumptions. Certain statistical packages given alternative solutions for the same question. For example, the standard output for a common *t*-test on the popular SAS or SPSS-X software include two answers: one for equal variances between groups and one for unequal variances. It also provides a test for which assumption is correct, an important item not to be overlooked. The advanced SPSS-X software includes options for tests of MANOVA. However, with careful attention to documentation, it becomes evident that the program does not control for or correct the alpha significance level for the repeated univariate analyses that it conducts as part of the default options. Therefore, knowledge of one's database and statistical theory cannot be replaced with the sophistication of automated computer and software devices.

Inadequate documentation of databases can lead to erroneous results. The use of coding manuals that specifically describe all available scoring options for each variable can prevent some of these errors. Log files that are produced by statistical programs often contain the procedures employed in an analysis. However, unless they are used as part of a batch program or are specifically requested in an interactive mode, these files are not saved. Then the only output is the statistical results. Without such a record of the analysis conducted, confirmation and replication is often difficult to achieve. In cases were subsampling of a database is conducted, the exact sample must be reproduced in future analyses. This may be extremely difficult if not impossible unless the cases chosen also are recorded as part of the analysis.

Several methods have been proposed for controlling certain attribute variables. Individual subject matching is the preferable method. However, this is often not the method employed. Many investigators instead elect to match subjects on a group mean performance level basis, which leads to an increased likelihood of unequal variances, and thus violation of the assumptions for use of parametric statistics. An additional method of statistical control is the use of analysis of covariance (ANCOVA). The ANCOVA method is often used when groups differ on a variable which is believed to be correlated to the dependent measure (e.g., Full Scale IQ and performance on WCST). However, this application of ANCOVA has been criticized (Adams, Brown, & Grant, 1984). Use of covariance analysis in this way will lead to inaccurate correlations. Take, for example, Full Scale IQ used as a covariate for WCST performance in an examination of the effects of head injury on WCST performance. Using Full Scale IQ as a covariate would partial out the portion of variance from the WCST that is common to both Full Scale IQ and head injury. Therefore, a portion of variance in WCST due to head injury would be removed.

INTERPRETATION OF THE LITERATURE

Level Versus Pattern of Performance

All too often investigations of neuropsychological functioning in clinical populations have focused on the level of performance on specific tests rather than the overall pattern that the test results represent. Over two decades ago, Luria (1973) discussed the importance of studying brain processes in terms of how discrete skill areas contribute to composition of a cognitive functional system. In this discussion he described three functional units that interact in behavioral or cognitive processes: a unit which regulates tone or waking, a unit which processes and stores information, and a unit which programs, regulates, and verifies mental processes. Since this description, relatively little neuropsychological research has been conducted that directly examines brain processes in relation to a functional system network. Instead, the majority of studies have attempted to localize cognitive processes to brain areas. Typically, studies examine specific areas or types of deficits resulting from localized lesions without regard to how these lesions interrupt information processing networks.

Clinical Significance

The focus on the level of performance is a potential source of interpretive problems when considering differences between groups in patient populations. Absolute differences in levels of a specific neuropsychological process can be quite large, with relatively little clinical relevance. For example, in an examination of neuropsychological functioning in Alzheimer's disease patients, Hom (1992) reported large differences between a group of patients and a group of age and education equated controls. However, on further examination of the data, it became evident that the control group was not a "normal" group of individuals. The mean Wechsler Intelligence Full Scale IQ of the control group was 123, placing them in the superior range of intellectual functioning. When comparing groups of nonclinical subjects with IQ discrepancies of this magnitude, significant differences in neuropsychological functioning will be apparent. Clinical significance, on the other hand, is lacking. Unless there is reason to believe that individuals of superior intelligence are more susceptible to Alzheimer's disease, a more clinically valid comparison would include a control group with mean IQs in the average range. Neuropsychological measures are highly correlated with IQ. A control group of patients with superior IQs will make statistically significant differences much easier to find, but difficult if not impossible to interpret.

Numerous studies demonstrate differences between groups with the mean performance of both groups in the clinically "normal" range. Again, in these instances clinical relevance is lacking. In a comparison of Korsakoff, alcohol-dependent, and control samples on a variety of neuropsychological measures, Joyce and Robbins (1991) reported significant differences in performance on the WAIS–R IQ measures. Control subjects had significantly higher Performance IQs than the Korsakoff and alcohol-dependent subjects. However, the mean Performance IQ for the control group was 111, whereas the mean IQs for the Korsakoff and alcohol-dependent subjects were 93 and 103, respectively, which are both within the average range. Their cognitive performance level cannot be considered to be impaired with reference to the population in general. It is only when reference is made to the specific control group used that statistically significant differences emerge. Therefore, although in many cases statistically significant differences may be achieved, clinically significant impairment, or performance falling in the impaired range, is more relevant to understanding the neuropsychological processes that are involved in the disorder.

The techniques employed in the classification or categorization of groups is an important factor in considering the significance of reported differences. This issue becomes extremely important when one is evaluating the sensitivity of neuropsychological tests. Numerous attempts have been made to distinguish Alzheimer's disease from multi-infarct dementia based on the performance on tests of memory and other neuropsychological processes. When one is determining whether the measure is specific to one or the other dementing process, a consideration of the base rate of the disorder is warranted. Alzheimer's disease is by far the most common type of cortical dementia. If, for example, we assume that the base rate of Alzheimer's disease is 90%, whereas the base rate of multi-infarct dementia is 10%, an overall hit rate of 80% would be achieved by assuming that all dementia patients are of the Alzheimer's type. Obviously, by assuming that all dementias are of the Alzheimer's type, the hit rate for multi-infarct dementia would be zero. Test specificity is only achieved if adequate identification of both groups is demonstrated, and if the use of the measure substantially improves on identification in relation to base rates.

Individual neuropsychological tests typically have an actuarial hit rate of about 71%, whereas the combination of several tests have a mean hit rate of approximately 80% (Spreen & Benton, 1965). However, simply identifying brain impairment is not the end point for a clinical neuropsychologist. Determination of specific processes that are involved in the impairment syndrome is more important. For this reason, test specificity is required in addition to test sensitivity.

SUMMARY

In summary, although clinical neuropsychology appears to be a potentially more exact science compared to many other subfields of psychology, it is still plagued by numerous research flaws. Whether one is conducting research in this field or evaluating research conducted by others, the following questions may serve as a basic guide to assist one in considering the soundness and limitations of the implications of the typical investigation:

1. *Exploratory Versus Confirmatory Analyses.* Does the study properly develop a hypothesis based on a theoretical discussion of research conducted on the topic to date?

2. *Sample Size.* Is the size of the sample employed large enough to conduct the investigation given the number and type of variables used and the type of statistical methodology that is employed?

3. *Homogeneous Samples.* Have samples been developed in a way to determine whether homogeneous groups are employed, or have subtypes been collapsed, thereby increasing within-group error variance?

4. *Demographic Variables.* Have appropriate demographic variables been controlled without changing the representativeness of the groups?

5. *Moderating Variables.* Has the influence of moderating variables been considered in selecting dependent measures and controls for demographic variables?

6. *Psychometric Reliability/Validity.* Have tests been selected that have data available on reliability of administration and validity of the constructs they propose to measure?

7. *Administration Procedure.* Has the test administration procedure, including the qualifications of the examiner and test order, been taken into account?

8. *Statistical Analysis.* Has the proper statistical analysis (i.e., parametric vs. nonparametric) been employed for the variables and populations of interest? Have raw or standard scores been used in these analyses? Have corrections or control for multiple comparisons been employed?

9. *Level or Pattern of Deficits.* Has an attempt been made to examine the pattern of test performance in addition to the level of performance on each test?

10. *Clinical Significance.* Are the results reported of clinical utility or does the performances of both the control and patient groups fall in the "normal" range of scores.

These questions should lead one to evaluate their own research design as well as the design, methodology, and implications of the research findings presented in the literature. Proper interpretation and recognition of the limitations of research findings is the responsibility of the reader as well as the investigator. It should be routine practice for academicians and practitioners alike.

REFERENCES

Adams, K., Brown, G., & Grant, I. (1984). Analysis of covariance as a remedy for demographic mismatch of research subject groups: Some sobering simulations. *Journal of Clinical and Experimental Neuropsychology, 7*(4), 445–462.

Alekoumbides, A., Charter, R., Adkins, T., & Seacat, G. (1987). The diagnosis of brain damage by the WAIS, WMS, and Reitan battery utilizing standardized scores corrected for age and education. *The International Journal of Clinical Neuropsychology, 9*(1), 11–28.

American Psychiatric Association. (1994). *Diagnostic and statistical manual of mental disorders* (4th ed.). Washington, DC: Author.

Barona, A., Reynolds, C., & Chastain, R. (1984). A demographically based index of premorbid intelligence for the WAIS–R. *Journal of Consulting and Clinical Psychology, 52*(5), 885–887.

Bryan, J., Weins, A., & Crossen, J. (1992). Estimating WAIS–R IQ from the National Adult Reading Test–Revised among normal adults. *Journal of Clinical and Experimental Neuropsychology, 14*(1), 64.

Cohen, M., & Duffner, P. (1989). Tumors of the brain and spinal cord including Leukemic involvement. In K. Swaiman (Ed.), *Pediatric neurology: Principles and practice* (pp. 661–714). St. Louis, MO: Mosby.

Crocker, L., & Algina, J. (1986). *Introduction to classical and modern test theory.* New York: Holt, Rinehart & Winston.

Dawson, D., Harford, T., & Grant, B. (1992). Family history as a predictor of alcohol dependence. *Alcoholism: Clinical and Experimental Research, 16*(5), 572–575.

Dodrill, C. (1979). Sex differences on the Halstead–Reitan neuropsychological battery and on other neuropsychological measures. *Journal of Clinical Psychology, 35,* 236–241.

Eppinger, M., Craig, P., Adams, R., & Parsons, O. (1987). The WAIS–R index for estimating premorbid intelligence: Cross-validation and clinical utility. *Journal of Consulting and Clinical Psychology, 55*(1), 86–90.

Fishman, M. (1989). Disorders primarily of white matter. In K. Swaiman (Ed.), *Pediatric neurology: Principles and practice* (pp. 755–776). St. Louis, MO: Mosby.

Graham, S. (1992). "Most of the subjects were white and middle class": Trends in published research on African-Americans in selected APA journals, 1970–1989. *American Psychologist, 47*(5), 629–639.

Heaton, R., Baade, L., & Johnson, K. (1978). Neuropsychological test results associated with psychiatric disorders in adults. *Psychological Bulletin, 85,* 141–162.

Heaton, R., Grant, I., & Matthews, C. (1986). Differences in neuropsychological test performance associated with age, education, and sex. In I. Grant & K. Adams (Eds.), *Neuropsychological assessment in neuropsychiatric disorders: Clinical methods and empirical findings* (pp. 100–120). New York: Oxford University Press.

Heaton, R., Grant, I., & Matthews, C. (1991). *Comprehensive norms for an expanded Halstead–Reitan Battery.* Odessa, FL: Psychological Assessment Resources.

Hegedus, A., Alterman, A., & Tarter, R. (1984). Learning achievement in sons of alcoholics. *Alcoholism: Clinical and Experimental Research, 8*(3), 330–333.

Hom, J. (1992). General and specific cognitive dysfunction in patients with Alzheimer's disease. *Archives of Clinical Neuropsychology, 7*(2), 121–133.

Joyce, E., & Robbins, T. (1991). Frontal lobe dysfunction in Korsakoff and non-Korsakoff alcoholics: Planning and spatial working memory. *Neuropsychologia, 29*(8), 709–723.

Kaufman, D. (1990). *Clinical neurology for psychiatrists.* Philadelphia: Saunders.

Krull, K., Scott, J., & Sherer, M. (1995). Estimation of premorbid intelligence from combined performance and demographic variables. *The Clinical Neuropsychologist, 9*(1), 83–88.

Krull, K., Sherer, M., & Adams, R. (1995). A comparison of indices of premorbid intelligence in clinical populations. *Applied Neuropsychology, 2*(1), 35–38.

Lezak, M. (1983). *Neuropsychological assessment* (2nd ed.). New York: Oxford University Press.

Lezak, M., & Gray, D. (1984). Sampling problems and nonparametric solutions in clinical neuropsychological research. *Journal of Clinical Neuropsychology, 6*(1), 101–109.

Luria, A. (1973). *The working brain: An introduction to neuropsychology.* New York: Basic Books.

Matarazzo, J., Matarazzo, R., Wiens, A., Gallo, A., Jr., & Klonoff, H. (1976). Retest reliability of the Halstead impairment index in a normal, a schizophrenic, and two samples of organic patients. *Journal of Clinical Psychology, 32,* 338–349.

Matthews, C., Shaw, D., & Klove, H. (1966). Psychological test performance in neurologic and "pseudo-neurologic" subjects. *Cortex, 2,* 244–253.

Mayeux, R., Williams, J., Stern, Y., & Cote, L. (1984). Depression and Parkinson's disease. *Advances in Neurology, 40,* 241–250.

Nelson, H. (1982). *National adult reading test (NART): Test manual.* Windsor, UK: NFER Nelson.

Newman, P., & Sweet, J. (1992). Depressive disorders. In A. Puente & R. McCaffrey (Eds.), *Handbook of neuropsychological assessment: A biopsychosocial perspective* (pp. 263–307). New York: Plenum.

Parsons, O., & Prigatano, G. (1978). Methodological considerations in clinical neuropsychological research. *Journal of Consulting and Clinical Psychology, 46*(4), 608–619.

Prigatano, G., & Parsons, O. (1976). Relationship of age and education to Halstead test performance in different patient populations. *Journal of Consulting and Clinical Psychology, 44*(4), 527–533.

Sattler, J. (1988). *Assessment of children.* San Diego: J. Sattler.

Scott, J., Krull, K., Williamson, D., Iverson, G., & Adams, R. (1995). *Oklahoma premorbid intelligence estimate (OPIE): Validation on clinical samples.* Manuscript in progress.

Seidenberg, M., Gamache, M., Beck, N., Smith, M., Giordani, B., Berent, S., Sackellares, J., & Boll, T. (1984). Subject variables and performance on the Halstead neuropsychological test battery: A multivariate analysis. *Journal of Consulting and Clinical Psychology, 52*(4), 658–662.

Silverstein, A. (1987). Accuracy of estimates of premorbid intelligence based on demographic variables. *Journal of Clinical Psychology, 43*(5), 493–495.

Spreen, O., & Benton, A. (1965). Comparative studies of some psychological tests for cerebral damage. *Journal of Nervous and Mental Disease, 140,* 323–333.

Starkstein, S., & Robinson, R. (1989). Affective disorders and cerebral vascular disease. *British Journal of Psychiatry, 154,* 170–182.

Stevens, J. (1986). *Applied multivariate statistics for the social sciences.* Hillsdale, NJ: Lawrence Erlbaum Associates.

Sweet, J., Moberg, P., & Tovian, S. (1990). Evaluation of Wechsler Adult Intelligence Scale–Revised premorbid IQ formulas in clinical populations. *Psychological Assessment, 2*(1), 41–44.

Sweet, J., Newman, P., & Bell, B. (1992). Significance of depression in clinical neuropsychological assessment. *Clinical Psychology Review, 12,* 21–45.

Tupper, D., & Rosenblood, L. (1984). Methodological considerations in the use of attribute variables in neuropsychological research. *Journal of Clinical Neuropsychology, 6*(4), 441–453.

Vega, A., Jr., & Parsons, O. (1967). Cross-validation of the Halstead–Reitan tests for brain damage. *Journal of Consulting Psychology, 31,* 619–623.

Walsh, K. (1987). *Neuropsychology: A clinical approach.* Edinburgh: Churchill Livingstone.

Wilson, R., Rosenbaum, G., Brown, G., Rourke, D., & Whitman, D. (1978). An index of premorbid intelligence. *Journal of Consulting and Clinical Psychology, 46*(6), 1554–1555.

Wragg, R., & Jeste, D. (1989). Overview of depression and psychosis in Alzheimer's disease. *American Journal of Psychiatry, 146,* 577–587.

Author Index

Numbers in italics indicate pages with complete bibliographic information.

A

D

H

I

J

K

M

S

U

V

W

Y

Z

Subject Index

C

E

F

G

M

O

P

Q

R

S

T

X

Z